NEURORADIOLOGY

The Core Curriculum

NEURORADIOLOGY

MAURICIO CASTILLO, M.D.

Professor of Radiology
Chief and Program Director, Neuroradiology
University of North Carolina School of Medicine
Chapel Hill, North Carolina

LIPPINCOTT WILLIAMS & WILKINS
A **Wolters Kluwer** Company
Philadelphia • Baltimore • New York • London
Buenos Aires • Hong Kong • Sydney • Tokyo

Developmental Editor: Denise Martin
Production Editor: Rakesh Rampertab
Manufacturing Manager: Tim Reynolds
Cover Designer: Karen Quigley
Compositor: Lippincott Williams & Wilkins Desktop Division
Printer: Edwards Brothers

530 Walnut Street
Philadelphia, PA 19106 USA
LWW.com

Printed in the USA

Library of Congress Cataloging-in-Publication Data

Castillo, Mauricio.
Neuroradiology / Mauricio Castillo.
p. cm.—(The core curriculum)
Includes bibliographical references and index.
ISBN 0-7817-3664-1
1. Central nervous system—Radiography. I. Title. II. Series.

RC349.R3 C367 2002
616.8'04757—dc21

2002075271

---

10 9 8 7 6 5 4 3 2 1

Para Hortensia, con amor

CONTENTS

Preface *ix*

Acknowledgments *xi*

1. Congenital Anomalies 1
2. Neurocutaneous Syndromes 41
3. White Matter Disorders 59
4. Metabolic, Toxic, and Degenerative Disorders 79
5. Disorders of Cerebral Spinal Fluid Flow 117
6. Intracranial Tumors 133
7. Pituitary Gland 177
8. Vascular Occlusive Disorders 193
9. Non-Occlusive Cerebral Vascular Disease 231
10. Cranial Trauma 257
11. Infectious and Inflammatory Processes 273
12. Effects of Therapy 301
13. Congenital Spinal Anomalies 315
14. Spinal Trauma 339
15. Inflammatory and Infectious Spinal Disorders 361
16. Spinal Tumors and Masses 387
17. Degenerative Disorders 413
18. Vascular Diseases of the Spinal Cord 433
19. The Post-Surgical Spine 443
20. Brachial and Lumbosacral Plexi 463

Subject Index *475*

PREFACE

The goal of this new book is to provide a concise review of modern imaging of the brain and the spine. It is hopefully short enough so that residents can read it entirely during their neuroradiology rotations, and complete enough to also serve as a fast reference source to fellows and others interested in imaging of the central nervous system. I have intended to keep the book balanced, with approximately one half of it dealing with the brain and other half on the spine. I have excluded head and neck imaging because I believe that this area of imaging is vast enough to deserve a separate textbook. I have tried to organize all of the chapters based on conferences that I gave, for which I have received good responses from the audience. As such, the reader will find that many of my personal beliefs are included in the text. In addition, the organization of some chapters vary somewhat from that found in other textbooks and reflects the way in which I think neuroradiology should be taught. It is my hope that this approach will encourage those who are curious to read the book completely and then to continue their studies onward with more detailed literature. I have avoided including chapters on physics and imaging protocols because these may be found elsewhere and would have increased the size of this book beyond what I think is reasonable. As always, I am solely responsible for any inadvertent mistakes. Neuroimaging is slowly adding biochemistry and physiology to its already strong anatomical basis. I hope that this book will reflect in some way those exciting changes.

ACKNOWLEDGMENTS

As with any other project, there are many people to thank for their direct and indirect help. My colleagues at the University of North Carolina, Drs. Smith, Solander, Kwock, and Jewells work hard in order to allow me the time for this and other projects. More important is that they are all true friends and a pleasure to work with. My office assistant, Ms. Barbal, is not only my "right hand" but is taking over the functions of my "left hand" too; my gratitude to her for making my days go smoothly. Our Chairman, Dr. Joseph Lee, is the main reason for my coming to North Carolina and not a day goes by without me thanking my "lucky stars" for his help and friendship. Our photographers, Mr. Strain and Mr. Nobel, have again provided invaluable assistance for this project. Joyce-Rachel John convinced me to do "one more book" and I am glad that she did. I have tried to acknowledge the sources of many of the illustrations that I have used in this book. If everyone was not credited, I apologize for this oversight. Lastly, on a personal basis, many thanks go to my sister, Denise, and her family for helping me sail through some rough waters.

NEURORADIOLOGY

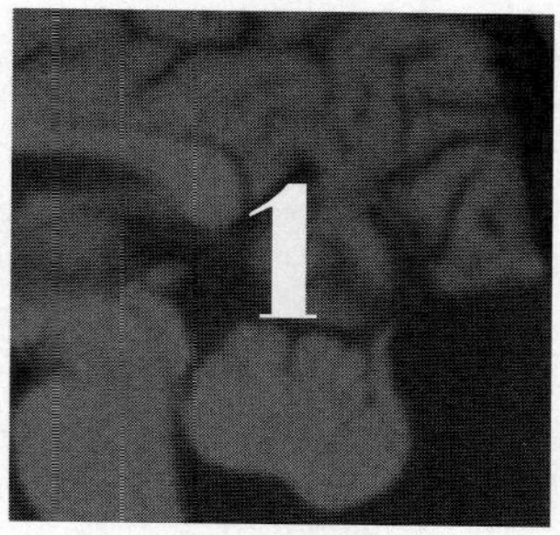

CONGENITAL ANOMALIES

- Infratentorial Congenital Anomalies
- Supratentorial Congenital Anomalies

INFRATENTORIAL CONGENITAL ANOMALIES

DANDY-WALKER SPECTRUM OF MALFORMATIONS

Recently, there have been attempts to classify mega cisterna magna (MCM), Dandy-Walker variant, and Dandy-Walker syndrome as points along a spectrum of a single malformation based on a unified embryologic theory. The embryology of the cerebellum is reviewed briefly here. The superior aspects of the future cerebellar hemispheres are formed by the alar plates and the inferiorly located rhombic lips (1). The dorsal aspect of the fourth ventricle is covered by a membrane consisting of ependyma and vascularized pia (called the *tela choroidea*). At approximately 50 days of gestation, the primitive hemispheres join in the midline. The most primitive structures of the cerebellum are the nodulus (inferior and central) and flocculus (inferior and lateral), together called the *flocculonodular lobule*. The midline fusion of the hemispheres gives rise to the superior aspect of the vermis. The vermis develops from superior to inferior and contains nine lobules separated by fissures. As the vermis grows inferiorly, it obliterates the membranous roof (anterior membranous area) of the fourth ventricle. At the same time, an invagination of the tela choroidea (future choroid plexus) begins the filtration of cerebrospinal fluid (CSF). CSF distends the fourth ventricle and results in fenestration of the posterior (and inferior) membranous area with formation of the midline (Magendie) and lateral (Luschka) foramina. Incomplete development of the vermis results in a persistent anterior membranous region that becomes dilated in a balloon-like configuration. Thus, when the vermis is significantly underdeveloped, the result is a full-blown Dandy-Walker malformation. Lack of development of only the inferior vermis results in a Dandy-Walker variant, whereas slight vermian hypoplasia gives rise to an MCM.

Mega Cisterna Magna

MCM is an entity that nearly always is an incidental finding and a normal variant. It is an expansion of the normal cisterna magna and is seen in approximately 1% to 3% of the population (2). It communicates freely with subarachnoid spaces and results in no or very little mass effect on the posterior vermis. The vermis is normally formed (has its nine lobules) (1). MCM (also known as *retrocerebellar arachnoid pouch* or *Blake's cyst*) accounts for over 50% of all posterior fossa cystic malformations. It can be distinguished from arach-

An MCM often is traversed by the falx cerebelli and arachnoid septa, and there may be scalloping of the inner table because of CSF pulsations.

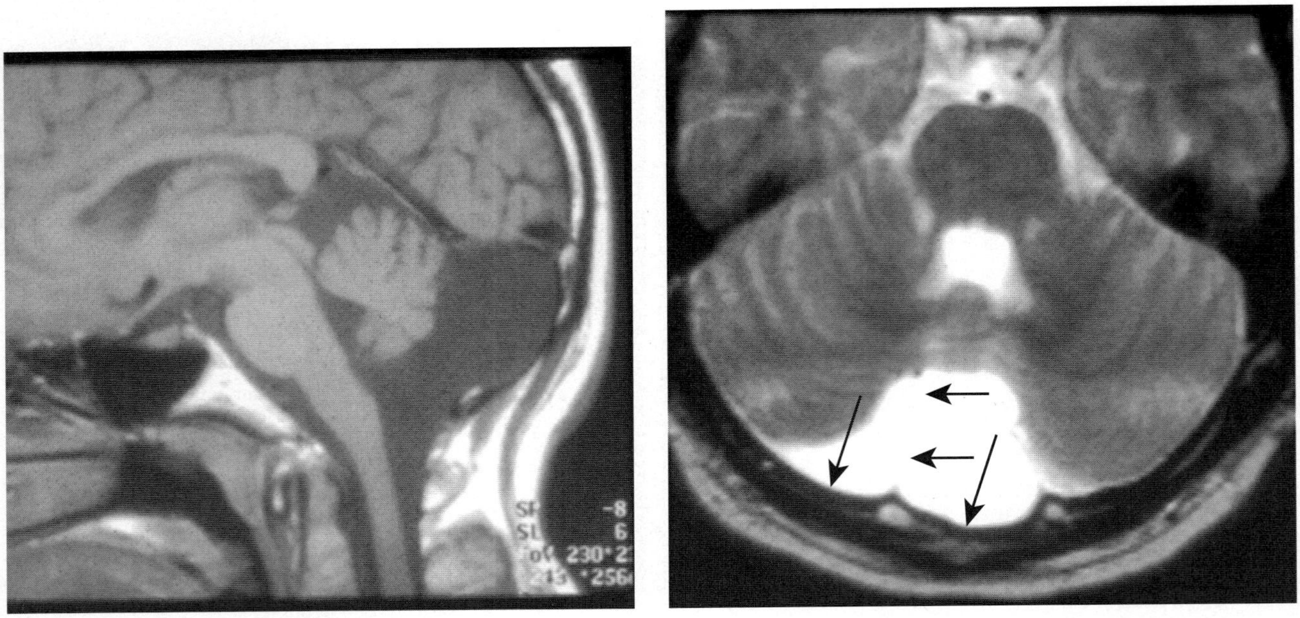

A B

Figure 1.1 *Mega Cisterna Magna.* Sagittal T1- *A* and axial T2-weighted *B* images show a large cisterna magna. Note mild compression of posterior vermis but no compression of the fourth ventricle. The inner table of the skull is mildly scalloped (*large arrows*) and the cistern is crossed by septa (*small arrows*).

noid cysts by its lack of mass effect on the fourth ventricle and the fact that it contains septa (Fig. 1.1). These septa often have a vein on their free edge. An arachnoid cyst displaces the septa, whereas an MCM is traversed by them. Occasionally, MCM results in scalloping of the inner table of the skull. This is likely to be the result of CSF pulsations. The overall size of the posterior fossa is normal. Some patients with MCM have hydrocephalus, and when this occurs I prefer to consider them as having a Dandy-Walker variant.

Dandy-Walker Variant

The Dandy-Walker variant is an intermediate entity characterized by expansion of an MCM and varying degrees of vermian hypoplasia (2). The large MCM is accompanied by

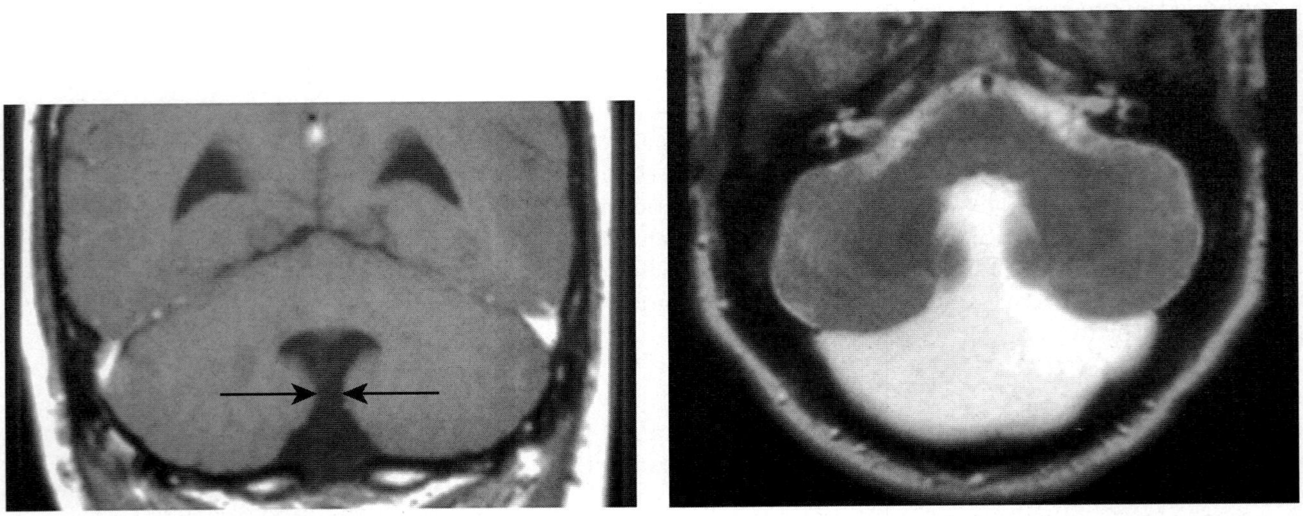

A B

Figure 1.2 *Dandy-Walker Variant.* Coronal T1- *A* and axial T2-weighted *B* images show a large cisterna magna, large vallecula (*arrows*), and prominent fourth ventricle. The inferior aspects of the cerebellar vermis are absent. The lateral ventricles are prominent.

dilation of the vallecula due to the absence of the inferior vermis (Fig. 1.2). The posterior fossa usually is of normal size. Approximately one third of these patients have some degree of hydrocephalus. The prognosis of these patients depends on the degree of hydrocephalus and is not directly related to the Dandy-Walker variant malformation.

Dandy-Walker Syndrome

The Dandy-Walker syndrome is a rare anomaly found in approximately 1:30,000 newborns (2,3). There is complete or partial vermian agenesis with only the superiormost lobules remaining intact. A cystlike fourth ventricle displaces and rotates the residual vermis anteriorly and superiorly (Fig. 1.3). The posterior fossa is large and venous sinuses do not descend normally. The straight sinus may be nearly vertical and the venous torcular is elevated (called a *torcular inversion*). The brainstem is hypoplastic. Most cases are diagnosed by *in utero* sonography. Hydrocephalus is found in most patients. The corpus callosum may be dysgenetic and anomalies of neuronal migration are not uncommon. An interhemispheric cyst may be present. The supratentorial abnormalities determine the patient's prognosis. Occasionally, Dandy-Walker syndrome may be accompanied by an occipitocervical meningoencephalocele.

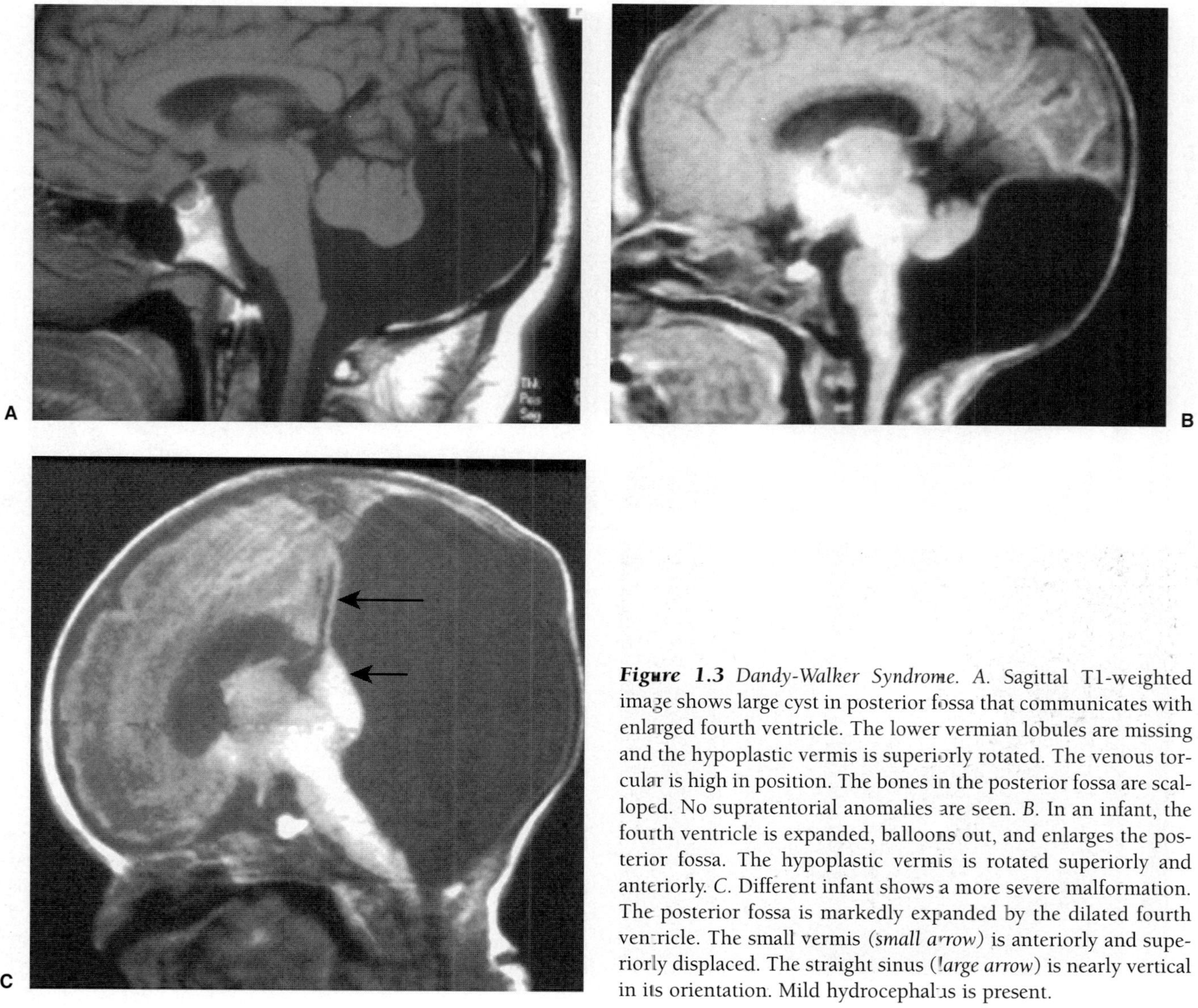

Figure 1.3 *Dandy-Walker Syndrome. A.* Sagittal T1-weighted image shows large cyst in posterior fossa that communicates with enlarged fourth ventricle. The lower vermian lobules are missing and the hypoplastic vermis is superiorly rotated. The venous torcular is high in position. The bones in the posterior fossa are scalloped. No supratentorial anomalies are seen. *B.* In an infant, the fourth ventricle is expanded, balloons out, and enlarges the posterior fossa. The hypoplastic vermis is rotated superiorly and anteriorly. *C.* Different infant shows a more severe malformation. The posterior fossa is markedly expanded by the dilated fourth ventricle. The small vermis (*small arrow*) is anteriorly and superiorly displaced. The straight sinus (*large arrow*) is nearly vertical in its orientation. Mild hydrocephalus is present.

Posterior Fossa Arachnoid Cysts

The most common locations for posterior fossa arachnoid cysts are the CPA cistern, the cisterna magna, and prepontine cistern, and the supravermian cistern.

Because posterior arachnoid cysts are included in the differential diagnosis of the Dandy-Walker spectrum of abnormalities, they are briefly addressed here. Arachnoid cysts are developmental anomalies of the meninx primitiva (2). This primitive and specialized tissue gives origin to the normal subarachnoid space. Its pluripotential cells may accumulate fat and their persistence results in formation of subarachnoid lipomas. Abnormal cavitation of the meninx primitiva may account for development of arachnoid cysts. The region of the cisterna magna is the second most common location for arachnoid cysts in the posterior fossa [the first being the cerebellopontine angle (CPA) cistern] (Fig. 1.4). Arachnoid cysts may compress the fourth ventricle, scallop adjacent bone, and contain no septa. They are rare in newborns but enlarge with time. At presentation, most are over 5 cm in diameter, and 30% to 100% of patients show hydrocephalus. They also occur in the prepontine region (third most common location in the posterior fossa), where they displace the brainstem posteriorly. The fourth most common location for posterior fossa arachnoid cysts is the supravermian cistern.

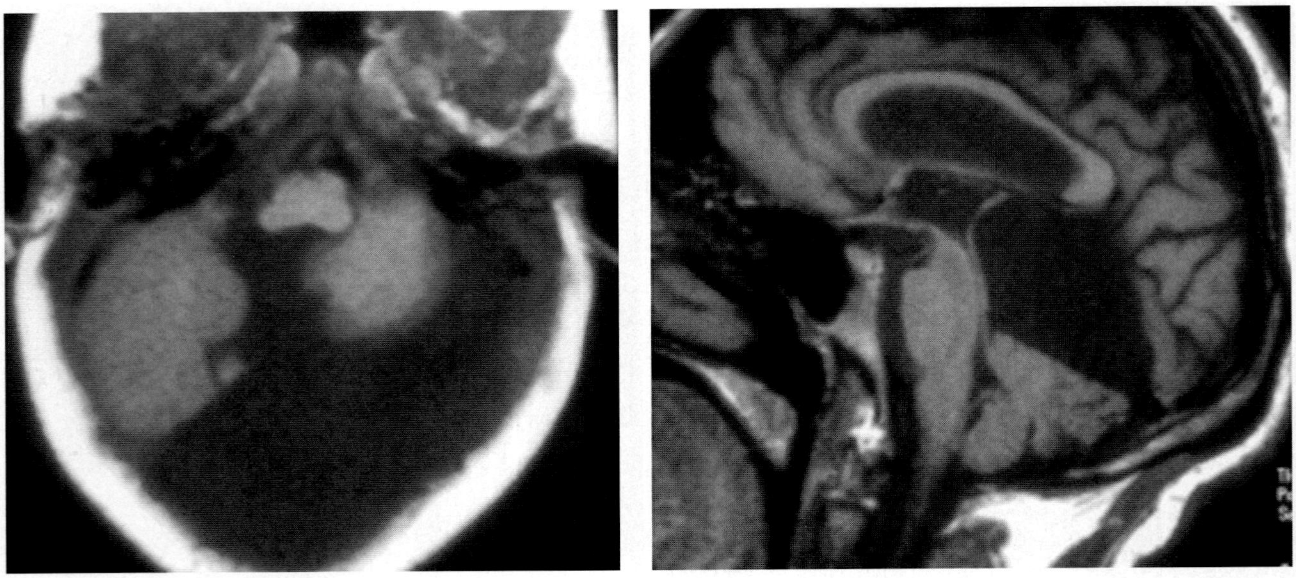

A

B

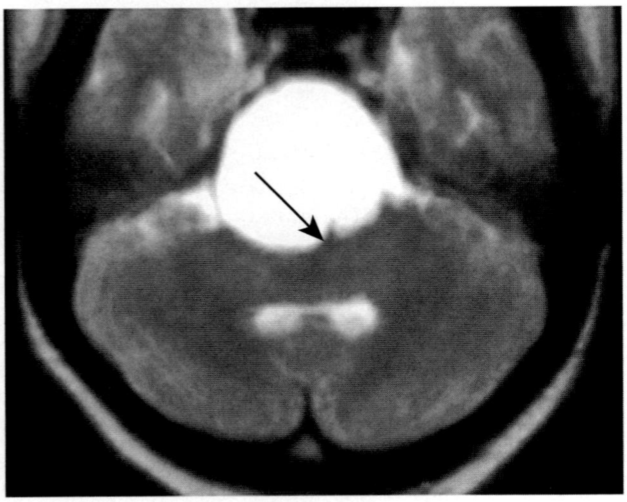

C

Figure 1.4 *Posterior Fossa Arachnoid Cysts. A.* An arachnoid cyst in the cisterna magna compresses the cerebellar hemispheres, particularly the left one. *B.* An arachnoid cyst in the supravermian cistern compresses the vermis and dorsal midbrain, resulting in moderate hydrocephalus. *C.* An arachnoid cyst in the prepontine cistern compresses the pons and basilar artery *(arrow)*.

CHIARI MALFORMATIONS

These three (four, in some classifications) malformations traditionally are grouped together, although they do not share an embryologic origin and have different imaging and clinical presentations. I address each one individually.

Chiari 1

This type of malformation is characterized by displacement of the cerebellar tonsils below the foramen magnum and is more common in girls (4). Its etiology is uncertain, but anomalies in expression of clustered (*Hox A–D*) and discontinuously expressed (*Gbx, Dbx*) homeobox genes may play an important role in its development (5). The symptoms depend on the degree of tonsillar herniation and most commonly include headaches, nystagmus, neck pain, and cranial nerve dysfunction. Most patients with herniations greater than 12 mm have symptoms, whereas only 30% of patients with herniations of 5 to 10 mm are symptomatic (most commonly, nystagmus, ataxia, and cranial nerve dysfunction) (4,6). Unilateral tonsillar herniation usually is not clinically significant. On mid-sagittal or slightly parasagittal T1-weighted magnetic resonance imaging (MRI), the normal tonsils are located above the foramen magnum. In newborns, a borderline position of the tonsils is not uncommon and usually disappears with age because of the differential growth between bone structures and the central nervous system (CNS). Tonsils inferiorly displaced less than 3 mm are normal (benign tonsillar ectopia); those displaced inferiorly 3 to 6 mm are suspect for a Chiari 1 malformation, but in the absence of symptoms, probably are not significant. Tonsils inferiorly herniated by more than 6 mm are compatible with a Chiari 1 malformation (Fig. 1.5). The shape of the tonsils also is important; most are triangular (peglike) in the Chiari 1 malformation (4). In this malformation, the foramen magnum also is small and cisterna magna is nearly absent. Approximately 30% to 55% of patients with a Chiari 1 malformation have a syringomyelia (4,7). Most spinal cord syrinxes in these patients occur in the cervical region. Accompanying bone abnormalities are found in 25% to 45% of patients with Chiari 1 malformation, and these include platybasia, basilar invagination, craniosynostosis (CS), and Klippel-Feil syndrome (4,6). Hydrocephalus also may develop. The flow of CSF at the level of the basal cisterns and foramen magnum is abnormal and may be evaluated using phase-contrast flow sensitive MRI. Phase-sensitive studies using prospective or (preferentially) retrospective cardiac gating show absence of caudal and cranial flow posteriorly, dissociation of CSF flow between cervical and cranial subarachnoid spaces, absence of flow and outlet foramina of the fourth ventricle, and downward displacement of tonsils during peak systole (7) (Fig. 1.6). After successful surgery, these abnormalities improve or disappear. Surgery entails augmentation of the foramen magnum, resection of the posterior arch of C1 (which tends to be small in these patients), resection of dural bands at the craniocervical junction, recreation of the cisterna magna, and, at times, resection of the tonsils.

Cerebellar tonsils displaced by more than 6 mm below the level of the foramen magnum and triangular in shape confirm the diagnosis of a Chiari 1 malformation.

Chiari 2

This is a complex malformation often detected *in utero* by sonography. It is more common in girls and practically all patients have a spinal myelomeningocele (most commonly in the lumbosacral region) (8). The intracranial anomalies are complex, but from a clinical point of view the most important one is the presence of hydrocephalus. Most patients undergo repair of the myelomeningocele shortly after birth, and their spine is not imaged acutely. Hydrocephalus is present in approximately 50% of neonates with Chiari 2 malformation, and develops in up to 80% of these patients eventually (9). Cranial sonography often is used to document hydrocephalus before the repair of the spinal dysraphism, and simultaneously dictates the need for ventricular shunting. The etiology of Chiari 2 malformation is not certain. A recent and unified hypothesis postulates that chronic leak of CSF through the open spinal dysraphism leads to lack of fluid accumulation and low intracranial pressure (10). The lack of distention of the CSF-containing spaces leads to

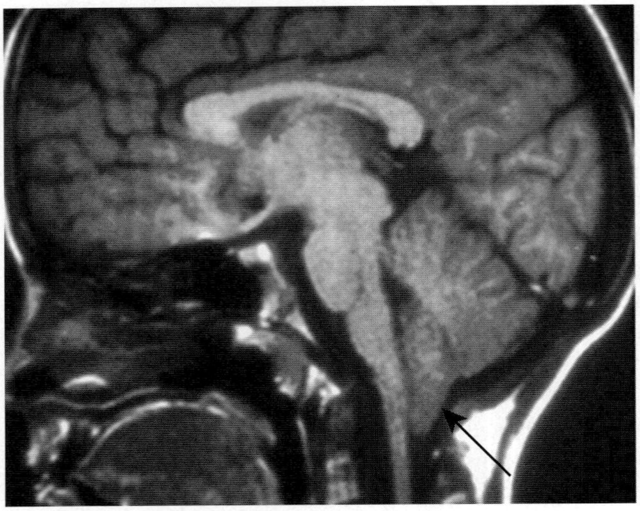

A

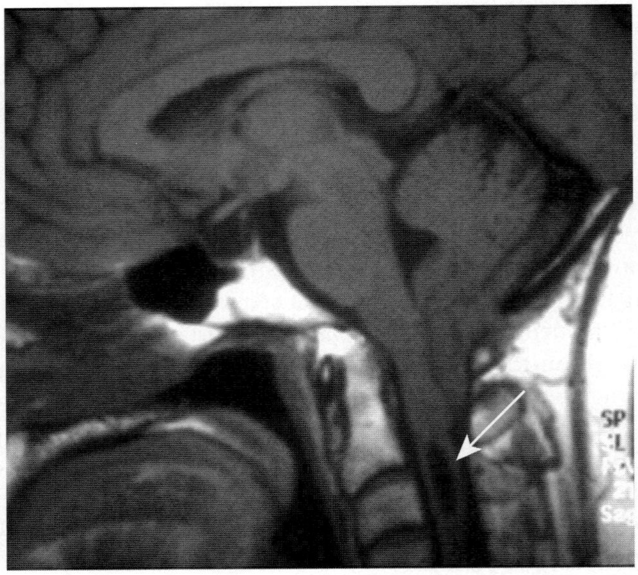

B

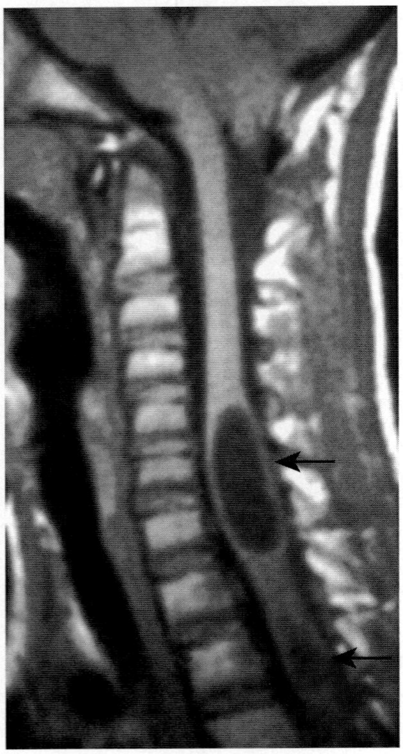

C

Figure 1.5 *Chiari 1 Malformation. A.* Child with a Chiari 1 malformation shows low-lying cerebellar tonsils *(arrow)* that are peg shaped. *B.* Different child shows inferiorly displaced and triangular cerebellar tonsils. Note reduction in size of cisterns about the foramen magnum and syrinx *(arrow)*. *C.* Different patient shows Chiari 1 malformation and spinal cord cysts *(arrows)* in the lower cervical and upper thoracic regions.

collapse and herniation of the posterior fossa structures, dysgenesis of the corpus callosum, anomalies of neuronal migration, and mesenchymal abnormalities. The most common symptoms are respiratory distress, apnea, and cranial nerve dysfunction thought to be due to an internal disorganization of the brainstem nuclei. Approximately 5% to 30% of patients with a Chiari 2 malformation are asymptomatic. The imaging features of this malformation have been extensively studied (3,9) (Table 1.1 and Fig. 1.7).

From a practical standpoint, most brain imaging in patients with Chiari 2 malformation is done to evaluate for hydrocephalus. Comparison with prior studies, if available, is imperative to detect early ventricular dilatation and shunt failure. The fourth ventricle always is small in patients with Chiari 2 malformation and working shunts. Distention of

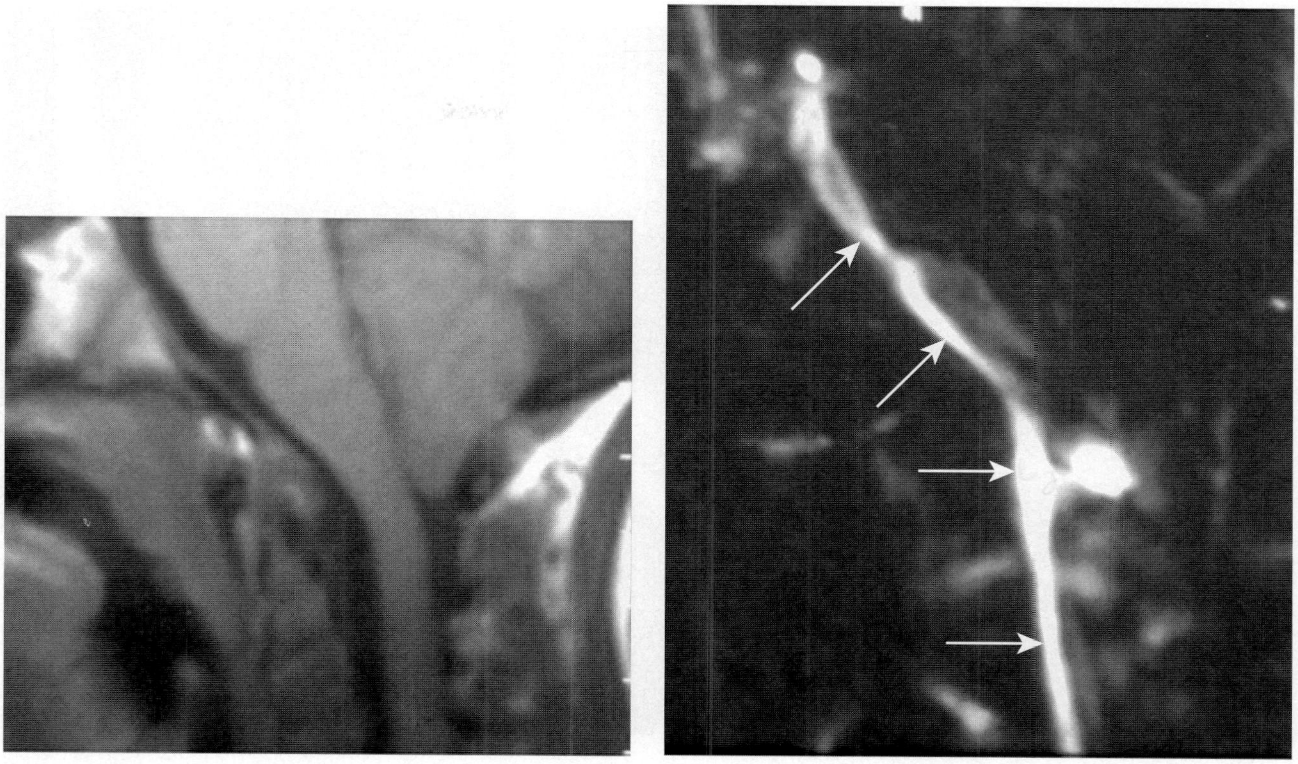

A B

Figure 1.6 *Cerberospinal Fluid (CSF) Flow Study in Chiari 1. A.* Sagittal T1-weighted image shows typical herniation of cerebellar tonsils. *B.* Phase-contrast CSF flow-sensitive study during systolic portion of cardiac cycle is abnormal because it shows downward *(arrows)* CSF flow in the ventral cisterns but none in the region of the cisterna magna or posterior cervical subarachnoid space.

the fourth ventricle is suspect for a malfunctioning shunt. Many patients with myelomeningoceles now are undergoing *in utero* repair of the defect. In our experience, these patients show intracranial changes of Chiari 2 malformation, but they are less severe. The incidence of hydrocephalus also is less after *in utero* repair of open spinal dysraphism.

Table 1.1: Magnetic Resonance Imaging Abnormalities in Chiari 2

Cerebral Hemispheres	*Cerebellum*	*Spinal Cord*	*Skull and Cervical Spine*
Hydrocephalus	Small fourth ventricle	Syrinx	Lukenschadel
Dysgenesis of corpus callosum	Overgrowth of hemispheres anterior to pons	Cervicomedullary kink	Hypoplasia or fenestration of falx cerebri
Frontal horn beaking	Herniation of the vermis below foramen magnum	Wide subarachnoid spaces	Wide interhemispheric fissure, particularly posteriorly
Stenogyria	Absent vermian folia		Clival scalloping
Aqueductal stenosis			Scalloping of posterior petrous bones
Beaked tectum			Anomalies of posterior arch of C1 and other vertebral segmentation anomalies
Neural migration anomalies			Small posterior fossa
Small or large third ventricle			Wide foramen magnum
Large massa intermeda			

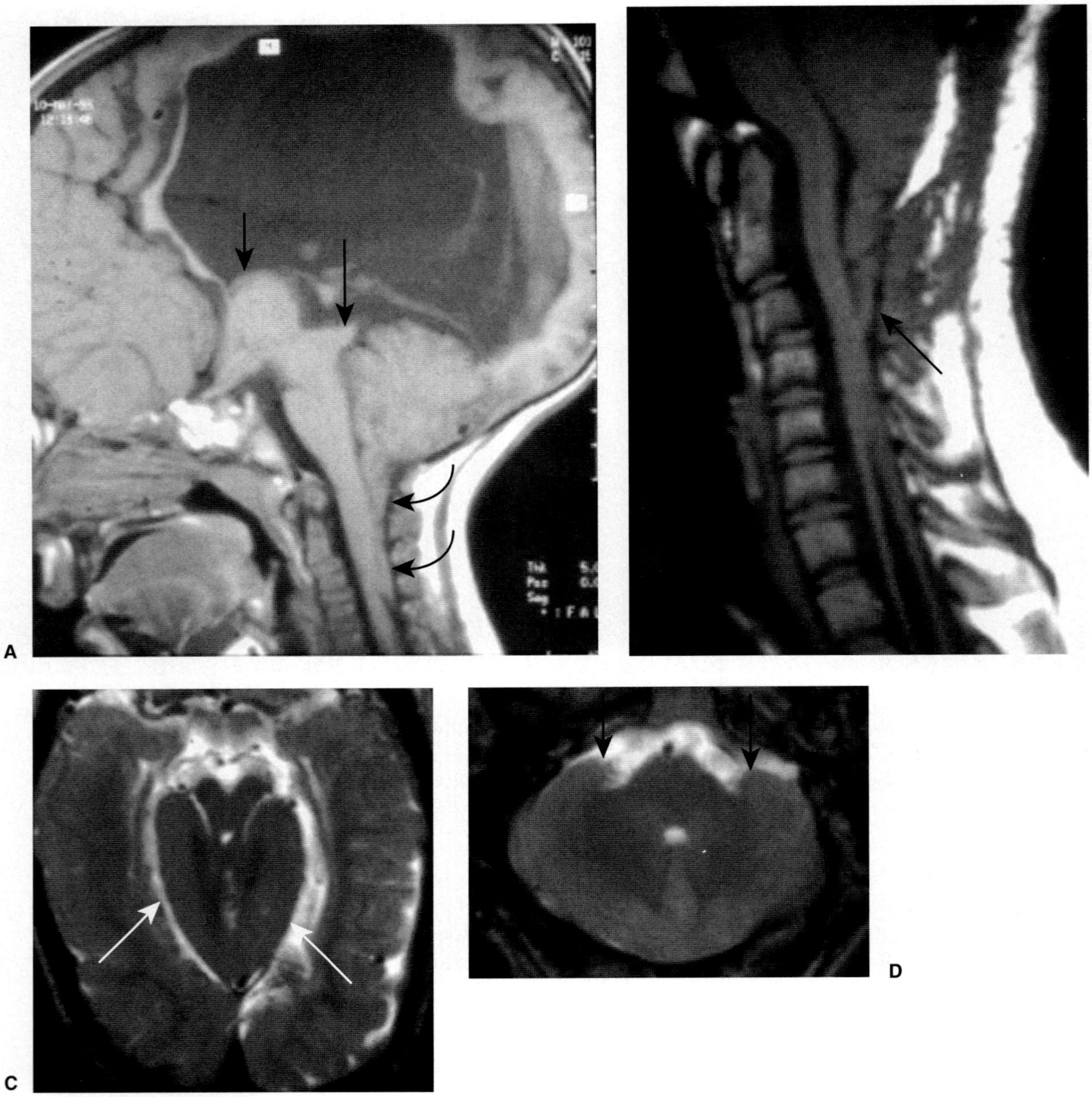

Figure 1.7 *Chiari 2 Malformation. A.* Sagittal T1-weighted image shows inferiorly displaced cerebellar vermis *(curved arrow)*, absent fourth ventricle, beaked tectum (*large arrow*), large massa intermedia *(small arrow)*, dysgenetic corpus callosum, and interhemispheric cyst. *B.* Different case shows inferiorly herniated vermis (*arrow*) and a cervical spinal cord cyst. *C.* Axial T2-weighted image shows heart-shaped (*arrows*) upward herniation of cerebellum due to an incompetent tentorial incisura. *D.* Axial T2-weighted image shows "anterior overgrowth" *(arrows)* of the cerebellar hemispheres.

To make the diagnosis of a Chiari 3 malformation, the encephalocele, which may be occipital, cervical, or parietal, needs to be accompanied by the intracranial findings seen in a Chiari 2 malformation.

Chiari 3

This is the most severe of all the Chiari malformations and is related to an anomaly of neural tube closure at the craniocervical junction. By definition, patients with a Chiari 3 malformation have a meningoencephalocele (occipital, parietal, cervical, or a combination of these locations) and the intracranial features of a Chiari 2 malformation (11). Not all posterior "celes" are Chiari 3 malformations; only those in combination with anomalies also seen in Chiari 2 malformation are classified as Chiari 3 (Fig. 1.8). The prognosis of these patients depends on the size of the meningoencephalocele; large ones are incompat-

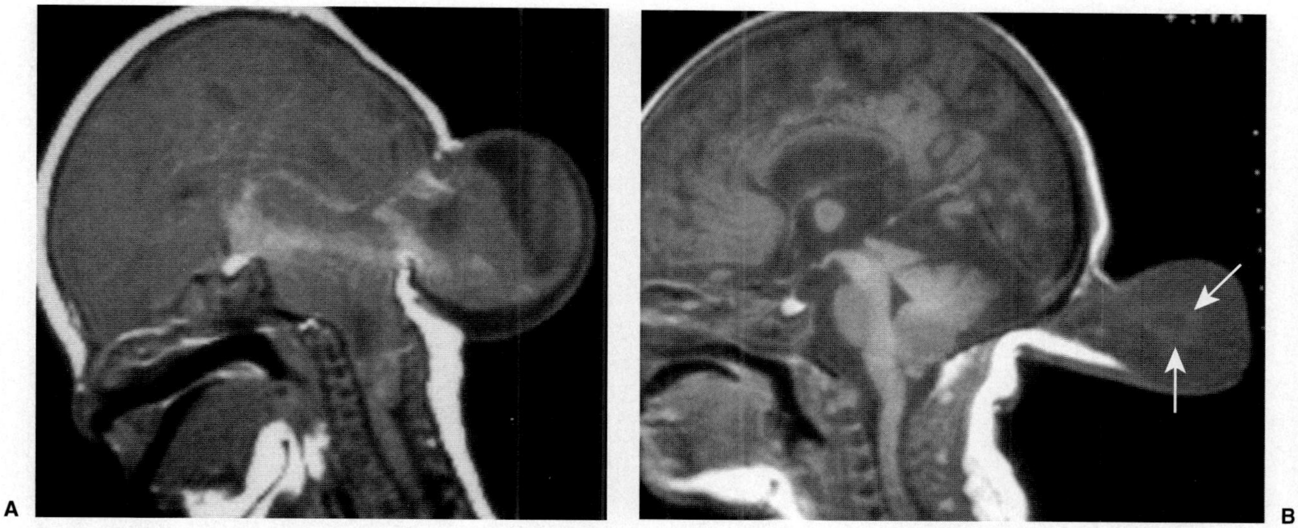

Figure 1.8 *Chiari 3 Malformation. A.* Sagittal T1-weighted image shows occipital encephalocele and inferior herniation of cerebellar structures through the foramen magnum. The corpus callosum is dysgenetic. *B.* In this patient, there is a suboccipital, mostly fluid-filled encephalocele [note tissues *(arrows)* contained in it]. Also note large massa intermedia and beaked tectum. The corpus callosum is dysgenetic.

ible with life. The encephaloceles often contain cerebellum, fourth ventricle, and occipital lobes. Most of the tissue in them is gliotic, malformed, and nonfunctional. It is imperative to determine the presence of venous sinuses inside the encephalocele to avoid their resection and subsequent development of intracranial hypertension. The brainstem also may extend into the herniated pouch. Most patients have severe supratentorial anomalies and hydrocephalus. Syringomyelia also may be present.

Chiari 4

I do not believe that this malformation exists as such. Chiari 4 describes a variety of anomalies whose end result is significant hypoplasia of the cerebellar vermis and hemispheres, a thin brainstem, a small posterior fossa, and normal or nearly normal cerebral hemispheres (12). Anomalies associated with cerebellar hypoplasia are shown in Table 1.2.

Table 1.2: Conditions in Which Cerebellar Hypoplasia is Present

Nearly Always	*Variable*
Dandy-Walker syndrome	Meckel-Gruber syndrome
Joubert's syndrome	Coffin-Siris syndrome
Walker-Warburg syndrome	Ellis-van Creveld syndrome
Pontocerebellar hypoplasia	Fraser's cryptophthalmos
Cerebrooculomuscular syndrome	Aicardi's syndrome
	Cornelia de Lange's syndrome
	Werdnig-Hoffman disease

JOUBERT'S SYNDROME

As used by radiologists, Joubert's syndrome refers to a group of imaging findings that may result in variable clinical findings. Strictly speaking, Joubert's syndrome is an autosomal recessive disease that may or may be not associated with retinal dystrophy (5). Symptoms are apnea, ataxia, nystagmus, and oculomotor apraxia. Facial anomalies and mental retardation also may be seen. On imaging, the findings are similar despite the varying symp-

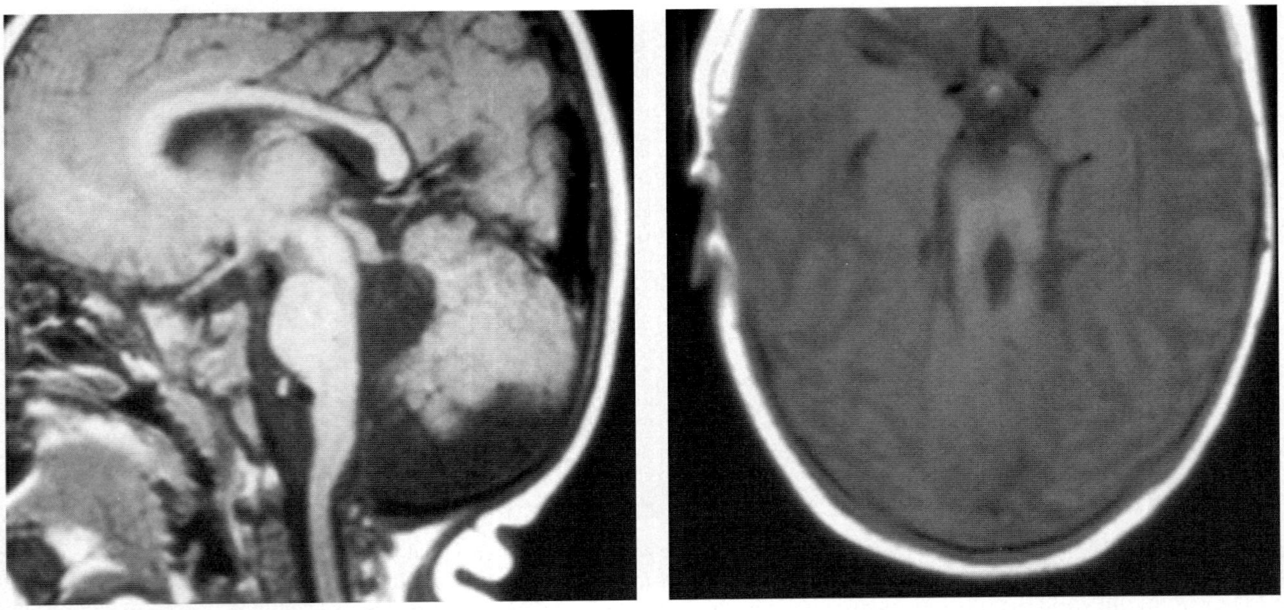

A B

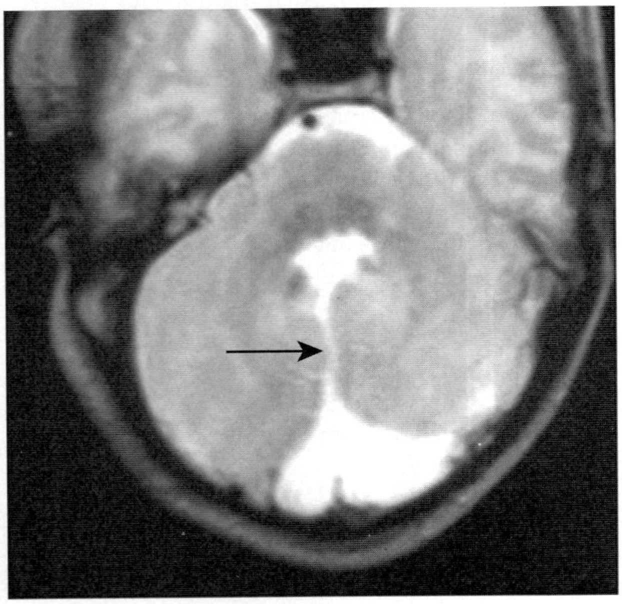

C

Figure 1.9 *Joubert's Syndrome. A.* Sagittal T1-weighted image shows superiorly enlarged fourth ventricle and dysplastic cerebellar vermis. *B.* Axial T1-weighted image shows parallel orientation of the superior cerebellar peduncles. *C.* Axial T2-weighted image shows cleft (*arrow*) where the vermis is expected.

toms. MRI shows complete or nearly complete agenesis of the cerebellar vermis (2) (Fig. 1.9). The fourth ventricle has an abnormal shape ("batwing" configuration on axial images) and is prominent superiorly on sagittal views. The cerebellar fissures are separated in the midline by a cleft where the vermis should be present. The superior cerebellar peduncles course parallel to each other (this is seen better on axial images). The brainstem may be hypoplastic. Joubert's syndrome may be associated with dysgenesis of the corpus callosum and occipital encephalocele. Cerebral atrophy is present in older patients. Cortical dysplasias, such as the perisylvian syndrome, also may be present.

Rhomboencephalosynapsis

Rhomboencephalosynapsis is extremely rare and is characterized by the absence of the cerebellar vermis and midline fusion of the cerebellar hemispheres (13). Most of the patients I have seen with this anomaly have significant supratentorial anomalies, and the

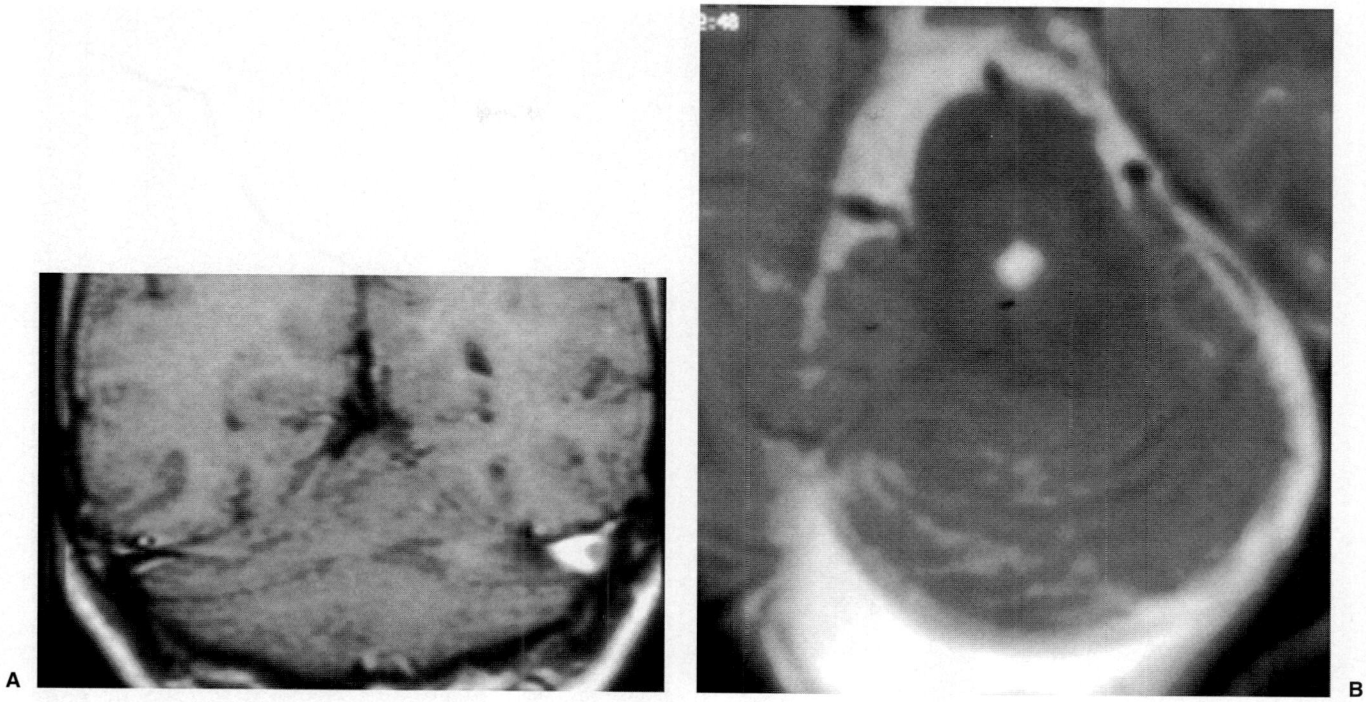

Figure 1.10 *Rhomboencephalosynapsis. A.* Coronal T1-weighted image shows midline fusion of the cerebellar hemispheres and absent vermis. *B.* In a different patient, axial T2-weighted image shows small cerebellum with absent vermis and midline fusion; note continuation of the folia and fissures across midline. The fourth ventricle and brainstem are small.

prognosis and symptoms depend on them rather than on the cerebellar abnormalities. MRI shows absence of the vermis with continuation of the folia and fissures across the midline (Fig. 1.10). The cerebellar cortex may appear thick, and the deep gray structures are fused. The fourth ventricle appears nearly normal on sagittal views but it is elongated in its anteroposterior dimension on axial images. The entire cerebellum may be small and the brainstem may be hypoplastic. The cerebral hemispheres may contain areas of abnormal neuronal migration, including gray matter heterotopias or cortical dysplasias. The hippocampi may be small or abnormally folded. Hydrocephalus, dysgenesis of the corpus callosum, and absence of the septum pellucidum also are seen with this anomaly.

Encephaloceles

Posterior "celes" are rare and found in 1 to 3:10,000 live births (14). In North America, 80% of all encephaloceles are posterior. Pure posterior meningoceles are rare. Most celes contain meninges as well as ectopic, nonfunctional brain tissues (and hence are encephaloceles). Most are occipital in location, but not uncommonly they extend into the upper cervical spine or parietal region (Fig. 1.11). The degree of intracranial anomalies is inversely proportional to the size and contents of the encephalocele The largest ones usually are accompanied by severe intracranial defects. Aventriculy (absence of the ventricles) often is seen in patients with large encephaloceles (15) (Fig. 1.12). The encephalocele usually contains cerebellum and occipital lobes. MR venography may be useful in assessing for sinuses inside the pouch (see section on Chiari 3 malformation). Occipital encephaloceles are seen in the following syndromes:

- Dandy-Walker syndrome
- Chiari 3 malformation
- Joubert's syndrome

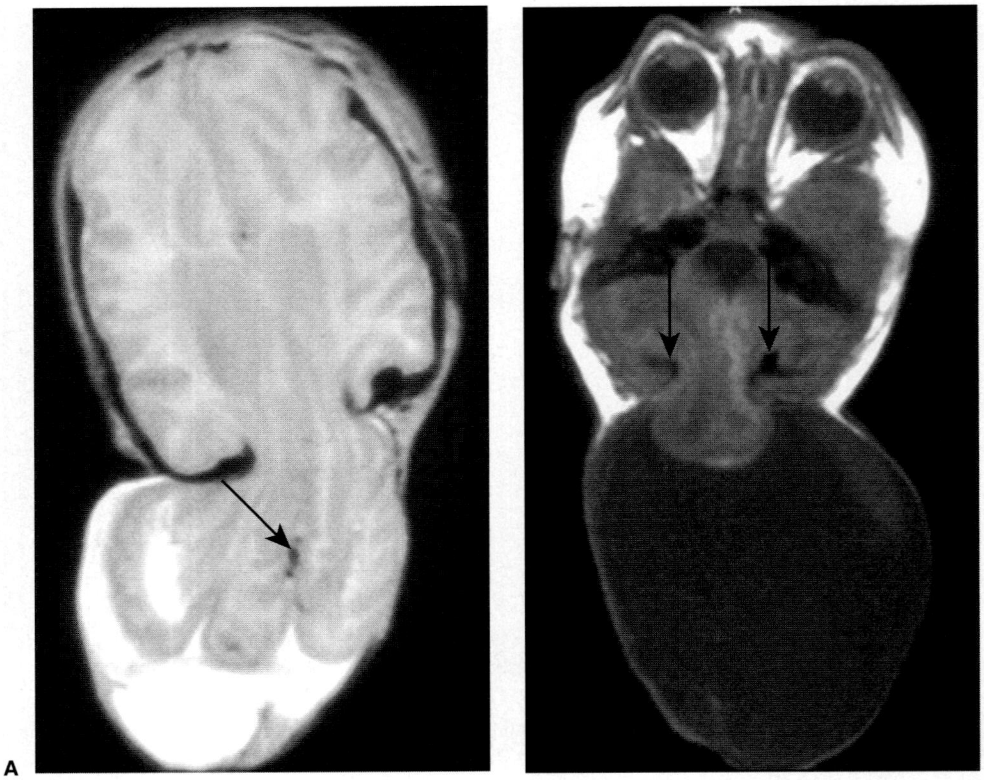

Figure 1.11 *Posterior Encephaloceles. A.* Axial T2-weighted image shows occipital encephalocele containing the superior sagittal sinus *(arrow). B.* Axial T1-weighted image (different case) shows occipital encephalocele containing mostly cisterns. The transverse sinuses (*arrows*) remain intracranially.

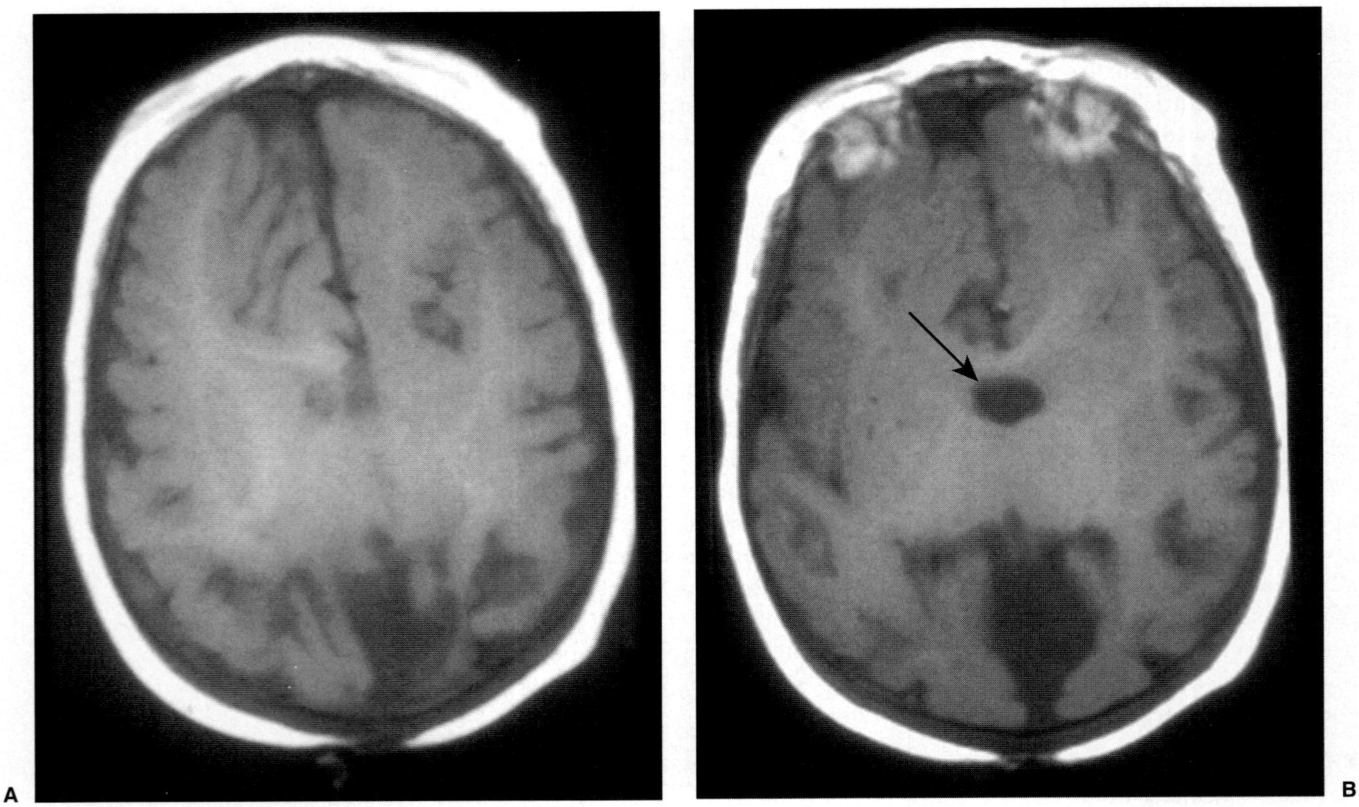

Figure 1.12 *Aventriculy*. Axial T1-weighted images in a patient status post repair of an occipital encephalocele shows absence of lateral ventricles *A* and only a rudimentary third ventricle (*arrow* in *B*).

- Klippel-Feil syndrome
- Walker-Warburg syndrome
- Meckel-Gruber syndrome
- Goldenhar-Gorlin syndrome
- Fraser's syndrome

Epidermoid and Dermoid

The most common location for posterior fossa epidermoid tumors are the CPA cistern, the vallecula and perimedullary cisterns, and the fourth ventricle.

Most epidermoid and dermoid tumors in children are found infratentorially. Both types of lesions contain ectodermal elements, but only dermoids contain skin appendages (e.g., sweat glands, hair follicles, sebaceous glands) (16). Both lesions presumably are the sequela of incomplete disjunction of the neural tube from the overlying ectoderm that results in entrapment of ectodermal elements in the CNS. Epidermoids are more common and are located off-midline, whereas intracranial dermoids are midline tumors. Outside the intracranial compartment, dermoids may be off-midline (lacrimal gland, intradiploic or frontozygomatic suture) or midline (submandibular space and anterior fontanelle). Nearly all epidermoids are located in the CPA cistern regions, followed by the suprasellar, pineal gland, and sylvian fissure regions. Epidermoids also may be found inside the fourth ventricle. Epidermoids may be found inside Meckel's cave or extending into it when the primary lesion is located in the CPA region. Dermoids are common in the spine (usually in association with dysraphism), but also may be found intracranially (17,18). The most common locations for dermoids are the fourth ventricle, vermis, and suprasellar and pineal gland regions. Both epidermoids and dermoids may be associated with dermal sinuses, especially when these sinuses are found in the occipital and suboccipital regions. Both tumors may compress adjacent structures and both may leak in the CSF-containing spaces, resulting in chemical meningitis. This aseptic meningitis may produce hydrocephalus.

Historically, epidermoids have been difficult to differentiate from arachnoid cysts using conventional MRI sequences. This is no longer the case. Although epidermoids may simulate arachnoid cysts on T1- and heavily T2-weighted images, there are many sequences that highlight their differences (16) (Fig. 1.13). On proton-density images, epidermoids show streaky or serpiginous areas of internal signal intensity not seen in arachnoid cysts. On CISS images (constructive interference in the steady state), epidermoids show internal areas of varying signal intensity not seen in arachnoid cysts. In addition, epidermoids are diffusely bright on diffusion-weighted imaging (DWI), whereas arachnoid cysts have a more heterogeneous appearance and overall lower signal intensity (18). Epidermoids do not enhance after contrast administration. I have seen two epidermoid tumors that were of very low signal intensity on DWI, but consider this finding to be very rare. Epidermoids and dermoids inside the ventricle are very rare (Fig. 1.14).

Dermoids nearly always are bright on T1-weighted images and simulate lipomas (16). It is difficult to differentiate a subarachnoid space lipoma from a dermoid, but the latter are very rare. The presence of fat droplets in the CSF-containing spaces is typical of a ruptured dermoid, but similar findings may be seen in those few remaining patients who underwent myelography with lipid-based contrast agents (e.g., Pantopaque) (17). In the presence of fat droplets, a search for a dermoid is indicated (18–20). If a tumor is not found intracranially, the spine should be studied. A dermoid also may appear similar to a teratoma. Teratomas do not rupture with resulting fat droplets, and unlike dermoids, nearly always show some enhancement.

Occasionally one encounters the so-called bright or white epidermoids and black dermoids (16). The signal intensity of both of these lesions depends on the presence of keratin and cholesterol and the way these substances are bound to water. In most epidermoids, these substances are in a solid state, which does not allow for shortening of the T1 relaxation time, whereas in dermoids they normally are found in a liquid form that allows for bright signal on T1-weighted sequences. Rare white epidermoids containing liquid cholesterol/keratin are bright on T1-weighted images, whereas the rare black dermoids contain these substances in a solid form and are dark on T1-weighted images.

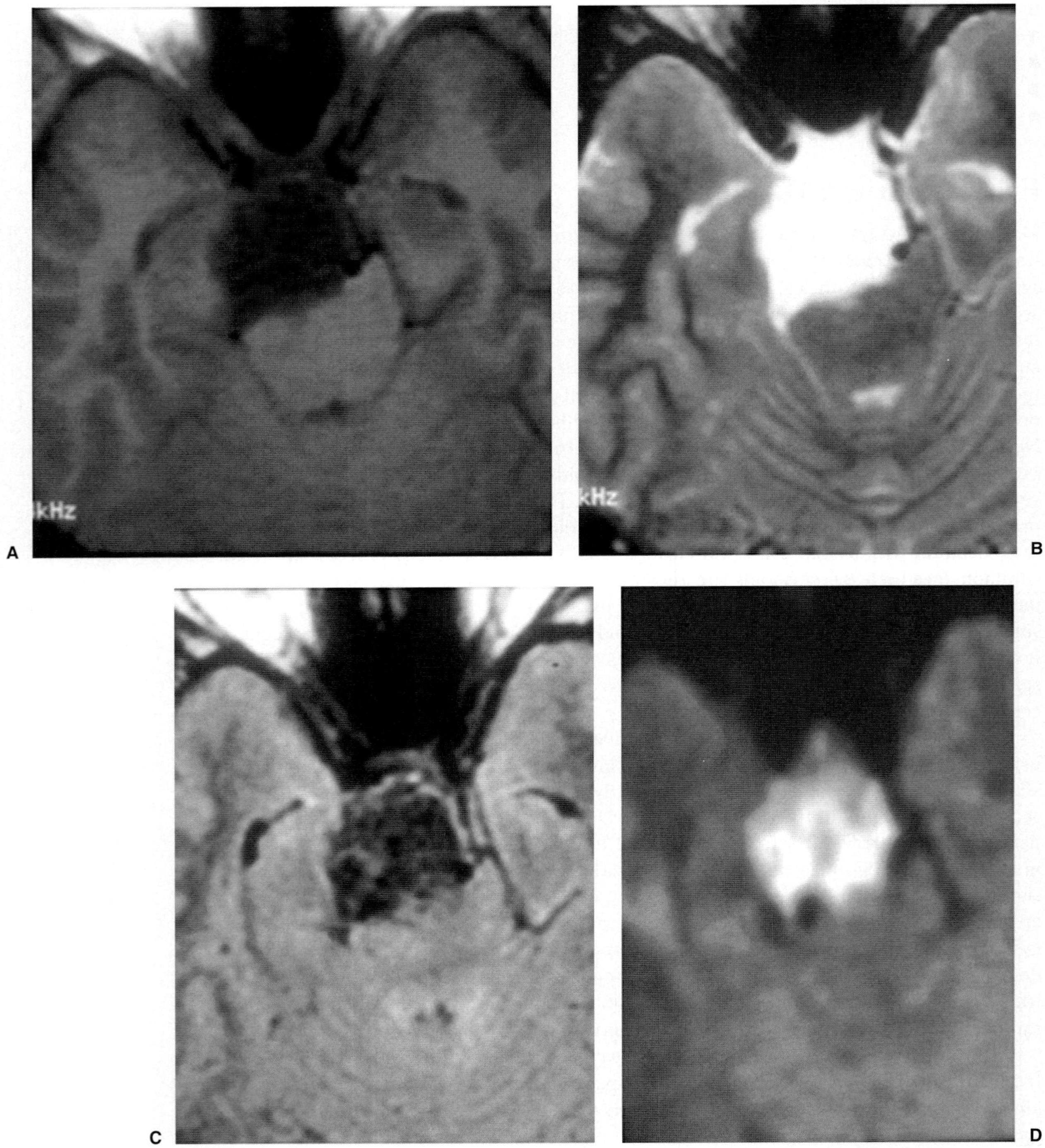

Figure 1.13 *Epidermoid.* Axial T1- *A* and T2-weighted *B* images show this prepontine epidermoid to be nearly identical in signal intensity to cerebrospinal fluid (CSF). Fluid attenuation inversion recovery image *C* shows it to be brighter than CSF and to contain areas of increased signal. Diffusion-weighted image *D* shows the lesion to the bright.

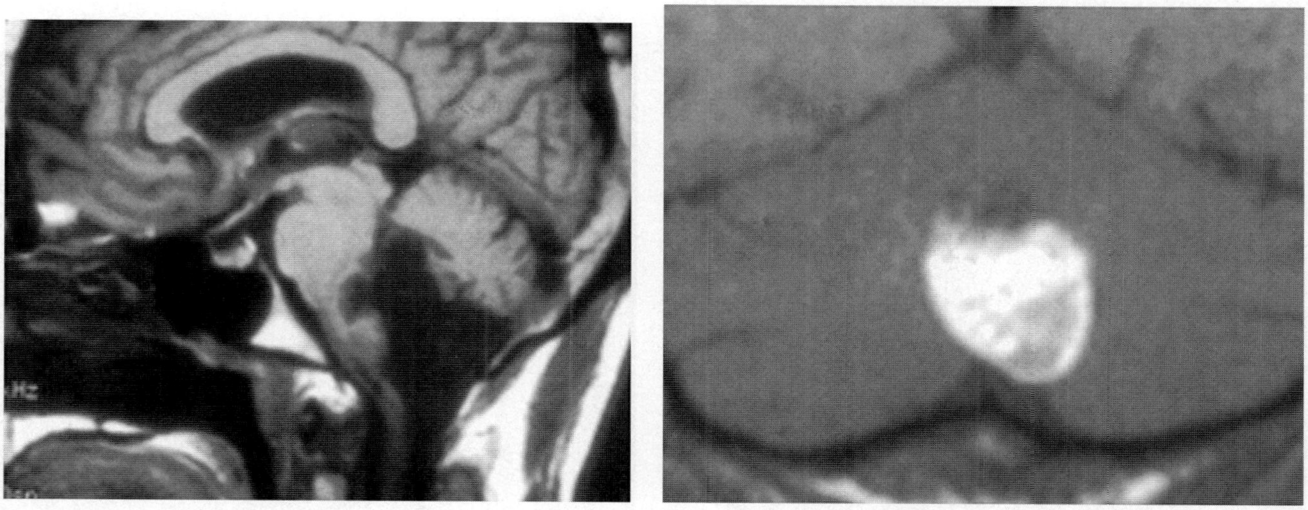

A B

Figure 1.14 *Fourth Ventricular Epidermoid and Dermoid. A.* Sagittal T1-weighted image shows epidermoid in an expanded fourth ventricle and extending through its outlet foramina to the cisterna magna. Note scalloped borders of the lesion. *B.* Coronal T1-weighted image shows a bright dermoid in the fourth ventricle.

Intracranial neuroenteric cysts may appear similar to dermoids, particularly in the posterior fossa (21). Intracranial neuroenteric cysts, however, are extremely rare. These cysts may be located inside the fourth ventricle or in the prepontine region. They tend to be bright on T1-weighted images because they contain mucin.

Supratentorial Congenital Anomalies

Dysgenesis of the Corpus Callosum

The pertinent embryology is reviewed briefly. The rostralmost aspect of the neural tube contains the lamina terminalis (1,3). At approximately 50 days of life, the lamina terminalis thickens and becomes the lamina reuniens (this is approximately the same time when the vermis is forming, and thus anomalies of the vermis commonly are associated with anomalies of the corpus callosum). The lamina reuniens has a midline groove that is filled with the meninx primitiva and also contains the glial cells that will guide the axons from one hemisphere to the next, eventually forming the corpus callosum. Incomplete formation of the corpus callosum results in differentiation of the persistent meninx primitiva into lipomas. Thus, many patients with a dysgenetic corpus callosum also harbor subarachnoid lipomas (mostly in the vicinity of the abnormal corpus callosum). The corpus callosum forms from front to back (genu, body, splenium), with the rostrum being the last portion to form. The junction between the body and splenium (isthmus) may be thin in up to 25% of individuals, and should not be interpreted as being abnormal (22). The corpus callosum myelinates from back to front (3) (Table 1.3).

Table 1.3: Myelination of the Corpus Callosum on T1-Weighted Images

Region of Corpus Callosum	*Time of Normal Myelination*
Splenium	3–4 mo
Body	4–5 mo
Genu	5–6 mo

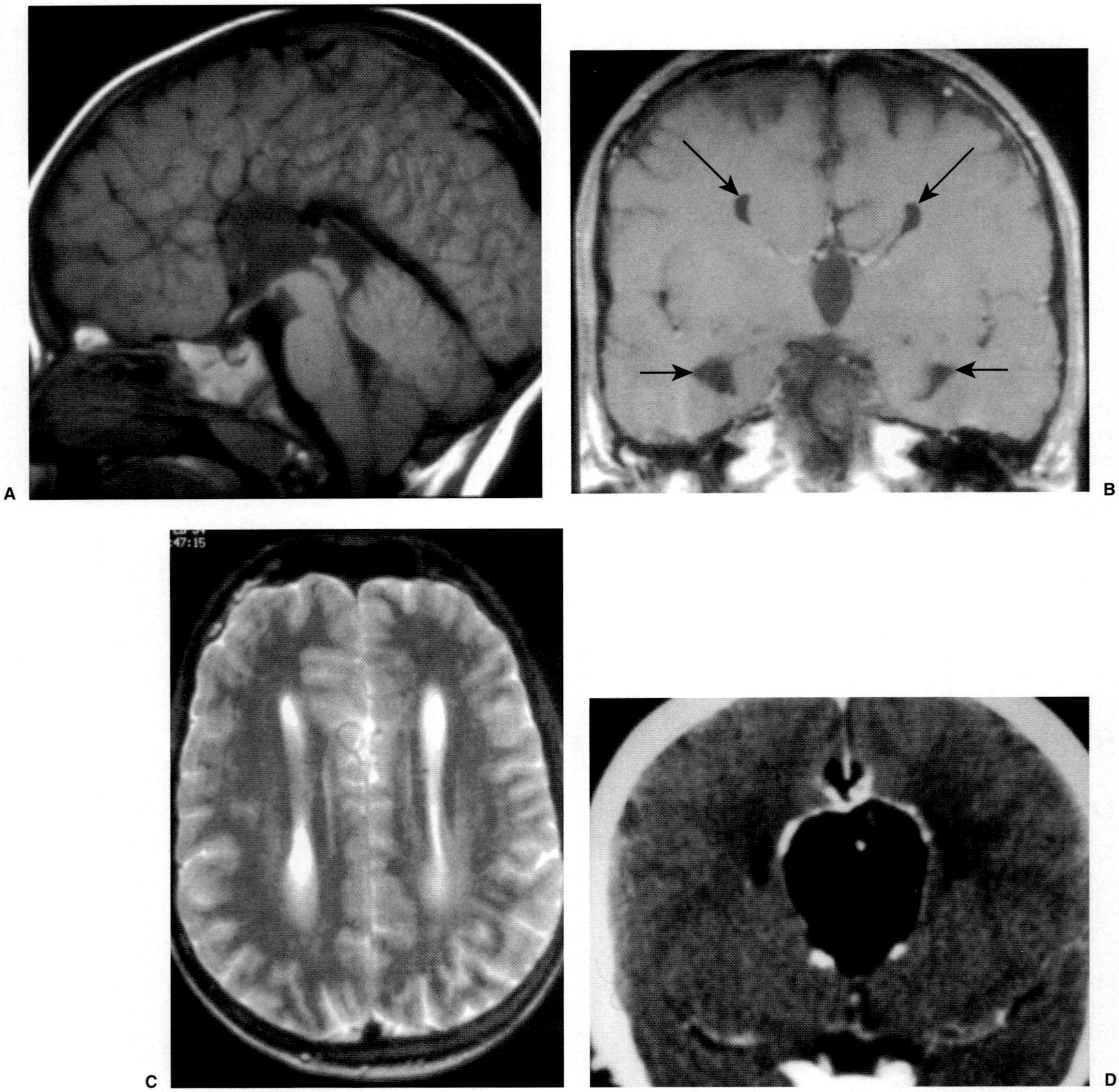

Figure 1.15 *Agenesis and Dysgenesis of the Corpus Callosum. A.* Sagittal T1-weighted image absent corpus callosum and a Chiari 1 malformation. *B.* On a coronal T1-weighted image, the frontal horns (*large arrows*) of the lateral ventricles have a "steer horn" appearance and the temporal horns (*small arrows*) are prominent due to abnormal folding of the hippocampi. *C.* On an axial T2-weighted image, the lateral ventricles have an abnormal orientation, parallel to each other, because of absence of the corpus callosum. *D.* Coronal computed tomography shows large nodular lipoma associated with agenesis of the corpus callosum.

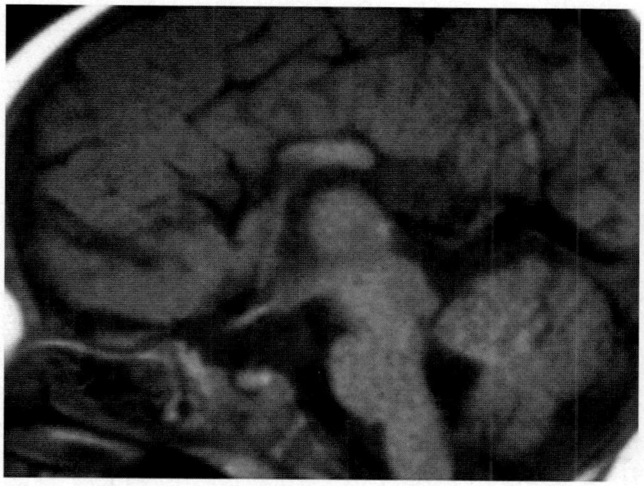

E

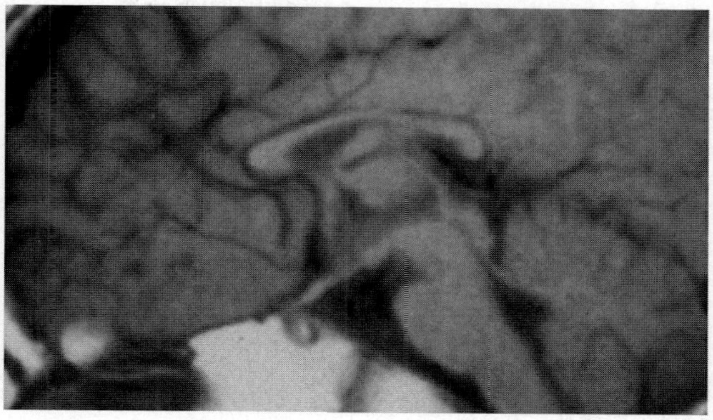

F

Figure 1.15 (continued) E. Sagittal T1-weighted image shows a tiny dysgenetic corpus callosum. F. In another patient, the corpus callosum has a normal shape but is very small.

The corpus callosum forms from front to back (with the exception of the rostrum, which is last to form) and myelinates from back to front.

If a portion of the corpus callosum is absent, it is most likely to be its posterior region (posterior body and splenium). At times, only the rostrum may be absent. The corpus callosum also may be completely absent (23) (Fig. 1.15A). In these cases, the third ventricle is high riding and may or may not communicate with an interhemispheric CSF-filled cyst. Most of these cysts are dorsal, but occasionally they are rostral in location. The cyst splays the lateral ventricles and may or may not communicate with them. On coronal images, the frontal horns are prominent and point superiorly and laterally ("steer horn" configuration; Fig. 1.15B). On axial images, the lateral ventricles assume a course parallel to each other (Fig. 1.15C). The sulci in the medial aspect of the hemispheres may assume a radial pattern, tending to converge in the region of the massa intermedia (interthalamic adhesion). The temporal horns of the lateral ventricles are prominent (even without hydrocephalus) because of an abnormal folding of the hippocampi (3,24). The atria of the lateral ventricles commonly are enlarged (called *colpocephaly*). Lipomas may be present (Fig. 1.15D). There are many syndromes associated with dysgenesis of the corpus callosum, and many patients with this anomaly have other cerebral malformations such as gray matter heterotopias and cortical dysplasias. The anterior aspect of the corpus callosum occasionally may be absent in the presence of the posterior corpus callosum. This usually is seen in patients with holoprosencephaly (HP), frontal schizencephaly (SC), and frontal congenital porencephalic cysts. Very rarely, the mid-portion of the corpus callosum is absent and its anteriormost and posteriormost regions are formed. This is most likely a variant of HP with midline hemispheric fusion (25). The corpus callosum may be thin but completely formed (3). This usually implies an insult after its formation has been completed, and the most common cause is periventricular leukomalacia that results in degeneration of its axons (Fig. 1.15E and F). Increased volume of the corpus callosum is rare and its significance is questionable, but this has been observed in patients with neurofibromatosis type 1 (NF-1) and in schizophrenia. Most patients with dysgenesis of the corpus callosum have developmental delay and seizures, but occasionally some are normal.

HOLOPROSENCEPHALY

HP is a spectrum of disorders involving midline fusion of the cerebral hemispheres. It is divided somewhat artificially into three types that may be difficult to separate. The most severe type is the alobar, but it has little significance to radiologists because most patients are stillborn or die shortly after birth. It is, however, important to establish the diagnosis

Table 1.4: Facial Features in Alober Holoprosencephaly

Malformation	*Components*
Cyclopia	Single median orbit, very rare and incompatible with life
Ethmocephaly	Hypotelorism with supraorbital single proboscis
Cebocephaly	Hypotelorism with infraorbital single proboscis
Absent intermaxillary segment	Hypoplastic nose, no nasal septum, midline facial cleft
Rudimentary intermaxillary segment	Small nose, midline cleft lip which may extend into the nose

for genetic counseling purposes. Alobar HP always is accompanied by facial malformations (by definition, hypotelorism always is present) (26) (Table 1.4).

In alobar HP, the falx cerebri and midline venous sinuses are absent (26). The brain shows midline continuation of gray/white matter and the interhemispheric fissure is absent (Fig. 1.16). The anterior cerebral arteries may be solitary (azygos). There is a single ventricle (monoventricle) that is horseshoe shaped and may communicate with a dorsal midline CSF-filled cyst. The septum pellucidum and fornices are absent. The third ventricle is not identified and the thalami are fused. The brainstem is small and the cerebellum is nearly normal in size. The patients are severely microcephalic.

In the intermediate form (semilobar), there is some differentiation of the hemispheres, particularly posteriorly (26). The occipital horns and atria of the lateral ventricles may be present, but the diencephalon and forebrain show midline fusion as well as the anomalies described for alobar HP (Fig. 1.17). Some patients with semilobar HP survive, but all are severely handicapped. The least severe variant is lobar HP. In these patients, the brain appears nearly normal. Imaging studies show absence of the septum pellucidum, an abnormal configuration of the frontal horns of the lateral ventricles, a shallow anterior interhemispheric fissure with hypoplasia of the falx cerebri in that

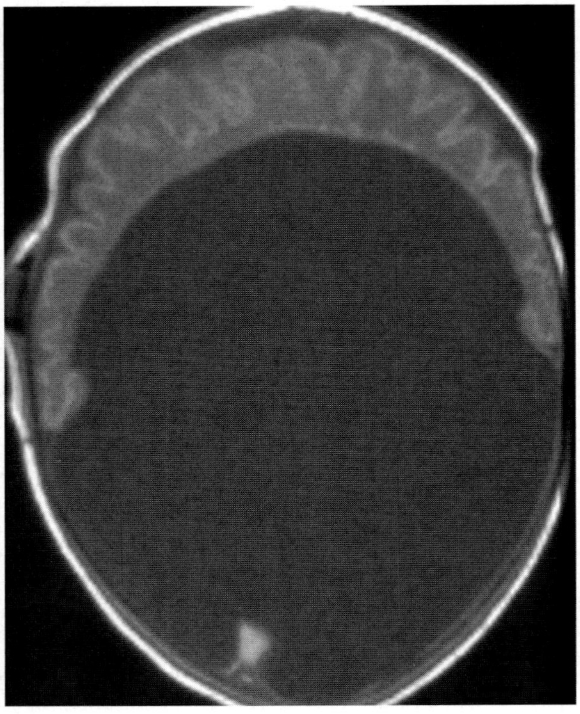

Figure 1.16 *Alobar Holoprosencephaly.* Axial T1-weighted image shows midline fusion of the frontal lobes and large horseshoe-shaped monoventricle communicating with a dorsal interhemispheric cyst.

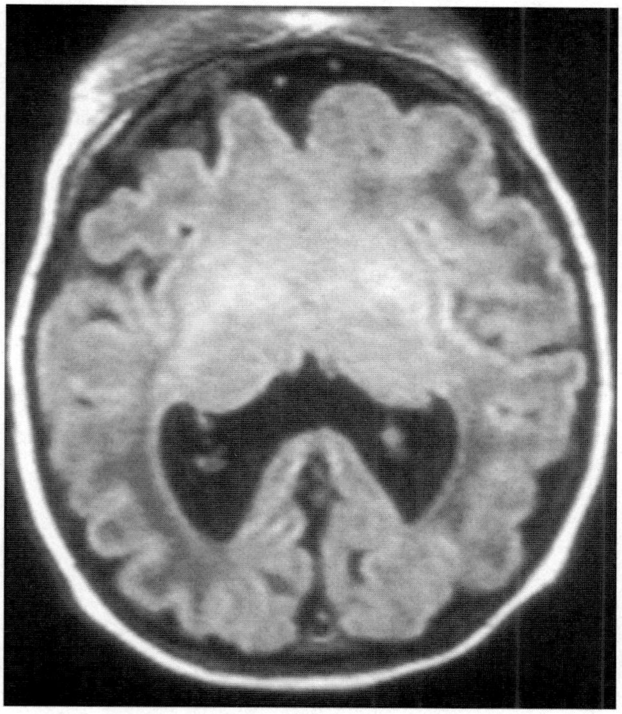

Figure 1.17 *Semilobar Holoprosencephaly.* There is fusion of the frontal lobes and thalami but posterior differentiation with two atria of the lateral ventricles and interhemispheric fissure.

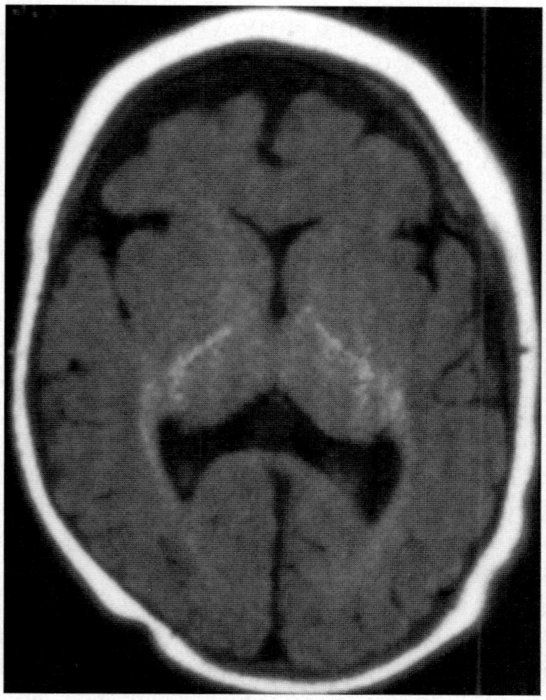

A

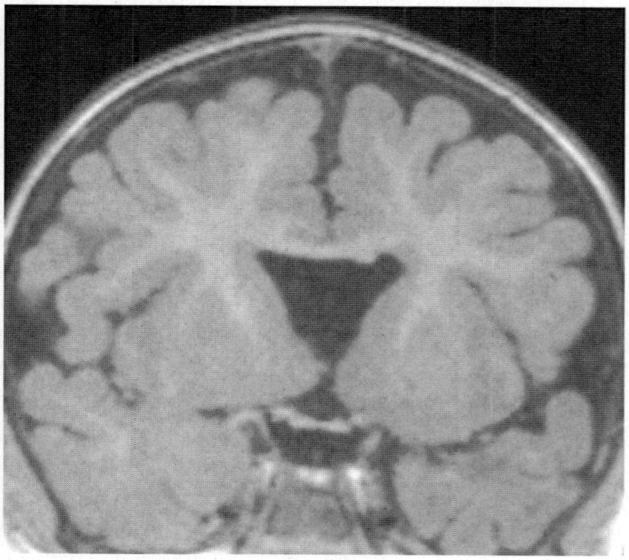

B

Figure 1.18 *Lobar Holoprosencephaly. A.* Axial T1-weighted image shows nearly normal-appearing brain with absence of the septum pellucidum, fused thalami, and diffuse pachygyria. *B.* In a different case, a coronal T1-weighted image shows absent septum pellucidum and a boxlike configuration of the roof the lateral ventricles.

Table 1.5: Brain Abnormalities in the Different Holoprosencephalies

Anatomic Structures	*Alobar*	*Semilobar*	*Lobar*
Forebrain	Fused in midline	Fused in midline	Nearly normal
Lateral ventricles	Horseshoe-shaped monoventricle	Atria and occipital horns present	Nearly normal
Septum pellucidum	Absent	Absent	Absent
Third ventricle	Absent	Variably present	Present
Corpus callosum	Absent	Absent anteriorly	Nearly normal
Thalami	Fused	Fused	Normal
Interhemispheric cyst	Present	None	None
Interhemispheric fissure	Absent	Absent anteriorly	Present but may be shallow anteriorly
Anterior cerebral artery	Azygos	Azygos	Azygos or normal
Venous sinuses	Absent	Variably present	Normal

region, and at times an azygos anterior cerebral artery (Fig. 1.18). In many instances, the brain anomalies are very similar to those seen in septooptic dysplasia (SOD), and many neuroradiologists consider lobar HP and SOD as related diseases. Midline cerebral (interhemispheric) fusion is, as its name implies, a form of HP at the level of the body of the corpus callosum (25). This anomaly is very rare. The features of the different holoprosencephalies are shown in Table 1.5.

Schizencephaly

SC refers to a cleft in the brain (usually a cerebral hemisphere, but very rarely also in the cerebellum) that extends from the surface of the cortex into a ventricle (27,28). The cleft may be separated and contain CSF (open-lip SC) or fused (closed-lip SC; Figs. 1.19A–C and 1.20). The lips are formed by dysplastic gray matter usually in the form of polymicrogyria (PMG). The lips are lined by pia laterally and ependyma medially. Most SCs are found the frontal and temporal regions. They are more commonly unilateral, but bilateral clefts also are found. It is not unusual to have an SC on one side and a lesser abnormality of neuronal migration in a mirror-like location on the opposite side. In some frontal SCs, the anterior aspect of the corpus callosum may be absent. Patients with open-lip SC have more severe symptoms than those with the closed-lip type. These patients show developmental delay, seizures, and varying degrees of hemiplegia on the side opposite the open-lip SC (27). Large, bilateral open-lip SCs are considered by some to be a variation of hydranencephaly (this observation is based on the assumption that both disorders may arise from a similar vascular insult; Fig. 1.19D). The cerebral hemisphere containing the SC usually is small and the corresponding lateral ventricle is large. In closed-lip SC, the outer wall of the corresponding lateral ventricle may show either a nipple-like protuberance of gray matter or a dimple. The septum pellucidum is absent in both types of SC. In both types of SC, there is a lack of condensation of the cortical veins on the outer surface of the defect and sometimes along their walls (particularly with the open-lip type). These prominent cortical veins should not be misinterpreted as a vascular malformation, although there is one case report showing an SC associated with a true arteriovenous malformation (29). In open-lip SC, the CSF spaces overlying the defect are prominent and occasionally a true cyst may present. When an arachnoid cyst is present, there usually is a mass effect and remodeling of the overlying skull. These cysts may need to be shunted.

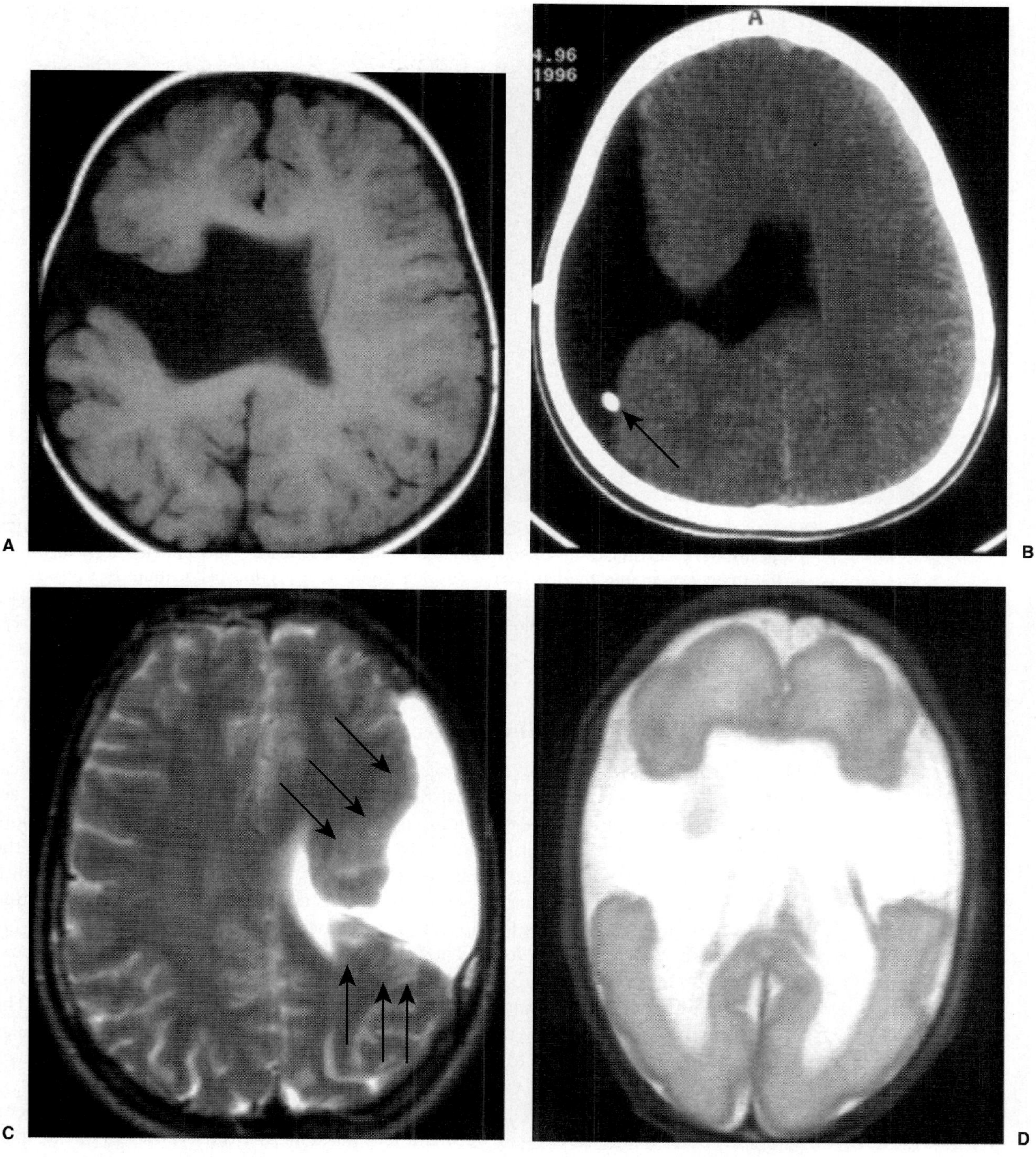

Figure 1.19 *Open-Lip Schizencephaly. A.* Axial T1-weighted image shows right open-lip schizencephaly. The right lateral ventricle is large, the right cerebral hemisphere is small, and the septum pellucidum is absent. *B.* In a different case, there is a cerebrospinal fluid–filled cyst overlying the schizencephaly. Note that this cyst had to be shunted *(arrow)* because of mass effect. *C.* Axial T2-weighted image shows a left side schizencephaly. Note that lips are lined by thick and abnormal-appearing gray matter (*arrows*). *D.* Axial T2-weighted image shows large bilateral open-lip schizencephalies, large ventricles, absent septum pellucidum, and diffuse pachygyria.

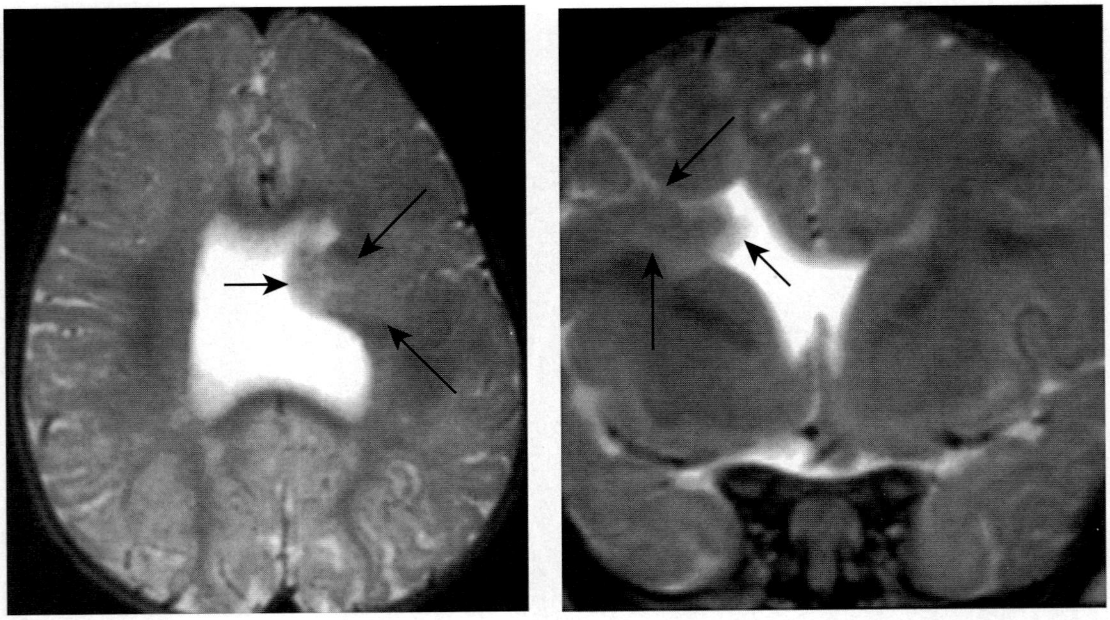

Figure 1.20 *Closed-Lip Schizencephaly. A.* Axial T2-weighted image shows band of gray matter *(large arrows)* extending from surface of brain to left lateral ventricle. Note protrusion *(small arrow)* of the brain matter into the left lateral ventricle and absent septum pellucidum. *B.* Coronal T2-weighted image shows right frontal band of gray matter *(large arrows)* extending from brain surface to lateral ventricle. Note nipple-like protrusion *(small arrow)* in right frontal horn and absent septum pellucidum.

Septooptic Dysplasia

There are two types of SOD, those associated with an SC and those without it.

The syndrome of SOD actually comprises different disorders with different imaging features, all of which have similar clinical findings. The classic manifestations of SOD are hypoplasia of the optic nerves on funduscopy and hypothalamic–pituitary dysfunction, but these are not present in all patients (30). In reality, SOD probably is a variant of the optochiasmatic–hypothalamic–pituitary dysplasias (30). By imaging, there are two well defined types of SOD, and a finding shared by both is absence of the septum pellucidum. In the first type, the brain has the appearance of lobar HP (see earlier) (3). This, in my opinion, is the most common form. The frontal horns of the lateral ventricles are "box-like" superiorly (flat roof) and point inferiorly. The septum pellucidum is absent (Fig. 1.21). The pituitary gland is small and its posterior lobe may be ectopic or absent. The optic nerves are hypoplastic. Hypoplasia of the optic nerves is a clinical diagnosis and may be confidently diagnosed by MRI in only approximately 50% of patients. The optic chiasm also may be small. The corpus callosum may be dysgenetic in these patients.

In the second form of SOD, an SC is present (3). The septum pellucidum is absent. The optic chiasm and nerves may be small. It is possible that the hypoplasia of the anterior optic pathways is a degeneration caused by the interruption of the posterior pathways by the cleft. The SC in these patients usually is more posteriorly located than in those without SOD. The pituitary gland nearly always is normal in these patients. I am not sure that this second type of the disease truly is SOD.

Lipomas

Subarachnoid space lipomas commonly encase cranial nerves and blood vessels, a finding that implies their developmental nature.

Although subarachnoid space lipomas may happen anywhere in the brain, they are more common supratentorially, and thus are discussed here. Lipomas now are considered true congenital abnormalities because they arise from an anomaly of development of the meninx primitiva (31), a layer of undifferentiated mesenchyme that surrounds the brain

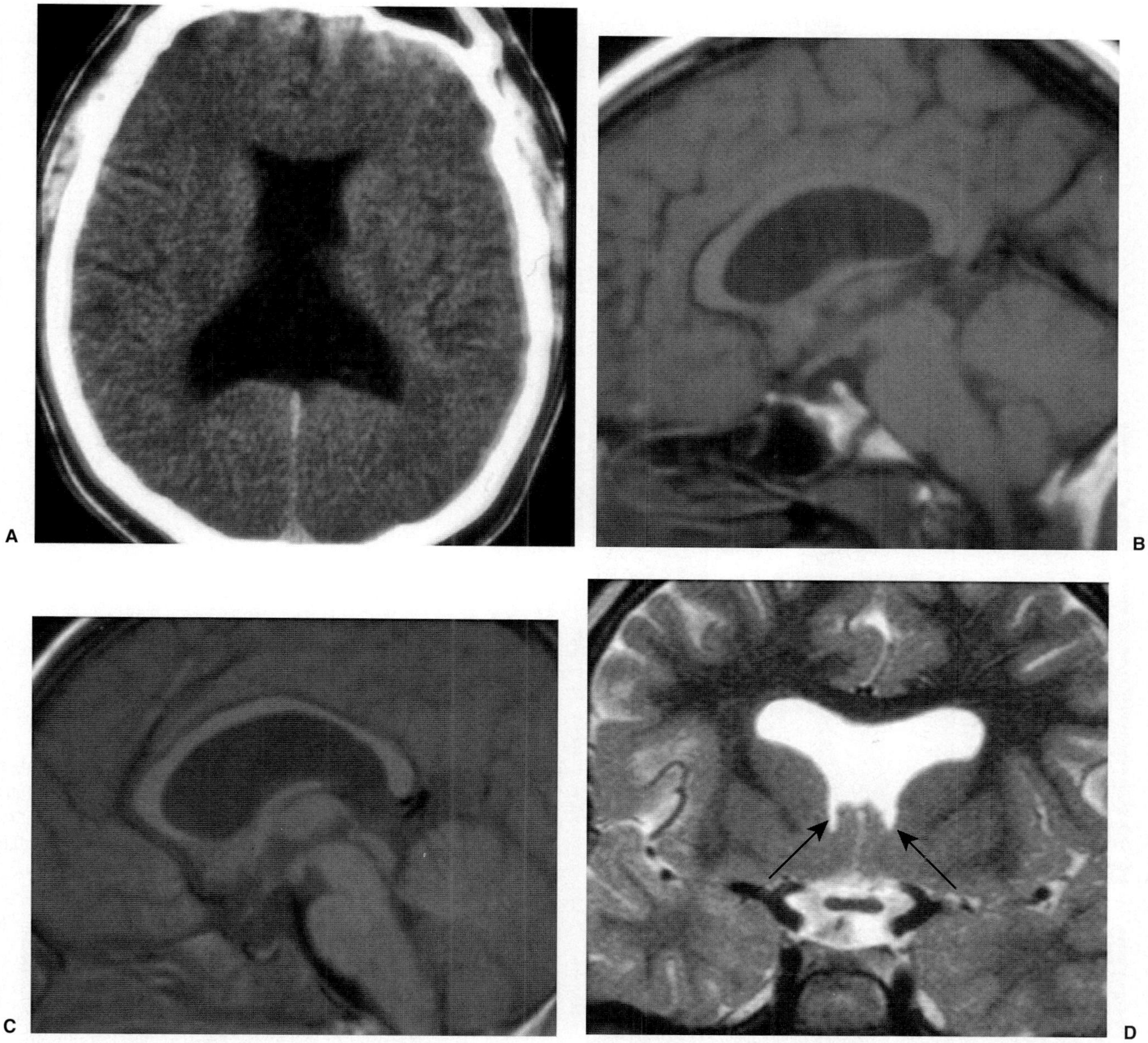

Figure 1.21 *Septooptic Dysplasia. A.* Axial computed tomography shows prominent lateral ventricles and absent septum pellucidum. *B.* Sagittal T1-weighted image (different case) shows small pituitary gland and stalk, normal-appearing optic chiasm, and prominent lateral ventricles. *C.* In a different patient, the pituitary gland and optic chiasm are small and the stalk is not seen. The lateral ventricles are prominent. *D.* Coronal T2-weighted image shows flat roof of the lateral ventricles, absent septum pellucidum, and inferior-pointing *(arrows)* of the frontal horns.

in early life. The meninx primitiva differentiates into the subarachnoid space in an organized fashion. The last portions of the meninx primitiva to involute are located in the foldings of the brain such as the interhemispheric fissure, the suprasellar and interpeduncular cisterns, and the quadrigeminal plate region. The most common locations for intracranial lipomas are listed in Table 1.6 (31–33) (Fig. 1.22).

Interhemispheric lipomas may be of two types. The so-called nodular (masslike) lipomas usually are associated with agenesis or dysgenesis of the corpus callosum, encephaloceles, and facial clefting syndromes. Nodular lipomas may contain calcifications. The linear (tubular) lipomas usually follow the course of the pericallosal sulci, and the

Table 1.6: Locations of Subarachnoid Space Lipomas

Location	*Incidence*
Interhemispheric fissure	40%–50%
Quadrigeminal plate region	20%–30%
Suprasellar cistern	10%
Interpeduncular cistern	10%
Cerebellopontine angle region (including the internal auditory canal)	10%
Sylvian regions	5%–10%
Pontomedullary junction	1%–3%
Choroid plexus	>1%
Meckel's cave	>1%

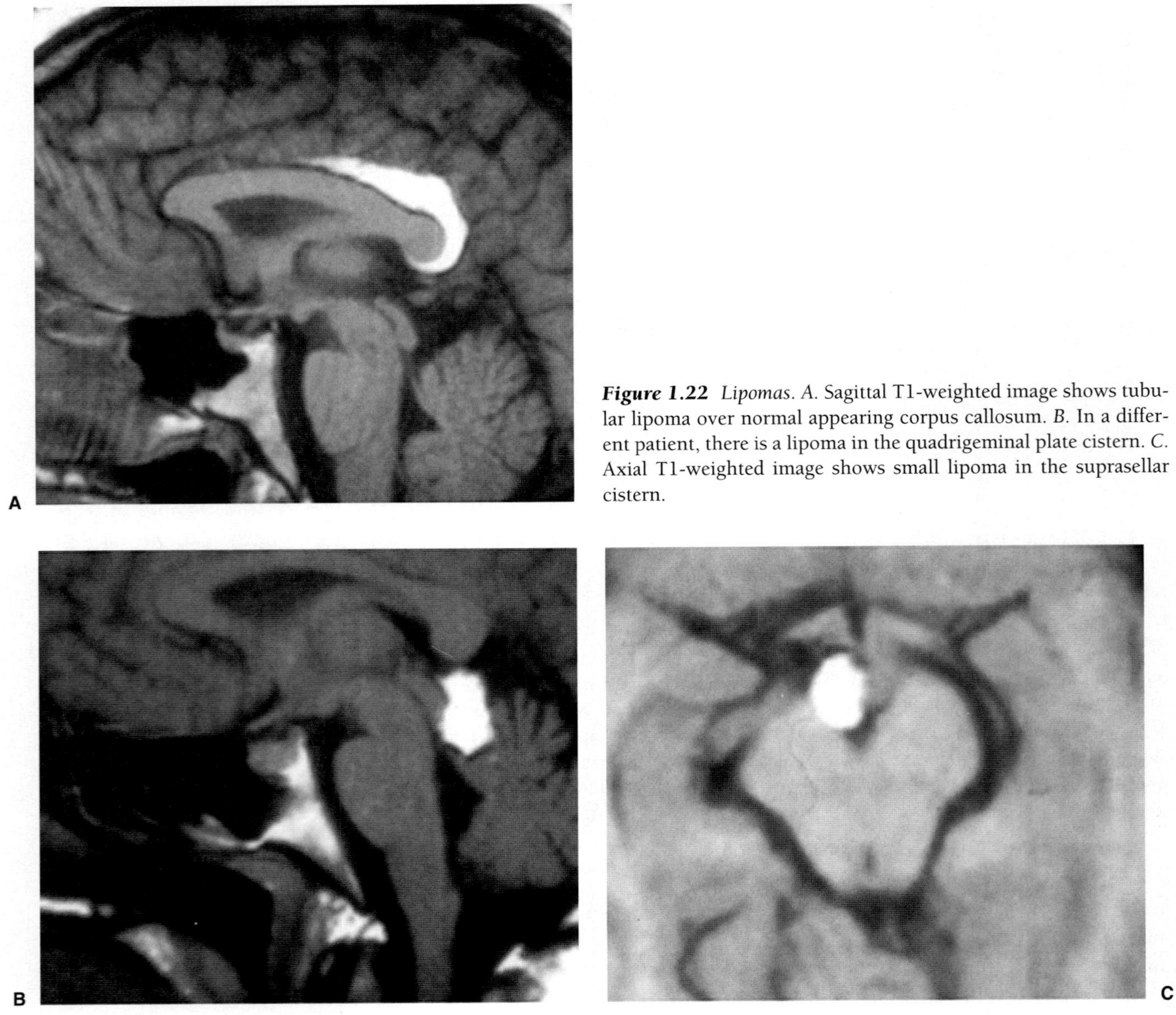

Figure 1.22 *Lipomas. A.* Sagittal T1-weighted image shows tubular lipoma over normal appearing corpus callosum. *B.* In a different patient, there is a lipoma in the quadrigeminal plate cistern. *C.* Axial T1-weighted image shows small lipoma in the suprasellar cistern.

underlying corpus callosum tends to be normal or only slightly dysgenetic. In other regions, lipomas may encircle the cranial nerves and blood vessels as they course in the subarachnoid spaces. Lipomas seldom result in symptoms. Occasionally, an arachnoid cyst becomes hemorrhagic and may appear identical to a lipoma. It is very difficult to differentiate a midline lipoma from a dermoid in the absence of fat drops in the CSF-containing spaces (although dermoids are much less common than lipomas, they may rupture in the subarachnoid spaces). The differential diagnosis of a suprasellar mass that is bright on T1-weighted MRI is as follows:

- Lipoma
- Ectopic posterior pituitary lobe
- Craniopharyngioma
- Suprasellar extension of hemorrhagic pituitary adenoma
- Dermoid
- Teratoma
- Thrombosed internal carotid artery or basilar tip aneurysm
- Cavernous angioma
- Metastases
- Bright epidermoid

Sincipital Encephaloceles and Related Anomalies

The main differential diagnosis of a mass on the glabella includes a dermoid, a "nasal glioma," and an encephalocele.

Posterior encephaloceles already have been addressed (see earlier), and now I address the anterior (sincipital) ones. The frontonasal region forms by a complex mechanism (3). Early in life, a small fontanelle (the fonticulus frontalis) separates the frontal from the nasal bones. Progressive growth of both bones obliterates this small fontanelle, leaving behind only the frontonasal suture. In addition, there is a potential space under the nasal bones and the developing nasal cartilage called the *prenasal space*. The prenasal space contains a diverticulum of dura that extends to the tip of the nose. This diverticulum regresses intracranially, the prenasal space obliterates, and the only evidence of this space left is the foramen cecum located anterior to the crista galli. If brain herniates through the fonticulus frontalis, the result is a frontonasal encephalocele. If brain herniates, but the fonticulus frontalis closes, a prenasal heterotopia (so-called nasal glioma) occurs. If the brain extends into the prenasal space and remains there, a nasoethmoidal encephalocele occurs. If the prenasal space closes and brain is trapped in it, an intranasal heterotopia (another form of nasal glioma) forms. Both types of nasal glioma may be completely detached from the brain (this type does not grow) or remain attached to the brain by a stalk (this type does grow) (34). The last types of malformation related to the development of the prenasal space are the sinus tracts and epidermoids/dermoids (Fig. 1.23). If the dural diverticulum in the prenasal space extends too anteriorly and makes contact with the dermis, as it retracts into the brain, dermal and ectodermal elements will be carried with it, forming a sinus dermal tract. The tract may remain as such or elements in it may grow, resulting in formation of dermoids or epidermoids. The tract may or may not communicate with the intracranial space.

Nasal gliomas (a misnomer because they are not tumors and have no malignant potential) appear as nonenhancing small masses anterior to the nasofrontal suture or anterior to nasal septum (Fig. 1.24). They usually are isointense to brain on T1-weighted images and hyperintense (reflecting gliosis) on T2-weighted sequences. When a dermal tract is present, a small sinus opening is seen on the nose (anywhere from the tip to the glabella). This tiny opening may contain hemangioma, hairs, and atrophic skin, and may become infected. If infection is suspected, contrast should be given to outline the course of the tract. Occasionally, subfrontal abscesses may be found in these patients. Dermoids and epidermoids may have varying signal intensities and may not be differentiated from each other when arising in the prenasal space. One of the most important aspects of the examination in these patients is to determine if a communication with the intracranial

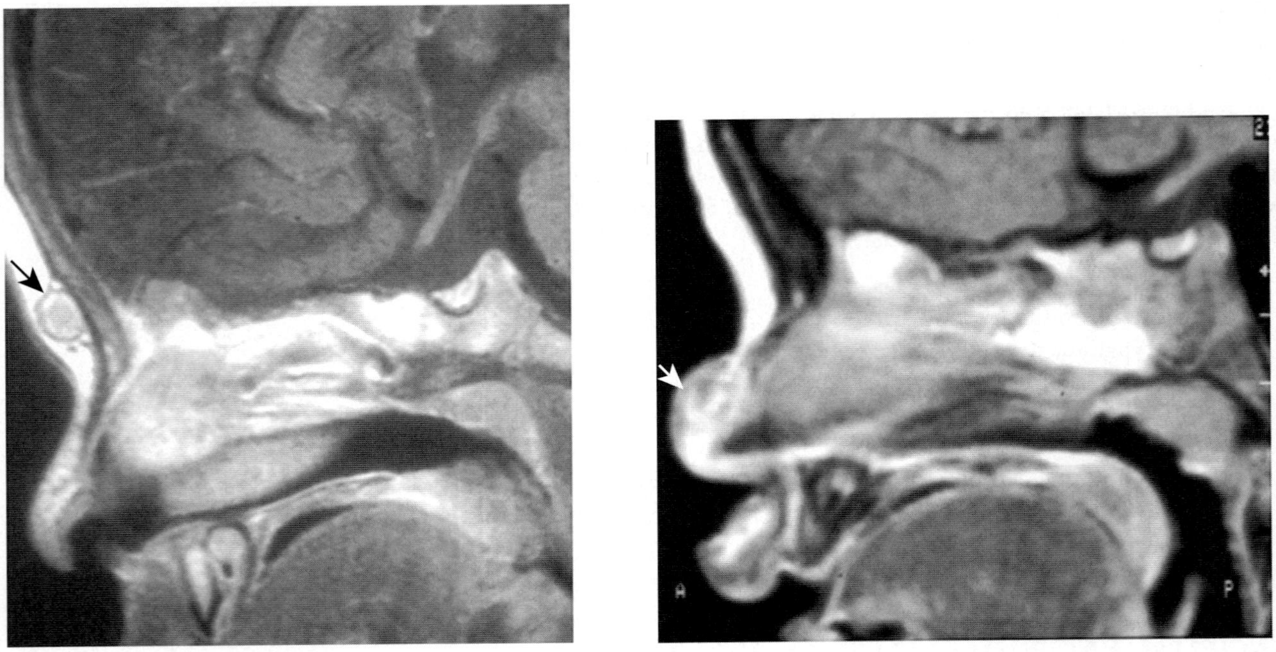

A B

Figure 1.23 *Nasal Dermoids. A.* Sagittal T1-weighted image shows small, bright *(arrow)* glabellar dermoid. *B.* In a different patient, postcontrast T1-weighted image shows enhancing and infected dermoid *(arrow)* close to the tip of the nose.

compartment exists. Findings suggesting communication are a wide foramen cecum or a crista galli that has a bifid configuration anteriorly. Enhancement of dura and leptomeninges in the frontobasal regions also is compatible with a patent communication.

Sincipital encephaloceles may be nasofrontal (through the fonticulus frontalis, 40% to 60%), nasoethmoidal (through the prenasal space, 20% to 30%) or nasoorbital (in the vicinity of the lacrimal bone, >10%) (3) (Figs. 1.25 and 1.26). Sincipital encephaloceles

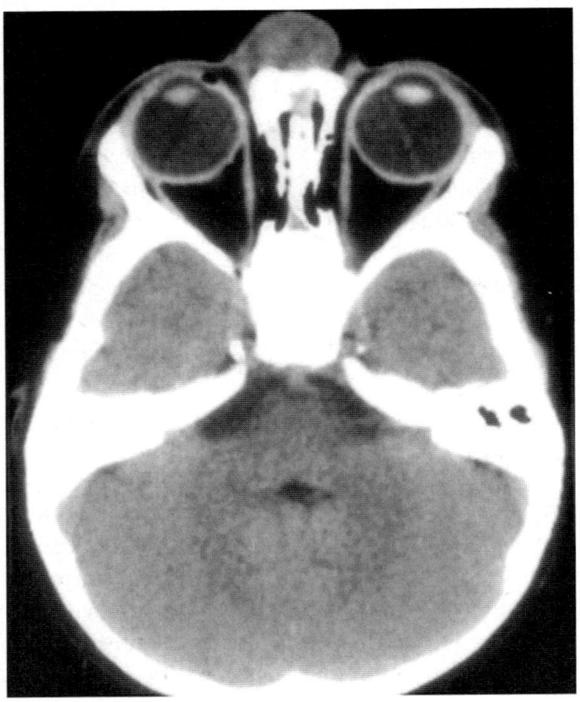

Figure 1.24 *Prenasal Heterotopia.* Axial computed tomography show nonspecific-appearing soft tissue mass in the nasofrontal region.

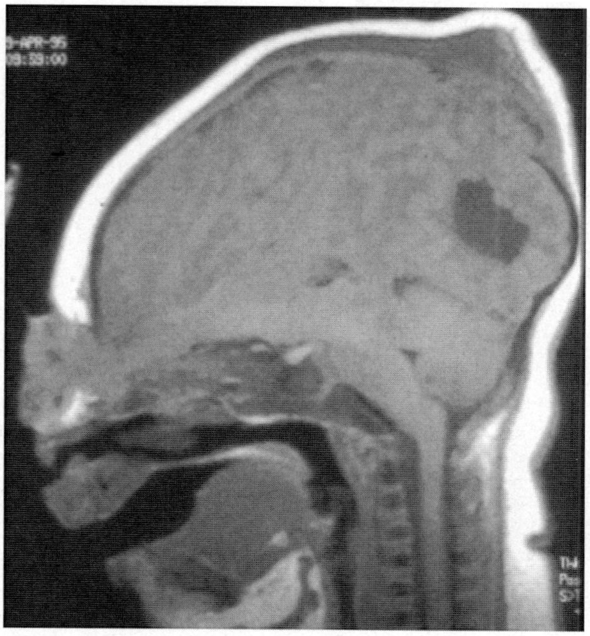

A

Figure 1.25 *Nasofrontal Encephalocele.* A. Sagittal T1-weighted image shows brain herniating between the frontal and nasal regions. The intracranial contents are dysplastic and the corpus callosum is not seen. *B.* Bone three-dimensional (3-D) reformation computed tomography (CT) shows large bone defect in the frontal and nasal regions. *C.* Soft tissue 3-D reformation CT shows appearance of the mass.

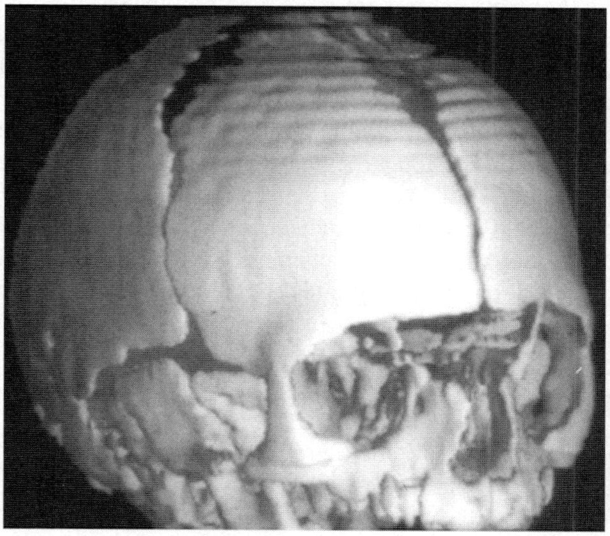

B

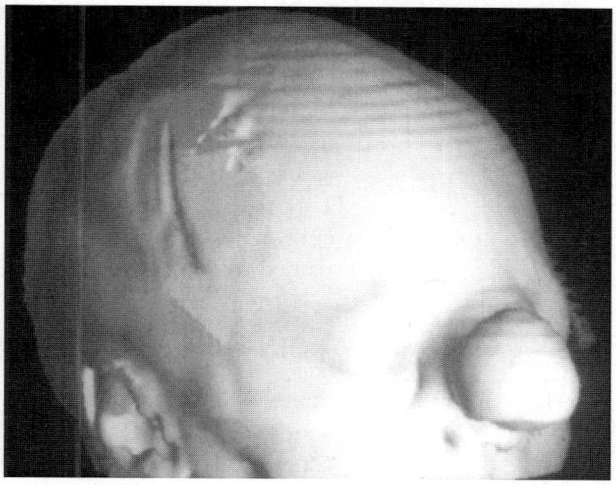

C

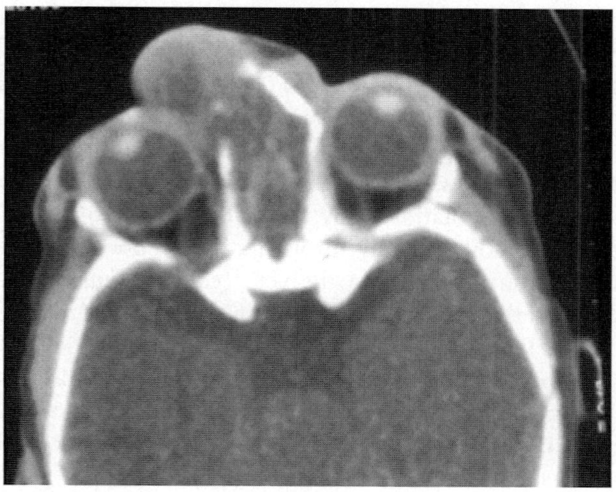

Figure 1.26 *Nasoorbital Encephalocele.* Axial computed tomography shows brain herniating between the nasal and lacrimal bones.

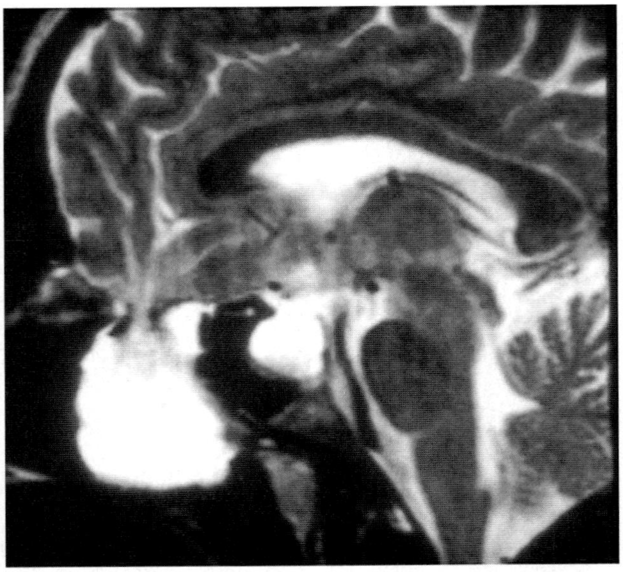

Figure 1.27 *Ethmoidal Encephalocele.* Sagittal T2-weighted image shows a mostly cerebrospinal fluid–filled sac herniating into the nasal cavities through a defect in the ethmoidal complex.

are rare in North America (1:40,000 live births) but are more common in Asia and Latin America. They are more common in boys and always are accompanied by hypertelorism. Most contain gliotic and nonfunctioning brain tissues. The degree of intracranial anomalies is proportional to the size of the encephalocele. Many patients with sincipital encephaloceles have severe facial dysraphism (midline facial clefts) (35). Anteriorly located encephaloceles also may be occult (no longer called *sincipital*; Fig. 1.27). These usually are through the anterior base of the skull and may be ethmoidal, sphenoethmoidal, central sphenoidal, and lateral sphenoidal (this last type may be seen on patients with NF-1 as part of the dysplasia of the greater wing of the sphenoid bone). Occult anterior encephaloceles may result in chronic leak of CSF. Sincipital encephaloceles may be accompanied by intracranial lipomas.

Vein of Galen Malformations

The most common type of VGM is supplied by multiple choroidal arteries and thus treatment usually is accomplished by occlusion of the feeding arteries and of the dilated venous pouch.

Vein of Galen malformations (VGM) is the name for a group of distinct disorders that result in increase in size of the vein of Galen. VGM is a misnomer because the vein of Galen usually does not form in these patients, and the dilated vein usually is a persistent prosencephalic vein (36) (Fig. 1.28). These are very rare malformations usually detected by *in utero* sonography or found in the neonatal period because of high-output heart failure. The most common type (>80%) is due to the presence of multiple choroidal vessels abnormally emptying in the vein of Galen (called a *choroidal VGM*) (36). It presents early in life with an intracranial bruit, congestive heart failure, and hydrocephalus. Regardless of treatment, these patients have a poor prognosis and eventually develop significant brain atrophy and intraaxial calcifications probably secondary to chronic arterial insufficiency and increased venous pressure. These malformations may be treated by diminishing the shunt by packing the vein of Galen with coils, usually through a transvenous approach. Occasionally, only a few or just one artery drains into the vein (called a *mural VGM*). These VGMs may be treated by transarterial occlusion of the feeding vessel(s). A different type of VGM usually found in older patients is due to the presence of an arteriovenous malformation in the midbrain or thalami draining in the vein of Galen. These children present with developmental delay, hydrocephalus, hemorrhage, and seizures. These VGMs may be treated by transarterial embolization. The third type of VGM represents a combination of a fistula and an arteriovenous malformation. VGMs are easily detected by sonography, computed tomography (CT), CT angiography, MRI, and MR angiography (MRA), but patients do need conventional angiography to establish clearly the type of malforma-

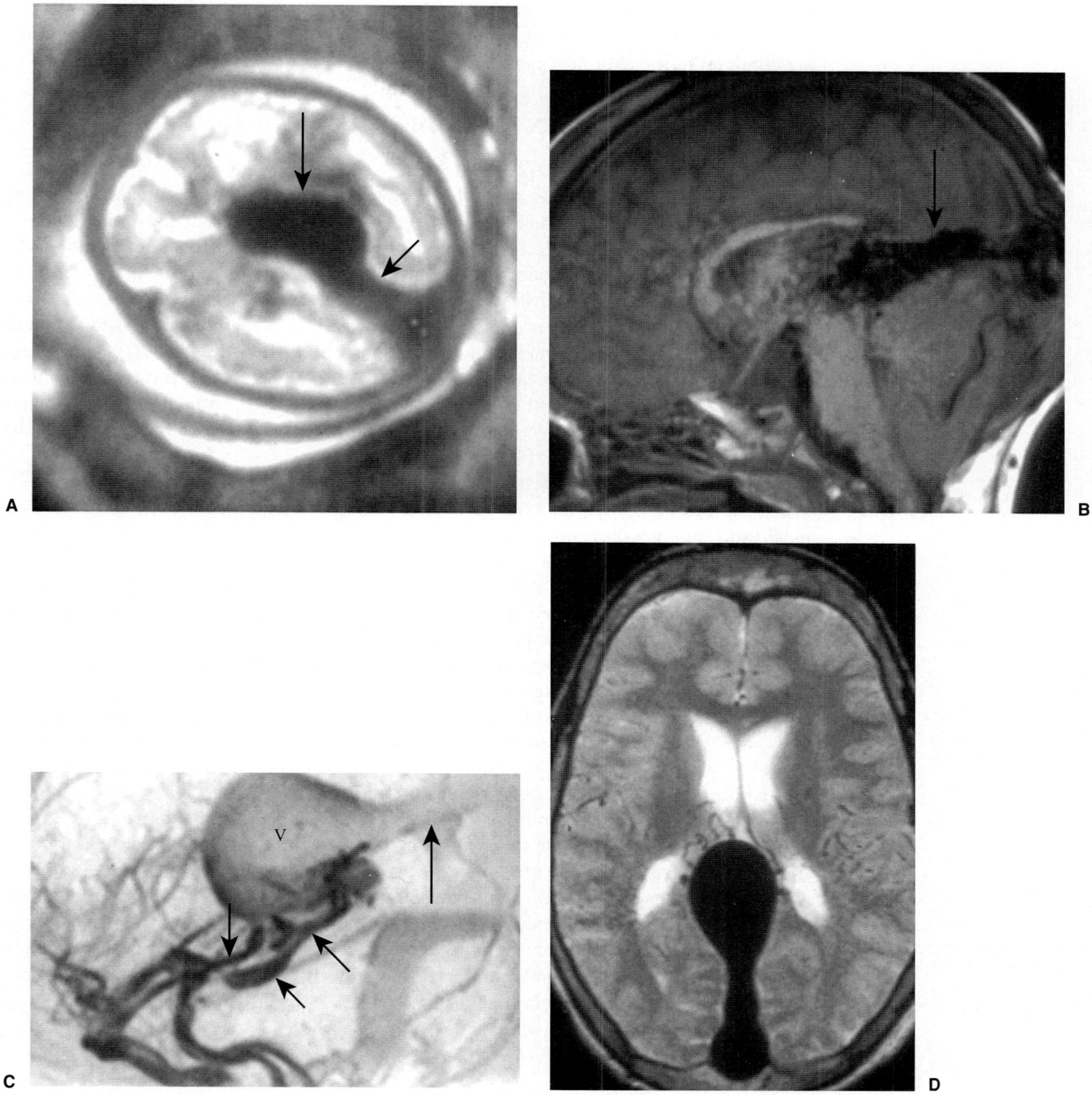

Figure 1.28 *Vein of Galen Malformations. A. In utero* HASTE axial image of the fetal brain shows a large vein of Galen *(large arrow)* and a dilated straight sinus *(small arrow). B.* Sagittal T1-weighted image (different patient) shows dilated vein of Galen and presence of a large falcine sinus *(arrow). C.* In a different patient, lateral magnetic resonance angiography view shows large vein of Galen (V) and dilated falcine sinus *(large arrow)*. Malformation is supplied by choroidal branches from the posterior cerebral arteries *(small arrows)*, which also are enlarged. *D.* Axial T2-weighted image in the same patient also shows the malformation.

tion. Occasionally, some VGMs clot and occlude spontaneously (37,38). Associated venous anomalies such as absence of the straight sinus and persistence of the falcine sinus are common in the choroidal type of VGM (39).

Neuronal Migration Disorders and Cortical Dysplasias

The germinal matrix is a zone containing young and proliferating neurons located along the outer borders of the ventricles. At approximately the 50th to 60th day of life, the neurons begin to migrate to the future cortex using the radial glial fibers as scaffolding (30). There is a high correlation between the site of neuronal proliferation in the germinal matrix and the destination of these neurons in the cortex. The first neurons to reach the outer plate (called *pioneering neurons*) establish layer 1, which guides the organization of the rest of the cortex. Subsequent neurons establish the cortex "inside out." Once all six layers are formed, connections are established through a process called *cortical organization*. The radial glial fibers then transform into astrocytes. Most errors in neuronal migration are genetic, ischemic, infectious, or due to toxins. Gray matter malformations may be divided as shown in Table 1.7 (40–42).

Table 1.7 is based on a classification proposed by Barkovich and colleagues (40–42). This classification is helpful because it separates the malformations into those that are focal (and thus possibly amenable to resection) versus those that are generalized (nonsurgical).

The most severe of the generalized malformations are the agyria (lissencephaly–pachygyria) complex and the band heterotopias (3,43) (Fig. 1.29). In lissencephaly, the brain is smooth and has a primitive appearance with wide sylvian fissures. To make things even more confusing, lissencephalies may be due to decreased (classic) or increased (cobblestone) migration of neurons (3) (Table 1.8).

Approximately 10% of patients with intractable seizures may have gray matter heterotopias, but occasionally patients with heterotopias may be asymptomatic.

Gray matter heterotopias are collections of dysplastic neurons in abnormal locations. It is assumed that an injury to the radial glial fibers results in arrested migration of the neurons. Most patients with heterotopias have seizures (44). There is an increased incidence of heterotopias in patients with chronic and medically intractable seizures. Heterotopias also may occur at or close to the hippocampus, resulting in partial complex epilepsy. Most heterotopias are subependymal, in white matter, or subcortical. They follow the signal intensity of gray matter in all MRI sequences, but they may be difficult to visualize in newborns (Fig. 1.30). Transmantle heterotopias, as their name implies, extend from the ventricle to the cortex (3). The overlying cortex always is thin in all heterotopias, and in the larger ones the corresponding cerebral hemisphere may be small. Occasionally one sees the so-called giant heterotopias, which basically are a hamartomatous malformation of most or all of one cerebral hemisphere (Figs. 1.31 and 1.32).

Table 1.7: Gray Matter Malformations

Mechanism	*Generalized*	*Focal*
Due to abnormal neuronal and glial proliferation	Lissencephaly	Schizencephaly, tuberous sclerosis, transmantle dysplasia, hemimegalencephaly, some tumors such as DNET
Due to abnormal neuronal migration	Agyria/pachygyria, cobblestone lissencephaly, band heterotopia, heterotopias	Focal agyria/pachygyria, heterotopia, cortical infolding
Due to abnormal cortical organization	Polymicrogyria, cortical dysplasia of Taylor (balloon cell type)	Polymicrogyria/schizencephaly

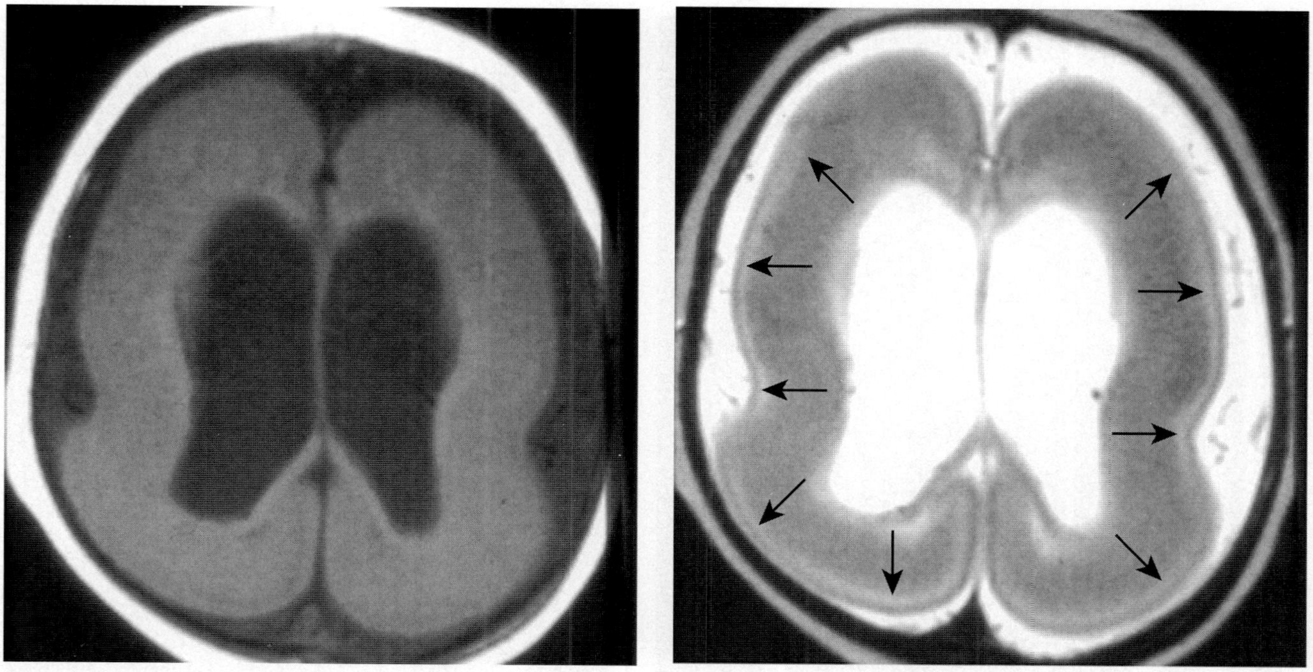

Figure 1.29 *Lissencephaly. A.* Axial T1-weighted image shows small and smooth brain with large lateral ventricles. *B.* Axial T2-weighted image shows a thin area of increased signal intensity *(arrows)* contained in the cortex. This area is the sparse neuronal cell layer and should not be confused with a band heterotopia.

Band heterotopias are a distinct and very rare anomaly (43). In these patients, a band of gray matter is located between a thin and dysplastic cortex (double cortex sign) and the ventricles (Fig. 1.33). In most instances, band heterotopias are generalized, but occasionally they are segmental. There may be areas of high T2 signal in the brain. The zone of white matter between the double cortex may be difficult to distinguish from the "sparse" neuronal layer present in some lissencephalies. This observation is important because of a specific type of X-linked lissencephaly/band heterotopia syndrome (45,46). This anomaly, inherited through a defect on chromosome 22, has different presentations according to the

Table 1.8: Differences between the Lissencephalies

	Classic	*Cobblestone*
Inheritance	Abnormalities in chromosome 17, may be X-linked	According to syndrome present
Appearance	May incompletely involve the brain and be more pronounced anteriorly	Diffuse, may have microophthalmos, dysgenesis of corpus callosum, encephalocele, dysgenetic vermis, hypomyelination
Cortex	Three layers, thin	Thick
Associated syndromes	Miller-Dicker	Congenital muscular dystrophy (Fukuyama's autosomal recessive, chromosome 9), Walker-Warburg, muscle–eye–brain disease (Finland)

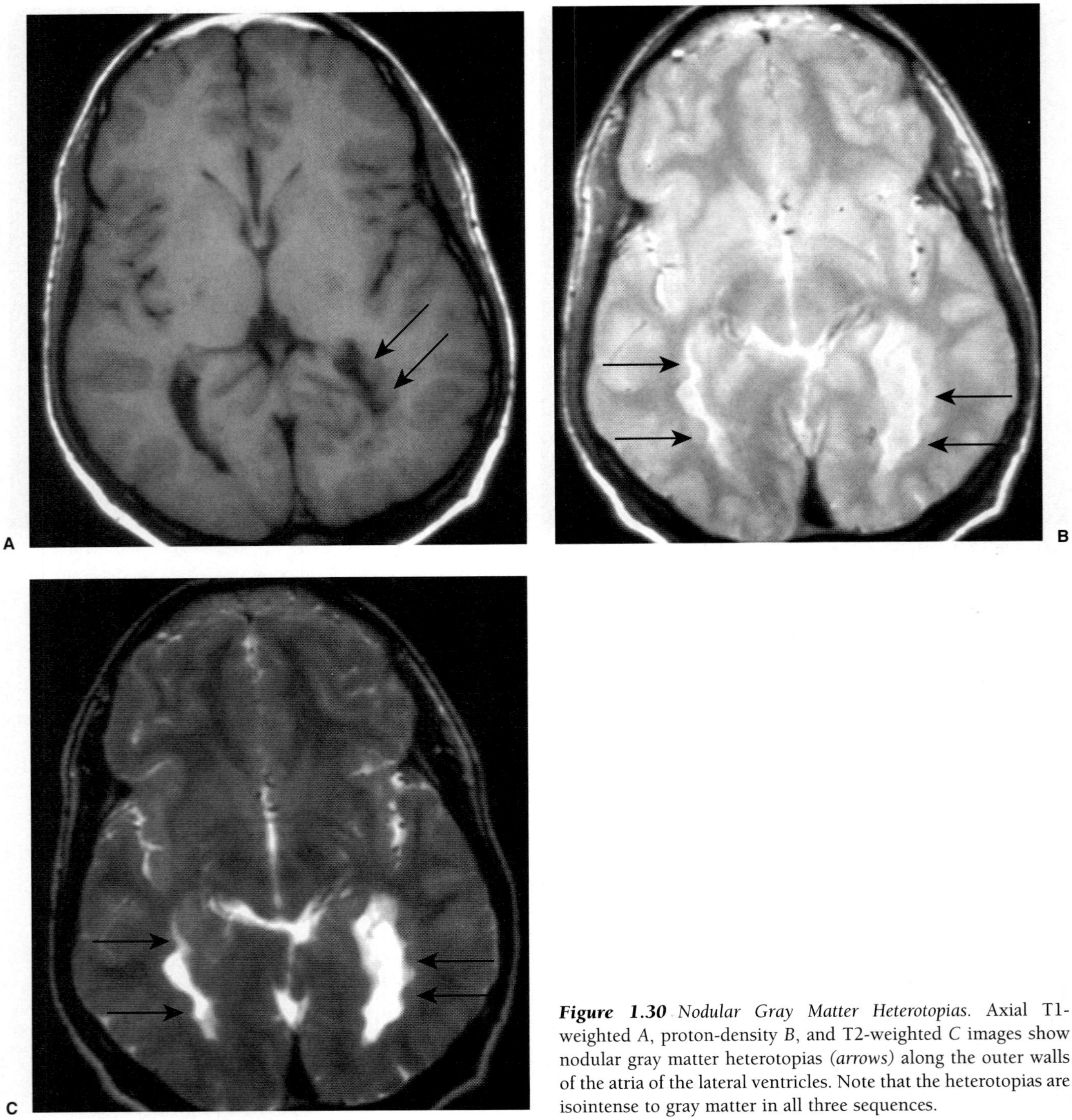

Figure 1.30 *Nodular Gray Matter Heterotopias.* Axial T1-weighted *A*, proton-density *B*, and T2-weighted *C* images show nodular gray matter heterotopias *(arrows)* along the outer walls of the atria of the lateral ventricles. Note that the heterotopias are isointense to gray matter in all three sequences.

penetrance of the trait. In boys, the manifestation is lissencephaly, whereas in girls it is band heterotopia.

PMG is a disorder not of neuronal migration but of cortical organization (3,47). It is characterized by a disorganization of the normal six-layered cortex. PMG is a term that encompasses many entities, and thus I prefer to refer to this group of anomalies simply as *cortical dysplasias*. The etiology is unknown, but because most cortical dysplasias occur in the region supplied by the middle cerebral artery, a vascular insult frequently is invoked as the responsible mechanism (Fig. 1.34). Despite this observation, cortical dysplasias may

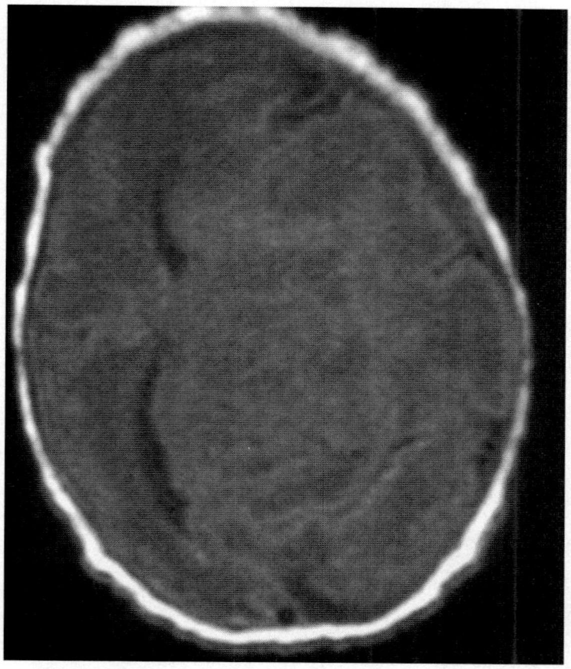

Figure 1.31 *Giant Heterotopia.* Axial T1-weighted image shows hamartomatous malformation of the entire left cerebral hemisphere, which also is somewhat large (unilateral hemimegalencephaly?). It is important to recognize this as a malformation because biopsy may show dysplastic neurons suggesting a ganglion cell tumor.

involve any part of the brain. Although PMG is grossly characterized by the presence of many small gyri and shallow sulci, these are not appreciated by MRI and the affected site appears as a patch of smooth cortex. Three-dimensional (3-D) reformations of the cortex may show an area of flat cortex containing a dimple (48). The underlying gray–white matter junction may appear lumpy or indistinct. Underlying high T2 signal intensity may be seen in nearly 20% of patients, and it is assumed to be related to gliosis secondary to ischemia. Large cortical veins may overlie the malformation. In the so-called perisylvian or opercular syndrome, zones of cortical dysplasia follow one or usually both sylvian fissures posteriorly (49) (Fig. 1.35).

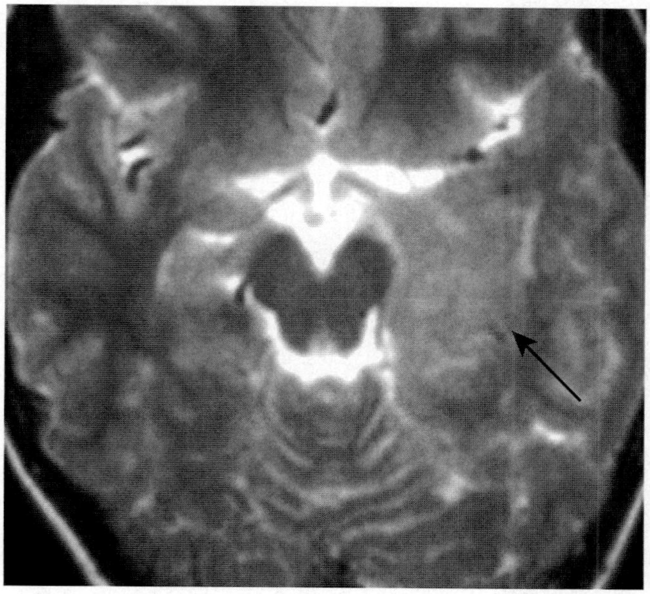

Figure 1.32 *Mesial Temporal Lobe Heterotopia Versus Cortical Dysplasia.* A large nodular area *(arrow)* of signal intensity equal to gray matter is seen in the left mesial temporal lobe of this patient with partial complex seizures of temporal lobe origin.

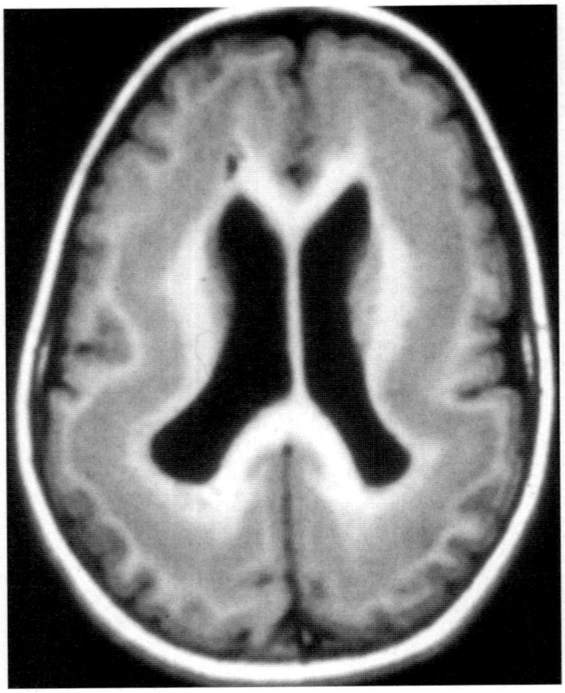

Figure 1.33 *Band Heterotopia.* Axial T1-weighted image shows thin and somewhat smooth outer cortex, a layer of white matter, a thick layer of gray matter (band heterotopia), and again white matter. The ventricles are large.

An abnormality that deserves brief mention here is the cortical dysplasia of Taylor, balloon cell type (50). Histologically, this lesion is identical to the subcortical hamartomas seen in tuberous sclerosis, but it is solitary. Most patients have seizures. On MRI, the overlying cortex appears flat, the involved gyrus is expanded, and there may be an underlying zone of high T2 signal extending from the lesion to the outer border of a ventricle (Fig. 1.36). This last observation has led some to postulate that the lesion may be an anomaly of neuronal migration.

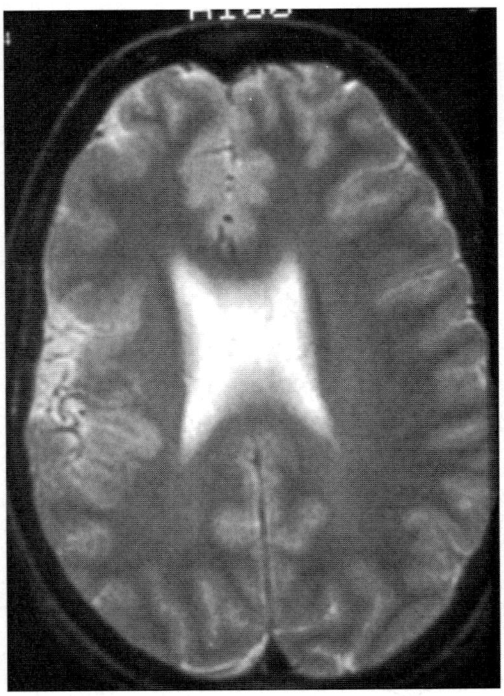

Figure 1.34 *Nonlissencephalic Focal Cortical Dysplasia.* Axial T2-weighted image shows a dimple in the cortex of the right temporal lobe. The underlying cortex is thick and the gray–white matter differentiation is not sharp. Overlying the malformation are several large cortical veins. This probably is polymicrogyria.

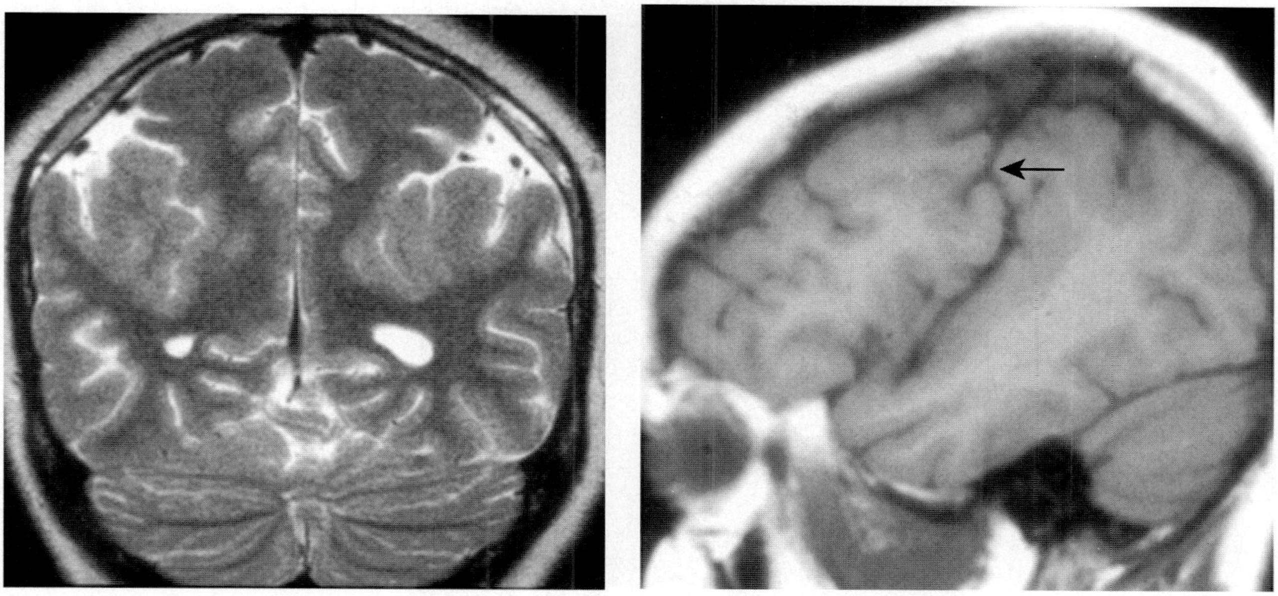

A B

Figure 1.35 *Perisylvian Syndrome. A.* Coronal T2-weighted image shows thick cortex in the posterior aspect of both sylvian fissures. The subarachnoid space over these regions is enlarged and contains prominent cortical veins. *B.* Sagittal T1-weighted image shows abnormal posterior extension *(arrow)* of the sylvian fissure, which is lined by thick cortex.

The last disorder I cover is hemimegalencephaly. Most megalencephalies are idiopathic or hereditary (parents with large heads). Other causes of generalized brain enlargement are pituitary gigantism, NF-1, mucopolysaccharidoses, and some rare leukodystrophies (14). Unilateral megalencephaly is a different disorder and represents a hamartomatous disorganization of one hemisphere (51) (Fig. 1.37),Patients present developmental delay, seizures, and hemiplegia. This disorder may be sporadic or associated with

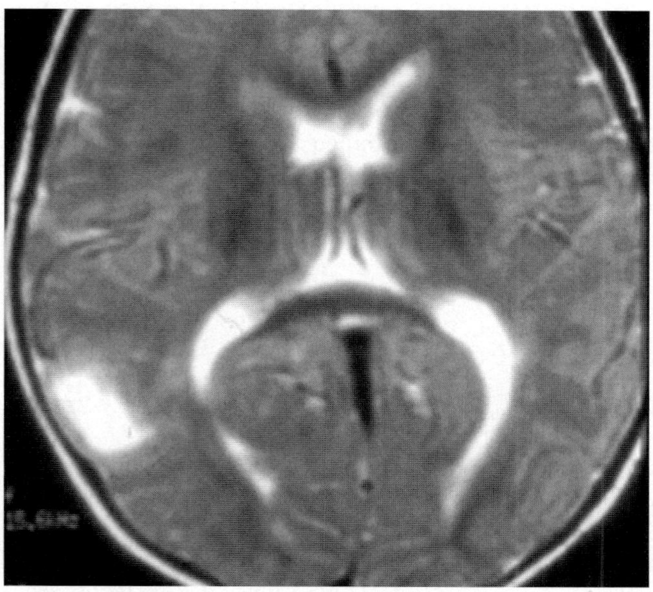

Figure 1.36 *Dysplasia of Taylor.* Axial T2-weighted image shows area of increased signal with expansion of the overlying cortex in the right parietal region. The appearance of this solitary lesion is identical to that of the cortical tubers seen in tuberous sclerosis.

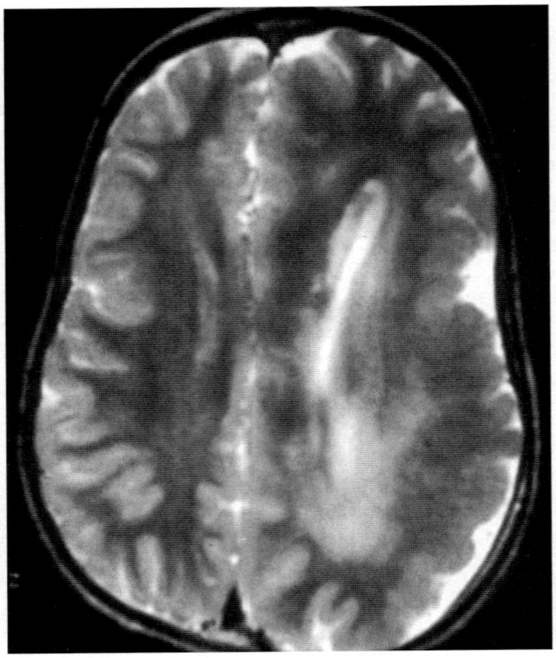

Figure 1.37 *Hemimegalencephaly.* Axial T2-weighted image shows enlarged left cerebral hemisphere containing multiple areas of cortical dysplasia and abnormally high signal in the white matter.

neurocutaneous syndromes (NF-1, hypomelanosis of Ito, and sebaceous nevus syndrome). The affected hemisphere is large, as is its lateral ventricle (particularly the frontal horn, which also has an abnormal shape). Multiple areas of thick gyri and shallow cortical sulci are present. The underlying white matter may show increased T2 signal intensity.

CRANIOSYNOSTOSES

The most common craniosynostoses are coronal, sagittal, lamboid, metopic, and generalized.

The growth of the skull occurs perpendicular to the axes of the major sutures (52). Most of the skull's growth depends on the coronal and sagittal sutures. CS refers to fusion (closure) of one (simple) or more (compound) sutures. CT is the imaging method of choice. We use 1- to 3-mm sections and process them through the high-resolution bone filter. Although 3-D reformations are helpful in assessing the overall shape of the head, the axial images provide better information to localize the fusion (53). CT is very good to diagnose bony CS, but poor in documenting the presence of fibrous CS. In bony synostosis, the suture is obliterated by bone and its edges may be prominent in a liplike fashion. Many patients with CS show mildly enlarged CSF spaces; the reason for this is not clear, although an abnormality of CSF absorption or compromised venous drainage (leading to increased venous pressure and decreased CSF absorption) may be the cause. Surgery is

Table 1.9: Imaging of Craniosynostosis

	Coronal CS	*Sagittal CS*	*Segmental CS*	*Metopic CS*	*Compound CS*
Suture affected	Entire coronal	All or part of the sagittal	Usually the coronal or lambdoid	Metopic	All
Shape of head	Dolichocephaly or scaphocephaly	Brachycephaly	Plagiocephaly	Trigonocephaly	Turricephaly or oxycephaly
Incidence	60%	20%–30%	5%–10%	1%–2%	1%–2%
Associated abnormalities	Increased intracranial pressure	Proptosis and optic nerve compression	Torticollis	Midline facial and brain anomalies	Severe brain, eye, and temporal bone anomalies

CS, craniosynostosis.

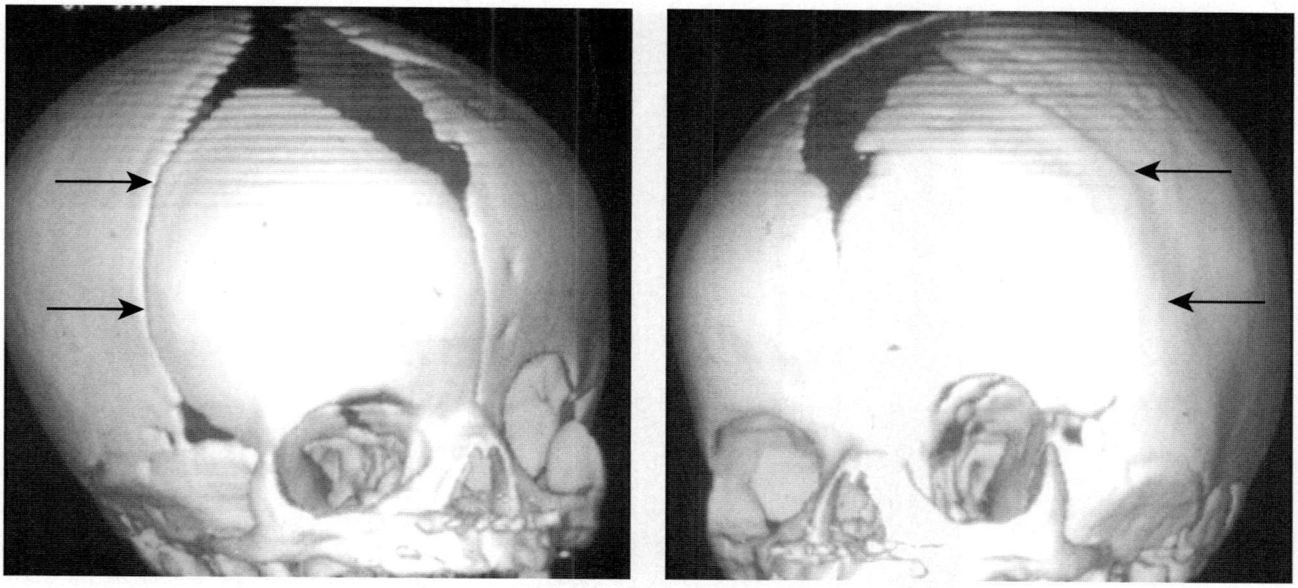
A B

Figure 1.38 *Coronal Suture Synostosis. A.* Bone three-dimensional reformation of computed tomography scan shows normal-appearing right coronal suture *(arrows). B.* There is bone fusion of the left coronal suture *(arrows)* and upward lifting (plagiocephaly) of the left orbit.

performed in patients with increased intracranial pressure or for cosmetic reasons. Postoperative evaluation is very difficult, and perhaps in those patients the 3-D images allow the shape of the head to be evaluated better. Table 1.9 describes the most common types of CS (52,53) (Figs. 1.38 to 1.40).

Many syndromes (e.g., Apert's, Carpenter's, and Crouzon's syndromes) are associated with CS. CS may be present in patients with delayed brain growth, such as those who have

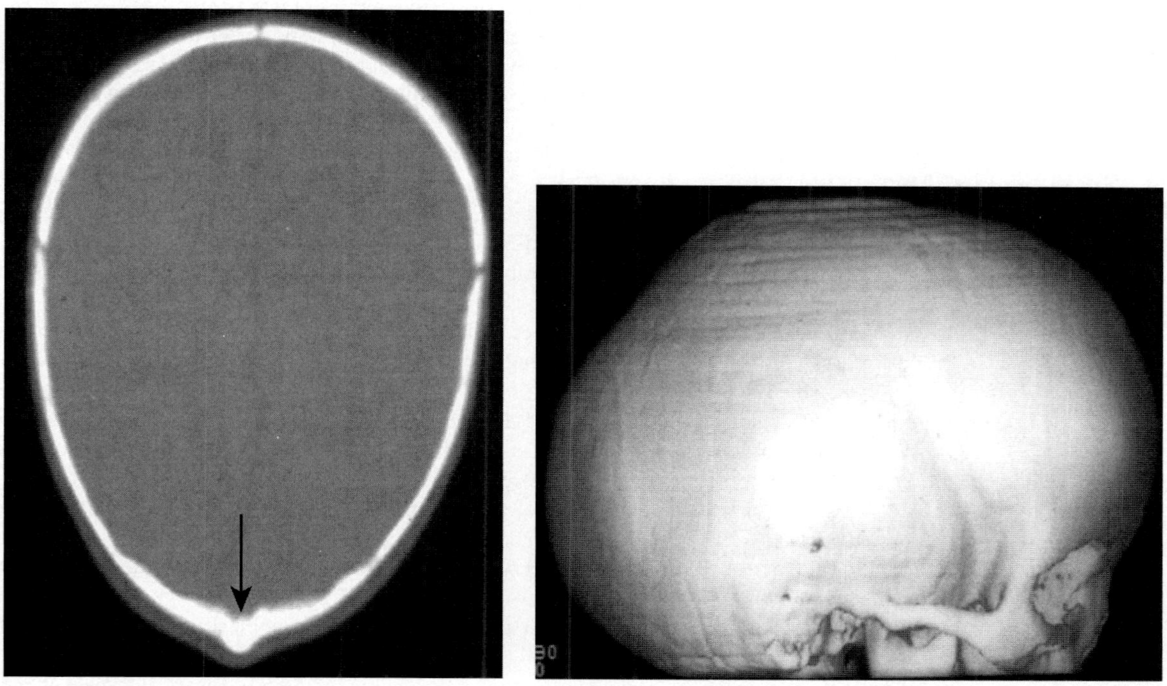
A B

Figure 1.39 *Sagittal Suture Synostosis. A.* Axial computed tomography (CT) shows fusion with formation of bone crest (*arrow*) in the posterior aspect of the sagittal suture. *B.* Bone three-dimensional reformation of CT scan shows elongation of the skull in its anteroposterior dimension (dolichocephaly or scaphocephaly).

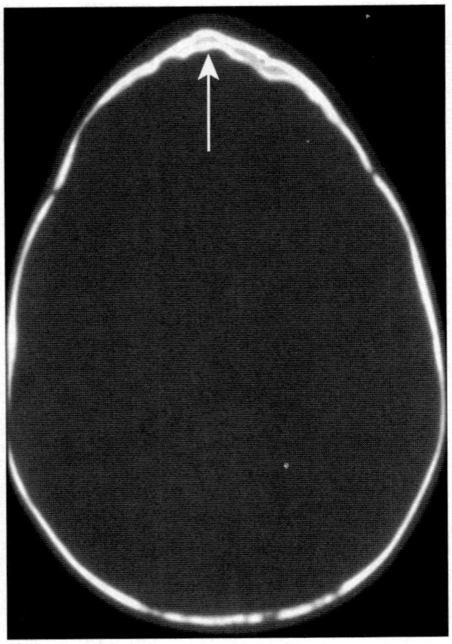

Figure 1.40 *Metopic Suture Synostosis.* Axial computed tomography shows fusion and formation of bone crest *(arrow)* in the region of the metopic suture. The head is pointed anteriorly (trigonocephaly).

received a ventricular shunt after severe hydrocephalus or those with Chiari 2 malformations, dysgenesis of the corpus callosum, severe periventricular leukomalacia, and HP. Segmental CS needs to the differentiated from postural flattening, in which the suture is open and its edges commonly overlap.

References

1. Larsen WJ. Human embryology, 2nd ed. New York: Churchill Livingstone, 1997.
2. Kollias SS, Ball WS, Prenger EC. Cystic malformations of the posterior fossa: differential diagnosis clarified through embryologic analysis. Radiographics 1993;13:1211–1231.
3. Barkovich AJ. Pediatric neuroimaging, 3rd ed. Philadelphia: Lippincott Williams & Wilkins, 2000:251–382.
4. Elster AD, Chen MYM. Chiari 1 malformations: clinical and radiologic reappraisal. Radiology 1992;183:347–353.
5. Ashwal S. Congenital structural defects. In: Swaiman KR, Ashwal S, eds. Pediatric neurology: principles and practice, 3rd ed. St. Louis: Mosby, 1999:234–300.
6. Ball WS, Crone KR. Chiari 1 malformation: from Dr. Chiari to MR imaging. Radiology 1995;195:602–604.
7. Nitz WR, Bradley WG, Watanabe AS, et al. Flow dynamics of cerebrospinal fluid: assessment with phase-contrast velocity MR imaging performed with retrospective cardiac gating. Radiology 1992;183:395–405.
8. Pittman HW. The Chiari crisis. BNI Q 1990;6:10–16.
9. Wolpert SM, Anderson M, Scott RM, et al. Chiari II malformation: MR imaging evaluation. AJNR Am J Neuroradiol 1987;8:783–792.
10. McClone DG, Knepper PA. The cause of Chiari II malformation: a unified theory. Pediatr Neurosci 1989;15:1–12.
11. Castillo M, Quencer RM, Dominguez R. Chiari III malformation: imaging features. AJNR Am J Neuroradiol 1992;13:107–113.
12. DeSouza N, Chaudhuri R. Bingham J, et al. MRI in cerebellar hypoplasia. Neuroradiology 1994;36:148–151.
13. Truwit CL, Barkovich AJ, Shanahan R, et al. MR imaging of rhomboencephalosynapsis: report of three cases and review of the literature. AJNR Am J Neuroradiol 1991;12:957–965.
14. Castillo M. Neuroradiology companion: methods, guidelines, and imaging fundamentals, 2nd ed. Philadelphia: Lippincott Williams & Wilkins, 1999.

15. Garfinkle WB. Aventriculy: a new entity? AJNR Am J Neuroradiol 1996;17:1649–1650.
16. Kalmes DF, Provenzale JM, Cloft HJ, et al. Typical and atypical MR imaging features of intracranial epidermoid tumors. AJR Am J Radiol 1997;169:883–887.
17. Gupta S, Gupta RK, Gujral RB, et al. Signal intensity patterns in intraspinal dermoids and epidermoid on MR imaging. Clin Radiol 1993;48:405–413.
18. Barsi P, Kenez J, Varallyay G, et al. Unusual origin of free subarachnoid fat drops: a ruptured spinal dermoid tumor. Neuroradiology 2001;34:343–344.
19. Tsuruda JS, Chew WM, Mosely ME, et al. Diffusion-weighted MR imaging of the brain: value of differentiating between extraaxial cysts and epidermoid tumors. AJNR Am J Neuroradiol 1990;11:925–931.
20. Cavazzani P, Ruelle A, Michelozzi G, et al. Spinal dermoid cysts originating intracranial fat drops causing obstructive hydrocephalus: case reports. Surg Neurol 1995;43:466–470.
21. Simon JA, Olan WJ, Santi M. Intracranial neuroenteric cysts: a differential diagnosis and review. Radiographics 1997;17:1587–1593.
22. Georgy BA, Hesselink JR, Jernigan TL. MR imaging of the corpus callosum. AJR Am J Radiol 1993;160:949–955.
23. Davidson HD, Abraham R, Steiner RE. Agenesis of the corpus callosum: magnetic resonance imaging. Radiology 1985;155:371–373.
24. Atlas SW, Zimmerman RA, Bilaniuk LT, et al. Corpus callosum and limbic system: neuroanatomic MR evaluation and developmental anomalies. Radiology 1986;160:355–362.
25. Barkovich AJ, Quint D. Middle interhemispheric fusion: an unusual variant of holoprosencephaly. AJNR Am J Neuroradiol 1993;14:431–440.
26. Smith MM, Thompson JE, Naidich TP, et al. Cebocephaly with single midline proboscis: alobar holoprosencephaly. Int J Neuroradiol 1996;2:251–263.
27. Barkovich AJ, Kjos BO. Schizencephaly: correlation of clinical findings with MR characteristics. AJNR Am J Neuroradiol 1992;13:85–94.
28. Bird CR, Gilles FH. Type I schizencephaly: CT and neuropathologic findings. AJNR Am J Neuroradiol 1987;8:451–454.
29. Hung PC, Wang HS, Yeh YS, et al. Coexistence of schizencephaly and intracranial arteriovenous malformation in an infant. AJNR Am J Neuroradiol 1996;17:1921–1922.
30. Brodsky MC, Glasier CM. Optic nerve hypoplasia: clinical significance of associated central nervous system abnormalities on magnetic resonance imaging. Arch Ophthalmol 1993;111:66–74.
31. Truwitt CL, Barkovich AJ. Pathogenesis of intracranial lipoma: an MR study in 42 patients. AJNR Am J Neuroradiol 1990;11:665–672.
32. Uchino A, Hasuo K, Matsumoto S, et al. Solitary choroid plexus lipomas: CT and MR appearance. AJNR Am J Neuroradiol 1993;14:116–118.
33. Ruocco MJ, Robles HA, Rao KC, et al. Intratentorial lipomas with Meckel's cave and cerebellopontine angle extension. AJNR Am J Neuroradiol 1995;16:1504–1506.
34. Castillo M, Mukherji SK. Imaging of facial anomalies. Curr Probl Diagn Radiol 1996;25: 169–188.
35. Castillo M, Mukherji SK. Imaging of orofacial clefting disorders. Neuroimaging Clin North Am 2000;10:253–270.
36. Seidenwurm D, Berenstein A, Hyman A, et al. Vein of Galen malformation: correlation of clinical presentation, arteriography, and MR imaging. AJNR Am J Neuroradiol 1991;12:347–354.
37. Hurst RW, Kagetsu NJ, Berenstein A. Angiographic findings in two cases of aneurysmal malformation of vein of Galen prior to spontaneous thrombosis: therapeutic implications. AJNR Am J Neuroradiol 1992;13:1446–1450.
38. Whitaker JB, Latack JT, Venes JL. Spontaneous thrombosis of a vein of Galen aneurysm. AJNR Am J Neuroradiol 1987;8:1134–1136.
39. Lasjaunias P, Ter Brugge K, Lopez Ibor L, et al. The role of dural anomalies in vein of Galen aneurysms: report of six cases and review of the literature. AJNR Am J Neuroradiol 1987;8: 185–192.
40. Barkovich AJ, Kuzniecky RI, Dobyns WB, et al. A classification scheme for malformations of cortical development. Neuropediatrics 1996;27:59–63.
41. Kuzniecky RI, Barkovich AJ. Pathogenesis and pathology of focal malformations of cortical development and epilepsy. J Clin Neurophysiol 1996;13:468–480.
42. Barkovich AJ, Kuzniecky RI. Neuroimaging of focal malformations of cortical development. J Clin Neurophysiol 1996;13:481–494.
43. Barkovich AJ, Jackson DE, Boyer RS. Band heterotopia: a newly recognized neuronal migration anomaly. Radiology 1989;171:455–458.

44. Smith AS, Weinstein MA, Quencer RM, et al. Association of heterotopic gray matter with seizures: MR imaging. Radiology 1988;168:195–198.
45. Ross ME, Allen KM, Srivastava AK, et al. Linkage and physical mapping of x-linked lissencephaly/SBH (XLIS): a gene causing neuronal migration defects in human brain. Hum Mol Genet 1997;6:555–562.
46. Dobyns WB, Andermann E, Andermann F, et al. X-linked malformations of neuronal migration. Neurology 1996;47:331–339.
47. Yagishita A, Arai N, Maehara T, et al. Focal cortical dysplasia: appearance on MR images. Radiology 1997;203:553–559.
48. Bronen RA, Spencer DD, Fulbright RK. Cerebrospinal fluid cleft with cortical dimple: MR imaging marker for focal cortical dysplasia. Radiology 2000;214:657–663.
49. Guerrini R, Dubeau F, Dulac O, et al. Bilateral parasagittal parietooccipital polymicrogyria and epilepsy. Ann Neurol 1997;41:65–73.
50. Bronen RA, Vives KP, Kim JH, et al. Focal cortical dysplasia of Taylor, balloon cell subtype: MR differentiation from low-grade tumors. AJNR Am J Neuroradiol 1997;18:1141–1151.
51. Kalifa GL, Chiron C, Sellier N, et al. Hemimegalencephaly: MR imaging in five children. Radiology 1987;165:29–33.
52. Castillo M, Mukherji SK. Imaging of the pediatric head, neck, and spine. Philadelphia: Lippincott-Raven, 1996.
53. Boyle CM, Rosenblum JD. Three-dimensional CT for pre- and postsurgical imaging of patients with craniosynostosis: correlation of operative procedure and radiology imaging. AJR Am J Radiol 1997;169:1173–1177.

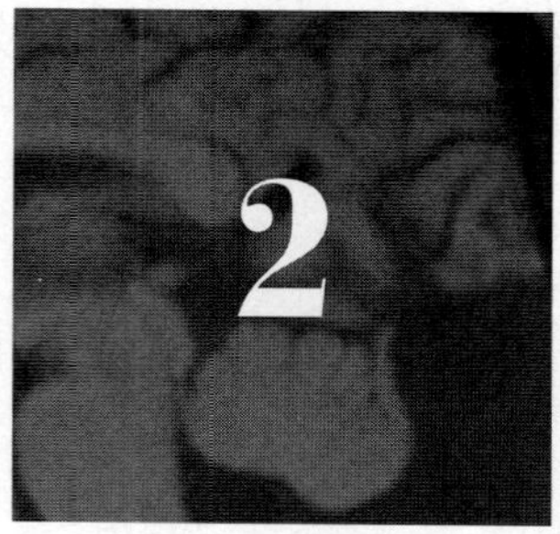

Neurocutaneous Syndromes

- Neurocutaneous Syndromes
- Neurofibromatosis
- Tuberous Sclerosis
- Sturge-Weber Syndrome
- Von Hippel-Lindau Disease
- Rare Neurocutaneous Syndromes

There are now more than 30 recognized phakomatoses (1). The most common are the neurofibromatoses, tuberous sclerosis (TS), von Hippel-Lindau disease (VHL), and Sturge-Weber syndrome (SW), and these are addressed here individually. The rare neurocutaneous disorders include Klippel-Trenaunay syndrome, Gorlin's syndrome, hypomelanosis of Ito, ataxia–telangiectasia, Cowden's syndrome, xeroderma pigmentosa, incontinentia pigmenti, Cockayne's syndrome, dysautonomia, Refsum's disease, Werner's syndrome, progeria, Chediak-Higashi syndrome, Sjögren-Larson syndrome, and neurocutaneous melanosis. I address only the most common of these disorders.

Neurofibromatosis

Most neurofibromatoses are type 1 (NF-1) or type 2 (NF-2), and both are autosomal dominant disorders (2). Rarely, there is some overlap among these two disorders (e.g., so-called NF-3) (1–3). Both NF-1 and NF-2 may be of the segmental type (NF-5). Other types of neurofibromatoses are hereditary spinal neurofibromatosis, schwannomatosis, familial intestinal neurofibromatosis, café-au-lait spots alone (NF-6), Watson's syndrome (pulmonary valvular stenosis, indeterminate; NF-4), late onset neurofibromatosis (NF-7; Lisch nodules, macrocephaly, and short stature), Noonan's/neurofibromatosis syndrome, LEOPARD syndrome (multiple lentigines syndrome), and a syndrome comprising the presence of multiple nevi, schwannomas, and vaginal leiomyomas (1–3).

Neurofibromatosis Type 1

Although traditionally NF-1 was believed to arise from an abnormality in chromosome 17, it is now known that in this disease 11 functional genes are missing and that up to 200 point mutations exist (1–3). The main defect is located on chromosome 17Q11.2, which includes a tumor suppressor gene (1–4). This gene encodes for a product named *neurofibrin*. This gene has complete penetrance but variable phenotypic manifestations. The incidence of NF-1 is 1 in 2,000 to 5,000 individuals and thus it is the most common neurocutaneous syndrome. The life span of patients with NF-1 is reduced by 10 to 15 years, and most die secondary to malignant tumors (most of these are due to degeneration of preex-

NF-1 is a disorder of the "substance" of the central nervous system, and thus its main lesions are astrocytomas, cerebral hamartomas (areas of vacuolar myelin), and neurofibromas.

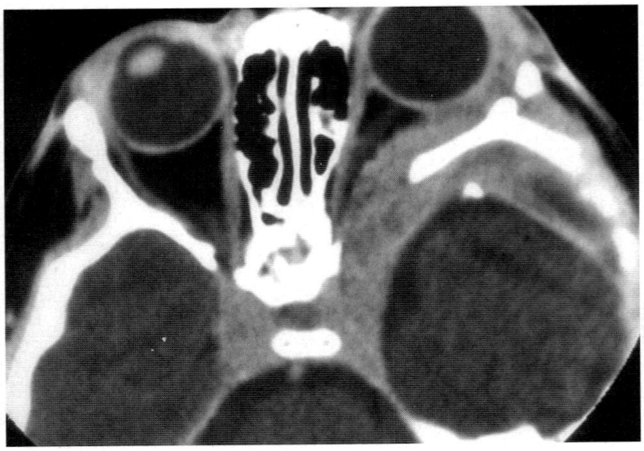

Figure 2.1 *Neurofibromatosis Type 1, Dysplasia of the Sphenoid Bone.* Axial computed tomography shows absence of a portion of the left greater sphenoidal wing with a plexiform and enhancing neurofibroma extending from the left cavernous sinus into the orbit. There is left proptosis.

isting tumors). The use of major and minor diagnostic criteria as established by the National Institutes of Health (NIH) is helpful only in patients older than 8 years of age. Bone lesions are the earliest sign of NF-1 and appear during the first year of life (long bone pseudoarthrosis and dysplasia of the sphenoid bone; Fig. 2.1). Many astrocytomas arise before 3 years of age, and most are diagnosed before 7 years of age. Before 4 years of age, only 46% of patients with NF-1 meet the established NIH diagnostic criteria (1) (Box 2.1).

The protein truncation test, which has been advocated for screening of the disease, is helpful but expensive, and its reliability has not been entirely proven. The hallmark of the disease is the presence of bilateral optic nerve gliomas, seen in 15% to 40% of patients (1) (Fig. 2.2). Only 50% of patients with these masses are symptomatic and only a very small number of them eventually need specific treatment. Most of these tumors arise in the optic nerves (in multifocal fashion) and secondarily involve the chiasm. These tumors are of the "pilocytic" type, but they diffusely infiltrate the visual apparatus. Some show contrast enhancement, whereas other do not. Some tumors show patchy areas of enhancement. Enhancement does not signify a greater degree of malignancy. These tumors also may extend along the optic radiations, and in this location they are very difficult to different from so-called hamartomas (areas of vacuolar myelination). Some of these tumors regress with advancing age, and some investigators therefore believe them to be more akin to a hamartoma than to a true tumor (5,6). The second most common site for astrocytomas in patients with NF-1 is the tectum (7) (Fig. 2.3). These tumors may result in hydrocephalus and show high T2 signal intensity, mass effect, and varying degrees of contrast enhancement. The third most common site of tumors in NF-1 is the brainstem. Hemispheric tumors also occur and may be of low or high histologic grades.

Box 2.1: National Institutes of Health Criteria for Diagnosis of Neurofibromatosis Type 1 (Two or More of the Findings Listed)

More than six café-au-lait spots before puberty, after puberty >15 mm in diameter
Freckles in axial or inguinal region
One plexiform neurofibroma
Two or more neurofibromas
Optic glioma
Two or more hamartomas in the iris (Lisch nodules)
Sphenoid wing dysplasia or long bone pseudoarthrosis
First-degree relative with neurofibromatosis type 1

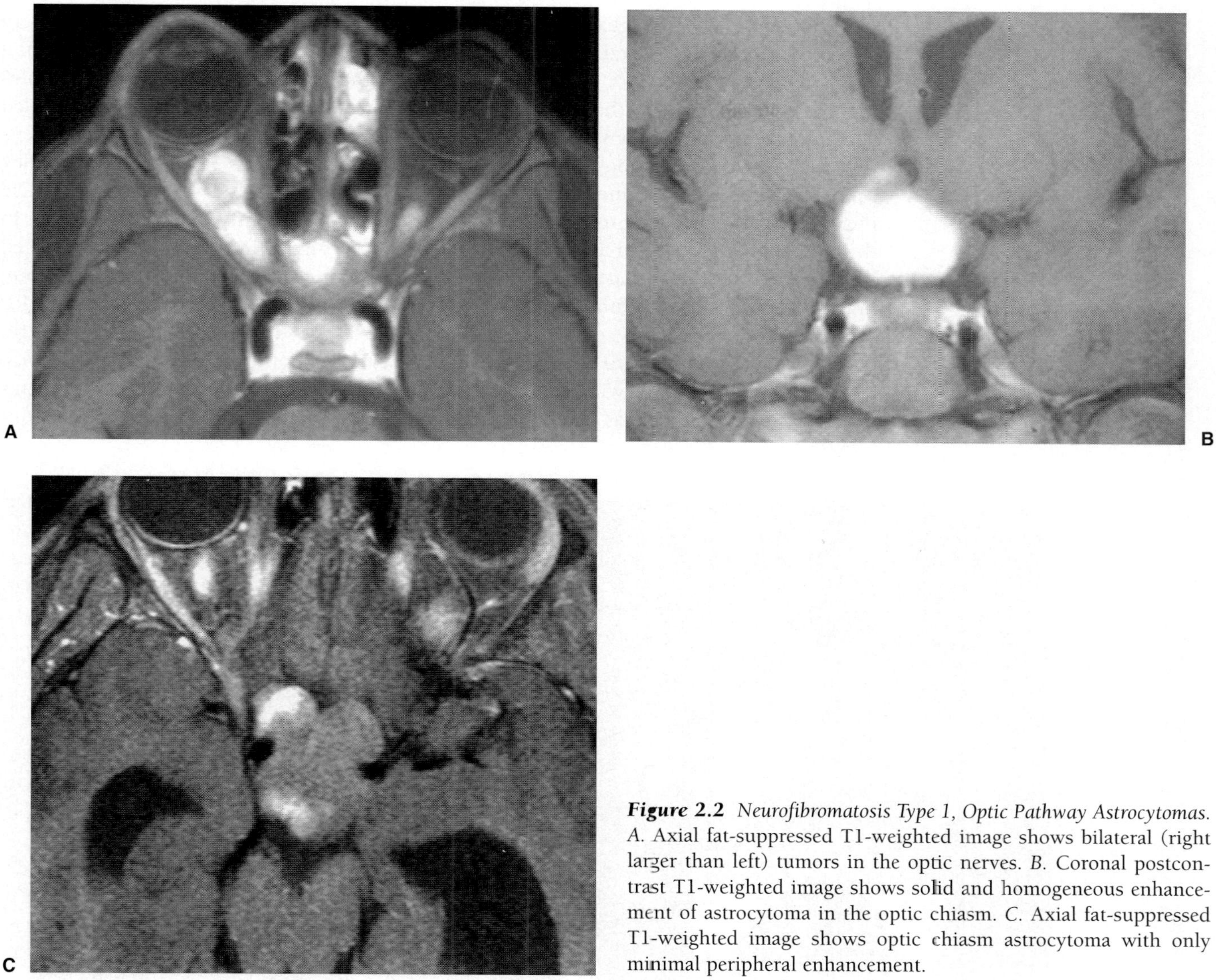

Figure 2.2 *Neurofibromatosis Type 1, Optic Pathway Astrocytomas. A.* Axial fat-suppressed T1-weighted image shows bilateral (right larger than left) tumors in the optic nerves. *B.* Coronal postcontrast T1-weighted image shows solid and homogeneous enhancement of astrocytoma in the optic chiasm. *C.* Axial fat-suppressed T1-weighted image shows optic chiasm astrocytoma with only minimal peripheral enhancement.

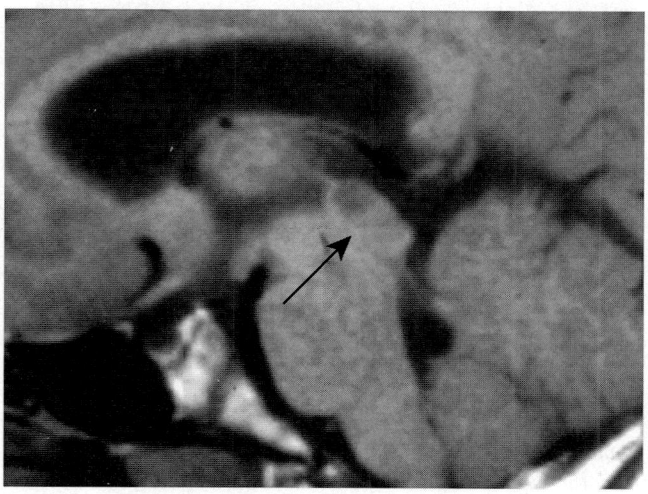

Figure 2.3 *Neurofibromatosis Type 1, Tectum Astrocytoma.* Sagittal noncontrast T1-weighted image show masslike thickening *(arrow)* of the tectal plate with effacement of the aqueduct of Sylvius.

Areas of high T2 signal intensity [including fluid attenuation inversion recovery (FLAIR) images] in the brain of these patients have been called *hamartomas* for lack of a better name (8) (Fig. 2.4). Some reports indicate that they represent areas of vacuoles (spongiform changes) in the myelin. As myelin maturation progresses, these fluid-filled vacuoles disappear and the signal intensity in the region returns to normal. Others believe that these areas are composed of dysplastic neurons. Regardless of their etiology, they probably are the most common abnormality in NF-1 seen on brain magnetic resonance imaging (MRI). They tend to occur in the basal ganglia, particularly in the globi pallidi. In this location, they also may show slightly increased signal intensity on T1-weighted images. They also are found along the optic radiations, internal capsules, corpus callosum, brainstem, medial cerebellum, cerebellar peduncles, medulla, and even the spinal cord (9). They usually have no mass effect and do not enhance. They usually are not seen at birth, tend to enlarge slightly until 10 to 12 years of age, and shrink thereafter. Their significance is uncertain, but patients with many of these areas demonstrate more pronounced cognitive difficulties. These areas show increased diffusion of extracellular water on diffusion-

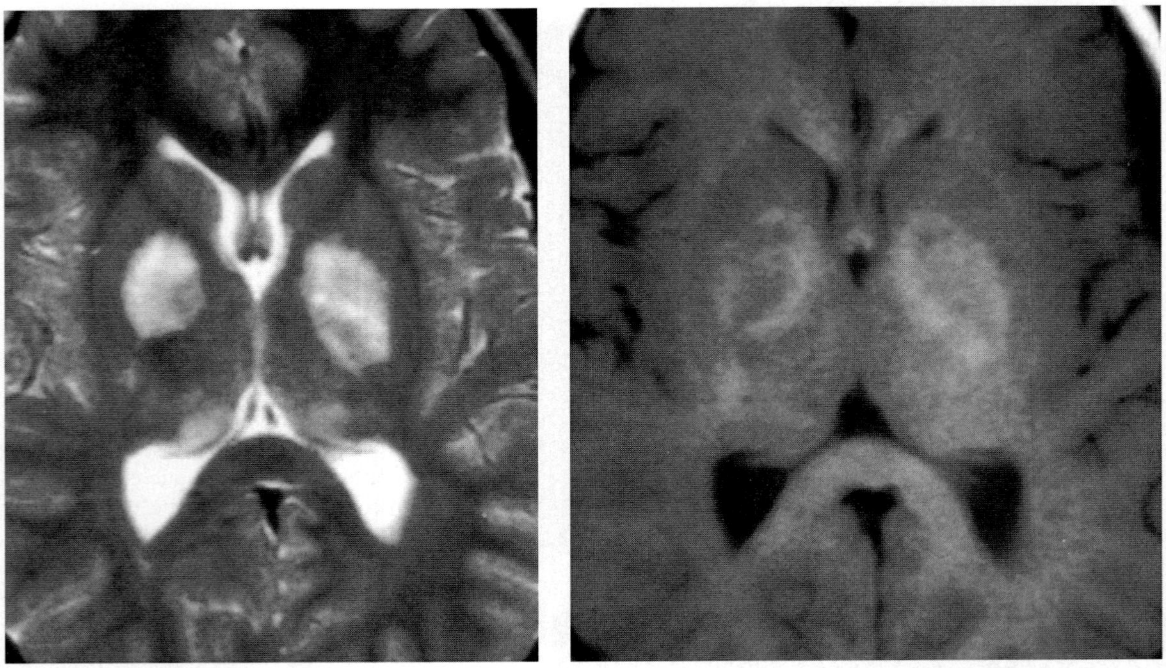

A B

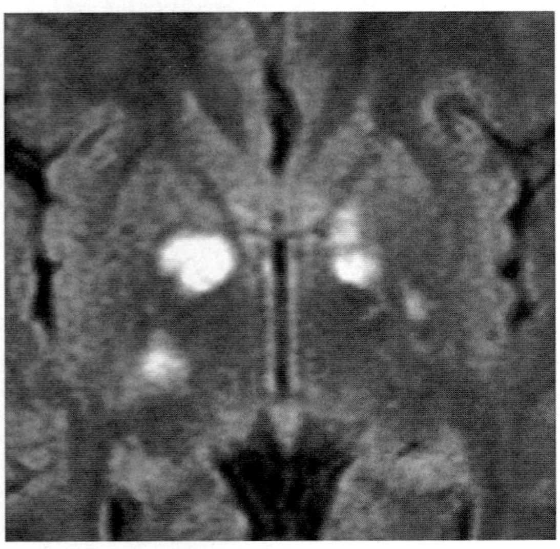

C

Figure 2.4 *Neurofibromatosis Type 1, Areas of Presumed Vacuolar Myelin.* Axial T2-weighted *A* and T1-weighted *B* images in the same patient show hamartomatous involvement of the lentiform nuclei. The lesions are T2-bright and also somewhat bright on T1. In a different patient, fluid attenuation inversion recovery (FLAIR) image *C* shows these hamartomas also to be bright.

weighted imaging. The overall size of the brain also is enlarged in patients with NF-1. This seems to be at the expense of more white matter. The brain may be diffusely enlarged, or only one hemisphere may be affected. The corpus callosum sometimes may appear thick. Intracranial neurofibromas also occur, particularly along the course of the cranial nerves. A neurofibroma in a purely motor cranial nerve is highly suspect for NF.

The spine is affected in approximately 60% of patients with NF-1 (1–3). Bone changes included remodeling and scalloping of the dorsal vertebral bodies (due to dural ectasia or neurofibromas) and the presence of arachnoid cysts (Fig. 2.5A). A lateral thoracic meningocele (which is a type of dural ectasia) is typical of NF-1. Kyphoscoliosis, which may be pronounced, may be secondary to a primary bone abnormality or to neurofibromata (Fig. 2.5B). In the spinal cord, hamartomas and astrocytomas occasionally are found (10).

Newly described and less common lesions seen in patients with NF-1 are arterial anomalies (moyamoya-like lesions, aneurysms, arteriovenous fistulas, spontaneous hematomas), Miller-Dicker syndrome, gray matter heterotopias, melanoma, hypothalamic hamartoma, glomus tumor, Triton tumor (a lesion with neurogenic and myogenic differentiation), ganglioneuromas, giant cell granulomas, gingival enlargement, Wilms' tumor, rhabdomyosarcoma, chronic myelogenous leukemia, and thyroid medullary cancer, as well as attention deficit/hyperactivity disorder and Tourette's syndrome (1). Other findings in NF-1 are large eyes (called *buphthalmos*, meaning "ox eye"), vasculopathy with cerebral infarctions, overgrowth of the choroid plexuses into the temporal horn of the lateral ventricles, and a skull defect at the junction of the temporal, parietal, and occipital bones. NF-1 is a disorder of the "substance" of the central nervous system (CNS) characterized by astrocytomas, cerebral hamartomas, and neurofibromas.

There is evidence that proton MR spectroscopy may be useful in patients with NF-1 (11,12). MR spectroscopy may be used to distinguish between hamartomas and gliomas. Hamartomas shows low *N*-acetyl aspartate, which implies neuronal dysfunction, whereas gliomas show low and elevated choline, which correlates with hypercellularity.

A

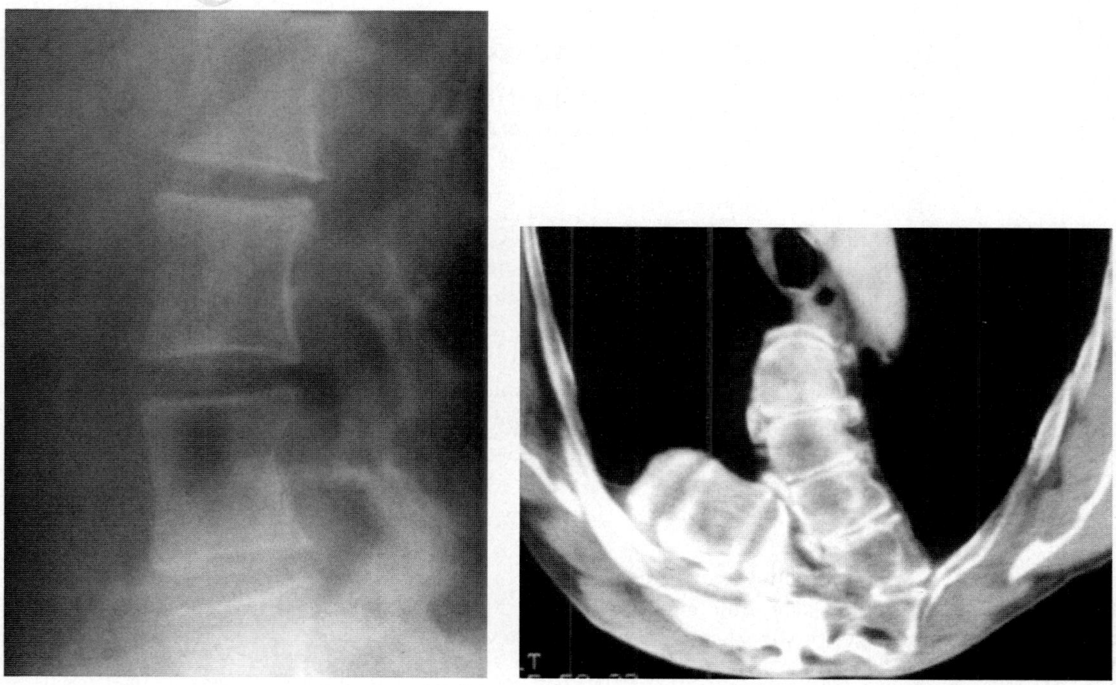

B

Figure 2.5 *Neurofibromatosis Type 1, Spinal Involvement. A.* Lateral radiograph shows scalloping of the posterior border of the vertebral bodies in this patient secondary to dural ectasia. *B.* Axial computed tomography shows acute-angle kyphoscoliosis.

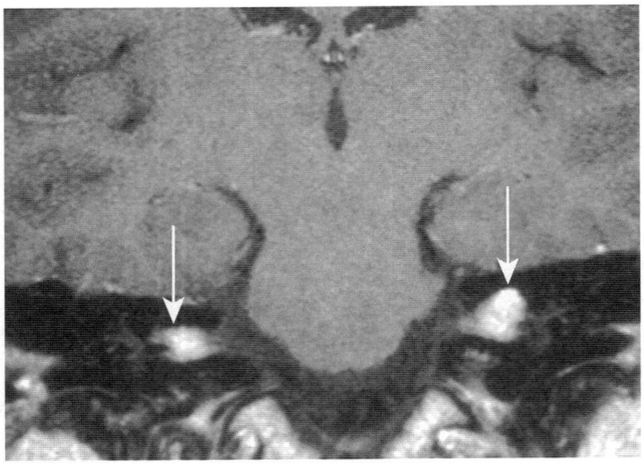

Figure 2.6 *Neurofibromatosis Type 2, Vestibular Schwannomas.* Postcontrast axial T1-weighted image shows enhancing masses *(arrows)* in the region of cranial nerve VIII.

Neurofibromatosis Type 2

NF-2 is a disorder of the coverings of the CNS, and thus its main lesions are meningiomas, schwannomas, and ependymomas.

This disorder is not related to NF-1, although occasionally one sees overlap of NF-1 and NF-2 syndromes (sometimes referred to as *NF-3*). NF-2 is relatively uncommon and is found in 1 in 20,000 to 50,000 individuals (1,13). It is a disorder characterized by lesions of the "linings" of the brain—that is, meningiomas, schwannomas, and ependymomas (Fig. 2.6). Other, less common lesions seen in patients with NF-2 are sarcoma, meningoangiomatosis, and pituitary adenoma. The main genetic defect is localized to chromosome 22 and results in decreased synthesis of "merlin," which is a tumor suppressor gene product (1,13). Merlin modulates cell morphology and cell growth. Most patients with NF-2 present during the third decade of life. Skin lesions are much less common than in NF-1. The NIH criteria for the diagnosis if NF-2 are shown in Box 2.2, and the types of tumors seen in patients with NF-2 are shown in Table 2.1 (1).

Box 2.2: Revised National Institutes of Health Criteria for the Diagnosis of Neurofibromatosis Type 2

Definite NF-2	Probable NF-2
Bilateral CN VIII schwannomas	Unilateral CN VIII schwannoma + a meningioma, glioma, schwannoma elsewhere, juvenile posterior subcapsular lenticular opacities
or	
First-degree relative with NF-2	Multiple meningiomas + 1 vestibular schwannoma in patient <30 years of age, or glioma, schwannoma elsewhere, juvenile posterior subcapsular lenticular opacities
plus	
Two of the following: meningioma, glioma, schwannoma, or juvenile posterior subcapsular lenticular opacities	

CN, cranial nerve; NF-2, neurofibromatosis type 2.

Table 2.1: Most Common Central Nervous System Tumors in Neurobibromatosis Type 2

Tumor	*Incidence*
Vestibular schwannomas	98%
Spinal cord tumors (most ependymoma)	67%
Meningioma(s)	50%
Other cranial nerve schwannomas	25%
Cerebral astrocytoma/ependymoma	>5%

With regard to Table 2.1, note that multiple meningiomas still are much more common in the absence of NF-2, and thus only a few patients with multiple meningiomas have this rare neurocutaneous syndrome. Meningiomas seen in NF-2 may be in atypical locations (e.g., intraventricular) and have atypical imaging features (Fig. 2.7). Meningiomas in children always are suspect for NF-2.

Spinal tumors are more common in NF-2 than in any of the other neurofibromatoses (14). Nearly 100% of patients with NF-2 have spinal schwannomas (Fig. 2.8). Unlike NF-1, kyphoscoliosis is not common. Intramedullary spinal cord ependymomas also are relatively common (15). Their imaging appearance is nonspecific, but the presence of a spinal cord tumor in the context of NF-2 always should raise the suspicion for an ependymoma.

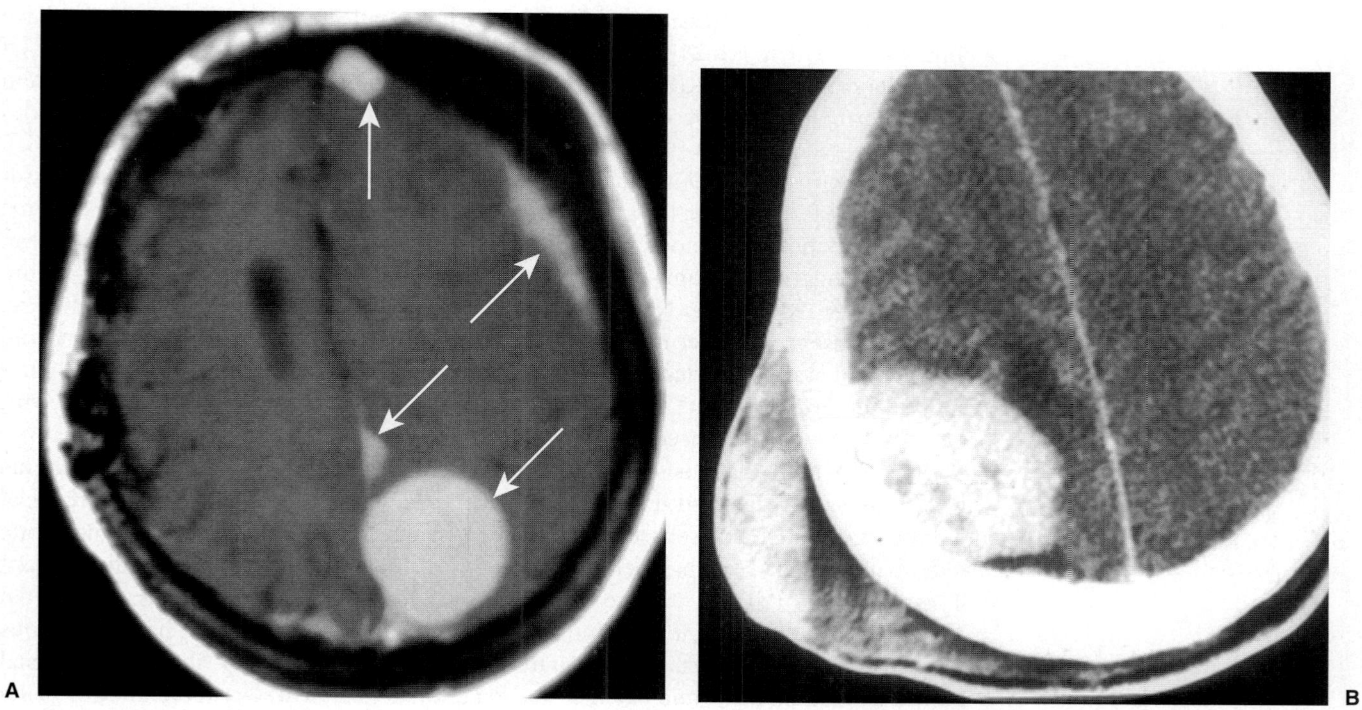

Figure 2.7 *Neurofibromatosis Type 2, Meningiomas. A.* Axial postcontrast T1-weighted image shows multiple enhancing meningiomas (*arrows*). *B.* In a different case, postcontrast computed tomography shows a large meningioma, and overlying it a large schwannoma arising in the scalp.

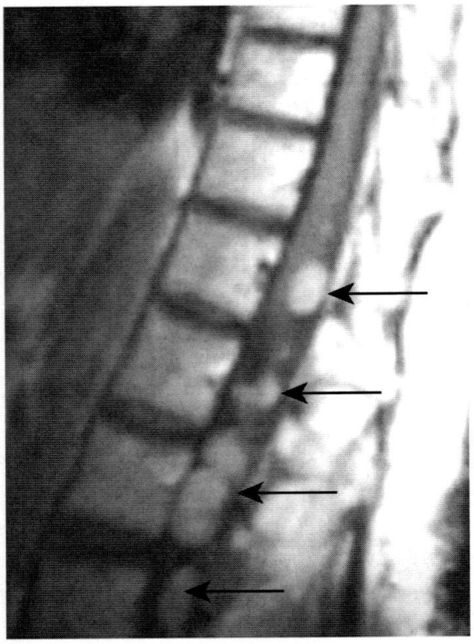

Figure 2.8 *Neurofibromatosis Type 2, Spinal Involvement.* Sagittal postcontrast T1-weighted image shows multiple enhancing intradural schwannomas *(arrows)* in the lower spine.

TUBEROUS SCLEROSIS

TS affects approximately 40,000 individuals in the United States, and approximately 2 million worldwide (16). The classic triad of adenoma sebaceum, seizures, and mental retardation is found in only one-third of patients with TS (17). Although it is inherited in an autosomal dominant fashion, its penetrance is variable and heterogeneous, accounting for different phenotypic expressions of the disease. For unaffected parents who already have a child with TS, there is a 2% to 3% incidence of subsequent children with the disease. Of the two abnormal genes, *TSC1* is found on chromosome Q19 and encodes for a protein called *hamartin* (18). The second gene, *TSC2*, is located on chromosome P16 and encodes for a protein called *tuberin* (18). These two proteins have tumor suppressor effects. Call lines for hamartin are found in the brain, heart, placenta, lung, liver, skeleton, muscle, kidney and pancreas. Call lines for tuberin are found in the brain, kidney, skin, liver, adrenal glands, colon, and white blood cells (18). Tuberin is a negative growth factor regulator, whereas the function of hamartin is not yet known. All complications of TS arise from defects in these two genes. New mutations do, however, result in more severe disease. Specifically, absence of tuberin gives rise to dominantly inherited renal cell carcinoma and subependymal and subcortical hamartomas. Part of the *TSC2* gene also encodes for polycystic kidney disease—that is, all patients with TS have renal lesions, but patients with polycystic kidney disease need not have TS.

The most common brain lesion in tuberous sclerosis is the subcortical hamartoma, followed by the periventricular hamartoma.

Prenatal genetic diagnosis is expensive but available and usually reserved for parents with the disease or those with a previously affected child. Major features of TS are facial angiofibromas (adenoma sebaceum), forehead plaque, ungual fibroma, hypomelanotic macules (more than 13), shagreen patches, cortical tubers, subependymal nodules, giant cell astrocytoma (GCA), cardiac rhabdomyoma, lymphangiomyomatosis, and renal angiomyolipoma (16) (Fig. 2.9). Minor features are pits in dental enamel, hamartomatous intestinal polyps, bone cysts, white matter migration lines, gingival fibromas, nonrenal hamartomas, retinal achromic patches, and renal cysts (16). These criteria are now being replaced by the investigation of hamartomas using imaging. Finding two or more hamartomas in different organs is so uncommon that it strongly suggests the diagnosis of TS. Hamartomas may be found in the face, forehead, ungual region, skin, retina, cortex, subependymal regions, heart, kidneys, and lungs. The criteria for the diagnosis of TS are shown in Box 2.3 (16).

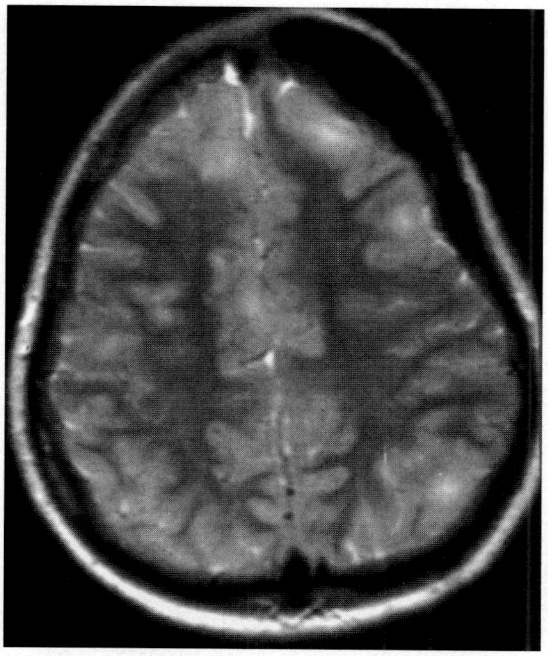

Figure 2.9 *Tuberous Sclerosis, Fibrous Plaque.* Axial T2-weighted image shows thick hypointense area in the left frontal bone.

Neuroimaging plays an important role in diagnosis and follow-up (19,20). MRI is better for patients known to have TS and for those who are symptomatic (19). Computed tomography is a cheaper screening test for asymptomatic patients, and although its sensitivity is less than that of MRI, its specificity (because of the calcified periventricular nodules) is somewhat greater. It is now believed that cortical tubers are more common than periventricular lesions and that they are the "hallmark" of TS in the brain, seen in over 90% of patients (Fig. 2.10). Histologically, they contain disorganized glial tissues, dysplastic and heterotopic neurons, and giant cells, and later in life they develop calcifica-

Box 2.3: Revised Criteria for Diagnosis of Tuberous Sclerosis

Major	Minor
Facial angiofibromas (adenoma sebaceum) or forehead plaque	Pits in dental enamel
Ungual or periungual fibromas	Hamartomatous rectal polyps
Hypomelanotic macules	Bone cysts
Connective tissue nevus (Shagreen patch)	More than three cerebral white matter migration lines
Retinal nodular hamartomas	Gingival fibromas
Cortical tubers	Nonrenal hamartomas
Subependymal nodules	Retinal achromic patch
Heart rhabdomyoma(s)	"Confetti" skin lesions
Lymphangiomyomatosis	Multiple kidney cysts
Kidney angiomyolipoma	

Definite TS: 2 major or 1 major + 1 minor
Pobable TS: 1 major + 1 minor
Possible TS: 1 major or 2 or more minors

TS, tuberous sclerosis.

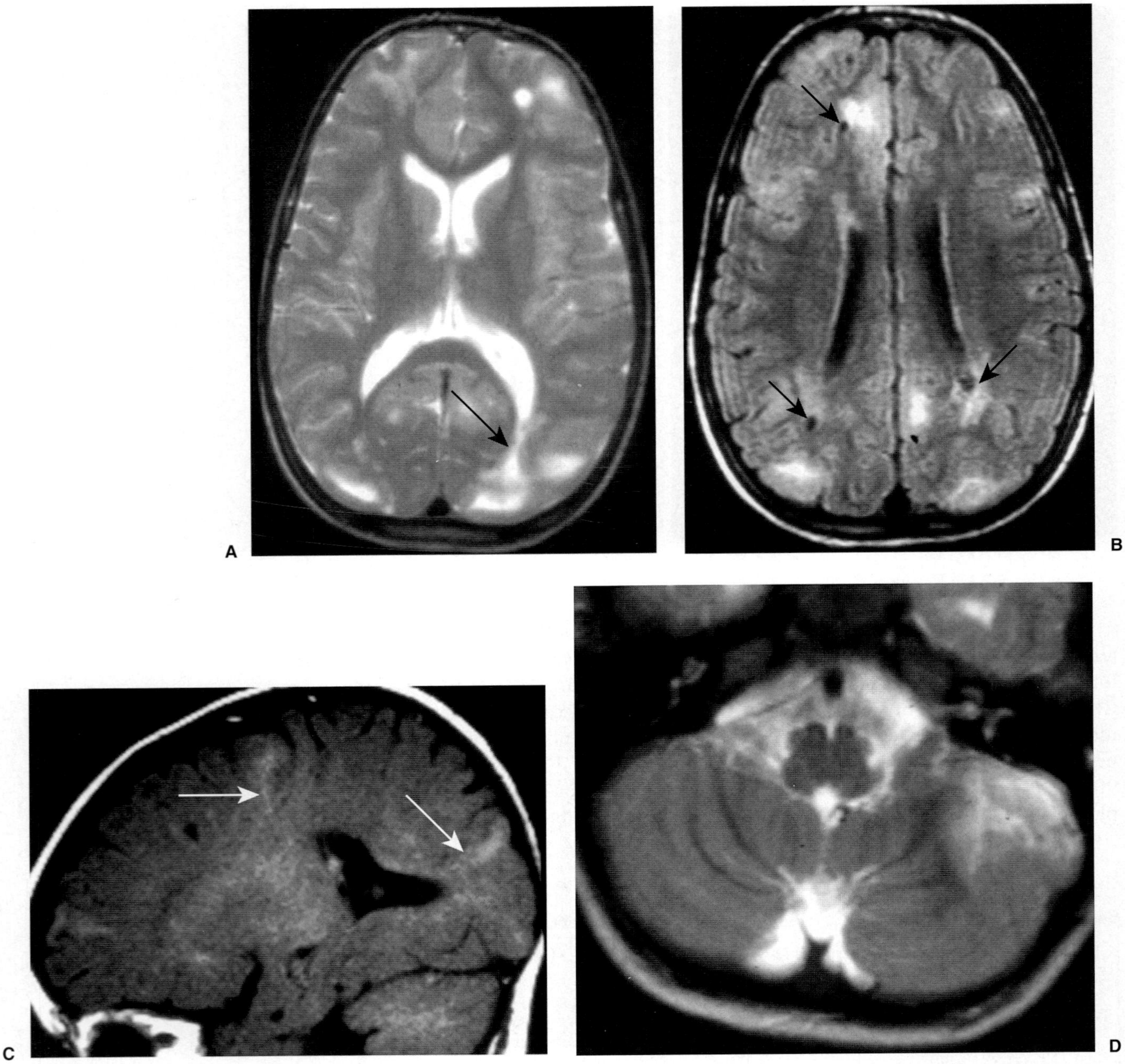

Figure 2.10 *Tuberous Sclerosis, Hamartomas. A.* Axial T2-weighted image shows several hyperintense hamartomas in subcortical regions. One hamartoma in the left occipital region has a linear hyperintensity *(arrow)* extending to the lateral ventricle. The cortex over the hamartomas appears expanded. *B.* Fluid attenuation inversion recovery (FLAIR) image (different patient) shows the hamartomas to be bright. Note brain cysts *(arrows)*. *C.* Sagittal T1-weighted image in a young patient shows that hamartomas are bright and have linear extensions *(arrows)* into the lateral wall of the ventricles. *D.* Axial T2-weighted image shows a bright hamartoma in the left cerebellar hemisphere.

tions. These hamartomas may be seen along the walls of the ventricles (curiously, mostly the lateral ones) and in the brain substance. Hamartomas are better seen using FLAIR sequences than other T2-weighted sequences (21). Subcortical hamartomas do not enhance, but the periventricular ones may show some enhancement on MRI (22). Some hamartomas are slightly bright on precontrast T1-weighted images, but most are isointense or hypointense. Subcortical hamartomas are T2-hyperintense lesions that expand the overlying gyrus. The zone of increased signal intensity commonly extends to the outer border of the ventricles (region of the germinal matrix) and has led some to postulate that they are anomalies of neuronal migration. Mental retardation and seizures are more severe in patients with a large number of lesions. Tubers (hamartomas) in the temporal lobes correlate with a high risk of autism. Other behavioral problems in patients with TS are attention deficit/hyperactivity disorder and increased aggression. Tubers in the temporal lobes also result in seizures of the infantile spasm type. This type of seizure in the very young should prompt the clinician to investigate for the possibility of TS. There is evidence that MRI may be of use in the diagnosis of TS in very young patients (<3 months of age). In these patients, the brain lesions are bright on T1- and dark on T2-weighted images, which is the opposite of the findings in older children and adults. Hamartomas may be found in the cerebellum, where they have an identical appearance to the supratentorial ones and have little clinical significance.

GCAs deserve special mention. These tumors are basically pathognomonic of TS and occur mostly at the level of the foramina of Monro (I have seen only one case of a GCA in a different location; Fig. 2.11). They are found in approximately 5% of patients with TS. They are presumed to arise from subependymal nodules, but the relationship between the two lesions is not certain. They are histologically benign masses that grow slowly and do not invade the adjacent brain. They are, however, one of the most common causes of death in patients with TS because of hydrocephalus and increased intracranial pressure (seizures are another common neurologic cause of death). Only growth on sequential imaging may be use to differentiate them from subependymal nodules. All GCAs show contrast enhancement (23). Rare features reported include malignant transformation and location in the fourth ventricle. Although GCAs commonly are bilateral (but asymmetric in size), when unilateral they tend to occur in the right side.

Giant cell astrocytomas are seen almost exclusively in patients with tuberous sclerosis.

Less common imaging abnormalities seen in patients with TS include multiple brain cysts (which probably are dilated perivascular spaces) found mostly in the white matter, and hemimegalencephaly (24,25).

Sturge-Weber Syndrome

SW also is known as *encephalotrigeminal angiomatosis* and is inherited as an autosomal recessive trait (26). It is a disorder involving the face, brain, and meninges. It is part of a group of disorders called the *phakomatoses pigmentovascularis*. SW is included in the type 2 classification of these disorders and is characterized by blue skin spots (nevus flammeus). A nevus in the distribution of the first division of one trigeminal nerve is typical of the disease and usually is ipsilateral to the pial angioma. Occasionally, there is no facial nevus or the pial angioma is contralateral to it. Only 2% of patients with a facial nevus flammeus have SW (27). A recently described association is that of giant oral pyogenic granulomas. Intraocular choroidal angiomas leading to glaucoma may be seen, which in young patients may result in enlargement of one or both eyes (buphthalmos) (28). Most patients are healthy at birth, but seizures eventually develop in over 90%. Other symptoms include developmental delay, hemiplegia, visual deficits, and dementia. The optic globes may be enlarged (buphthalmos), and choroidal hemangiomas are present in over 70% of patients, but are small and difficult to see on imaging studies.

A facial nevus flammeus in the distribution of the ophthalmic (V1) division of the trigeminal nerve is suggestive of Sturge-Weber syndrome.

There is an angioma of the leptomeninges, absence of cortical veins, recruitment of deep medullary veins, and enlargement of the ipsilateral choroid plexus as an alternate route for blood drainage (29,30) (Fig. 2.12). When this occurs, the ipsilateral choroid

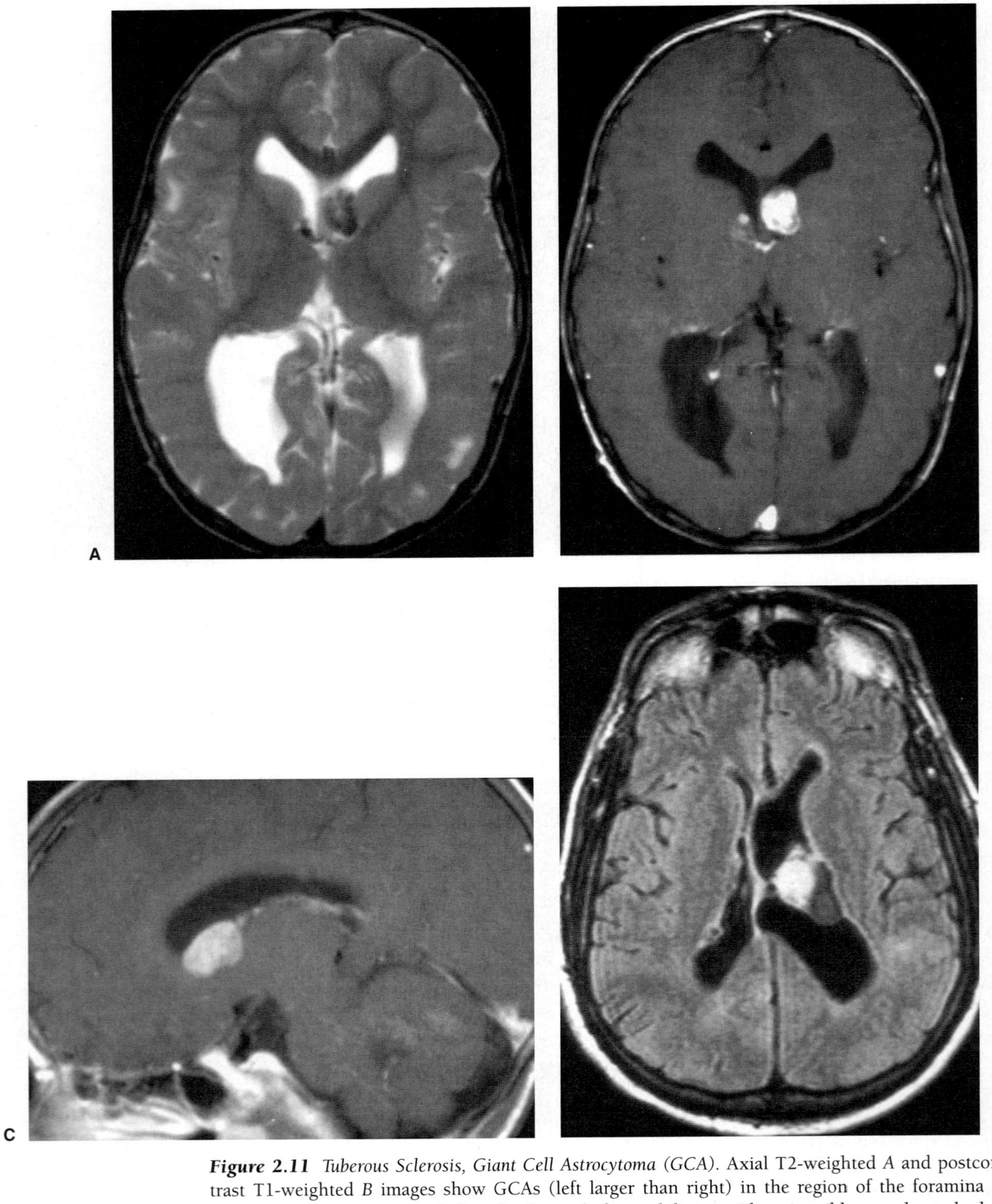

Figure 2.11 *Tuberous Sclerosis, Giant Cell Astrocytoma (GCA)*. Axial T2-weighted *A* and postcontrast T1-weighted *B* images show GCAs (left larger than right) in the region of the foramina of Monro. The tumors are T2-dark and enhanced after gadolinium. There is mild to moderate hydrocephalus. Sagittal postcontrast T1-weighted image *C* shows the enhancing tumor on the left. Fluid attenuation inversion recovery (FLAIR) image *D* shows GCA in the mid-portion of the lateral wall of the left lateral ventricle.

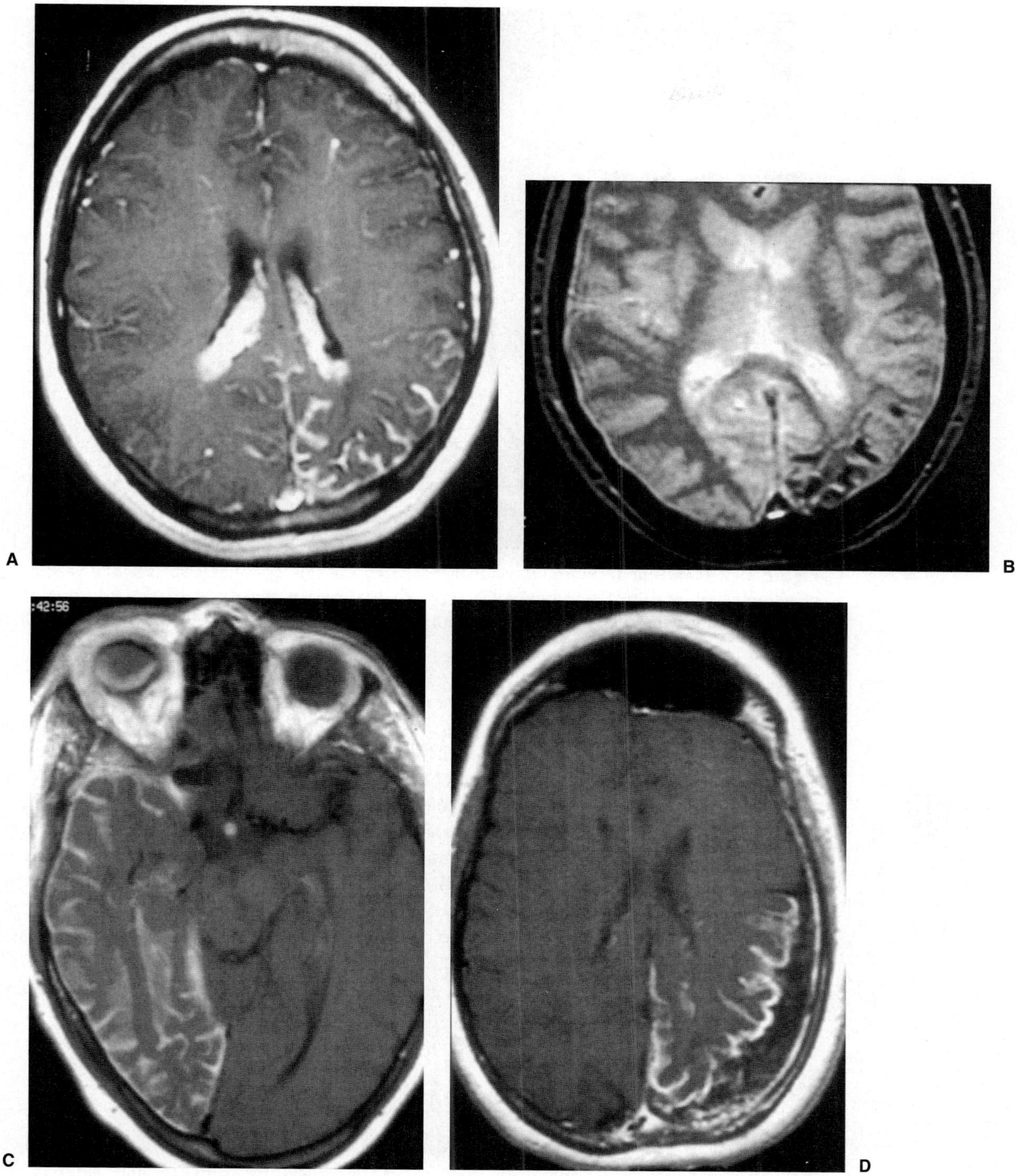

Figure 2.12 *Sturge-Weber Disease. A.* Postcontrast axial T1-weighted image shows enhancing pial angioma in the left occipitoparietal region and hypertrophy of both choroid plexuses. *B.* Different patient, axial T2*-weighted image shows dark calcification in the cortex of the left occipitoparietal region, which also is atrophied. *C.* In this patient, the enhancing pial angioma involves most of the right cerebral hemisphere as well as the right eye. *D.* This study shows chronic changes with an enhancing pial angioma and cerebral atrophy. *(continued on next page)*

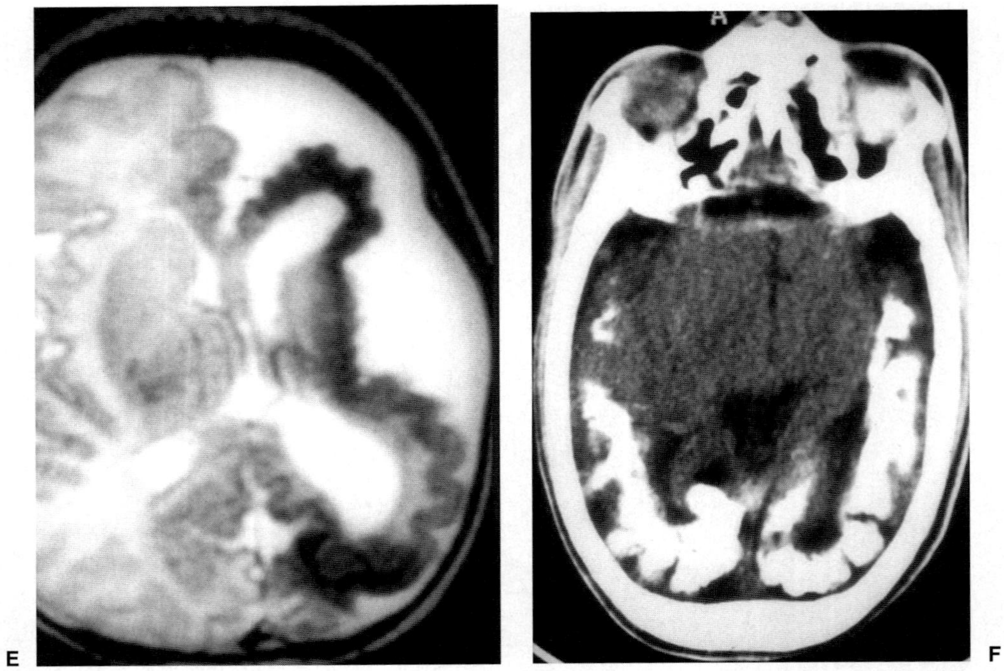

Figure 2.12 (continued) *E.* End-stage changes are seen in this T2-weighted image as a very atrophied and dark (calcified) left cerebral hemisphere. *F.* Unusual chronic changes are seen in this patient as extensive bilateral cortical calcifications.

plexus becomes enlarged. The imaging method of choice is MRI, which shows pial enhancement even before brain substance abnormalities develop. Venous infarctions in the distribution of the pial angioma may occur (31). The involved hemisphere becomes progressively atrophied and shows cortical dystrophic calcifications (uncommon before 2 years of age). Bilateral involvement is rare (<7%). More recently, it has been noted that MRI may show accelerated myelination on T2-weighted images in the region of involvement even before the pial enhancement from the angioma becomes evident. It is rare to observe the pial angioma before 1 year of age. Afterward, the affected regions becomes atrophic, T1 and T2 hypointensity (due to calcium) develops in the cortex, and the underlying white matter becomes bright on T2-weighted images owing to gliosis (32,33). The cortical calcifications are seen better with gradient-echo T2 (T2*) sequences, but this finding is of secondary importance if contrast is used.

Von Hippel-Lindau Disease

VHL belongs to a group of disorders called the *neurocutaneous angiomatoses*. Other diseases in this group are Klippel-Trenaunay, Osler-Weber-Rendu, and Louis-Bar syndromes, and Fabry's disease. VHL is an autosomal dominant disease linked to a defect in a tumor suppressor gene in chromosome 3p25,26 (34). Its incidence is approximately 1 in 35,000 to 50,000 individuals. Most patients become symptomatic between 20 and 50 years of age. There two distinct types of patients with VHL, some who have pheochromocytoma and others who do not. The classification for VHL proposed by the National Cancer Institute is shown in Box 2.4 (34).

Multiple hemangioblastomas are pathognomonic of von Hippel-Lindau disease.

Hemangioblastoma is the hallmark of the disease and is found in one-half of patients (Fig. 2.13). Over 10% of patients with VHL have multiple hemangioblastomas. The hemangioblastomas involve the cerebellum (65%), brainstem (20%) cerebrum, spinal cord (15%), and retina (35). Most hemangioblastomas (60% to 80%) have a cystic component,

Box 2.4: National Cancer Institute Classification of Von Hippel-Lindau Disease

VHL without pheochromocytomas
- Pheochromocytomas + retinal angiomas + CNS hemangioblastomas

VHL with pheochromocytomas
- Pheochromocytomas + retinal angiomas + CNS hemangioblastomas + renal cell carcinoma + pancreas lesions

CNS, central nervous system; VHL, von Hippel-Lindau disease.

A

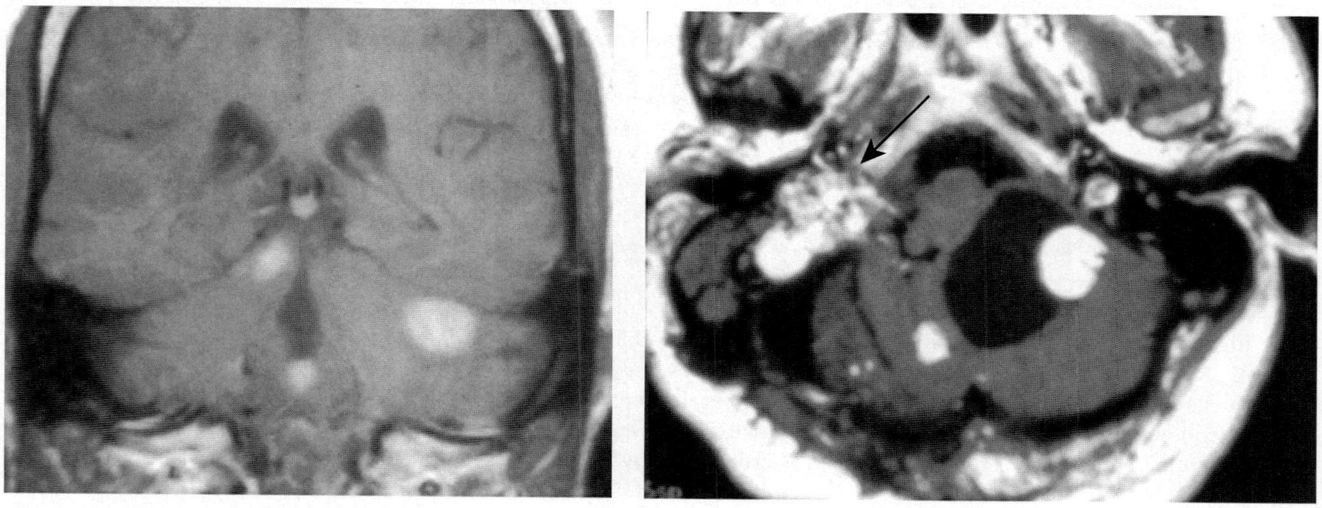

B

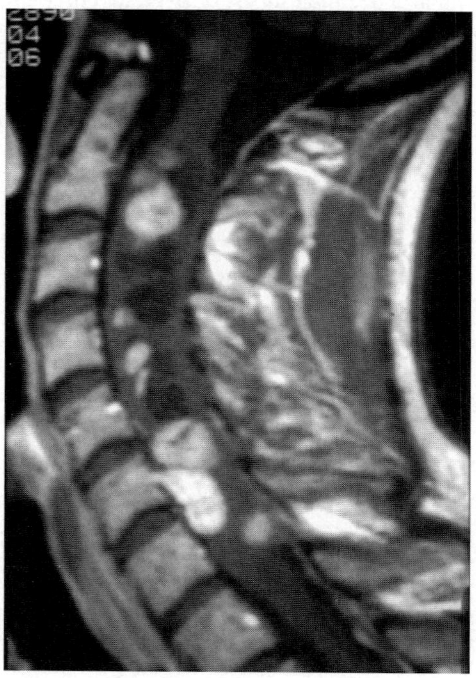

C

Figure 2.13 *Von Hippel-Lindau Disease. A.* Coronal postcontrast T1-weighted image shows multiple solid and enhancing cerebellar hemangioblastomas. *B.* In a different case, there is cystic hemangioblastoma in the left cerebellar hemisphere containing a peripheral enhancing nodule. Small, solid hemangioblastomas are seen in the right hemisphere. In addition, an endolymphatic sac tumor *(arrow)* is present. *C.* Sagittal postcontrast T1-weighted image shows multiple enhancing tumors with associated cysts in the spinal cord. The spinal canal is expanded.

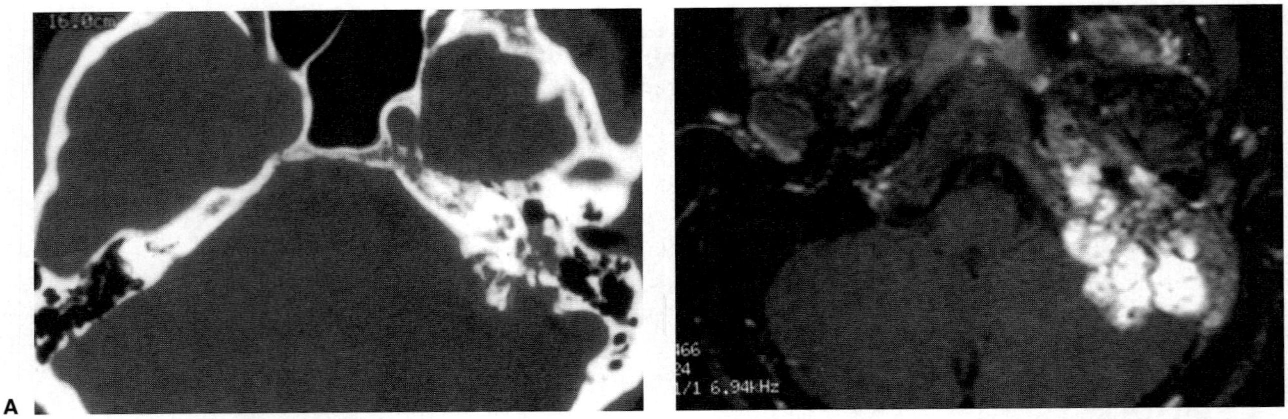

Figure 2.14 *Von Hippel-Lindau Disease, Endolymphatic Sac Tumor.* Axial computed tomography *A* and axial postcontrast fat-suppressed T1-weighted image *B* show typical bone destruction, location in the posterior aspect of the petrous bone, and enhancement of the tumor. These tumors usually have areas of T1 hyperintensity before contrast is given.

Table 2.2: Neuroimaging Features of Rare Neurocutaneous Diseases

Syndrome	*Major Imaging Findings*[a]
Gorlin's (basal cell nevus syndrome)	Cysts in mandible/maxilla, intracranial dural calcifications, vertebral anomalies, medulloblastoma in 5%
Hypomelanosis of Ito (incontinentia pigmenti acromians) (37,38)	Hemimegalencephaly, neuronal migration anomalies, nonspecific white matter T2 changes, delayed myelination
Incontinentia pigmenti	Microcephaly, hydrocephalus, neuronal heterotopias, cortical dysplasias, dysgenesis of corpus callosum, cysts
Neurocutaneous melanosis	Bright T1 areas in mesial temporal and occipital lobes, delayed myelination, vermian dysgenesis, arachnoid cysts
Cowden's disease	Lhermitte-Duclos disease (dysplastic cerebellar gangliocytoma), macrocephaly
Ataxia–telangiectasia (Louis-Bar syndrome)	Cerebellar and vermian atrophy, cerebellar bleeds, cerebral infarctions due to emboli shunted by lung vascular malformations, marked basal ganglia calcification, pachygyria (?), medulloblastomas
Xeroderma pigmentosa	No specific central nervous system disease
Klippel-Trenaunay syndrome	Sturge-Weber syndrome, vascular occlusions
Cockayne's syndrome	Calcifications in basal ganglia, cerebellum, and elsewhere, hydrocephalus, abnormal white matter, thick skull
Refsum's disease	Cerebellar atrophy, abnormal signal intensity in dentate nuclei, optic nerve atrophy, thick peripheral nerve
Werner's syndrome (adult progeria)	Brain atrophy
Progeria	Wormian bones, brain atrophy
Chédiak-Higashi syndrome	Brain atrophy, abnormal-appearing periventricular white matter
Cerebellopontine angle lipomas, multiple pigmented nevi, temporal lobe hypoplasia (39)	Anomalies as the name implies, not well established
Sjögren-Larson syndrome	Hydrocephalus, abnormal-appearing white matter, hypertelorism, basilar invagination, vermian dysgenesis

[a]Not listed in any specific order.

but up to 40% may be entirely solid. There is an increased incidence of solid tumors when they are multiple. Solid hemangioblastomas are more in patients with VHL and in sporadic ones. Multiple hemangioblastomas may give rise to elevated erythropoietin and its complications. In all hemangioblastomas, the tumor nodule is pial based, enhances, and may contain dilated blood vessels. Patients with this disease have an increased incidence of endolymphatic sac tumors (cystadenomas), and young patients with these tumors should be suspected of having VHL (Fig. 2.14). Retinal angiomas commonly are seen on funduscopy, but are difficult to detect on imaging studies. Patients with VHL have an increased incidence of renal cell carcinoma and pancreatic islet cell tumors. The former may result in metastases to the CNS that may be difficult to distinguish from solid hemangioblastomas on imaging studies.

Rare Neurocutaneous Syndromes

Table 2.2 addresses the most salient neuroimaging findings of the rare neurocutaneous syndromes (36).

References

1. Friedman JM, Gutman DH, MacCollin M, et al. Neurofibromatosis: phenotype, natural history, and pathogenesis, 3rd ed. Baltimore: Johns Hopkins University Press, 1999.
2. Aoki S, Barkovich AJ, Nishimura K, et al. Neurofibromatosis types 1 and 2: cranial MR findings. Radiology 1989; 172:527–534.
3. Neurofibromatosis—Conference Report. Arch Neurol 1988;45:575–578.
4. Roos KL, Dunn DW. Neurofibromatoses. CA Cancer J Clin 1992;42:241–254.
5. Kim G, Mehta M, Kucharczyk W, et al. Spontaneous regression of a tectal mass in neurofibromatosis 1. AJNR Am J Neuroradiol 1998;19:1137–1139.
6. Parazzini C, Triulzi F, Bianchini E, et al. Spontaneous involution of optic pathway lesions in neurofibromatosis type 1: serial contrast MR evaluation. AJNR Am J Neuroradiol 1995;16: 1711–1718.
7. Leisti EL, Pyhtinen J, Poyhonen M. Spontaneous decrease of a pilocytic astrocytoma in neurofibromatosis type 1. AJNR Am J Neuroradiol 1996;17:1691–1694.
8. Mirowitz SA, Sartor K, Gado M. High-intensity basal ganglia lesions on T1-weighted MR images in neurofibromatosis. AJNR Am J Neuroradiol 1989;10:1159–1163.
9. Shu HH, Mirowitz SA, Wippold FJ. Neurofibromatosis: MR findings involving the head and spine. AJR Am J Radiol 1993;160:159–164.
10. Egelhoff JC, Bates DJ, Ross JS, et al. Spinal MR findings in neurofibromatosis types 1 and 2. AJNR Am J Neuroradiol 1992;13:1071–1077.
11. Gonen O, Wang ZJ, Viswanathan AK, et al. Three-dimensional multivoxel proton MR spectroscopy of the brain in children with neurofibromatosis type 1. AJNR Am J Neuroradiol 1999; 20:1333–1341.
12. Castillo M, Green C, Kwock L, et al. Proton MR spectroscopy in patients with neurofibromatosis type 1: evaluation of hamartomas and clinical correlation [published erratum appears in AJNR Am J Neuroradiol 1995;16:808]. AJNR Am J Neuroradiol 1995;16:141–147.
13. Starshak RJ. Chromosome 22: a model with implications for diagnostic imaging. AJR Am J Radiol 1996;167:315–324.
14. Mautner VF, Tatagiba M, Lindenau M, et al. Spinal tumors in patients with neurofibromatosis type 2: MR imaging study of frequency, multiplicity, and variety. AJR Am J Radiol 1995;165: 951–955.
15. Patronas NJ, Courtcoutsakis N, Bromley CM, et al. Intramedullary and spinal canal tumors in patients with neurofibromatosis 2: MR imaging findings and correlation with genotype. Radiology 2001;218:434–442.
16. Hyman MH, Whittemore VH. National Institutes of Health consensus conference: tuberous sclerosis complex. Arch Neurol 2000;57.
17. Seidenwurm DJ, Barkovich AJ. Understanding tuberous sclerosis. Radiology 1992;183:23–24.
18. O'Callaghan FJ, Osborne JP. Advances in the understanding of tuberous sclerosis. Arch Dis Child 2000;83:140–142.

19. Nixon JR, Houser OW, Gomez MR, et al. Cerebral tuberous sclerosis: MR imaging. Radiology 1989;170:869–873.
20. Altman NR, Purser RK, Post MJ. Tuberous sclerosis: characteristics at CT and MR imaging. Radiology 1988;167:527–532.
21. Takanashi J, Sugita K, Fujii K, et al. MR evaluation of tuberous sclerosis: increased sensitivity with fluid-attenuated inversion recovery and relation to severity of seizures and mental retardation. AJNR Am J Neuroradiol 1995:16:1923–1928.
22. Braffman BH, Bilaniuk LT, Naidich TP, et al. MR imaging of tuberous sclerosis: pathogenesis of this phakomatosis, use of gadopentetate dimeglumine, and literature review. Radiology 1992; 183:227–238.
23. Shepherd CW, Houser OW, Gomez MR. MR findings in tuberous sclerosis and correlation with seizure development and mental impairment. AJNR Am J Neuroradiol 1995;16:149–155.
24. Van Tassel P, Cure JK, Holden KR. Cystlike white matter lesions in tuberous sclerosis. AJNR Am J Neuroradiol 1997:18:1367–1373.
25. Griffiths PD, Gardner SA, Smith M, et al. Hemimegalencephaly and focal megalencephaly in tuberous sclerosis complex. AJNR Am J Neuroradiol 1998;19:1935–1938.
26. Jay V. Sturge-Weber syndrome. Pediatr Dev Pathol 2000;3:301–305.
27. Griffiths PD. Sturge-Weber syndrome revisited: the role of neuroradiology. Neuropediatrics 1996;27:284–294.
28. Griffiths PD, Boodram MB, Blaser S, et al. Abnormal ocular enhancement in Sturge-Weber syndrome: correlation of ocular MR and CT findings with clinical and intracranial imaging findings. AJNR Am J Neuroradiol 1996;17:749–754.
29. Benedikt RA, Brown DC, Walker R, et al. Sturge-Weber syndrome: cranial MR imaging with Gd-DTPA. AJNR Am J Neuroradiol 1993;14:409–415.
30. Stimac GK, Solomon MA, Newton TH. CT and MR of angiomatous malformations of the choroid plexus in patients with Sturge-Weber disease. AJNR Am J Neuroradiol 1986;7:623–627.
31. Cure JK, Holden KR, Van Tassel P. Progressive venous occlusion in a neonate with Sturge-Weber syndrome: demonstration with MR venography. AJNR Am J Neuroradiol 1995;16:1539–1542.
32. Elster AD, Chen MY. MR imaging of Sturge-Weber syndrome: role of gadopentetate dimeglumine and gradient-echo techniques. AJNR Am J Neuroradiol 1990;11:685–689.
33. Chamberlain MC, Press GA, Hesselink JR. MR imaging and CT in three cases of Sturge-Weber syndrome: prospective comparison. AJNR Am J Neuroradiol 1989;10:491–496.
34. Choyke PL, Glenn GM, Walther MM, et al. Von Hippel-Lindau disease: genetic, clinical and imaging features. Radiology 1995;194:629–642.
35. Chu BC, Terae S, Hida K, et al. MR findings in spinal hemangioblastoma: correlation with symptoms and with angiographic and surgical findings. AJNR Am J Neuroradiol 2001;22:206–217.
36. Taybi H, Lachman RS. Radiology of syndromes, metabolic disorders, and skeletal dysplasias, 4th ed. St. Louis: Mosby, 1996.
37. Malherbe V, Pariente D, Tardieu M, et al. Central nervous system lesions in hypomelanosis of Ito: an MRI and pathological study. J Neurol 1993;240:302–304.
38. Bhushan V, Gupta RR, Weinreb J, et al. Unusual brain MRI findings in a patient with hypomelanosis of Ito. Pediatr Radiol 1989;20:104–106.
39. Amonkar PP, KK U, Patil JA, et al. Cerebellopontine angle lipomas, multiple pigmented nevi, and temporal lobe hypoplasia: a new neurocutaneous syndrome? AJR Am J Radiol 1997;169: 1429–1430.

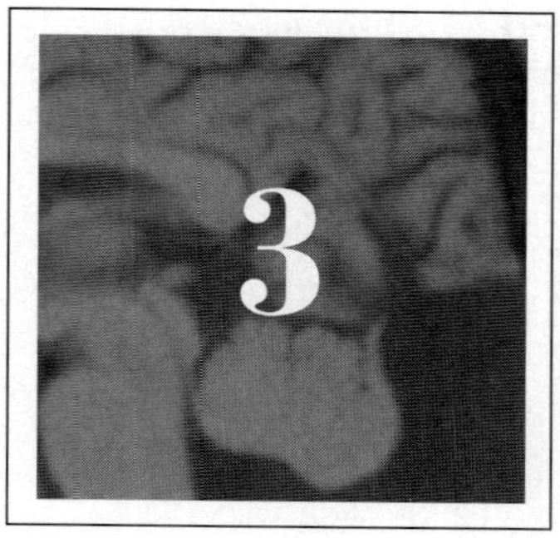

White Matter Disorders

- Classification
- Normal Myelination
- Congenital White Matter Disorders (Leukodystrophies)
- Acquired White Matter Disorders

Classification

White matter disorders have been divided into the traditional categories of dysmyelinating and demyelinating diseases, but because in reality most disorders of white matter probably are demyelinating, I have chosen not divide them in this fashion. I divide the leukodystrophies into those that present with large or normal/small head circumferences and then correlate this finding with the pattern of the white matter abnormalities as seen on magnetic resonance imaging (MRI). This approach is particularly helpful because the head circumference is readily available. The size of the head, the patient's age, and the distribution of abnormalities on MRI are the most helpful parameters in formulating a differential diagnosis. However, most referring physicians often are satisfied if the neuroradiologist simply tells them that the findings are suggestive of a leukodystrophy, and based on that observation they will order the appropriate biochemical tests. In many of these disorders, both white and gray matter eventually are affected. This chapter begins with a very brief review of normal myelination.

Normal Myelination

The following are general guidelines with regard to normal myelination using conventional MRI (1–3):

1. The brain myelinates from caudal to cephalad, posterior to rostral, and sensory to motor.
2. T1-weighted images depict myelination first. Brightness on T1 probably is due to deposition of lipids in myelin sheaths and correlates with a tightening of the myelin sheaths. When we say that "myelination has occurred" based on the images, we are not entirely correct because myelin already was present.
3. T2-weighted images depict mature myelin with little water content. Changes on T2-weighted images occur 3 to 4 months after those seen T1 images. T2 images are used to evaluate the progression of myelination after 6 months of age.
4. Myelination begins during the fifth month of intrauterine life. The terminal zones of myelination (around the atria of the lateral ventricles) myelinate during approximately the second to third decades of life, or may remain unmyelinated for life. These regions

show slight and somewhat fuzzy high T2 signal intensity. More than just a mildly increased in T2 signal probably is abnormal.

5. At term birth, the following structures are myelinated (bright) on T1-weighted images: medial cerebellum, dorsal brainstem, posterior limb of internal capsules, and pericentral white matter.
6. The corpus callosum forms from front to back and myelinates from back to front: splenium (4 months), body, genu (6 months), and rostrum (8 months) on T1-weighted images.
7. The brain should have an adult-like appearance by 12 months of age on T1-weighted images (except for the terminal zones of myelination, which were addressed previously).

Normally, the corpus callosum should be completely myelinated on T1-weighted images by 8 months of age.

There is preliminary evidence that diffusion-weighted imaging is helpful in assessing the brain even before myelination is seen on T1- or T2-weighted images (4–7). Increased diffusion anisotropy precedes not only MRI-visible changes but changes seen on histologic myelin stains (7). Diffusion tensor imaging probably is even more sensitive than apparent diffusion coefficient maps (4–6). Tensor imaging may show the direction of unmyelinated white matter tracts and shows marked differences in the anisotropy of the white matter according to the age of the patient. Thus, it seems that use of conventional MRI at best grossly evaluates myelination milestones.

Congenital White Matter Disorders (Leukodystrophies)

Disorders with Macrocephaly

Alexander's Disease

This very rare disorder also is called *fibrinoid leukodystrophy* (8) (Fig. 3.1). There is no identifiable biochemical defect, and its diagnosis requires a brain biopsy. It has been

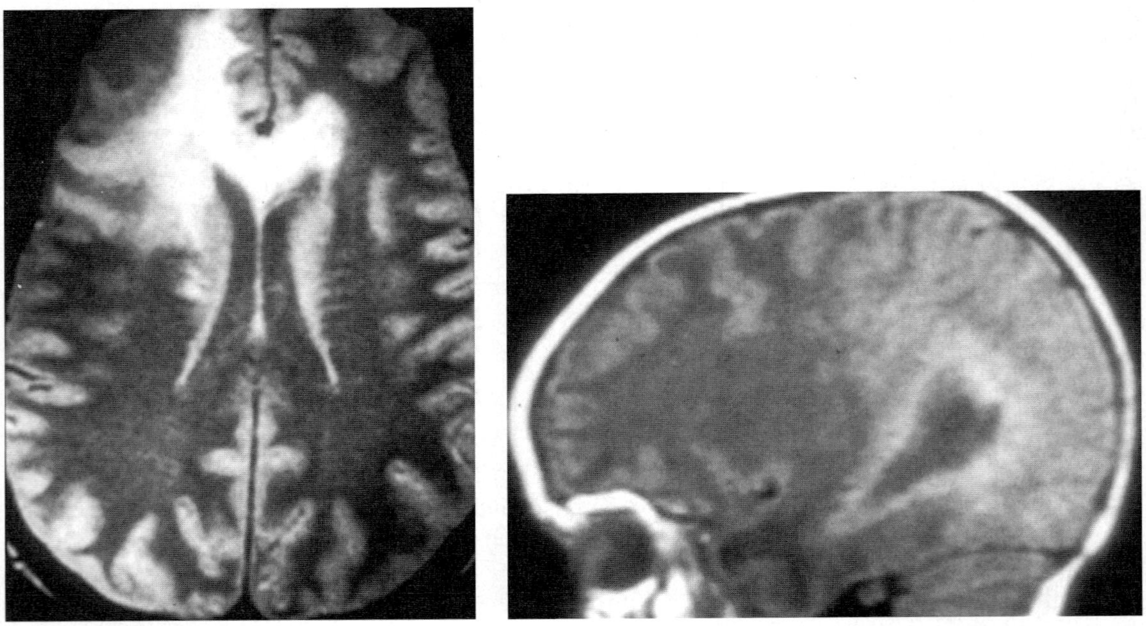

A B

Figure 3.1 *Alexander's Disease. A.* Axial T2-weighted image shows large bright area in the white matter of the right frontal lobe crossing the genu of the corpus callosum and extending into the white matter of the left frontal lobe. *B.* Sagittal T1-weighted image (different patient) shows hypointensity in the white matter of the frontal and temporal lobes.

divided arbitrarily into infantile, juvenile, and adult forms. Macrocephaly is typical and the manifestations include progressive spastic quadriparesis and intellectual failure, leading to death (in general, all patients are dead by their teenage years). It usually presents in infancy or adolescence, and death occurs as early as 2 to 3 years after diagnosis. There are increased astrocytic eosinophilic Rosenthal fibers (these are the most important finding for the histologic diagnosis), with sparing of neurons and active demyelination in the late part of the disease. The disease begins in the frontal regions and then extends posteriorly. Contrast enhancement may occur, but is rare. The subcortical u-fibers initially are spared but rapidly become affected. In end-stage disease, brain cysts may form.

Canavan's Disease

Canavan's disease (spongiform leukoencephalopathy) is included here, although it is now recognized as being a disorder of both white and gray matter (Fig. 3.2). It is more common in Ashkenazi Jews and patients usually die 2 to 3 years after the diagnosis (9). Many patients with macrocephaly and imaging findings identical to those of Canavan's

Canavan's disease and van der Knaap's disease appear very similar, but involvement of the basal ganglia is much more common in Canavan's disease.

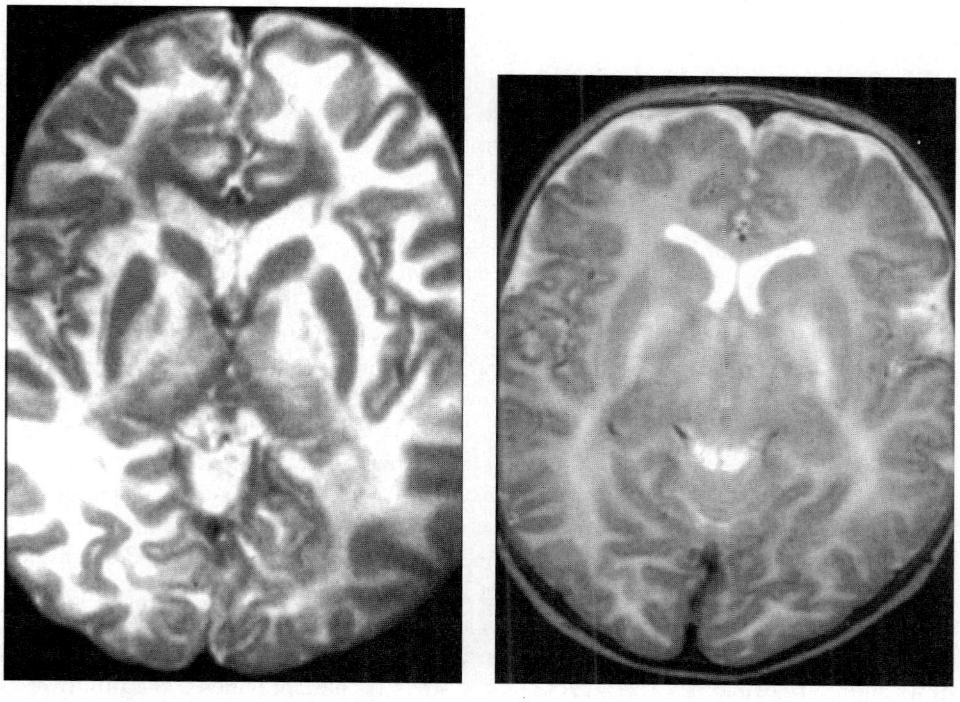

A B

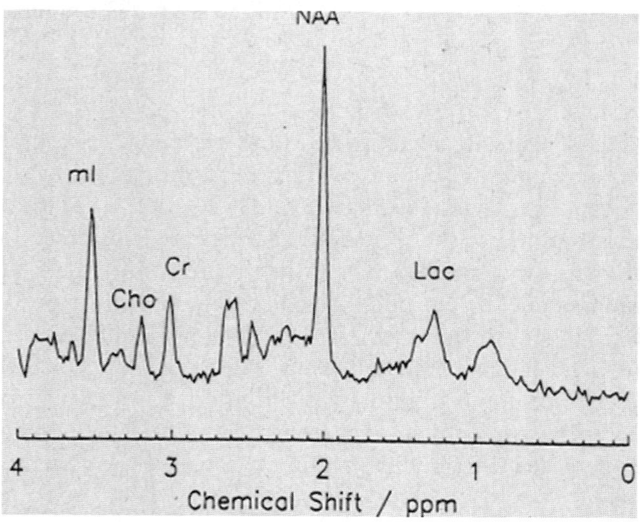

C

Figure 3.2 *Canavan's Disease. A, B.* Axial T2-weighted images show extensive hyperintensity in the white matter of both hemispheres and in the globi pallidi and thalami. *C.* Proton magnetic resonance spectroscopy shows marked elevation of the NAA, which is typical of this disorder. mI, myoincsitol; Cho, choline; Cr, creatine; NAA, *N*-acteyl aspartate; Lac, lactate.

disease probably have "van der Knaap's disease" (10). In patients with van der Knaap's disease, the clinical course is milder and usually only the white matter is diffusely affected. Canavan's disease is a very rare disorder characterized by a deficiency of the enzyme *N*-acetylaspartylase [which breaks down *N*-acetyl aspartate (NAA)], and therefore proton MR spectroscopy shows markedly elevated NAA (note that NAA may be mildly elevated in patients with van der Knaap's disease). The accumulation of NAA is toxic to the brain (11). Canavan's disease usually begins during the first 6 months of life and involves all of the white matter in a diffuse fashion, including the subcortical u-fibers. In addition, the globi pallidi and thalami nearly always are affected (they show high T2 signal). No contrast enhancement is present. As the disease progresses, the size of the head begins to decrease.

Another disease that needs to be included in the differential diagnosis of Canavan's disease is Cree leukoencephalopathy. The imaging findings are identical to those of Canavan's disease, but Cree has been reported only in northern Quebec and Manitoba in Canada (12).

Krabbe's Disease

This also is a very rare disorder, although perhaps somewhat more common than Alexander's and Canavan's diseases. It also is called *globoid cell leukodystrophy*. It is a lysosomal disorder characterized by a deficiency of the enzyme galactocerebroside β-galactosidase and is inherited as an autosomal recessive trait (13). The enzymatic defect blocks the degradation of β-galactocerebroside, which is a critical component of the myelin sheath. The presence of end products such as psychosine is toxic to the oligodendrocytes. The diagnosis is confirmed by establishing the levels of leukocyte lysosomal β-galactosidase (13). Krabbe's disease usually affects infants and young children, and most patients are diagnosed between the third and sixth months of life (one of the earliest leukodystrophies). The head initially is large and then becomes small (at presentation, most patients are microcephalic). Computed tomography (CT) may show increased density in the thalami (Fig. 3.3), but this study seldom is obtained for patients suspect of leukodystrophies, so this finding is uncommon (14). MRI shows increased signal intensity around the ventricles in a nonspecific pattern (15). High T2 signal also may be seen in the pyramidal tracts and in the medial aspect of the cerebellar hemispheres. In the late-onset variant, the splenium of the corpus callosum may be involved. Atrophy ensues in most patients, particularly late in the disease. The brain abnormalities usually do not show contrast enhancement. Krabbe's disease may result in hypertrophy of the cranial and spinal nerves (simulating Guillain-Barré syndrome) (16). These large nerves may show contrast enhancement. Bone marrow transplantation may be helpful in the treatment of the disease. Diffusion tensor imaging may be the best way to evaluate these patients. Tensor imaging shows more abnormalities than T2-weighted imaging and provides a quantitative measurement of the severity of the disease, making it an optimal way to study the response to therapy.

Mucopolysaccharidoses

Patients with mucopolysaccharidoses commonly have abnormalities of the cerebrospinal fluid–containing spaces, such as dilated perivascular spaces, large ventricles, prominent subarachnoid spaces, and arachnoid cysts.

Although this group of disorders also affects the white and gray matter, they are included here because children may present with an enlarged head (in reality, the diagnosis is well established in most patients by the time of imaging evaluation; Figs. 3.4 and 3.5). They are not true leukodystrophies, but mucopolysaccharides are deposited along the perivascular spaces, leading to focal changes mostly in the periventricular white matter. The mucopolysaccharidoses may be considered as disorders of lysosomes (17). Initially there is macrocephaly, but progression of these disorders eventually results in brain atrophy. The skull is thick and there is dolichocephaly and a thick and somewhat keel-shaped frontal bone (these are prominent features in Hurler's disease). Ventricular dilatation with or without increased intracranial pressure is common (18). It often is very difficult to tell if there is increased intracranial pressure because of the ventricular

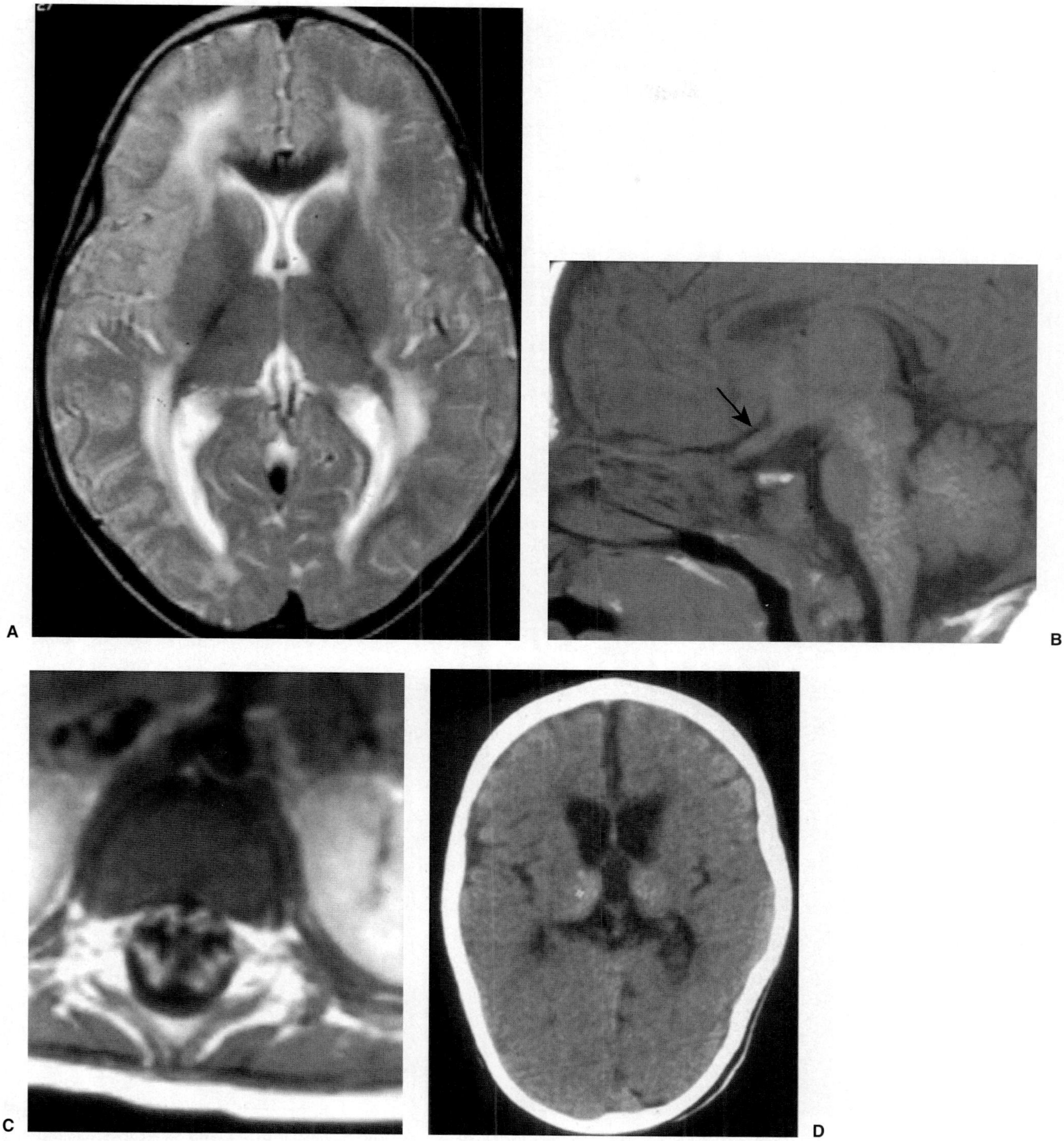

Figure 3.3 *Krabbe's Disease. A.* Axial T2-weighted image shows confluent hyperintensities in the deep white matter bilaterally. The lesions spare the subcortical u-fibers. *B.* In a different patient with neonatal Krabbe's disease, the optic chiasm (*arrow*) is enlarged. *C.* Axial postcontrast T1-weighted image (different patient) shows enhancement of ventral and dorsal nerves of the cauda equina in a pattern similar to Guillain-Barré syndrome. *D.* Computed tomography shows hyperdense thalami in a patient with Krabbe's disease.

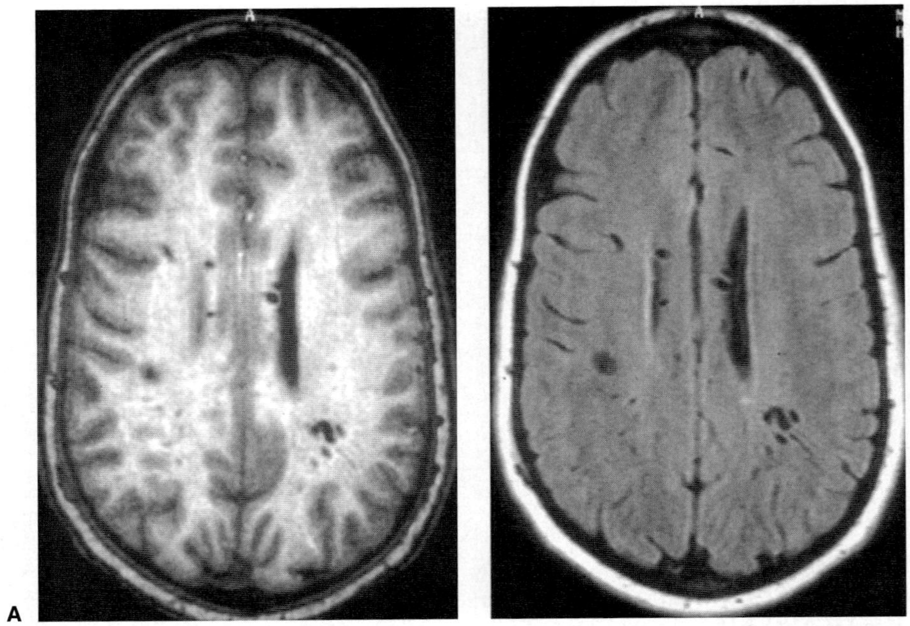

Figure 3.4 *Hunter's Disease.* Axial T1-weighted *A* and fluid attenuation inversion recovery (FLAIR) *B* images show cysts presumably representing perivascular spaces presumably filled with mucopolysaccharides. The shape of the head is dolichocephalic.

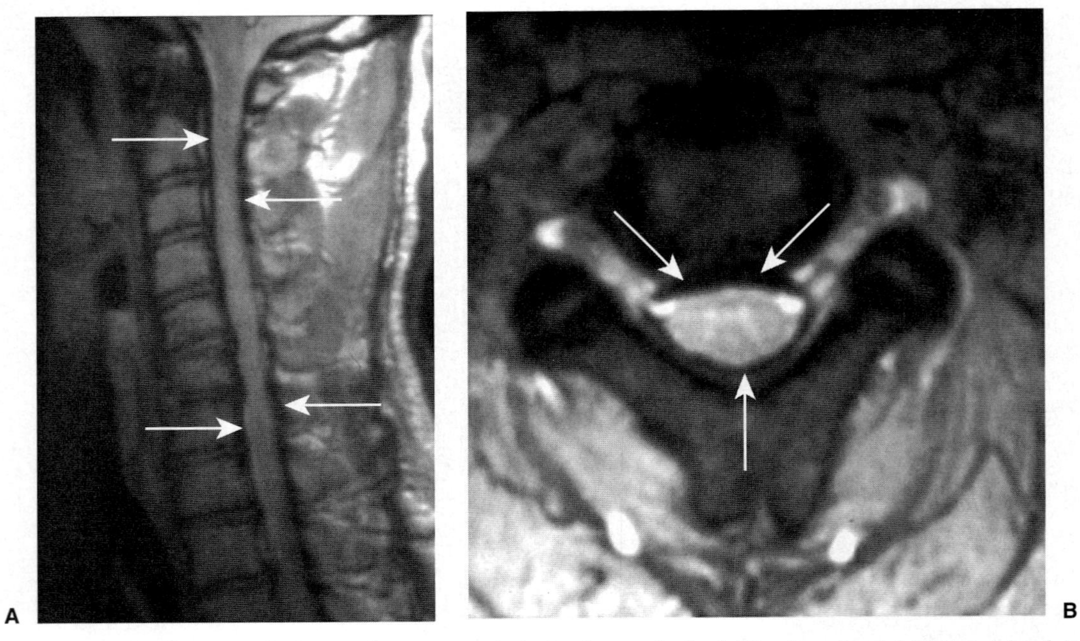

Figure 3.5 *Spinal Abnormalities in Hurler's Syndrome.* Sagittal T1- *A* and axial T2*-weighted *B* images show hypointense and diffusely thickened meninges *(arrows)* resulting in narrowing of the spinal canal.

Table 3.1: Genetics and Biochemical Defects in the Mucopolysaccharidoses

Disorder	*Inheritance*	*Material (Sulfate) Stored*
Hurler's syndrome (MPS1)	Autosomal recessive	Dermatan and heparan
Hunter's syndrome (MPS2)	X-linked	Dermatan and heparan
Scheie's syndrome (MPS1)	Autosomal recessive	Dermatan and heparan
Morquio's syndrome	Autosomal recessive	Keratin and chondroitin
Sanfilippo's syndrome	Autosomal recessive	Heparan

Table 3.2: Imaging Abnormalities in the Mucopolysaccharidoses

Disorder	*Neuroimaging Abnormalities*
Hurler's syndrome	Macrocrania, brain cysts (dilated perivascular spaces), hydrocephalus, dolichocephaly, vertebral beaks
Hunter's syndrome	Same as Hurler's + thick spinal dura + retrodental increased soft tissue
Scheie's syndrome	Same as Hurler's and Hunter's + arachnoid cysts
Morquio's syndrome	Hypoplastic or absent dens, thick spinal dura, atrophy, nonspecific white matter abnormalities, central vertebral beaks
Sanfilippo's syndrome	Atrophy, nonspecific white matter abnormalities, hydrocephalus

dilatation. Expansion of the skull may lead to multiple cranial nerve deficits. All mucopolysaccharidoses are autosomal recessive except for Hunter's syndrome, which is X-linked. Table 3.1 addresses the inheritance and biochemical abnormalities in the mucopolysaccharidoses, and Table 3.2 describes some of the imaging findings for specific mucopolysaccharidoses.

Disorders with Normocephaly

Adrenoleukodystrophy

Adrenoleukodystrophy (ALD) is the most important peroxisomal disorder and one of the most common primary white matter disorders in children (Fig. 3.6). It is inherited as an X-linked recessive trait (Xq28) and thus is seen only in boys (19). The affected gene encodes for the formation of coenzymes derived from the fatty acids in peroxisomes. The neonatal form of ALD is inherited as an autosomal recessive trait and is very rare. Very-long–chain fatty acids are not correctly metabolized and become elevated in serum and other tissues. The defect is at the level of the lignoceroyl coenzyme A ligase. The long-chain fatty acids are toxic to myelin and result in active demyelination and inflammation. ALD occurs in boys 3 to 10 years of age, and a vegetative state or death may occur as soon as 2 years after the diagnosis (20). In adults (30 to 40 years of age), a milder form of the disease is seen that preferentially involves the spinal cord (adrenomyeloneuropathy). Adrenomyeloneuropathy probably accounts for approximately 25% of all cases of ALD (21). The most common symptoms of ALD are shown in Table 3.3 (20).

In 80% of cases, CT and MRI show abnormalities in the white matter of the occipital regions that also involve the splenium of the corpus callosum and extend anteriorly. The location of the abnormalities closely correlates with the symptoms (22). The anterior border of these abnormalities may enhance after contrast administration, and this finding implies breakdown of the blood–brain barrier due to active demyelination and inflammation. The pathologic changes seen in ALD are listed in Table 3.4 (23).

Proton MR spectroscopy obtained at the level of the disease front (zones B and C) shows significant elevation of choline secondary to the presence of inflammatory cells. On MR spectroscopy, NAA (a neuronal marker) is decreased and lactate and lipids (from cellular breakdown) may be elevated (24,25). Patients with an inflammatory component have a more rapid and severe course and a worse prognosis. Early in the disorder, only the corticospinal tracts or the medial lemnisci may be affected (26). Rarely, ALD begins in the frontal regions. In the chronic stage of the disease, dystrophic calcifications may be seen in the white matter (27). This finding not only is unusual but is seldom seen because CT no longer is commonly obtained in patients with ALD.

Proton MR spectroscopy obtained at the level of the demyelinating front shows high choline, implying an inflammatory response, and elevated lactate, implying ischemia at that level.

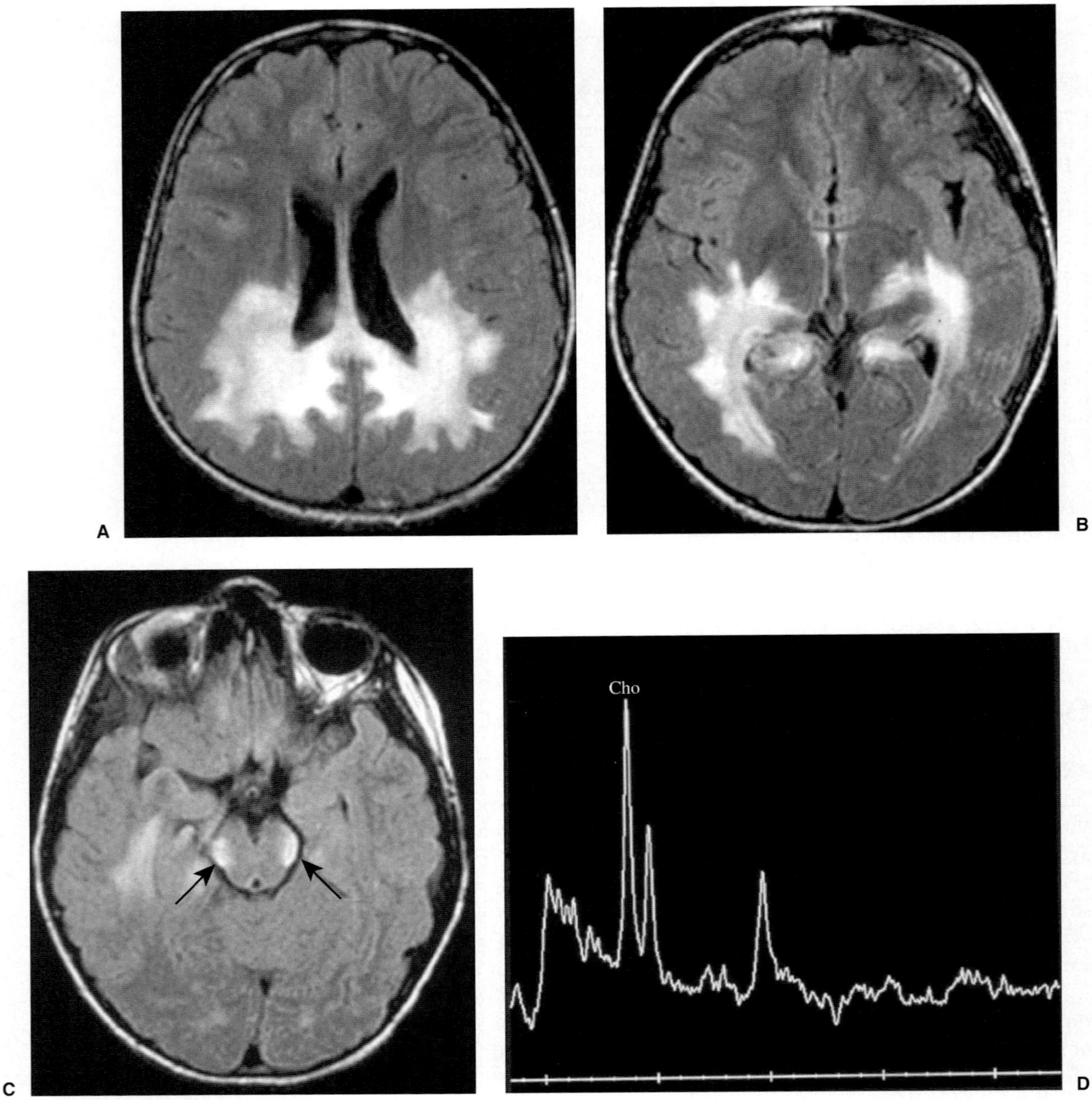

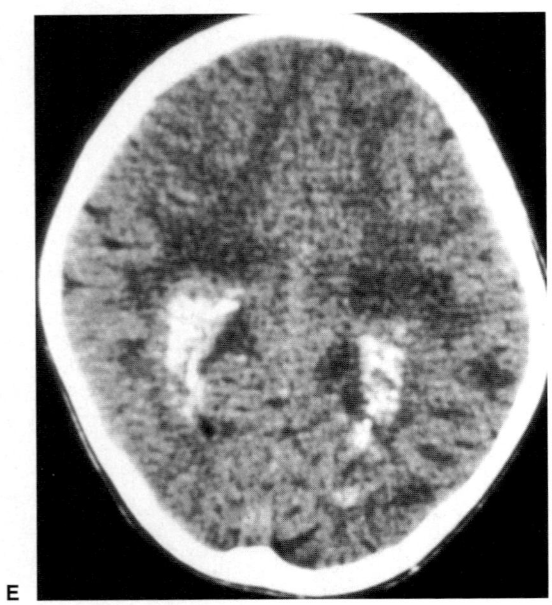

Figure 3.6 *Adrenoleukodystrophy*. Axial fluid attenuation inversion recovery (FLAIR) images *A–C* show hyperintense white matter in both occipital lobes and crossing the splenium of the corpus callosum. There is involvement of the medial lemnisci (*arrows* in *C*). Proton magnetic resonance spectroscopy (different patient) *D* obtained with long echo time and with voxel centered over enhancing anterior border shows elevation of the choline (Cho) peak. Computed tomography *E* in a patient with end-stage adrenoleukodystrophy shows calcification in the white matter.

Table 3.3: Symptoms in Adrenoleukodystrophy

Symptom	*Incidence*
Auditory problems	87%
Pyramidal tract symptoms	53%
Visual abnormalities	39%
Bizarre behavior	33%
Seizures	6%

Table 3.4: Pathologic Zones and Imaging Correlation in Adrenoleukodystrophy

Zone	*Pathology*	*Imaging*
A (inner)	Scar and gliosis	No enhancement, low T1 and high T2 signal
B (mid)	Inflammatory cells, demyelination, axons are preserved	Enhancement, low T1 and high T2 signal
C (outer)	Active destruction of myelin and no inflammatory cells	This region is very thin and not clearly visualized

Metachromatic Leukodystrophy

Metachromatic leukodystrophy is a lysosomal disorder characterized by a deficiency in arylsulfatase A (or one of its cofactors) and accumulation of sulfatides that are toxic to the white matter (28). There is lack of breakdown and reutilization of myelin, and the sulfatides impair the function of macrophages and of Schwann cells. It is the most common leukodystrophy. Most patients become symptomatic at 1 to 2 years of age (infantile form). There is a less common juvenile form in which the patients usually present at 5 to 7 years of age. Death occurs 1 to 4 years after the diagnosis. On imaging studies, the white matter is diffusely affected, but the subcortical u-fibers are spared (28) (Fig. 3.7). The medial regions of the cerebellum may be involved early in the course of the disease. No contrast enhancement is present. Eventually, all of the brain (including the corpus callosum and brainstem) becomes involved and atrophy ensues (29).

The most common variant of metachromatic leukodystrophy is the late infantile type, which presents approximately the end of the second year of life.

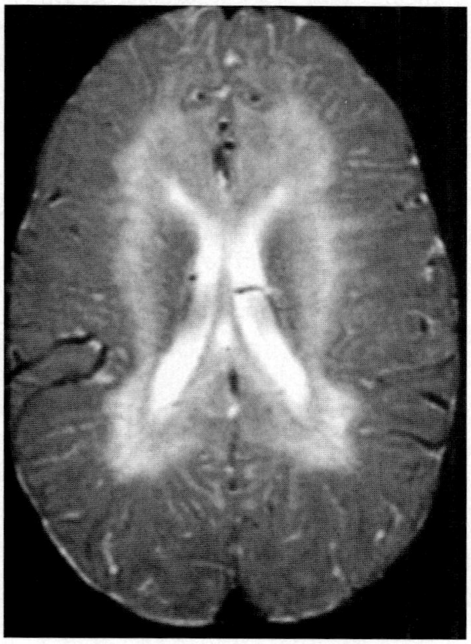

Figure 3.7 *Metachromatic Leukodystrophy.* Axial T2-weighted image shows diffuse white matter hyperintensity with sparing of the subcortical u-fibers.

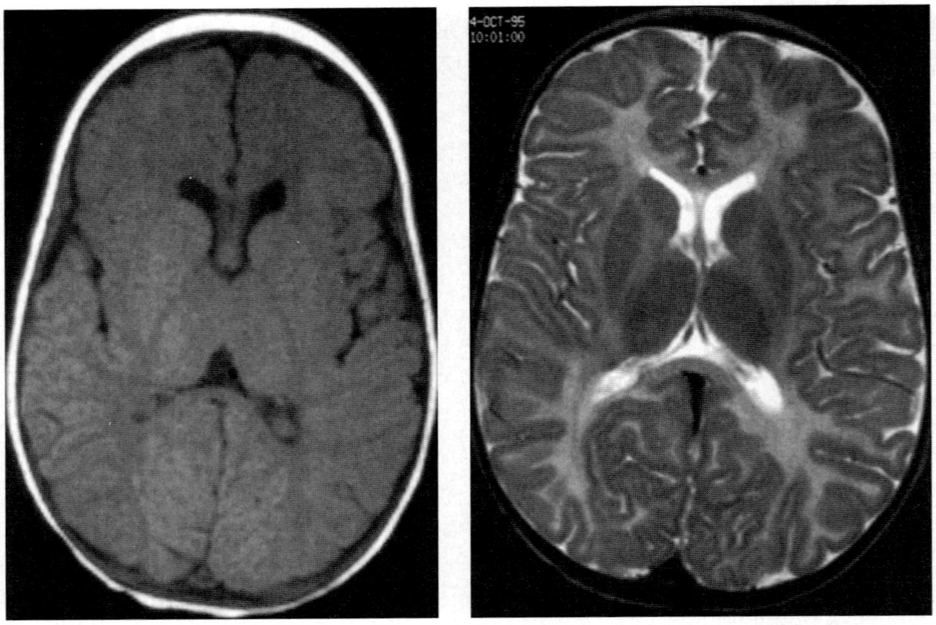

Figure 3.8 *Pelizaeus-Merzbacher Disease*. Axial T1- *A* and T2-weighted *B* images show complete lack of normal-appearing myelinated white matter at 2 years of age.

Disorders with Microcephaly

Pelizaeus-Merzbacher Disease

Pelizaeus-Merzbacher disease (PMD) is an X-linked disorder (classic form) that is characterized by a lack of myelin-specific lipids, leading to abnormal function of oligodendrocytes and hypomyelination. It belongs to a group of disorders called *sudanophilic* leukodystrophies (30). PMD presents very early in life. All of the patients I have seen presented with abnormal eye movements and cerebral palsy–like symptoms. The patients then show developmental delay, seizures, and spasticity, and all die a few years after the diagnosis (30). The white matter never forms normally because of a defect on the gene that encodes for a "proteolipid" protein that is essential for the development if myelin. On histologic study, the white matter has a "tigroid" appearance (31). On imaging studies, the white matter is diffusely abnormal and the brain retains an "in utero" appearance (the abnormalities may be so diffuse and symmetric that at first glance the studies may even be interpreted as normal). There is lack of mature myelin throughout most of white matter (Fig. 3.8). The basal ganglia may be dark owing to increased iron deposition. The cerebellum may be small, and eventually the brain shows atrophy. On proton MR spectroscopy, the NAA is low.

Trichothiodystrophy deserves to be briefly mentioned here because the brain may show abnormalities similar to those seen PMD on MRI. These patients have ectodermal defects such as brittle hair and abnormal dental enamel (32). In addition to the usual neurologic findings seen in most white matter disorders, patients with trichothiodystrophy have a peripheral neuropathy and abnormal hearing. This disease is extremely rare.

Acquired Disorders of White Matter

Osmotic Myelinolysis

This is an acute demyelinating disorder most often seen 2 to 3 days after the rapid correction of hyponatremia (<15 mmol/L), but it also may occur in hypernatremic states or

Table 3.5: Clinical Symptoms of Hyponatremic Encephalopathy

Early Symptoms	*Advanced Symptoms*	*Severe Symptoms*
Anorexia, headache, nausea, vomiting, muscle cramps, weakness	Impaired responses to verbal commands and pain, bizarre behavior, hallucinations, obtundation, respiratory distress	Decortication, bradycardia, hypertension or hypotension, altered temperature regulation, seizures, respiratory arrest, coma

in the absence of sodium concentration abnormalities (33). The current thinking is that rapid influx of water into the cells results in their damage. The neurologic symptoms of hyponatremia are given in Table 3.5.

Most patients with osmotic myelinolysis are chronic alcoholics or have extensive burns, sepsis, Hodgkin's disease, or other malignancies. Osmotic myelinolysis has a high mortality rate, but currently many patients survive. On imaging, most patients show abnormalities in the pontomedullary junction (called *central pontine myelinolysis*, or CPM) (34) (Fig. 3.9). Histologically, CPM shows acute demyelination (particularly of the pon-

Central pontine myelinolysis is more common in the presence of hyponatremia, but may occur with hypernatremia and even normonatremia.

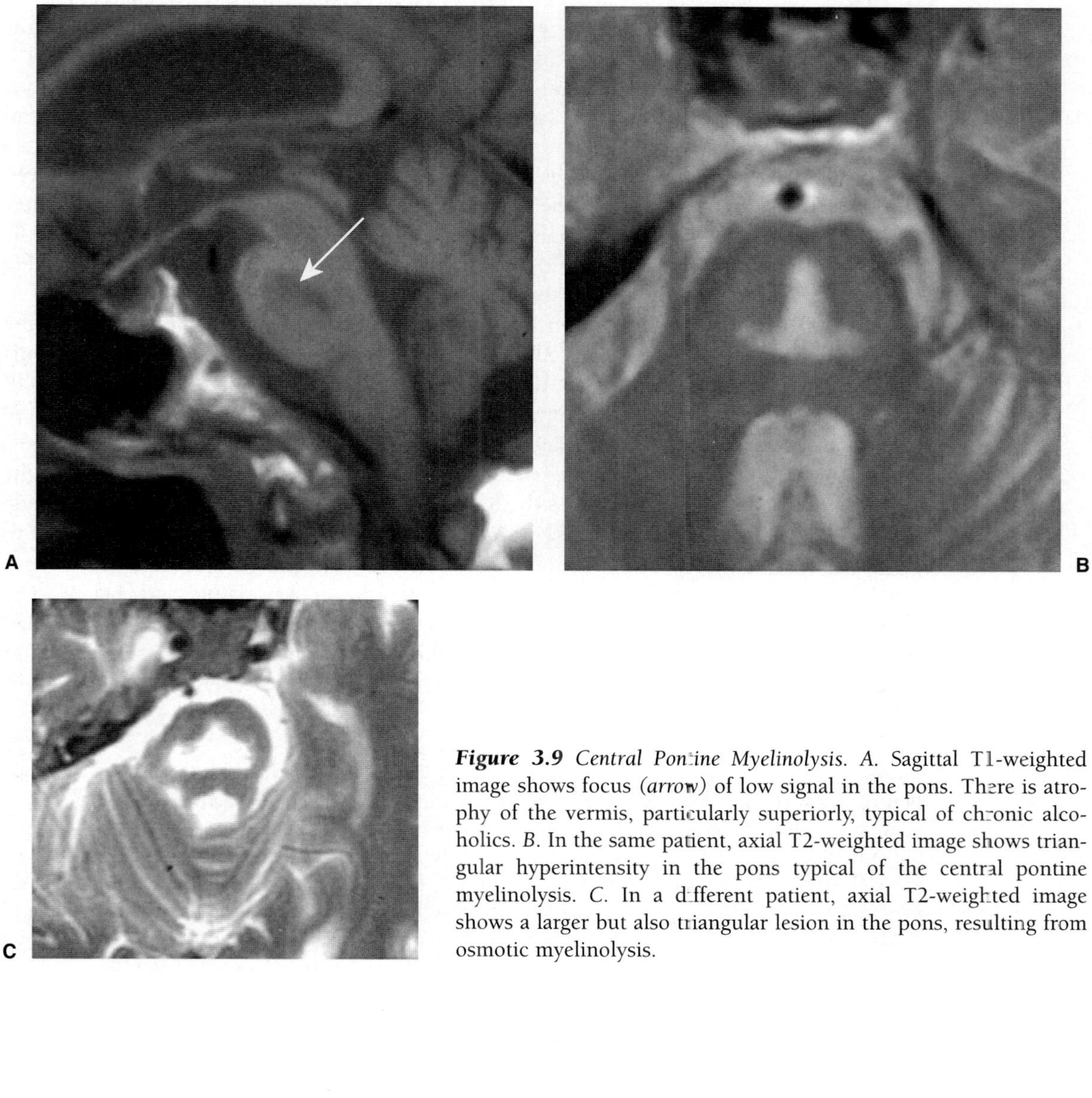

Figure 3.9 *Central Pontine Myelinolysis. A.* Sagittal T1-weighted image shows focus *(arrow)* of low signal in the pons. There is atrophy of the vermis, particularly superiorly, typical of chronic alcoholics. *B.* In the same patient, axial T2-weighted image shows triangular hyperintensity in the pons typical of the central pontine myelinolysis. *C.* In a different patient, axial T2-weighted image shows a larger but also triangular lesion in the pons, resulting from osmotic myelinolysis.

tine transverse fibers) with preservation of the neurons and axons. Patients with CPM present with lethargy, cranial nerve abnormalities, and problems swallowing, and may progress to quadriparesis, including a "lock-in" syndrome.

Results of imaging studies are reported as normal in up to 85% of patients with the clinical syndrome of CPM. MRI shows an area of high T2 signal centered in the lower pons (35,36). Sometimes the lesion has a triangular appearance on axial images, with its apex located in the midline and pointing forward (pontine infarcts may be triangular, but the lesion nearly always is off midline and its apex points posteriorly). In most patients, CPM has a nonspecific appearance and involves the entire cross-section of the brainstem. The lesion is devoid of mass effect and contrast enhancement. Although the cerebellar cortex commonly is affected, this finding usually is not appreciated on MRI. In 10% of patients, the supratentorial gray matter structures that are surrounded by white matter may be affected (extrapontine myelinolysis). The regions most commonly affected are the lentiform nuclei and the thalami. Occasionally, supratentorial white matter structures such as the internal capsule and corpus callosum may be involved. If the patients survive, a slow and gradual decrease in the size of the lesions is noted on follow-up studies, but the lesion never resolves completely (37).

Multiple Sclerosis

Multiple sclerosis (MS) is the most common demyelinating brain disorder, yet its etiology remains uncertain. It is more common in women than in men by approximately a 5:1 to 10:1 ratio, and usually begins at approximately 20 to 40 years of age (38). Occasionally it is seen in children, and in this age group there is a predilection for involvement of the structures in the posterior fossa. MS is more common in the northern hemisphere, but is now seen worldwide. MS is a clinical diagnosis, and not a radiographic or histologic one. Pathologically, the features of the disease include acute demyelination, presence of lymphocytes and monocytes, and phagocytosis, particularly at the edge of the lesion and in a perivascular location (these findings are not specific for MS). The axons are preserved until late in the disease. These are the same features seen in other demyelination disorders such as acute disseminated encephalomyelitis (ADEM), and the diagnosis of MS can be made only by a combination of the histologic findings and the appropriate clinical setting (including laboratory and imaging studies).

Perfusion MRI may help to differentiate tumefactive MS from neoplasias by showing increased perfusion in the latter.

The most common presentation is optic neuritis (39). Cranial neuropathies also are common, and many patients have only mild and often "bizarre" symptoms. Most patients have the relapsing/remitting type of the disease (70%) or the chronic-progressive form of MS (in which the spinal cord is severely affected; 25%). In a small number of patients, the disease takes the strange form of Balo's concentric sclerosis, which is considered to be a type of tumefactive MS. Overall, the patient's life span is not affected. Although MRI is the single most reliable test, it may miss the lesions in up 25% of affected patients. Less than 10% of all lesions seen on MRI are symptomatic. All lesions are of high signal intensity in proton-density, T2-weighted, and fluid attenuation inversion recovery (FLAIR) images (39) (Fig. 3.10). On diffusion-weighted imaging, the active plaques are bright. The plaques are ovoid in shape in the periventricular regions, but also commonly are rounded (40). The ovoid lesions usually follow the course of the periventricular white matter venules and are referred to as *Dawson fingers* (40). They may, however, involve all regions

Figure 3.10 *Multiple Sclerosis. A, B.* Axial fluid attenuation inversion recovery (FLAIR) images show typical hyperintense, oval lesions in the periventricular white matter and along the course of the optic radiations. *C, D.* Sagittal FLAIR images show hyperintensity in the undersurface of the corpus callosum (*arrows*, callososeptal interface) and extending into the periventricular white matter (*arrows*). *E.* In a different patient, axial postcontrast T1-weighted image shows incomplete ring of enhancement typical of active plaques. *F.* Axial T2-weighted image (different patient) shows plaque with rim of slightly low signal intensity. This lesion enhanced after contrast (not shown).

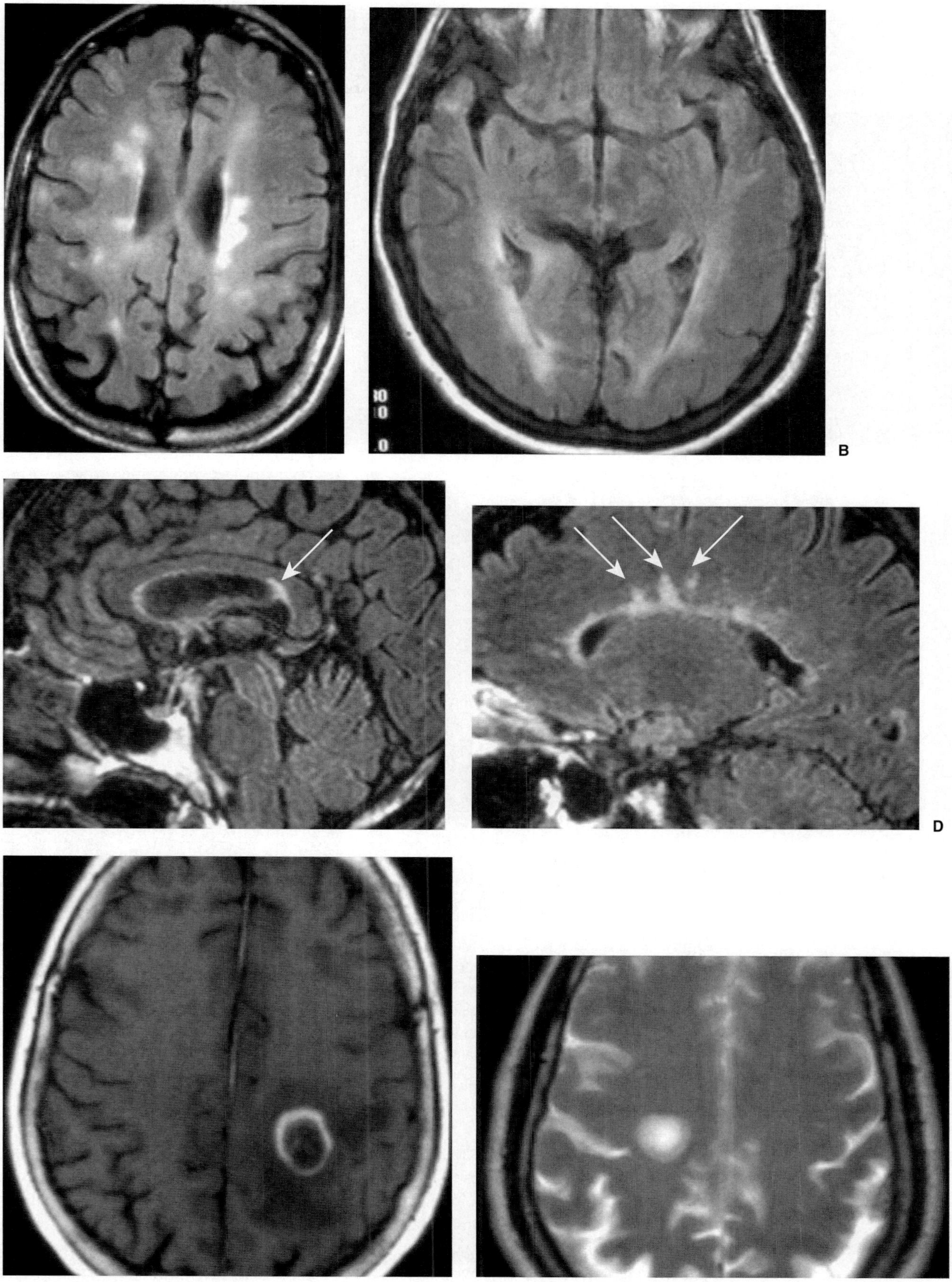

A B C D E F

(continued on next page)

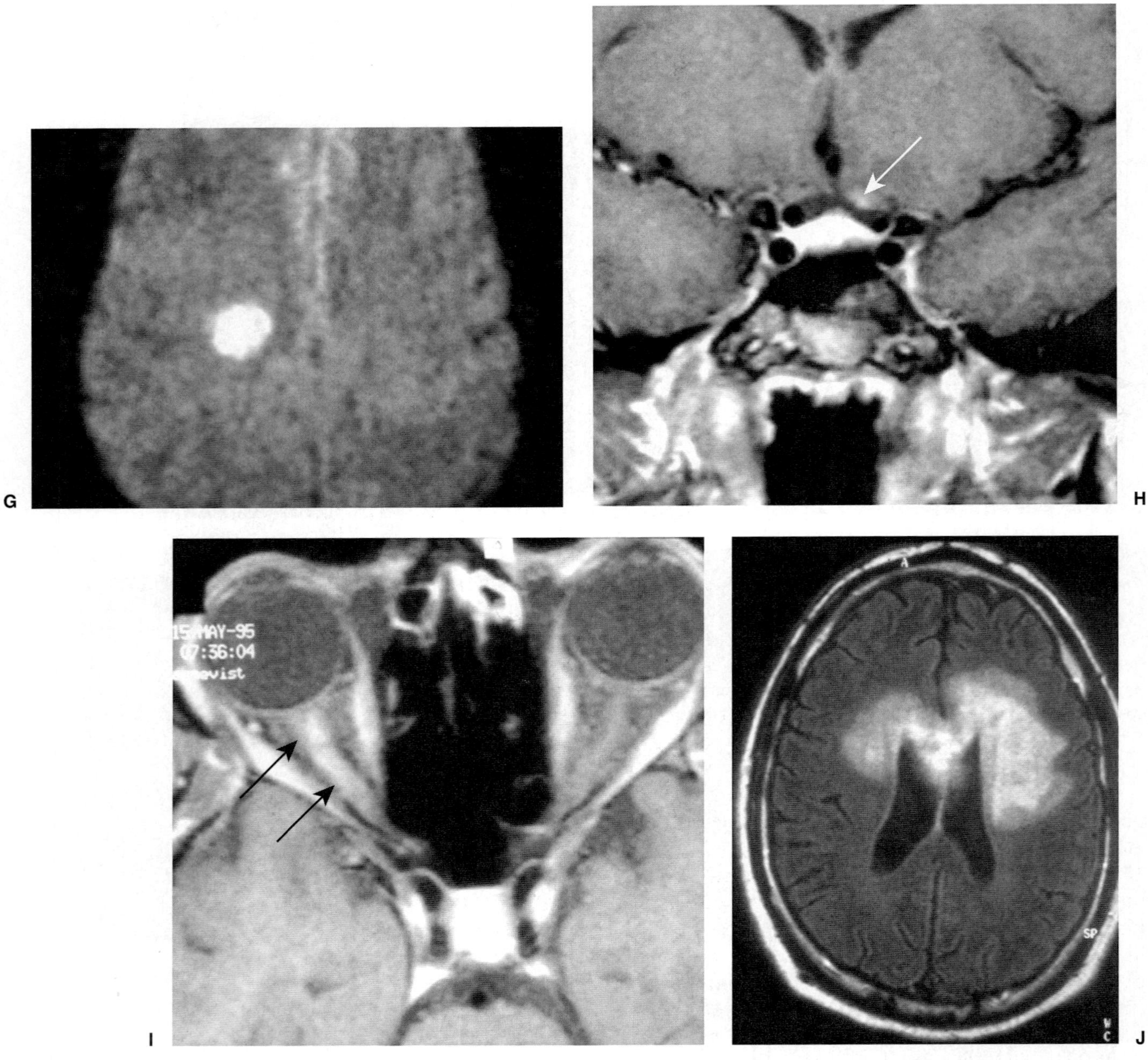

Figure 3.10 (continued) *G.* On diffusion-weighted imaging (trace image), a plaque is bright secondary to restriction of water motion in the extracellular space. *H.* In a patient with left optic neuritis, coronal postcontrast T1-weighted image shows enhancement of the left prechiasmatic optic nerve *(arrow)*. *I.* Axial postcontrast fat-suppressed T1-weighted image (different patient) shows diffuse enhancement of the right optic nerve *(arrows)*. *J.* Axial FLAIR image (different patient) shows tumefactive multiple sclerosis plaque with the appearance of "butterfly glioma."

of the brain. In 93% of patients, the callososeptal interface is affected, and this is better seen on sagittal FLAIR images (41). The callososeptal interface is the undersurface of the corpus callosum immediately continuous with the septum pellucidum. Note that many normal subjects show very tiny areas of increased signal intensity in the undersurface of the corpus callosum, particularly on FLAIR images (so-called subcallosal striations). Occasionally, the plaques show a rim of relatively low T2 signal intensity, and sometimes they are somewhat bright on precontrast T1-weighted images. After contrast administra-

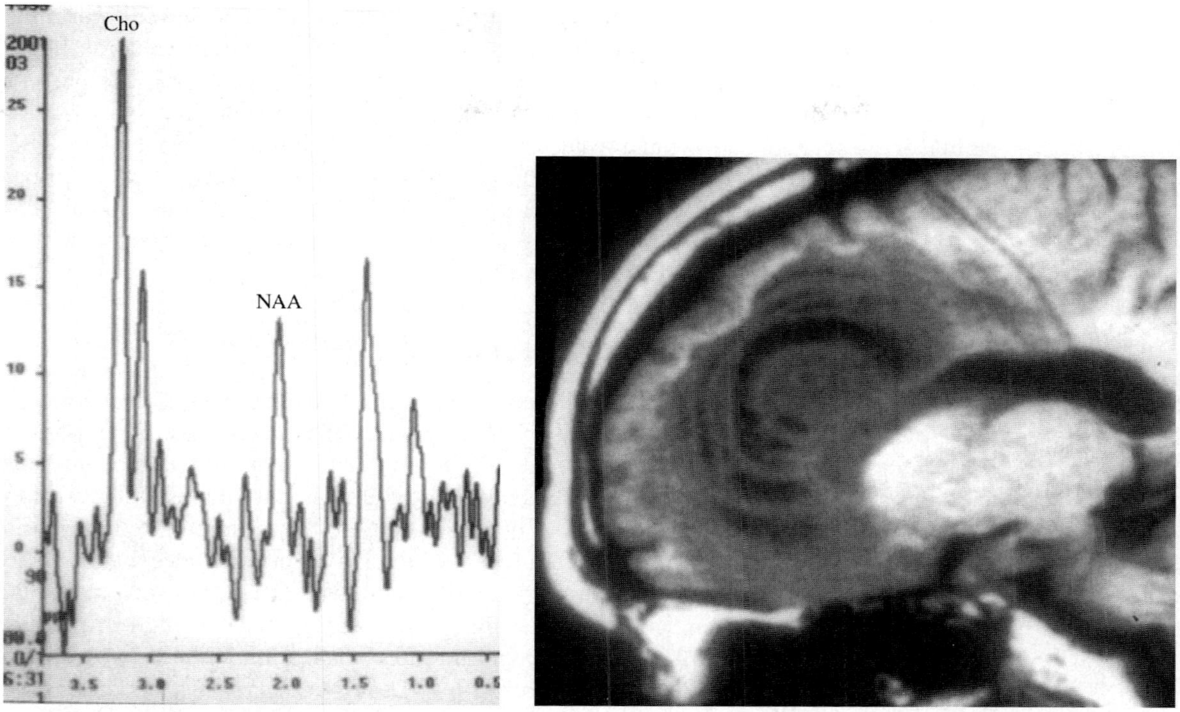

K L

Figure 3.10 (continued) *K.* In the same patient, proton magnetic resonance spectroscopy shows elevation of choline (Cho) and low *N*-acteyl aspartate (NAA). The level of Cho is somewhat less than that seen in high-grade astrocytomas, and the tissues in the immediate vicinity of the lesion were normal (they are not normal in infiltrating lesions). *L.* Sagittal T1-weighted image shows typical concentric rings in a lesion of the Balo's concentric sclerosis.

tion, the active plaques may enhance homogeneously or show a partial rim of enhancement that is typical of MS. Although MS is predominantly a white matter disorder, 10% to 15% of patients have lesions in the gray matter. This is because most gray matter structures in the brain contain myelinated white matter fibers. In the chronic stage, there is diffuse brain atrophy (particularly of the corpus callosum) and increased deposition of iron in the basal ganglia. MR proton spectroscopy may show elevated choline during the acute phase, reflecting the inflammatory cellular infiltration (42). Chronically, the NAA is low and this probably correlates with damage to the axons. Very sensitive techniques, such as magnetization transfer ratios, show that even the normal-appearing white matter is affected (43,44). Approximately 10% of all patients present with isolated spinal cord lesions, and this topic is addressed in Chapter 15.

I briefly address some of the variants of MS. Tumefactive MS is, as its name implies, an acute large plaque that is indistinguishable from a tumor by imaging studies but usually has an acute clinical presentation (45). Most of the cases of tumefactive MS that I have seen occurred in younger men. We have found proton MR spectroscopy very helpful for evaluation of tumefactive MS. Although these lesions look exactly like a tumor, the brain tissues immediately outside of the area of abnormality show normal spectra (in malignant tumors, there is infiltration of the surrounding tissues). In addition, using a short echo time (<35 milliseconds), the peak of myoinositol is elevated, and this is not seen in malignant tumors. The choline peak is high in acute MS and in tumors. Balo's concentric sclerosis is a very rare type of tumefactive MS. The lesions are large and preferentially located in the frontotemporal regions. The MRI features of Balo's, however, are considered nearly pathognomonic (46). On T1- and T2-weighted images, the lesion contains concentric rings of hypointensity and hyperintensity (47). This correlates with a type of "lamellar" demyelination seen histologically. Unlike MS, the prognosis of patients with Balo's is poor, and many die 3 to 5 years after the onset of the disease. Devic's disease (neuromyelitis optica) traditionally is discussed with MS despite the fact that their only relationship is historical. It previously was thought that Devic's disease was a type of MS (Marburg or acute type), but now it is known that it actually is a necrotizing myelitis that may be idiopathic or associated with viral infections, tuberculosis, or lupus erythematosus (48). Patients with Devic's disease usually are young and present with striking and acute visual deficits and signs of a transverse myelitis. MRI shows high T2 signal in the spinal cord (involvement may be holocord) and optic nerves, and these lesions may enhance after contrast is administered.

Acute Disseminated Encephalomyelitis

There is early evidence that the lesions related to ADEM appear during the recovery period and not the initial period of the disease.

I have chosen to address ADEM here because histologically it is similar to MS, although its clinical manifestations differ. It is believed that ADEM represents an abnormal immunologic reaction to a virus (or a viral particle), inducing the production of antibodies that cross-react with myelin (49). Attempts to culture the inciting agent have been fruitless, and a viral particle is thought to be responsible for the immune reaction. In the laboratory, identical lesions may be produced by inducing an allergic encephalitis (50). ADEM is primarily a disease of children (5 to 10 years of age) but also is seen in adults. Most patients recall an often trivial upper respiratory tract infection occurring 1 to 3 weeks before the onset of ADEM. ADEM also may occur after vaccinations. The most common clinical manifestations are headache, seizures, fever, transverse myelitis, optic neuritis, cranial neuropathy, and ataxia. The disease occasionally is fulminant, leading rapidly to coma and death. Histologically, there is acute demyelination and inflammation in a predominantly perivascular location (similar to MS). The major difference between ADEM and MS is that the former usually follows a monophasic course (49). Some patients initially thought to have ADEM go on to develop MS. To make things even more confusing, some authors speak of recurrent ADEM, although I am not exactly sure what this term means.

The imaging features of disease are better appreciated on MRI (CT may be negative in many; Fig. 3.11). The lesions usually are large and hypointense on T1 and bright on T2 and FLAIR (49,50). Lesions usually are found in the white matter of the hemispheres, but also may be seen in the cerebellum and brainstem. They are well demarcated and have little mass effect for their size. They often do not enhance, and many think that this finding is a function of the time in which the MRI study is obtained during the course of the disease (51). Enhancement is seen in 10% to 25% of lesions. Although ADEM is a white matter disease, approximately 10% to 60% of patients show gray matter involvement (remember that myelinated fibers are found throughout the gray matter) (52). The gray matter lesions (as well as the white matter lesions) tend to be bilateral but asymmetric in size and shape. Although we usually think of ADEM as a benign disease, and many patients do well and show resolution of the lesion on consecutive MRI studies, many also do poorly. Permanent neurologic abnormalities develop in approximately 20% of patients. Mild brain atrophy may develop.

Acute Hemorrhagic Leukoencephalopathy

Acute hemorrhagic leukoencephalopathy (AHL) may be considered a variant of ADEM and is very rare. A histologic difference is that AHL shows perivascular hemorrhage, whereas ADEM does not. AHL may occur at any age. The presentation is similar to that in ADEM (many patients also have a history of a prior viral illness), but the course of the disease is more severe and the prognosis is worse. If the patient survives, significant cerebral atrophy may ensue. The MRI findings are similar to those seen in ADEM, but the lesions are preferentially located in the centra semiovale, and there is diffuse brain swelling (Fig. 3.12). At times, large and confluent hemorrhages are seen in the cerebral hemispheres, cerebellum, and brainstem.

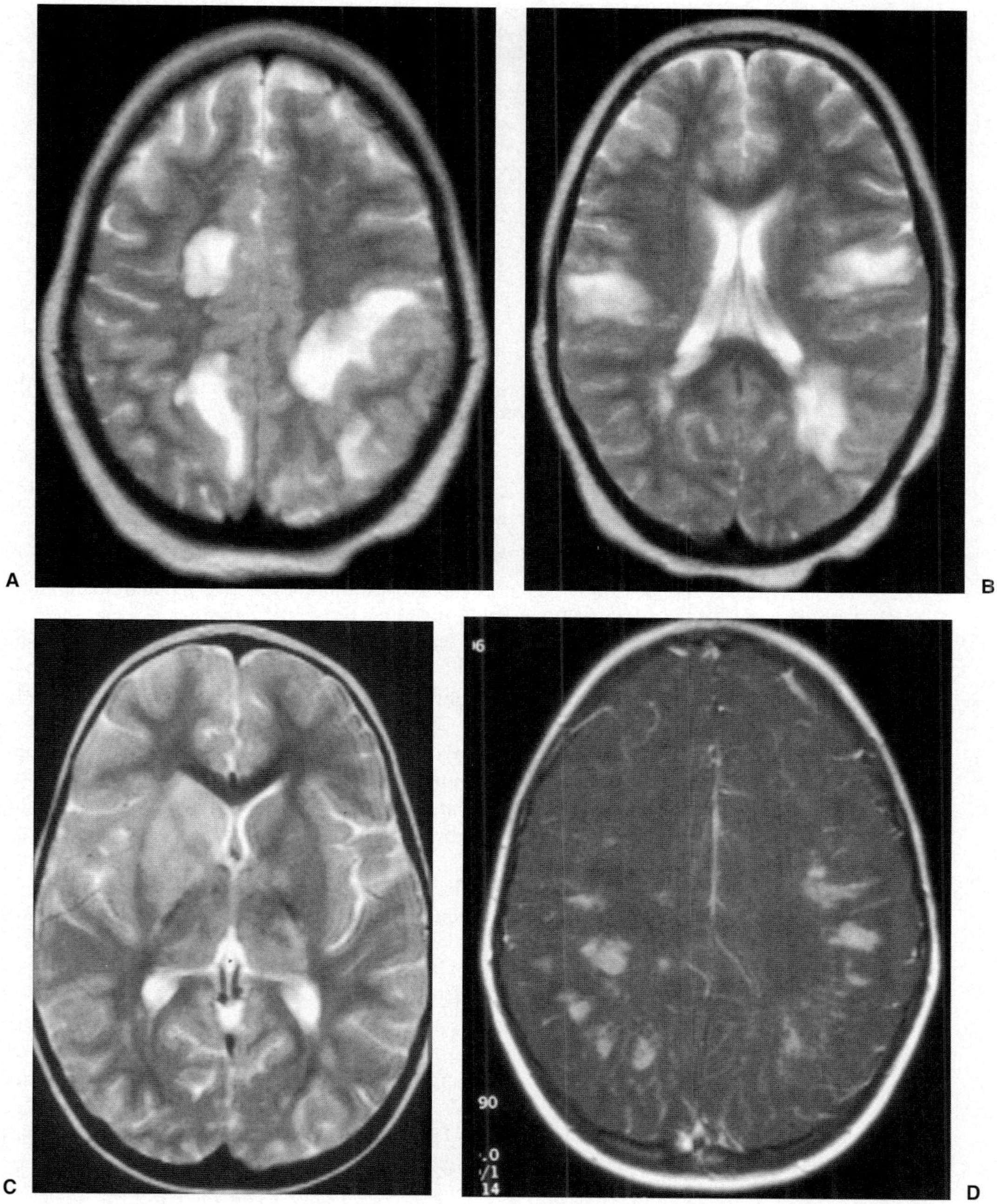

Figure 3.11 *Acute Disseminated Encephalomyelitis (ADEM). A, B.* Axial T2-weighted images show well defined, large, hyperintense lesions. Note lack of significant mass effect from the lesions. *C.* In a different patient, axial T2-weighted image shows hyperintense lesions in the right basal ganglia, medial left globus pallidus, and thalami. *D.* Postcontrast axial T1-weighted image (different patient) shows multiple enhancing lesions in the white matter.

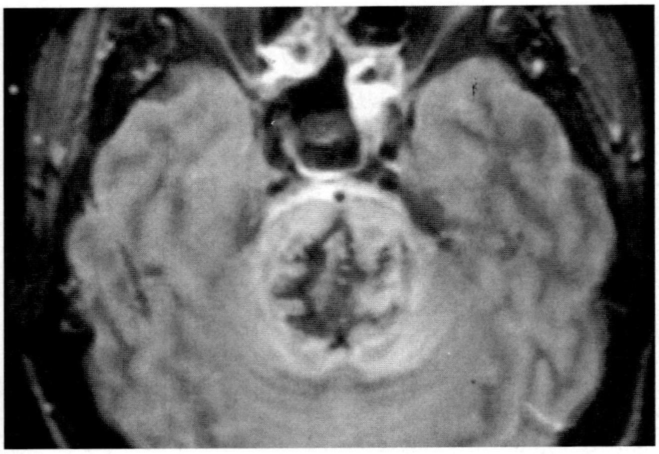

***Figure* 3.12** *Acute Hemorrhagic Leukoencephalopathy.* Axial T2-weighted image shows large hemorrhagic lesion in the brainstem.

References

1. Barkovich AJ, Kjos BO, Jackson DE, et al. Normal maturation of the neonatal and infant brain: MR imaging at 1.5 T1. Radiology 1988;166:173–180.
2. Hayakawa K, Konishi Y, Kuriyama M, et al. Normal brain maturation in MRI. Eur J Radiol 1990;12:208–215.
3. Ballesteros MC, Hansen PE, Soila K. MR imaging of the developing human brain. Radiographics 1993;13:611–622.
4. Sakuma H, Nomura Y, Takeda K, et al. Adult and neonatal human brain: diffusional anisotropy and myelination with diffusion-weighted MR imaging. Radiology 1991;180:229–233.
5. Neil JJ, Shiran SI, McKinstry RC, et al. Normal brain in human newborns: apparent diffusion coefficient and diffusion anisotropy measured by using diffusion tensor MR imaging. Radiology 1998;209:57–66.
6. Hüppi PS, Maier SE, Peled S, et al. Microstructural development of human newborn cerebral white matter assessed in vivo by diffusion tensor magnetic resonance imaging. Pediatr Res 1998;44:584–590.
7. Wimberger DM, Roberts TP, Barkovich AJ, et al. Identification of "premyelination" by diffusion-weighted MRI. J Comput Assist Tomogr 1995;19:28–33.
8. van der Knaap MS, Naidu S, Breiter SN, et al. Alexander disease: diagnosis with MR imaging. AJNR Am J Neuroradiol 2001;22:541–552.
9. McAdams HP, Geyer CA, Done SL, et al. CT and MR imaging of Canavan disease. AJNR Am J Neuroradiol 1990;11:397–399.
10. van der Knaap MS, Breiter SN, Naidu S, et al. Defining and categorizing leukoencephalopathies of unknown origin: MR imaging approach. Radiology 1999;213:121–133.
11. Brismar J, Brismar G, Gascon G, et al. Canavan disease: CT and MR imaging of the brain. AJNR Am J Neuroradiol 1990;11:805–810.
12. Alorayni IA, Patenaude YG, O'Gorman AM, et al. Cree leukoencephalopathy: neuroimaging findings. Radiology 1999;213:400–406.
13. Vanhanen SL, Raininko R, Santavuori P. Early differential diagnosis of infantile neuronal ceroid lipofuscinosis, Rett syndrome, and Krabbe disease by CT and MR. AJNR Am J Neuroradiol 1994;15:1443–1453.
14. Choi S, Enzmann DR. Infantile Krabbe disease: complementary CT and MR findings. AJNR Am J Neuroradiol 1993;14:1164–1666.
15. Finelli DA, Tarr RW, Sawyer RN, et al. Deceptively normal MR in early infantile Krabbe disease. AJNR Am J Neuroradiol 1994;15:167–171.
16. Hittmair K, Wimberger D, Wiesbauer P, et al. Early infantile form of Krabbe disease with optic hypertrophy: serial MR examinations and autopsy correlation. AJNR Am J Neuroradiol 1994;15:1454–1458.
17. Lee C, Dineen TE, Brack M, et al. The mucopolysaccharidoses: characterization by cranial MR imaging. AJNR Am J Neuroradiol 1995;16:1402–1403.
18. Johnson MA, Desai S, Hugh-Jones K, et al. Magnetic resonance imaging of the brain in Hurler syndrome. AJNR Am J Neuroradiol 1984;5:816–819.

19. Kumar AJ, Rosenbaum AE, Naidu S, et al. Adrenoleukodystrophy: correlating MR imaging with CT. Radiology 1987;165:495–504.
20. Jensen ME, Sawyer RW, Braun IF, et al. MR Imaging appearance of childhood adrenoleukodystrophy with auditory, visual, and motor pathway involvement. Radiographics 1990;10:53–66.
21. Snyder RD, King JN, Keck GM, et al. MR imaging of the spinal cord in 23 subjects with ALD-AMN complex. AJNR Am J Neuroradiol 1991;12:1095–1098.
22. Loes DJ, Hite S, Moser H, et al. Adrenoleukodystrophy: a scoring method for brain MR observations. AJNR Am J Neuroradiol 1994;15:1761–1776.
23. Melhem ER, Breiter SN, Ulug AM, et al. Improved tissue characterization in adrenoleukodystrophy using magnetization transfer imaging. AJR Am J Radiol 1996;166:689–695.
24. Rajanayagam V, Grad J, Krivit W, et al. Proton MR spectroscopy of childhood adrenoleukodystrophy. AJNR Am J Neuroradiol 1996;17:1013–1024.
25. Rajanayagam V, Balthazor M, Shapiro E, et al. Proton MR spectroscopy and neuropsychological testing in adrenoleukodystrophy. AJNR Am J Neuroradiol 1997;18:1909–1914.
26. Barkovich AJ, Ferreiro DM, Bass N, et al. Involvement of the pontomedullary corticospinal tracts: a useful finding in the diagnosis of X-linked adrenoleukodystrophy. AJNR Am J Neuroradiol 1994;15:1767–1771.
27. Inoue Y, Fukuda T, Takashima S, et al. Adrenoleukodystrophy: new CT findings. AJNR Am J Neuroradiol 1983;4:951–954.
28. Kim TS, Kim IO, Kim WS, et al. MR of childhood metachromatic leukodystrophy. AJNR Am J Neuroradiol 1997;18:733–738.
29. Stillman AE, Krivit W, Shapiro E, et al. Serial MR after bone marrow transplantation in two patients with metachromatic leukodystrophy. AJNR Am J Neuroradiol 1994;15:1929–1932.
30. Silverstein AM, Hirsch DK, Trobe JD, et al. MR imaging of the brain in five members of a family with Pelizaeus-Merzbacher disease. AJNR Am J Neuroradiol 1990;11:495–499.
31. van der Knaap MS, Valk J. The reflection of histology in MR imaging of Pelizaeus-Merzbacher disease. AJNR Am J Neuroradiol 1989;18:99–103.
32. Wetzburger CL, Van Regemorter N, Szliwowski HB, et al. Gray matter heterotopia and acute necrotizing encephalopathy in trichothiodystrophy. Pediatr Neurol 1998;19:392–394.
33. Ho VB, Fitz CR, Yoder CC, et al. Resolving MR features in osmotic myelinolysis (central pontine and extrapontine myelinolysis). AJNR Am J Neuroradiol 1993;14:163–167.
34. Sztencel J, Baleriaux D, Borenstein S, et al. Central pontine myelinolysis: correlation between CT and electrophysiologic data. AJNR Am J Neuroradiol 1983;4:529–530.
35. Korogi Y, Takahashi M, Shinzato J, et al. MR findings in two presumed cases of mild central pontine myelinolysis. AJNR Am J Neuroradiol 1993;14:651–654.
36. Price DB, Kramer J, Hotson GC, et al. Central pontine myelinolysis: report of a case with distinctive appearance on MR imaging. AJNR Am J Neuroradiol 1987;8:576–577.
37. Rosenbloom S, Buchholz D, Kumar AJ, et al. Evolution of central pontine myelinolysis on CT. AJNR Am J Neuroradiol 1984;5:110–112.
38. Guttmann CR, Ahn SS, Hsu L, et al. The evolution of multiple sclerosis lesions on serial MR. AJNR Am J Neuroradiol 1995;16:1481–1491.
39. Yousry TA, Filippi M, Becker C, et al. Comparison of MR pulse sequences in the detection of multiple sclerosis lesions. AJNR Am J Neuroradiol 1997;18:959–963.
40. Horowitz AL, Kaplan RD, Grewe G, et al. The ovoid lesion: a new MR observation in patients with multiple sclerosis. AJNR Am J Neuroradiol 1989;10:303–305.
41. Bastianello S, Bozzao A, Paolillo A, et al. Fast spin-echo and fast fluid-attenuated inversion-recovery versus conventional spin-echo sequences for MR quantification of multiple sclerosis lesions. AJNR Am J Neuroradiol 1997;18:699–704.
42. Grossman RI, Lenkinski RE, Ramer KN, et al. MR proton spectroscopy in multiple sclerosis. AJNR Am J Neuroradiol 1992;13:1535–1543.
43. Tomiak MM, Rosenblum JD, Prager JM, et al. Magnetization transfer: a potential method to determine the age of multiple sclerosis lesions. AJNR Am J Neuroradiol 1994;15:1569–1574.
44. Loevner LA, Grossman RI, McGowan JC, et al. Characterization of multiple sclerosis plaques with T1-weighted MR and quantitative magnetization transfer. AJNR Am J Neuroradiol 1995;16:1473–1479.
45. Rusin JA, Vezina LG, Chadduck WM, et al. Tumoral multiple sclerosis of the cerebellum in a child. AJNR Am J Neuroradiol 1995;16:1164–1166.
46. Caracciolo JT, Murtagh RD, Rojiani AM, et al. Pathognomonic MR imaging findings in Balo concentric sclerosis. AJNR Am J Neuroradiol 2001;22:292–293.
47. Korte JH, Bom EP, Vos LD, et al. Balo concentric sclerosis: MR diagnosis. AJNR Am J Neuroradiol 1994;15:1284–1285.

48. DeLara F, Tartaglino L, Friedman D. Spinal cord multiple sclerosis and Devic neuromyelitis optica in children. AJNR Am J Neuroradiol 1995;16:1557–1558.
49. Mader I, Stock KW, Ettlin T, Probst A. Acute disseminated encephalomyelitis: MR and CT features. AJNR Am J Neuroradiol 1996;17:104–109.
50. Grossman RI, Lisak RP, Macchi PJ, et al. MR of acute experimental allergic encephalomyelitis. AJNR Am J Neuroradiol 1987;8:1045–1048.
51. Kuharik MA, Edwards MK, Farlow MW, et al. Gd-enhanced MR imaging of acute and chronic experimental demyelinating lesions. AJNR Am J Neuroradiol 1988;9:643–648.
52. Baum PA, Barkovich AJ, Koch TK, et al. Deep gray matter involvement in children with acute disseminated encephalomyelitis. AJNR Am J Neuroradiol 1994;15:1275–1283.

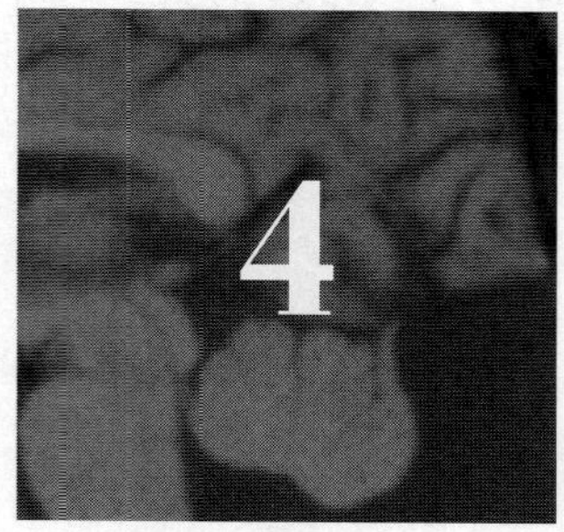

Metabolic, Toxic, and Degenerative Disorders

- Liver Failure, Parenteral Nutrition, and Alper's Syndrome
- Bilirubin Encephalopathy (Kernicterus)
- Mitochondriopathies
- Amino Acidurias
- Disorders of Copper Metabolism
- Disorders of Iron Metabolism
- Hypoglycemia
- Disorders Related to Ethanol Abuse
- Carbon Monoxide Intoxication
- Glycol-Related Products Intoxication
- Lead Intoxication
- Methanol Intoxication
- Mercury Intoxication
- Inhalant Abuse
- Huntington's Disease
- Hyperglycemia
- Amyotrophic Lateral Sclerosis
- Alzheimer's Disease
- Parkinson's Disease
- Pick's Disease
- Clivopontocerebellar Degeneration
- Amyloidosis
- Diseases Affecting the Kidneys and the Brain
- Thyroid Gland Disorders Affecting the Brain
- Effects of Miscellaneous Systemic Disorders on the Brain
- Hippocampal Sclerosis

Liver Failure, Parenteral Nutrition, and Alper's Syndrome

It is well known that hepatic insufficiency leads to abnormalities on brain magnetic resonance imaging (MRI) (1). T1-weighted images show increased signal in the caudate nucleus, tectum (particularly the inferior colliculi), globus pallidus, putamen, subthalamic nucleus, red nucleus, adenohypophysis, and substantia nigra (Fig. 4.1). The abnormalities are bilateral, symmetric, and of homogeneous signal intensity, and their differential diagnosis is as follows (2):

- Chronic liver failure
- Total parenteral nutrition
- Manganese (Mn) poisoning
- Normal calcifications
- Neurofibromatosis type 1

Despite the abnormalities on T1 images, there are no corresponding abnormalities on T2 images, and computed tomography (CT) scans are negative (note that when magnetization transfer is applied, the basal ganglia normally may be slightly bright on T1 images). The MRI findings are believed to be due to increased amounts of Mn and other factors leading to a shortening of the relaxation time, as follows (3):

- Increased concentrations of Mn
- Overabundance of lipofuscin in mitochondria, endoplasmic reticulum, and vacuoles of Alzheimer type II astrocytes
- Unidentified paramagnetic substances
- Spongiform changes and myelin vacuolization

The most common cause of increased T1 signal intensity in the basal ganglia is the deposition of hydrated calcium that occurs normally with aging.

Increased plasma levels of Mn may be found in chronic liver failure, patients receiving long-term parenteral nutrition, and occupational toxicity. Approximately 95% of Mn

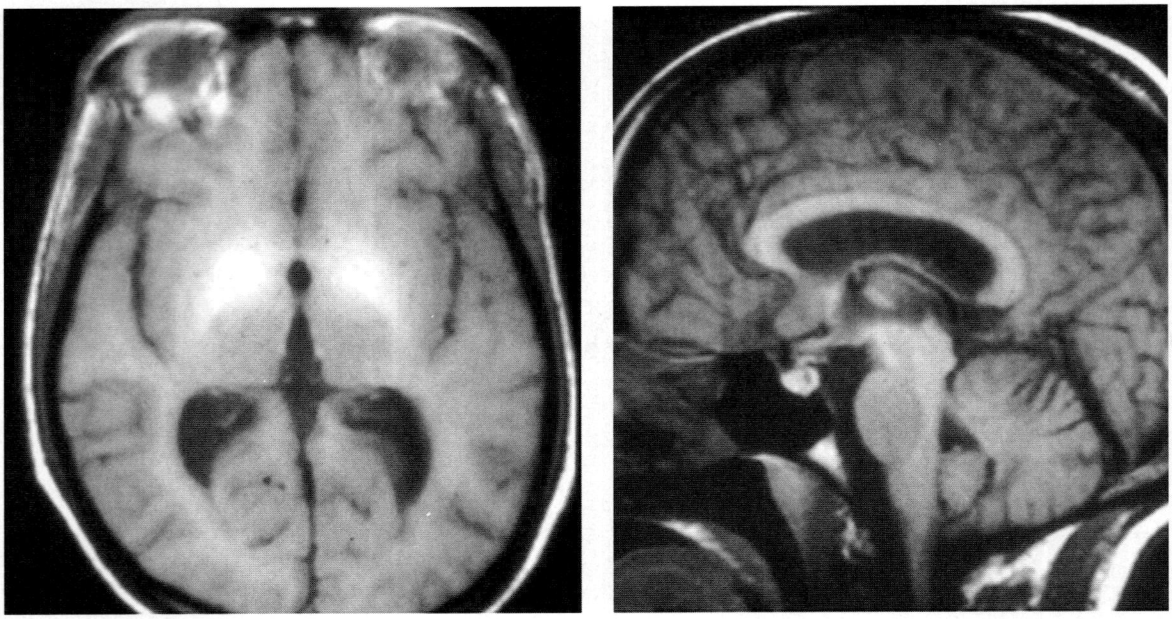
A B

Figure 4.1 Basal Ganglia in Liver Failure. Axial *A* and sagittal *B* T1-weighted images show increased signal in the lentiform nuclei, dorsal brainstem, and anterior pituitary lobe.

is excreted in bile. Mn is involved in some enzymatic cell cycles, including superoxide dismutase and glutamine synthetase. Mn reaches the brain by way of erythrocytes and plasma. Transferrin and albumin are its carriers in plasma. The half-life of blood Mn is 10 to 42 days, but when it reaches the brain, it may remain there for prolonged periods. Astrocytes have specific transport systems for Mn. Mn is neurotoxic and results in striatal dopamine depletion, *N*-methyl-D-aspartate (NMDA) excitotoxicity, and oxidative stress. Thus, Mn may play a role in the development of hepatic encephalopathy that is clinically characterized by pyramidal and extrapyramidal dysfunction, brisk tendon reflexes, and tremors. The concentration of Mn in the pallidus of cirrhotic patients is threefold higher compared with control subjects. The frequency of MRI abnormalities in the brain of cirrhotic patients is approximately 73% (4).

Long-term total parenteral nutrition also results in increased T1 signal intensity in the same regions. These solutions are rich in Mn and lead to development of neurologic symptoms. Once the parenteral nutrition is discontinued, MRI finding may revert to normal (5). The amount of time required for these abnormalities to resolve is not clear, but most do so within 1 year after cessation of parenteral nutrition. Similar findings are noted in patients after liver transplantation. Although the clinical and imaging abnormalities are reversible in adults, their long-term effects on the child's brain are not known.

Other MR techniques may be more sensitive to the effects of liver disease on the brain than just imaging. Magnetization transfer contrast ratios are abnormal not only in the previously named brain regions but in the white matter (6). With liver failure, there is an increased proliferation of Alzheimer type II astrocytes in the affected brain regions. The etiology for the proliferation of these cells may be hyperammonemia. These cells are characterized by cytoplasmic hypertrophy and increased water content. This relatively large amount of water may decrease magnetization transfer by virtue of protein dilution. Proton MR spectroscopy (MRS) of the brain also may show abnormalities in patients with liver failure. Studies have shown that MRS may be able to show abnormalities in patients with subclinical and clinical hepatic encephalopathy (7,8). These abnormalities include reduced levels of choline, reduced levels of myoinositol, and increased glutamine/glutamate. In patients with Wilson's disease, MRS may be able to distinguish between portosystemic encephalopathy and primary neurodegeneration by virtue of demonstrating low N-acetyl aspartate (NAA) in the latter. Proton MRS also may be helpful in assessing the effects of treatment in patients with hepatic encephalopathy (9). Oral lactulose is given to these patients in an attempt to restore their nitrogen balance. Proton MRS is able to detect brain metabolite changes in the patients undergoing this type of treatment.

Repeated episodes of hepatic failure may lead to the development of acquired (non-Wilsonian) hepatocerebral degeneration. The clinical symptoms are permanent and death commonly follows. By MRI, these patients no longer show the typical T1 hyperintensities in the basal ganglia described previously for chronic hepatic encephalopathy. Patients with acquired hepatocerebral degeneration show areas of increased T2 signal intensity, particularly in the middle cerebellar peduncles. These zones correspond to spongiform myelinolytic changes that most likely are the sequelae of ischemia. These changes are not secondary to osmotic myelinolysis.

Alper's syndrome is a rare childhood disorder characterized by progressive neuronal degeneration with liver disease (10). Seizures and liver failure develop in these patients. Pathologically, there may be necrosis of the deep gray nuclei and of the cortex. MRI shows increased T2 signal intensity in the basal ganglia and thalamus. There is atrophy and increased T2 signal intensity in the cortex, predominantly in the occipital lobes. The abnormalities are bilateral but may be asymmetric. It has been suggested that these abnormalities also may reflect a mitochondrial dysfunction that is present is patients with Alper's syndrome.

Bilirubin Encephalopathy (Kernicterus)

The sequelae of kernicterus are due to neuronal necrosis in the basal ganglia and in the cranial nerve nuclei in the brainstem.

Kernicterus has become a rare disorder because of the rapid control and effective treatment of hyperbilirubinemia. Currently, most cases are the result of isoimmunization to Rh factor or from ABO blood group incompatibility. As such, it almost always still is a disease of neonates. Later in life, most cases are due to genetic hematologic or liver diseases such as defects of glucose-6-phosphate dehydrogenase, Crigler-Najjar disease, and Gilbert's disease, and in rare cases is secondary to breast-feeding or severe sepsis (11). In kernicterus, the liver is unable to conjugate bilirubin. The enzyme uridine diphosphate glucuronyltransferase does not function well and albumin-bound (insoluble) bilirubin cannot be deconjugated into bilirubin diglucuronide or "water-soluble" bilirubin. Initially, the child appears hypotonic, then becomes hypertonic; after approximately 1 week, the hypotonia returns. On gross brain examination, there is yellow staining of the globi pallidi, mamillary bodies, subthalamic nuclei, and the indusium griseum. In the brainstem, the substantia nigra and some of the cranial nerve nuclei may be involved. The histologic findings are identical to those caused by hypoxia or hypoglycemia and reflect tissue necrosis. Surrounding inflammatory changes are common. There is neuronal necrosis in the basal ganglia, particularly the globi pallidi, subthalamic nuclei, dentate nuclei, hippocampi, and cranial nerve nuclei. Acutely, there are signs of liver failure, and this may account for the findings seen on MRI during this period of the disease.

MRI has been used mostly to evaluate the sequelae of kernicterus. Acutely, infants with kernicterus may show increased T1 signal intensity in the basal ganglia without corresponding T2-weighted abnormalities. I speculate that this finding probably is related to acute hepatic insufficiency and may be similar to that seen in adults with chronic liver disease (Fig. 4.2A). In the chronic stage there is increased T2 signal intensity in the globus pallidus and in the cerebellar dentate nucleus. These structures also are atrophic (Fig. 4.2B).

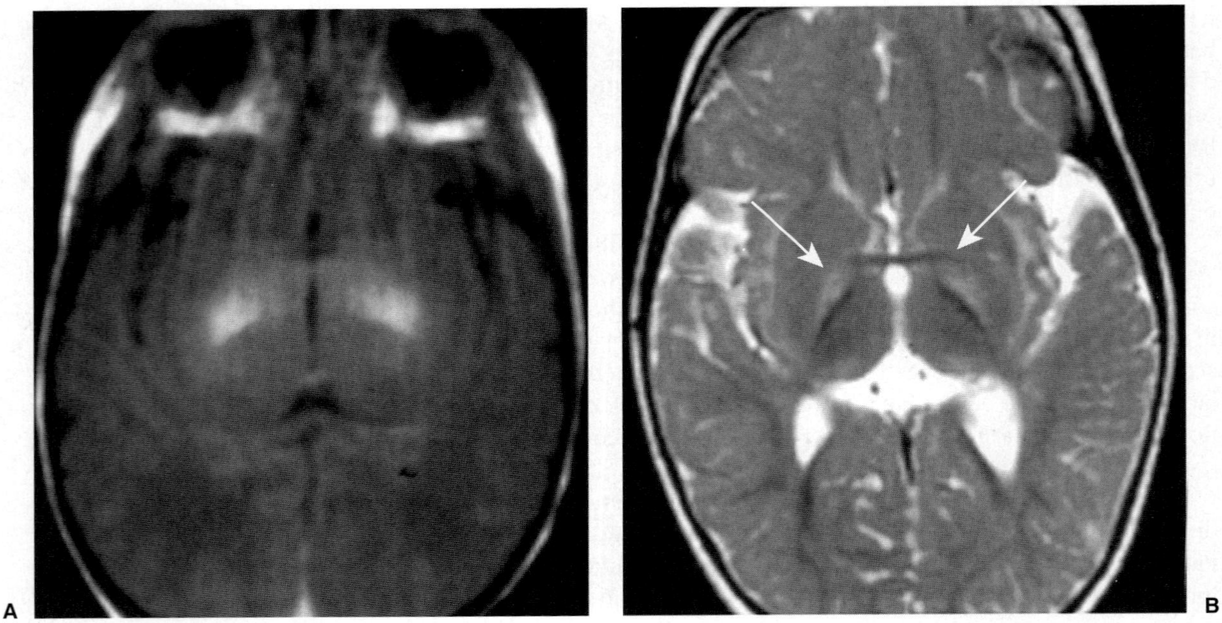

Figure 4.2 *Kernicterus. A.* Axial T1-weighted image during acute phase shows bright basal ganglia probably secondary to liver failure. *B.* Axial T2-weighted image shows the sequela of bilirubin encephalopathy. There is high signal in the medial globi pallidi *(arrows)*.

MITOCHONDRIOPATHIES

There are some mitochondrial disorders in which proton MRS does not show elevation of the lactate peak.

Mitochondrial encephalopathies are relatively rare disorders involving a defect in the oxidative respiratory mechanism (due to impaired production of adenosine triphosphate) that leads to accumulation of lactic acid. Lactic acid then may be detected in serum or cerebrospinal fluid (CSF) on laboratory studies or by proton MRS (12). Although most patients begin to have symptoms during childhood, some may present when they are adults. Most mitochondrial disorders affect the skeletal muscles and brain, and most present with weakness and seizures (due to ischemia) (13). Mitochondrial disorders and organic acidurias share many biochemical and clinical features. The most common mitochondrial disease is MELAS syndrome (mitochondrial myopathy, encephalopathy, lactic acidosis, and strokes), which results in large, nonterritorial cerebral infarctions (including the basal ganglia and thalami) (14) (Fig. 4.3A and B). It manifests more commonly during the second decade of life, and strokes are the result of impaired function of the muscle in the walls of cerebral arteries. Pathologically, there is spongy degeneration, neuronal loss, gliosis, and microcystic liquefaction in the affected regions. Proton MRS is helpful in the evaluation of these patients. Even in normal-appearing regions, lactate may be present. NAA is low acutely and chronically (Fig. 4.3C). Unfortunately, there are mitochondrial disorders in which MRS shows no elevation of the lactate peak.

Myoclonic epilepsy and ragged red fibers (MERFF) is characterized by myoclonic epilepsy and its imaging findings are identical to those described for MELAS syndrome. Leigh's disease (subacute necrotizing encephalomyelopathy) is due to pyruvate and cytochrome C oxidase deficiencies (15). This disease usually is diagnosed during the first year of life. It produces abnormalities in the basal ganglia, the periaqueductal gray matter, and the subcortical white matter (16). As in MELAS syndrome, proton MRS shows elevated lactate (particularly during the acute period) and low NAA. Kearns-Sayre syndrome is characterized by abnormalities in the basal ganglia and the white matter (which are extensive) (17). The typical clinical findings in these patients are ophthalmoplegia and cardiac conduction abnormalities. Pathologically, there is capillary proliferation, necrosis, vacuolization, and demyelination of the affected areas. The MRI findings are extensive and

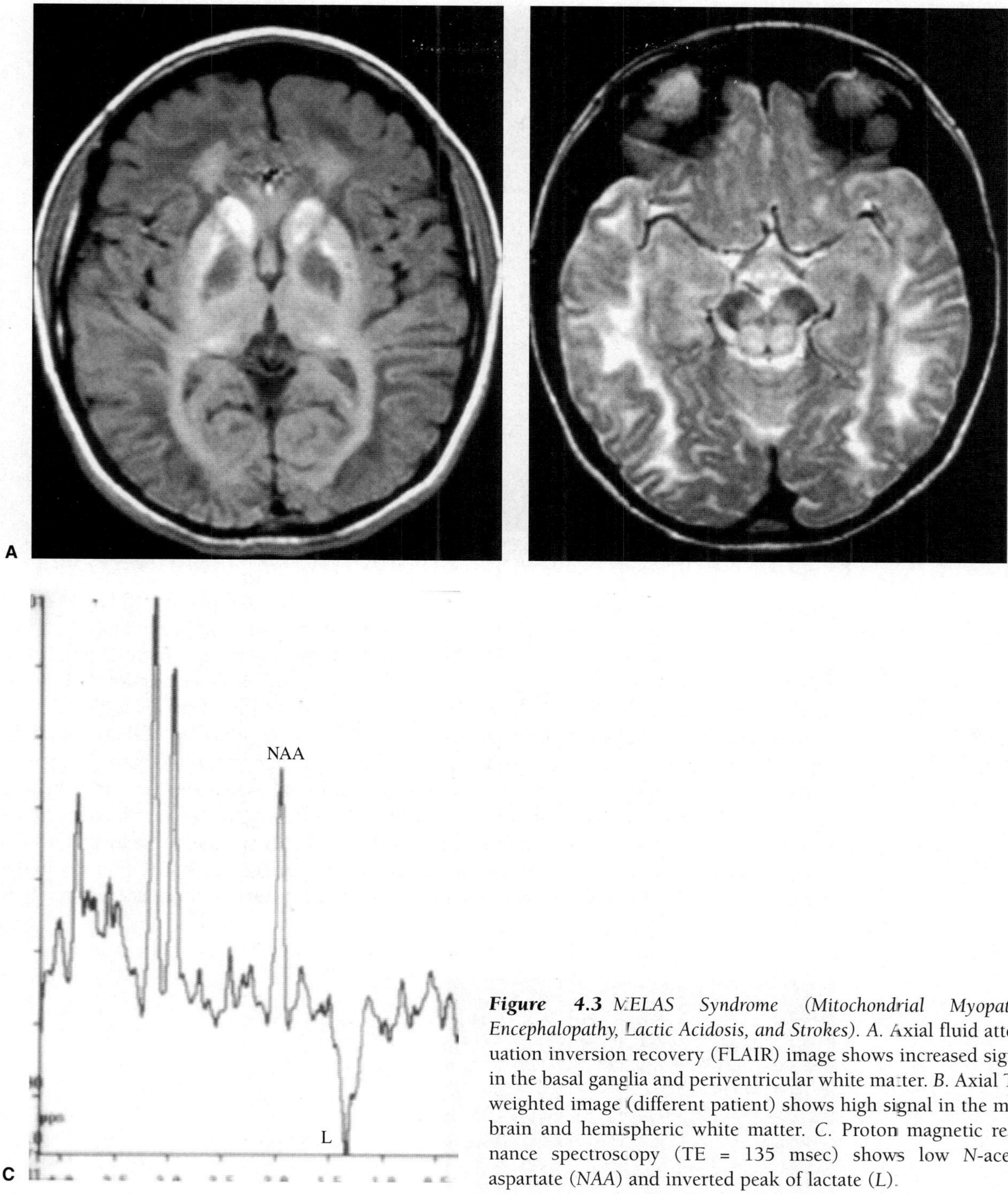

Figure 4.3 *MELAS Syndrome (Mitochondrial Myopathy, Encephalopathy, Lactic Acidosis, and Strokes). A.* Axial fluid attenuation inversion recovery (FLAIR) image shows increased signal in the basal ganglia and periventricular white matter. *B.* Axial T2-weighted image (different patient) shows high signal in the midbrain and hemispheric white matter. *C.* Proton magnetic resonance spectroscopy (TE = 135 msec) shows low *N*-acetyl aspartate (*NAA*) and inverted peak of lactate (*L*).

include involvement of all deep gray matter structures (high T2 signal intensity) and extensive increased T2 signal in the white matter.

Amino Acidurias

Although amino acid disorders are not true leukodystrophies, they predominantly affect the white matter. In these disorders, there is an abnormal formation of proteolipids that are needed to form normal myelin. The most common disorders in this group are phenylketonuria (PKU; nonspecific white matter changes and atrophy on MRI), maple syrup disease (white matter and basal ganglia show high T2 signal on MRI), homocystinuria (strokes and

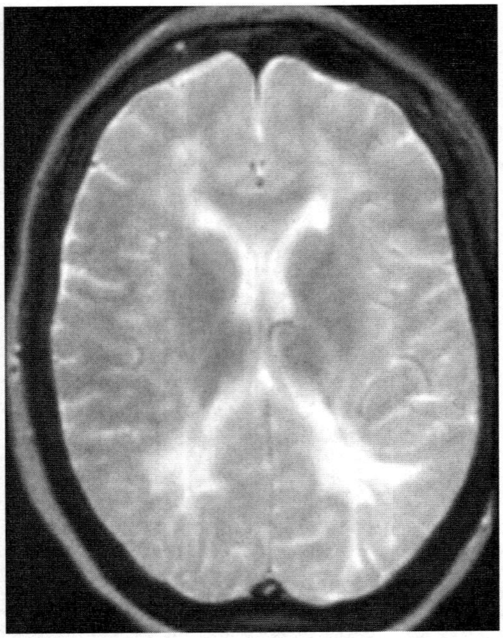

Figure 4.4 *Phenylketonuria.* Axial T2-weighted image shows nonspecific periventricular white matter increased signal intensity with sparing of subcortical u-fibers.

arterial occlusions on MRI and MR angiography, respectively), and glutaric (dilated sylvian fissures and increased T2 signal in the basal ganglia and thalami), methylmalonic, and propionic acidurias (both show increased T2 signal in the deep gray matter structures and hemispheric white matter) (18–24) (Fig. 4.4). Because of the neonatal screening for PKU mandated by law, this disorder no longer is as severe as it used to be. Patients with PKU are started promptly on a special diet and the imaging findings are mild (18). Glutaric aciduria type 1 (type 2 is very rare) is the one that classically results in cyst formation in the regions of the sylvian fissures (some believe that these are arachnoid cysts, whereas others believe that they are the reflection of underlying temporal lobe hypoplasia), white matter abnormalities, and basal ganglia abnormalities (21,22) (Fig. 4.5). Methylmalonic acidemia results in extensive white matter abnormalities and characteristically high T2 signal intensity in the globi pallidi (24). The findings in propionic aciduria are similar to those seen in methyl-

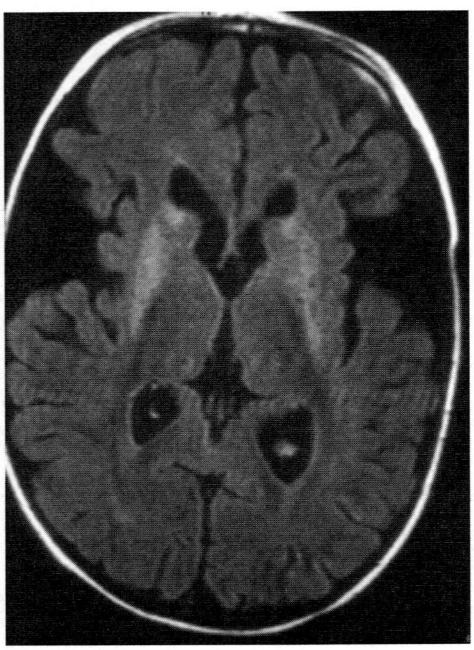

Figure 4.5 *Glutaric Aciduria Type 1.* Axial fluid attenuation inversion recovery (FLAIR) image shows high signal in both basal ganglia and enlarged sylvian fissures (arachnoid cysts?).

malonic aciduria (23). Many of these disorders show a dramatic improvement on MRI after a few weeks of treatment. The myelination milestones are delayed in all of these disorders. Proton MRS usually shows several peaks between 1.5 and 2.5 parts per million, which are thought to represent abnormal accumulation of amino acids and low NAA. In my opinion, it is extremely difficult to suggest these diagnoses based on imaging findings.

Disorders of Copper Metabolism

Wilson's Disease

The ophthalmologic lesions seen in patients with Wilson's disease are Kayser-Fleischer rings (common) and the sunflower cataract (uncommon).

Wilson's disease or hepatolenticular degeneration is a genetic disorder of copper metabolism that is characterized by failure to incorporate copper into ceruloplasmin in the liver, failure to excrete copper by the liver into the bile, and toxic accumulation of copper in multiple organs (25). Its defect has been mapped to chromosome 13q14.3, and several mutations exist. In addition, concentrations of other heavy metals such as zinc, iron, silver, and aluminum also are increased. Most children present with hepatic failure, whereas most adults present with neurologic symptoms. Accumulation of copper in Descemet's membrane results in the Kayser-Fleischer rings. Accumulation of copper in the lens results in the rare "sunflower" cataracts. Pathologically, there is cell loss and cavitation in the lentiform nucleus. Copper concentration at these sites is markedly increased. Other regions involved include the thalamus, subthalamus, red nucleus, substantia nigra, dentate nucleus, and the brainstem (26). Microscopically, these regions contain large cells with small nuclei (termed *Opalski cells*), and these are thought to be typical for Wilson's disease. Similar to effects of other liver disorders on the brain (see earlier), Alzheimer type II cells also are found in the affect areas. The brain is diffusely atrophic.

MRI shows abnormalities even in absence of clinical neurologic findings (27). The paramagnetic effects of copper are visible by MRI only in untreated patients. Basal ganglia lesions most often are bilateral and symmetric. The putamina show striking increased T2 signal intensity (Fig. 4.6A). This is present to a lesser degree in other deep gray matter

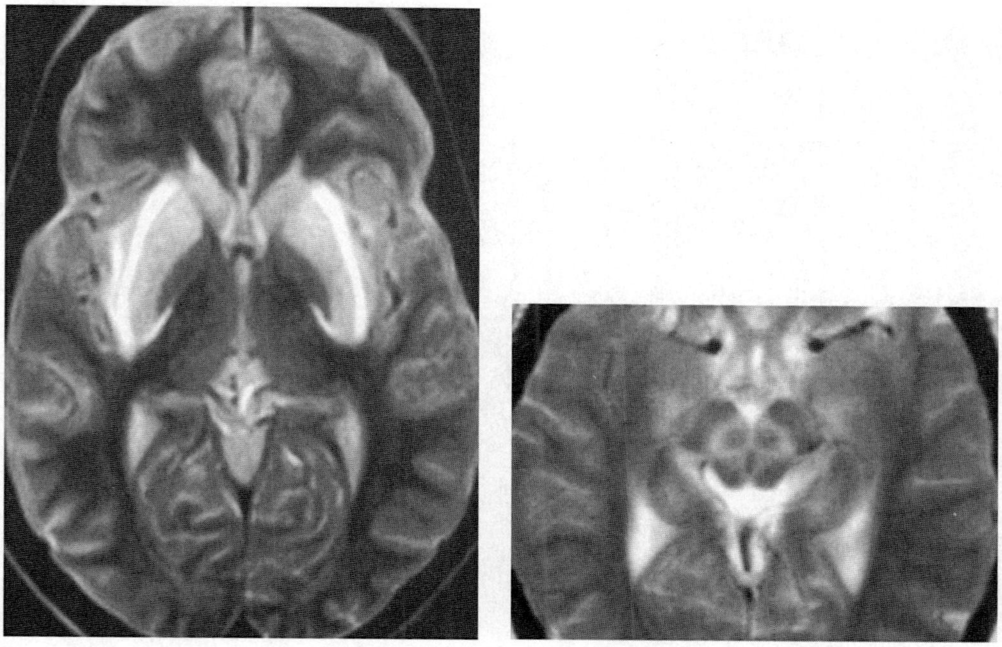

A B

Figure 4.6 *Wilson's Disease. A.* Axial T2-weighted image shows abnormal high signal intensity in the lentiform nuclei and the subinsular regions. *B.* Axial T2-weighted image shows high signal in the midbrain that is superimposed on the dark signal of the substantia nigra and red nuclei, giving the "panda face" appearance.

structures. Thalamic lesions often are present but typically spare the dorsomedial nuclei. White matter tracts, including the dentatothalamic, corticospinal, and pontocerebellar tracts, commonly are involved (26). The claustrum may show high T2 signal intensity. The midbrain is bright on T2-weighted images with relative sparing of its deep nuclei, giving rise to the so-called panda face sign (Fig. 4.6B). Although it is attractive to postulate that high copper concentrations are responsible for the MRI abnormalities, this probably is not true. Copper results in T1 and T2 shortening; hence, the imaging findings in Wilson's disease probably are secondary to spongy degeneration, cavitation, neuronal loss, and reactive astrocytosis. There is a correlation between the clinical and MRI findings (27): An abnormal-appearing striatum correlates with pseudoparkinsonism, an abnormal dentatothalamic tract with cerebellar signs, and an abnormal pontocerebellar tract with pseudoparkinsonism. The presence of portosystemic shunting may correlate with abnormalities seen in the globus pallidus. The abnormal T2 signal intensity may improve after copper trapping therapy. Contrast enhancement is rare, but may be seen when patients are receiving treatment with penicillamine. Positron emission tomography (PET) shows diffusely reduced glucose metabolism that is particularly marked in the caudate nucleus, frontoparietal cortex, and lentiform nucleus (28). These findings correlate with the severity of the disease and may be reversed after adequate therapy. Proton MRS shows that NAA/Cr and choline/Cr ratios are decreased in patients with Wilson's disease compared with control subjects. In addition, patients with Wilson's disease and portosystemic shunting have lower myoinositol/Cr ratios than such patients with no portosystemic shunting.

Menkes' Syndrome

Imaging findings in Menkes' syndrome include wormian bones, areas of delayed myelination, hydrocephalus, brain atrophy, and subdural hematomas.

Menkes' syndrome is a rare disease linked to chromosome 13 (Xq13.3) and in close proximity to the genetic defect found in Wilson's disease (29). Although the phenotype is variable, 90% to 95% of patients show the classic form of the disease. The gene abnormality leads to absent or decreased production of a specific protein involved in removing copper from the cells. The lack of this protein results in abnormalities involving the following pathways: cytochrome C oxidase, dopamine β-hydroxylase, monoamine oxidase, ascor-

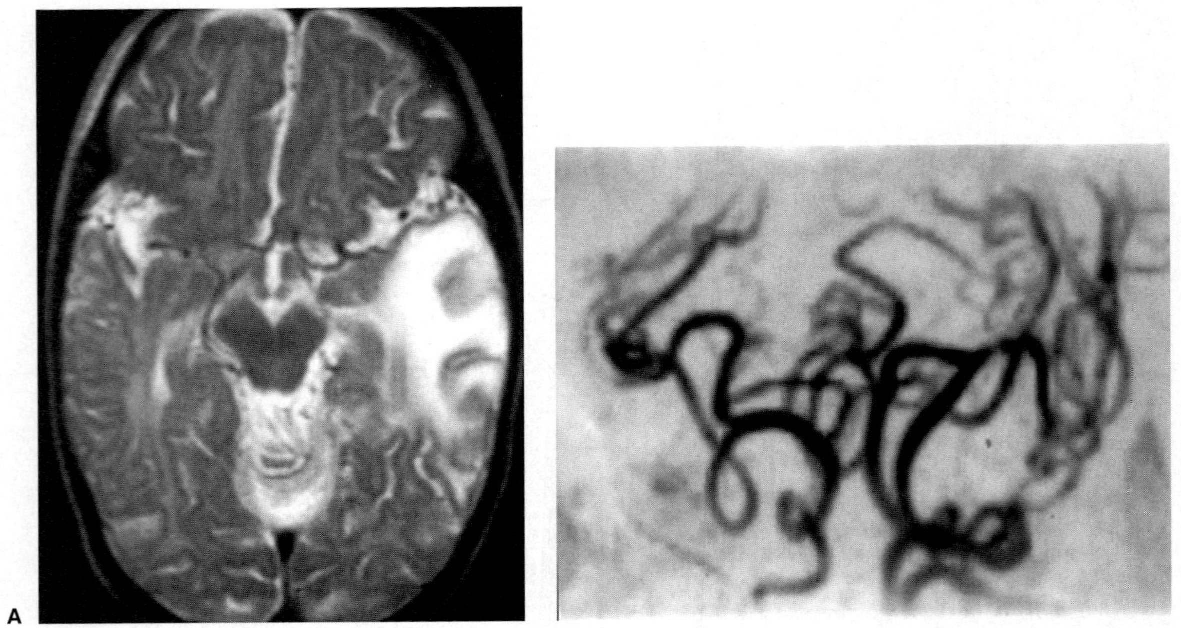

Figure 4.7 *Menkes' Syndrome. A.* Axial T2-weighted image shows high signal intensity in the white matter of the left temporal lobe. *B.* Frontal view from magnetic resonance angiogram shows extremely tortuous intracranial arteries.

bate oxidase, superoxide dismutase, lysyl oxidase, tyrosinase, and nicotinamide adenine dinucleotide CoQ reductase. All of these abnormalities are prevalent throughout the body, but less severely present in the liver. Low levels of copper in plasma, urine, and hair as well as a low level of plasma ceruloplasmin are typical. Clinical symptoms are developmental delay and regression of milestones, temperature instability, feeding difficulties, hypotonia, ataxia, progressive spasticity, irritability, and failure to thrive. The skin is depigmented and the hair has a "steel wool" appearance (so-called kinky hair syndrome). Radiographs show wormian (intrasutural) bones and MRI shows delayed myelination and cerebral atrophy (30) (Fig. 4.7A). CT and MRI may show subdural hematomas. Catheter angiography and MR angiography show marked elongation and tortuosity of the intracranial circulation (31) (Fig. 4.7B). These bizarre-appearing vessels are strongly suggestive of Menkes' syndrome. PET shows decreased blood flow and oxygen metabolism in the cerebellum, cerebral hemisphere, and brainstem. Single-photon emission CT (SPECT) shows reduced blood flow in the frontotemporal and parietal regions.

Disorders of Iron Metabolism

Disorders of iron (Fe) metabolism are common and may occur owing to deficiency or overload of this element (32) (Table 4.1).

Although these disorders are relatively common (particularly those related to iron deficiencies), their effects on the central nervous system (CNS) are few. It is well known that anemia related to chronic and debilitating disorders such as acquired immunodeficiency syndrome (AIDS) may result in a spinal bone marrow that appears hypointense on T1-weighted images (33). This presumably is due to a compensatory mechanism that leads to storage of iron in the bone marrow. The presence of increased iron results in a diffuse hypointense appearance of the bone marrow.

Disorders of iron overload are less common than anemias but occasionally give rise to interesting, albeit uncommon, imaging findings. Iron overload occurs when the iron-binding capacity of transferrin is exceeded or when increased catabolism of erythrocytes leads to accumulation of iron in the reticuloendothelial system and organ cells. Patients with hereditary hemochromatosis have an increased iron intestinal absorption. In the CNS, iron gets deposited in the pituitary gland and may give rise to abnormal and low endocrine functions. In these patients, the adenohypophysis may appear as an area of very low or no signal in both T1- and T2-weighted images (34). The ratio of the signal intensity of the pituitary gland to fat correlates with gland function. Reductions in this ratio correlate with hypogonadotropic hypogonadism and higher ferritin levels. In addition, in these patients the liver is damaged and the brain may show findings related to chronic hepatic encephalopathy (35). Juvenile hemochromatosis is nearly identical to the hereditary type, but manifests earlier in life and most patients die young from heart failure. Transfusional siderosis occurs only after chronic and repeated whole-blood transfusions and is seen more commonly in patients with cancer and those with sickle cell anemia. Aceruloplasminemia is different from Wilson's disease (see earlier) in that

In patients with hemochromatosis who are not alcoholics, liver function is surprisingly good regardless of the size of their liver.

Table 4.1: Disorders of Iron Metabolism

Disorders of Fe Deficiency	*Disorders of Fe Overload*
Iron deficiency anemia	Hereditary hemochromatosis
Anemia of chronic inflammation	Other hemochromatoses (including juvenile and neonatal forms)
	African iron overload
	Aceruloplasminemia
	Transfusional siderosis

ceruloplasmin is completely absent, not just low. Ceruloplasmin has ferroxidase action that is partly responsible for the release of iron from many cells. In the absence of ceruloplasmin, iron accumulates in the basal ganglia and dentate nuclei of the cerebellum and gives rise to progressive extrapyramidal signs, cerebellar ataxia, and eventually dementia.

Hallervorden-Spatz Disease

The eye of the tiger sign is virtually pathognomonic for Hallervorden-Spatz disease.

Hallervorden-Spatz disease (HS) and Friedreich's ataxia are also related to iron overload and degenerative brain disease (36). Little is known about the biochemical abnormalities of HS, but it has been linked to an abnormality in chromosome 20p12.3-p13. Large amounts of iron are deposited in the globus pallidus and pars reticulata of the substantia nigra. Iron deposition leads to axonal swelling and decreased myelin. Microscopy demonstrates the presence of abnormal spherical bodies that contain superoxide dismutase and are believed to be typical for HS. Eventually, these regions of the brain are destroyed. Patients with HS demonstrate dystonia, muscle rigidity, hyperreflexia, and choreoathetosis. Mental retardation is variable and death occurs 1 or 2 years after the diagnosis. Because laboratory findings are nonspecific, the combination of clinical symptoms and imaging findings is used to establish a diagnosis. The findings on CT are nonspecific and MRI is the imaging method of choice. Initially, only hypointensity (more pronounced on T2- than on T1-weighted sequences) is seen in the globi pallidi. When gliosis ensues, the globi pallidi become hyperintense on T2-weighted images but remain surrounded by hypointensity (Fig. 4.8). This abnormality is called the *eye of the tiger sign* and is said to be characteristic for HS.

Friedreich's Ataxia

Friedreich's ataxia is a rare autosomal recessive disorder. It is part of the hereditary ataxic syndromes and is discussed here because of its possible relation to abnormal iron metabolism (37). In 97% of patients it is caused by an abnormality located in chromosome 9 that encodes a protein called *frataxin*, which has been localized to mitochondria although its function is unknown. Increased iron deposition is found in the heart, liver, and spleen in

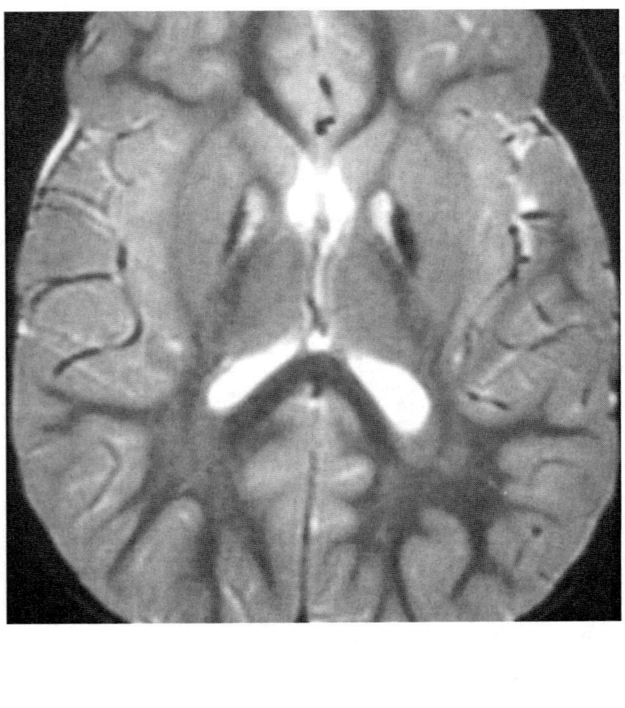

Figure 4.8 *Hallervorden-Spatz Disease.* Axial T2-weighted image shows high signal in the medial globi pallidi and low signal laterally ("eye of the tiger" appearance).

a pattern consistent with a mitochondrial location. There is iron accumulation, mitochondrial respiratory chain dysfunction, and mitochondrial DNA depletion. The spinal cord is pathologically atrophic with damaged white matter tracts. The lumbar and sacral nerves also are atrophic. The cerebellar cortex and the brainstem also may show atrophy. Atrophy of the gray matter in the central sulcus occasionally is evident on gross and imaging examinations. Unfortunately, the findings of imaging studies are subtle and nonspecific.

Hypoglycemia

Most cerebral insults due to hypoglycemia occur in young children (38). Oxygen and glucose are the major substrates needed for normal brain metabolism, and absence of either or both leads to significant injury. Hypoglycemia uncommonly affects the neonatal brain, which normally is fairly resistant to it. Acute symptoms of hypoglycemia include jitteriness, seizures, and vomiting. Hypoglycemia is diagnosed when the whole-blood glucose concentration falls below 20 mg/dL in preterm infants, 30 mg/dL in term infants, and 45 mg/dL in adults. Sequelae of hypoglycemia are mental retardation, spasticity, visual abnormalities, and microcephaly. In neonates, hypoglycemia leads to diffuse edema and infarctions (39). Typically, the occipital regions are affected more severely, but the basal ganglia also may be involved (38,40) (Fig. 4.9). The reason for this is not clear, but it may be related to the fact that in neonates the visual cortex is relatively more mature and metabolically more active than other regions because during the neonatal period it experiences intense axonal migration and synaptogenesis. Other reasons include diffuse hypoxia secondary to heart failure, loss of cerebral vascular autoregulation, and excitatory toxicity. Although the gray matter is especially affected, the occipital white matter and posterior thalamus also may be injured. Chronically, the cortex of the occipital lobes becomes thin and malacia develops, and these findings correlate with visual abnormalities. In adults, hypoglycemia also may induce occipital infarctions in addition to infarctions elsewhere (which usually are multiple), laminar necrosis, and transient imaging abnormalities.

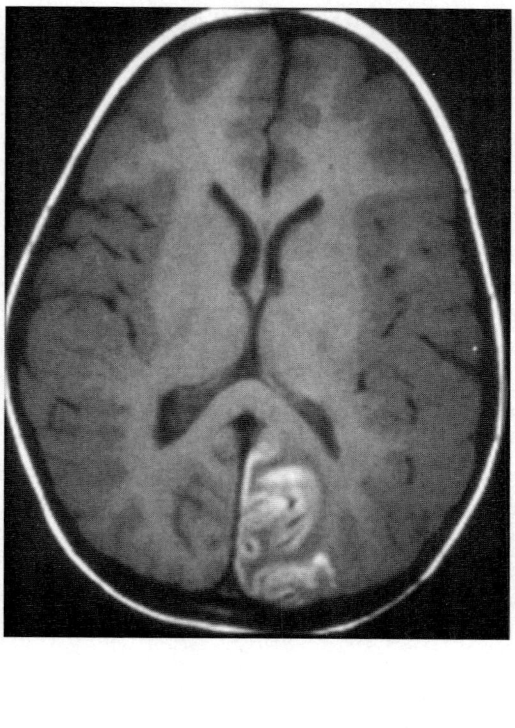

Figure 4.9 *Hypoglycemia.* Axial T1-weighted image in a child shows a left occipital infarction with areas of high signal in the cortex presumably due to laminar necrosis.

Disorders Related to Ethanol Abuse

Alcohol abuse is common and thus here discussed (however, I address liver failure at the beginning of this chapter). The sequelae of alcohol abuse include direct toxicity, dangerous behavior leading to cerebral and spinal trauma, nutrition (including vitamin deficiencies) abnormalities, and teratogenicity [including the fetal alcohol syndrome (FAS)] (41). Chronic alcohol consumption results in ataxia and lower limb incoordination that correlates well with cerebellar atrophy. Cerebellar atrophy is present in over 60% of alcoholics. There is shrinkage of the folia particularly in the superior vermis, reflecting a loss of Purkinje cells. Alcoholic myelopathy and peripheral neuropathy probably are related to a deficiency of thiamine. Other disorders associated with alcoholism are central pontine and extrapontine myelinolysis and the Marchiafava-Bignami syndrome (MB).

Clinical findings in acute Wernicke's encephalopathy mainly include impaired memory, confusion, hallucinations, abnormal eye movements, and ataxia.

The acute symptoms of the Wernicke-Korsakoff syndrome (WK) include lethargy, confusion, altered memory, nystagmus, ophthalmoplegia, and ataxia (42). Although WK is seen mostly in alcoholics, other related conditions include anorexia, protracted vomiting secondary to chemotherapy, digitalis toxicity, gastric plication procedures, starvation, and AIDS. The common underlying factor in all of these conditions is a deficiency of thiamine. After treatment, the patient may develop chronic memory problems (Korsakoff psychosis). Thiamine metabolism plays a role in brain glucose oxidation and membrane permeability to chloride ions. There is little reserve of thiamine, so its deficiency manifests early. Cerebral lactic acidosis occurs early. Glutamate (an excitatory amino acid) is found in high concentrations in thiamine-depleted brain regions. Acutely there is vascular dilatation and endothelial swelling, mostly involving small arteries. There is neuronal damage and swelling of astrocytes. This leads to ischemia of the mamillary bodies, the dorsomedial thalamic nuclei, the pulvinars, the walls of the third ventricle, periaqueductal gray matter, colliculi, third cranial nerve nuclei, inferior olives, and the superior cerebellar vermis (43). On MRI T2-weighted images, all of these regions may show abnormally high signal intensity (Fig. 4.10A and B). These findings are typical and in the correct clinical situation, they enable the diagnosis of acute Wernicke's encephalopathy. Contrast enhancement of the mamillary bodies or of the lateral walls of the third ventricle may be seen and is highly suggestive of this condition (44–46) (Fig. 4.10C and D). Hemorrhage is found only in approximately 20% of autopsy cases and usually is not seen on imaging studies. Absence of the aforementioned imaging abnormalities, however, does not exclude the diagnosis of Wernicke's encephalopathy. CT is of no utility in these patients. In the chronic stage of thiamine deficiency, vascular damage no longer is present. There is diffuse brain atrophy that is more prominent at the level of the fornices and mamillary bodies. MRI abnormalities reflect these findings.

Although central pontine myelinolysis may be seen in alcoholics, it also is the result of other conditions and is addressed in Chapter 3. MB is, however, seen mostly in alcoholics and is discussed here. MB is a rare disorder seen in chronic alcoholics (47,48). Although it initially was described in drinkers of Italian red wine, it may be seen in persons ingesting other types of alcoholic beverages. There is cystic necrosis of the corpus callosum, particularly of the genu and body. Similar lesions may be observed in the optic chiasm, anterior commissure, centrum semiovale, and brachium pontis. Histologically, there is demyelination with relative axonal preservation similar to that seen in cases of cyanide and carbon monoxide poisoning. MRI shows that the anterior region of the corpus callosum is of low T1 and high T2 signal intensity. Areas of abnormal increased T2 signal intensity also may be seen in the centrum semiovale. PET studies using fluorodeoxyglucose show diffusely decreased metabolism that is more pronounced in the frontal and parietal lobes, the frontobasal regions, and the thalamus. Cerebral perfusion studies show decreased perfusion corresponding to the regions of low glucose metabolism. These findings imply that MB is a diffuse brain disorder not localized only to the corpus callosum.

Alcoholics show atrophy of the cerebellum due to loss of Purkinje cell layer.

Alcohol is the most common teratogenic agent to which human beings are exposed. FAS was first described in the United States and France, but now is prevalent in other countries such as Russia (49). It is clinically characterized by mental retardation, anom-

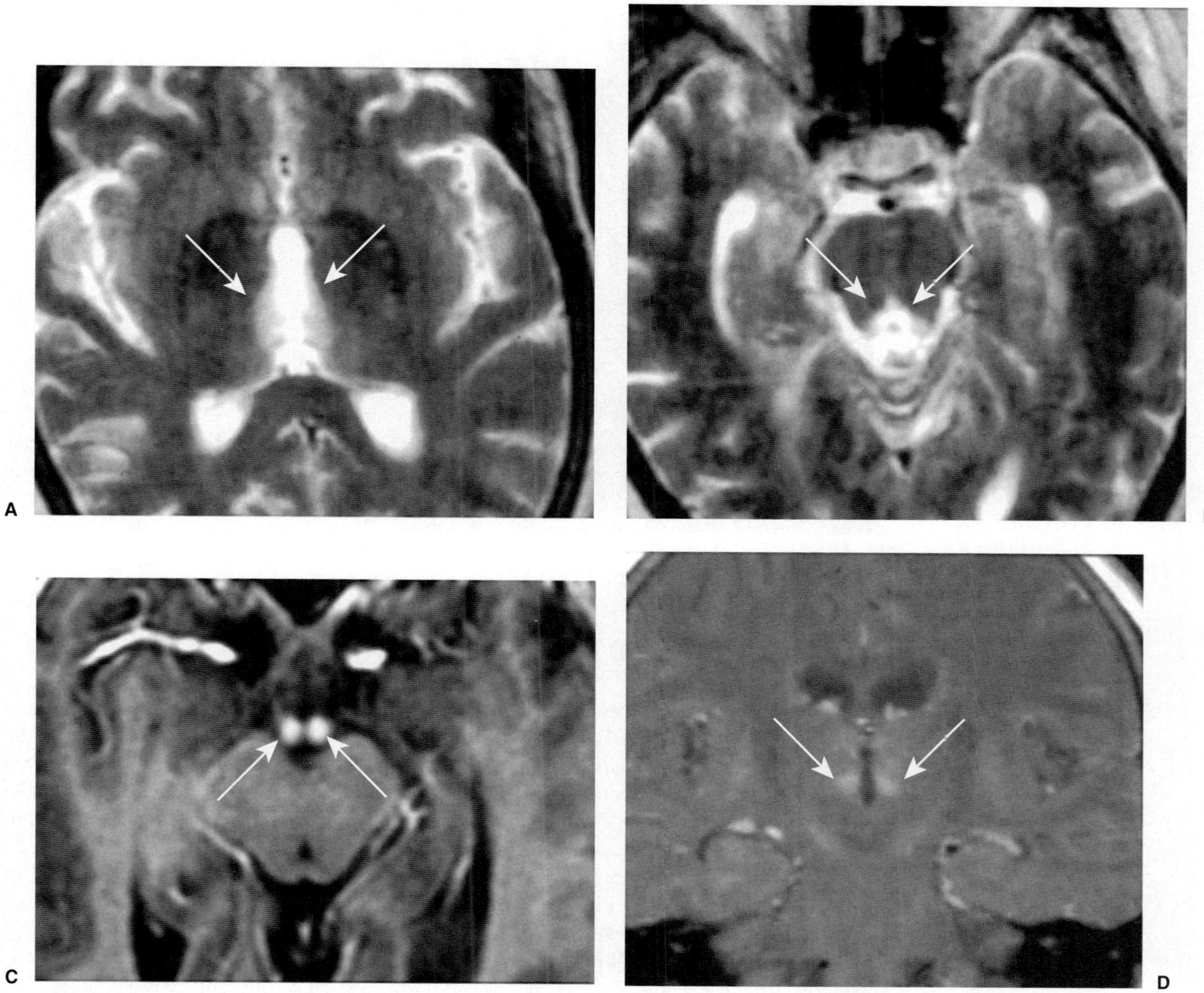

Figure 4.10 *Wernicke's Encephalopathy. A.* Axial T2-weighted image shows increased signal *(arrows)* in medial thalami. *B.* In the same patient, there is high T2 signal in the periaqueductal gray matter *(arrows)*. *C.* Axial postcontrast T1-weighted image shows enhancement of the mamillary bodies *(arrows)*. *D.* Coronal postcontrast T1-weighted image (different patient) shows enhancement *(arrows)* along the walls of the third ventricle.

alies of the CNS, dysmorphic facial features, and skeletal, cardiac, and urogenital abnormalities. Unfortunately, the mentation deficits are permanent and do not improve with age. The most common brain abnormalities include microcephaly, dysgenesis (and agenesis) of the corpus callosum, dysgenesis of the cerebellum and the brainstem, occipital meningoencephalocele, myelomeningocele, and holoprosencephaly. Facial anomalies include thin lips, small mandible and maxilla, and cleft lip and palate. Alcohol or its metabolites have adverse effects on the gastrulation stage of embryonic development by causing a reduction in the number of cells in the early neural plate and increased cell death (apoptosis) at the margins of the anterior neural folds. This mechanism explains the coexistence of brain and facial anomalies in FAS. Other common teratogens include carbamazepine, valproic acid, tretinoin, phenytoin, toluene, trimethadione, warfarin, cocaine, and probably benzodiazepines.

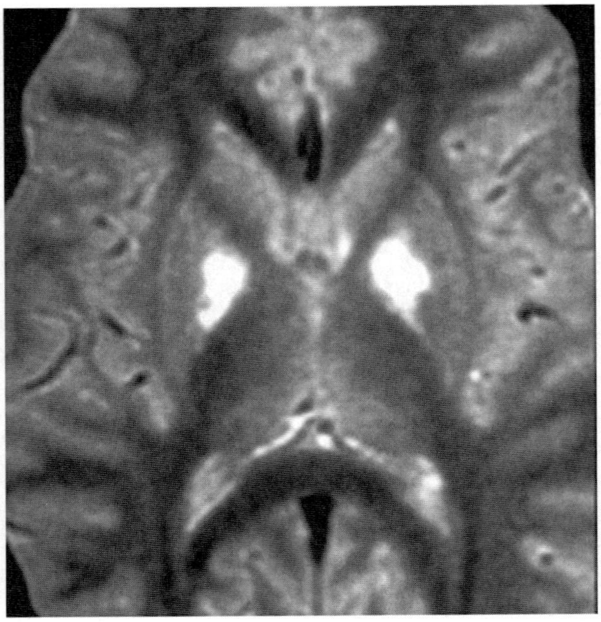

Figure 4.11 *Carbon Monoxide Intoxication.* Axial T2-weighted image shows high signal in the globi pallidi.

Carbon Monoxide Intoxication

Carbon monoxide (CO) results in nearly 6,000 accidental and suicide deaths per year in the United States alone (50). The most common causes of increased levels of CO are the burning of gasoline, kerosene, wood, coal, and, more recently, propane. Individuals working in enclosed spaces ("warehouse worker's headache") are particularly prone to acute CO intoxication. The incidence of CO intoxication is higher during the winter. Hemoglobin has a 200- to 250-fold greater affinity for CO than it does for carbon dioxide. CO affects the cytochrome oxidase system, impairs release of oxygen from tissues, and results in brain lipid peroxidation. Although symptoms tend to occur early, their severity has no correlation with the blood levels of CO. The early symptoms include headache, impaired vigilance, and abnormal audition and vision (50). Severe symptoms are nausea, vomiting, seizures, syncope, coma, and death. Classic findings such as the "cherry red" mucosa are rare. CO is directly responsible for the brain abnormalities. CO has two effects in the brain. First, it binds to regions that have a high oxygen demand (selective vulnerability mechanism) such as the globi pallidi (51) (Fig. 4.11). CO also binds to normal iron-containing structures such as the substantia nigra. It also is possible that systemic hypotension contributes or in some cases is mostly responsible for the brain lesions. MRI and CT show lesions confined mostly to the globi pallidi. These lesions are of low density on CT and high T2 signal intensity on MRI (51,52). The lesions are not hemorrhagic. If the patient survives, diffuse brain atrophy may ensue.

Glycol-Related Products Intoxication

Ethylene glycol is metabolized by the enzyme alcohol dehydrogenase; ethyl alcohol competes for this enzyme and may be used to treat ethylene glycol intoxication.

Ethylene glycol, a compound found in automobile antifreeze, hydraulic fluid, and industrial solvents, is a common cause of poisoning and suicide death (53). Other compounds, such as diethylene glycol and propylene glycol, also are toxic. The latter two compounds have been used to contaminate medications such as acetaminophen and resulted in toxic epidemics in Haiti, India, and Nigeria. After the ingestion of ethylene glycol, metabolic acidosis ensues that results in kidney damage owing to accumulation of calcium and oxalate crystals in urine and in acute renal failure that secondarily affects the CNS. A typ-

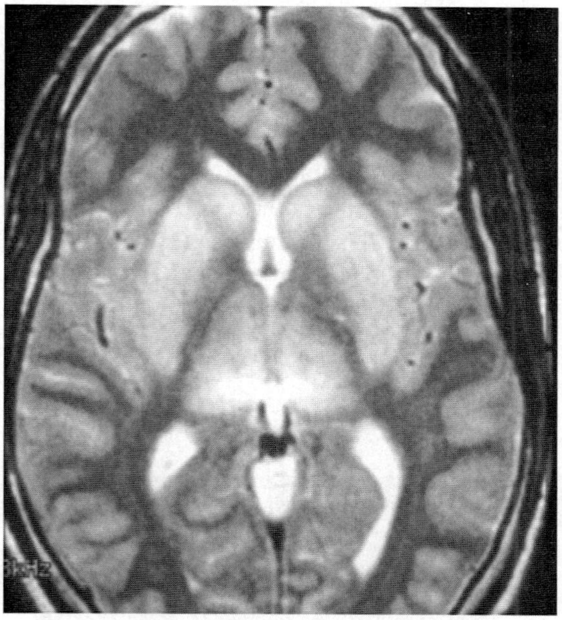

Figure 4.12 Ethylene Glycol Intoxication. Axial T2-weighted image shows high signal in the lentiform nuclei and the thalami.

ical clinical symptom of ethylene glycol poisoning is blindness. I have seen one patient in whom MRI performed within 6 hours of antifreeze ingestion showed abnormal increased T2 signal intensity in the putamen, globus pallidus, caudate nucleus, and thalamus (Fig. 4.12). No hemorrhages were present. The clinical manifestations of intoxication with diethylene glycol and propylene glycol include fever, vomiting, diarrhea, cough, abdominal pain, altered mentation, dyspnea, and acute renal failure.

Lead Intoxication

Acute lead poisoning in the United States is rare (54). Most cases of lead poisoning occurred in children secondary to the ingestion of peeling paint chips. Since 1978, lead-based paint has been banned for interior painting. Acute lead poisoning results in encephalopathy and diffuse cerebral edema. On gross examination, the brain shows congestion, petechial hemorrhages, thrombosis, and demyelination. In adults, most lead poisoning cases are chronic. Chronic lead intoxication occurs as a consequence of gasoline sniffing, inhalation of automobile exhaust fumes, lead smelting, and consumption of "moonshine" whiskey, and may be associated with battery manufacturing and lead glazing of pottery and crystal. Chronic exposure to lead results in intracranial calcifications, particularly in the cerebellum. It is thought that these calcifications are dystrophic secondary to underlying vascular damage. CT scanning and skull radiographs also may show widening of the cranial sutures in cases of chronic lead poisoning. I have seen one case of acute lead intoxication in which CT showed abnormal hypodensity in the subinsular regions, but in most cases there are no imaging abnormalities in the brain. Proton MRS may show substantially reduced NAA/Cr ratios in the white and gray matter (55). This finding may reflect a diffuse process affecting the neurons.

Methanol Intoxication

Methanol (methyl alcohol) is used in the production of antifreeze solution, in illegal drinks (as a substitute for ethanol), and in poor-quality cologne (56). After the ingestion of methanol, there is a latent period that ranges from 1 to 72 hours. Thereafter, metabolic acidosis and cortical blindness ensue. Other symptoms are parkinsonism, inebriation, headache, dizziness, seizures, and coma. Methanol and its byproducts (formaldehyde and formic acid) are toxic to the CNS. Putaminal hemorrhagic necrosis is a typical histologic feature. Imaging studies correlate well with this finding. CT shows the putamina to be of low density, swollen, and to contain small hemorrhages (57) (Fig. 4.13A). MRI shows these regions to be of either low or high T1 signal intensity and hyperintense on T2-weighted images (58) (Fig. 4.13B and C). Other patients also show cortical necrosis, particularly in the paramedian aspects of the frontal lobes. This finding results in high T2 signal intensity in the affected cortex. The cerebellum and occipital regions typically are spared. Optic atrophy may be seen, but the signal intensity in these structures remains within normal limits. The white matter may be diffusely edematous.

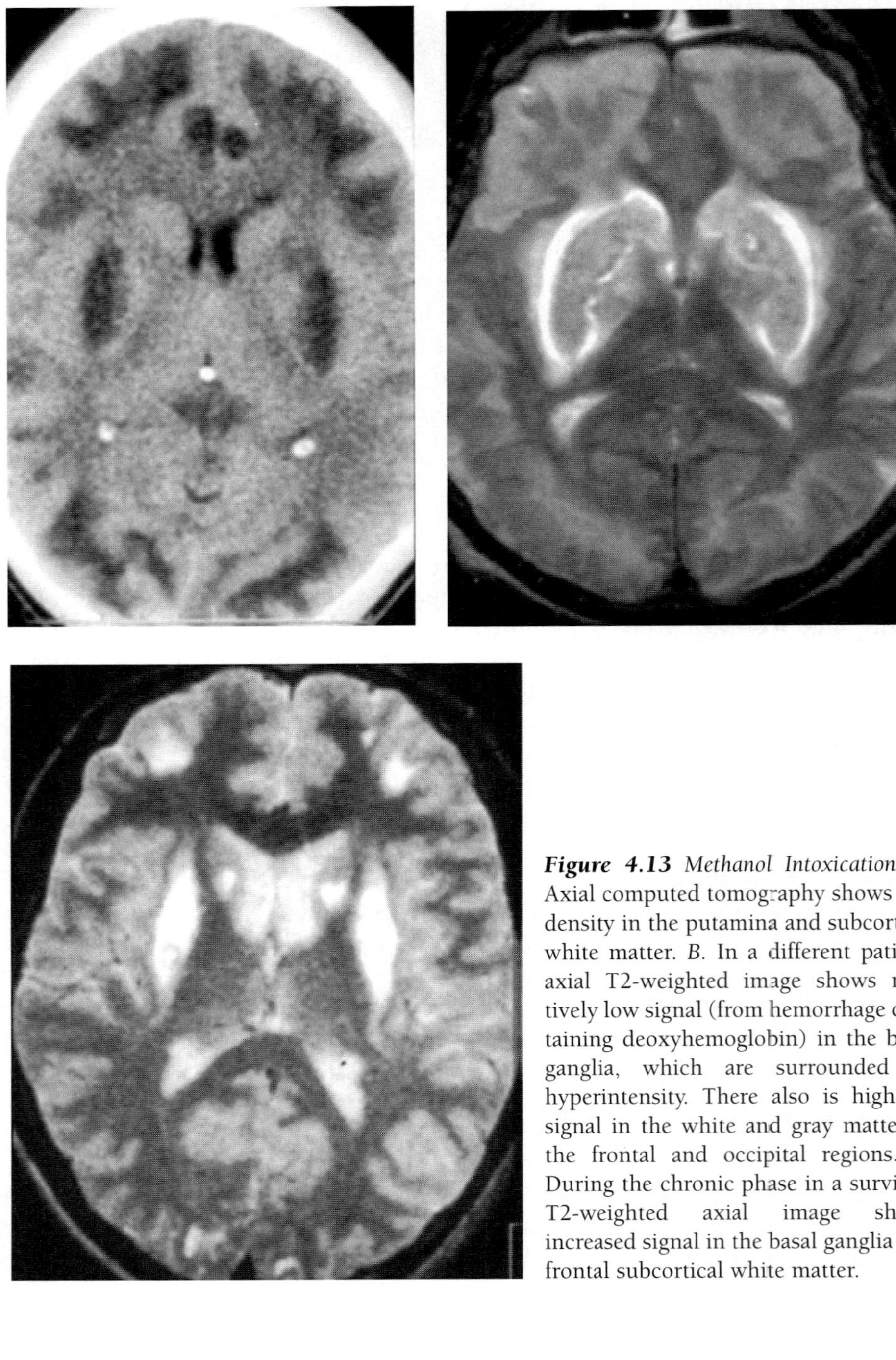

A B C

Figure 4.13 *Methanol Intoxication. A.* Axial computed tomography shows low density in the putamina and subcortical white matter. *B.* In a different patient, axial T2-weighted image shows relatively low signal (from hemorrhage containing deoxyhemoglobin) in the basal ganglia, which are surrounded by hyperintensity. There also is high T2 signal in the white and gray matter of the frontal and occipital regions. *C.* During the chronic phase in a survivor, T2-weighted axial image shows increased signal in the basal ganglia and frontal subcortical white matter.

Mercury Intoxication

Mercury intoxication usually is the result of the ingestion of contaminated fish and is more common in Japan and the Amazon River basin.

Mercury poisoning is rare and may occur after the ingestion of organic or inorganic mercury (59). Organic mercury intoxication results from the consumption of contaminated fish or pork (as a sequela of the use of mercury-based fungicides). Symptoms include ataxia, neuropathy, choreoathetosis, visual loss, confusion, and coma. Chronic ingestion of mercury-laden fish was first described in Japan (Minamata disease), but has now been found in other parts of the world, such as the Amazon River, where fish is a dietary staple (60). In these patients, MRI shows atrophy of the calcarine and postcentral cortex as well as the cerebellar vermis. These areas are slightly hypointense on T1-weighted images and of high T2 signal intensity. It is thought that these findings reflect underlying spongiotic changes and that they correlate well with the symptoms of visual field deficits, sensory abnormalities, and ataxia. Inorganic mercury poisoning is not addressed here because it usually results in gastrointestinal symptoms without neurologic complications.

Inhalant Abuse

Inhaling solvents, volatile substances, and glue vapors results in a transient euphoric state. Inhalant abuse most commonly occurs in teenagers (61). The most commonly abused substances are listed in Table 4.2 (61).

The fumes of these substances may be inhaled directly or by placing them in a bag or rag. After an initial euphoric state, drowsiness and sleep ensue. Because the brain is a lipid-laden organ, these compounds have a great affinity for it. Suffocation, aspiration, and dangerous behavior are common causes of death. The neuropathologic and imaging features of toluene abuse ("spray heads") are well known. Chronic abuse of toluene results in cognitive impairment, cerebellar ataxia, tremor, and anosmia. MRI shows diffuse cerebral, cerebellar, and brainstem atrophy. T2-weighted images show an abnormal increase in the signal intensity of the white matter reflecting underlying gliosis (62). Hypointensity in the basal ganglia and thalamus is seen on both T1- and T2-weighted images and is believed to be the result of iron deposition (a nonspecific finding appreciable in many degenerative brain disorders) (63). It has been suggested that partitioning of toluene into the lipid membranes of cells in the brain may be responsible for this finding. *In vitro* experiments show that toluene-tainted lipid bilayers dramatically shorten T2 relaxation times. Other reported MRI findings in toluene abuse include loss of the cerebral and cerebellar gray–white matter discrimination, scattered foci of abnormal signal intensity in the white matter, thinning of the corpus callosum, and generalized atrophy.

The effects of nitrous oxide on the CNS have been documented (64). Nitrous oxide commonly is used in dental anesthesia and as a propellant in certain foods such as whipped cream. Contrary to other inhalants, nitrous oxide is not readily available to children and teenagers and its abuse is more common in the adult population. Nitrous oxide causes damage by irreversibly oxidizing vitamin B_{12}. On a chronic basis, this results in formation of abnormal substrates for fatty acid synthesis that eventually are incorporated

Table 4.2: Commonly Abused Inhalants

Aerosols	*Liquids*
Paint	Model-building glue and contact cement
Butane	Gasoline
Cooking sprays	Laquers
Cosmetics and toiletries	Dry cleaning fluids
Nitrous oxide	Typewriter correction fluid
	Lighter fluids

into the formation of myelin. The clinical manifestations of chronic nitrous oxide toxicity are thus identical to those of vitamin B_{12} deficiency. There is involvement of the posterior columns of the spinal cord beginning at the thoracic level. This eventually leads to subacute spinal cord degeneration. On T2-weighted images, there may be abnormal increased signal intensity that usually is confined to the posterior columns. After appropriate therapy, this abnormality may resolve completely. In some patients, a peripheral neuropathy also develops.

Huntington's Disease

This autosomal dominant (complete penetrance) inherited disorder is characterized by onset of choreiform movements during the fourth decade of life and death 10 to 30 years after onset (65). The abnormal gene is in chromosome 4. The juvenile form of the disease begins during the second decade of life but accounts for only 5% of all patients with Huntington's disease. There is neuronal loss and gliosis predominantly affecting the heads of the caudate nuclei, which become symmetrically small (Fig. 4.14). The globi pallidi also are affected, but to a lesser degree. Unfortunately, these changes are evident only late in the course of the disease. Most patients have been diagnosed with Huntington's disease by the time of imaging, or it is well known that their parents had it. With progression of the disease, there may be increased iron deposition in the lentiform nuclei and diffuse atrophy (65,66).

Hyperglycemia

Lesions that affect the subthalamic nuclei or the globus pallidus may result in increased cortical outflow and hemiballismus.

Hyperglycemia also has adverse affects on the CNS (67). Hyperglycemia may lead to increases in cerebral lactic acid that may damage the brain primarily or worsen the outcome of patients with underlying infarctions. A typical manifestation and, at times the initial one of hyperglycemia is hemichorea–hemiballism (HH) (68–70). The clinical manifestation of HH are random and fast jerking motion in the distal extremities (chorea) and violent flinging and kicking mainly involving the proximal joints (ballismus). In these

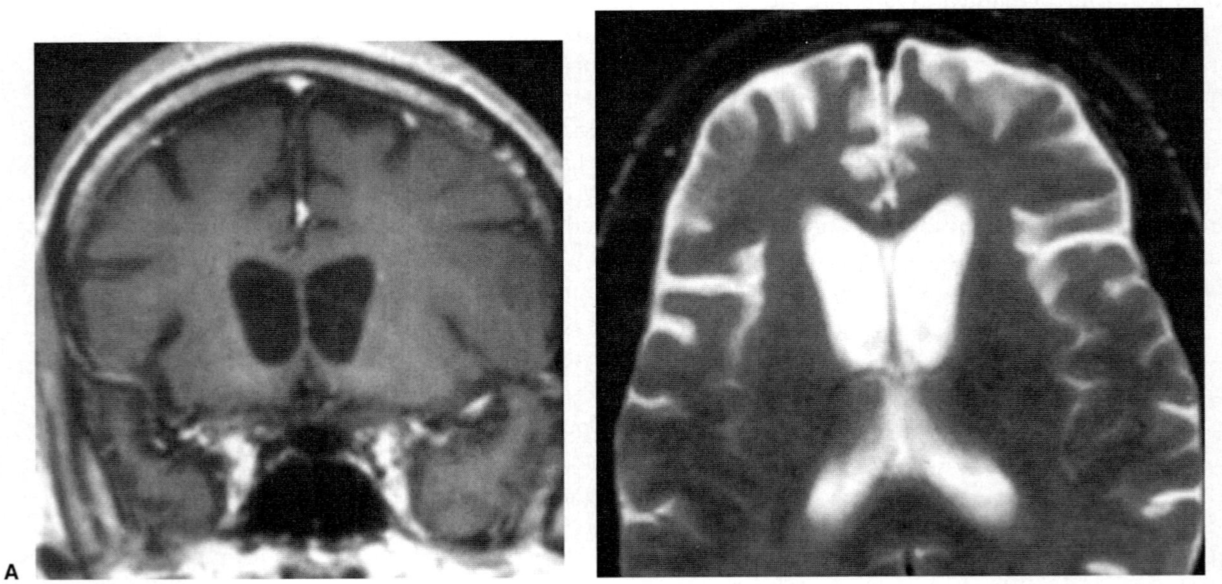

Figure 4.14 *Huntington's Chorea.* Coronal T1- *A* and axial T2-weighted *B* images shows significant atrophy of the head of the caudate nuclei, leading to prominent frontal horns of the lateral ventricles.

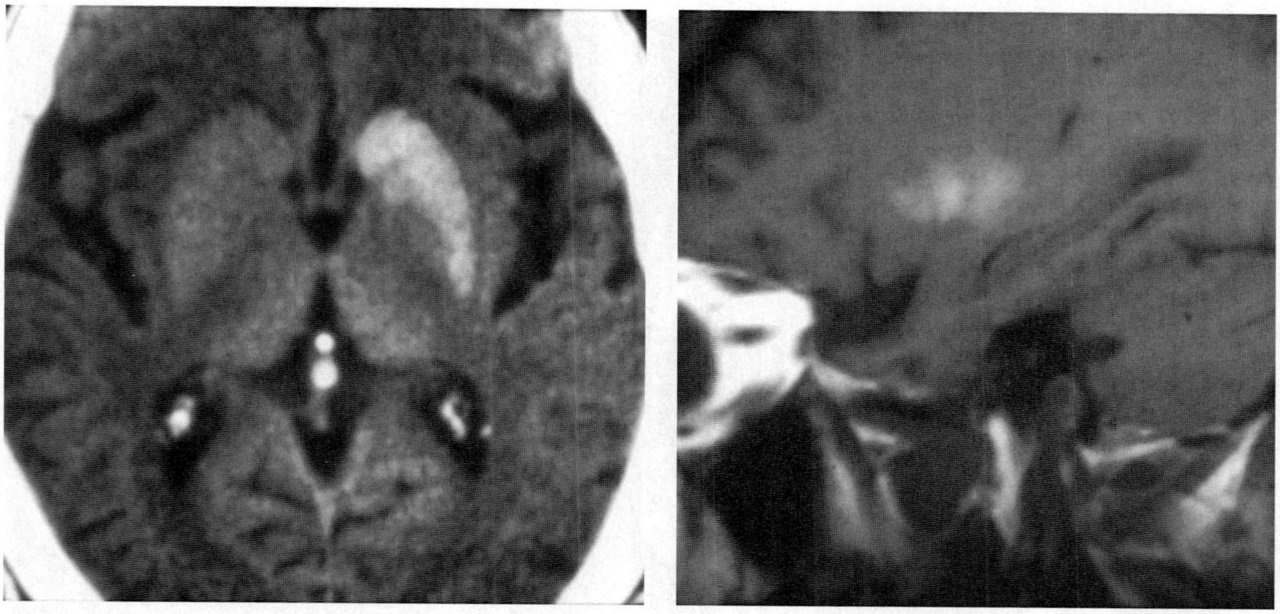

A B

Figure 4.15 *Hyperglycemia.* Axial computed tomography *A* and sagittal T1-weighted image *B* in a patient with hemichorea–hemiballismus shows increased density and signal intensity in the left basal ganglia.

patients, CT shows high density conforming to one lentiform nucleus and the head of the ipsilateral caudate nucleus. These regions are of increased signal intensity on MRI T1-weighted images, and the corresponding T2-weighted images are normal (Fig. 4.15). Occasionally, the ipsilateral cerebral peduncle also may show T1 hyperintensity in its anteromedial region. Hemorrhage or calcifications are not present in HH and the findings are thought be due to the presence of gemistocytes. Proton MRS obtained from the region of T1 signal intensity abnormality demonstrates elevated lactic acid and decreased creatine. These features have been interpreted as being due to depletion of energy, leading to neuronal malfunction. Although the aforementioned MRI abnormalities are fairly typical for HH, they also have been noted in a patient with lupus erythematosus and chorea.

Amyotrophic Lateral Sclerosis

Amyotrophic lateral sclerosis (ALS) is the most common motor neuron disorder. It is seen predominantly in men between 50 and 70 years of age. There are three clinical subtypes of the disease: upper and lower motor neurons, upper motor neurons, and lower motor neurons (71). The symptoms are muscle weakness, fasciculations, hyperreflexia, spasticity, and muscle atrophy. Dementia occurs late in the disease. ALS usually is sporadic, but in some instances it is inherited as an autosomal dominant trait. Histologically, there is loss of neurons and their axons with little reactive gliosis. Axonal spheroids (representing degenerating and swollen axons) are typical of ALS. Thereafter, there is antegrade degeneration of the pyramidal and corticospinal tracts. It predominantly affects the cortex (particularly the perirolandic regions) and ventral gray matter horns of the spinal cord, with subsequent degeneration of the corresponding white matter tracts (72). There is atrophy of the cortex, increased T2 and fluid attenuation inversion recovery (FLAIR) signal intensity in corticospinal tracts (this is well seen on coronal T2-weighted images), and atrophy of the ventral spinal nerve roots (73) (Figs. 4.16A and B). Increased iron deposition in the affected cortex may be seen (but in many older patients this occurs normally and should not be misinterpreted as abnormal; Fig. 4.16C).

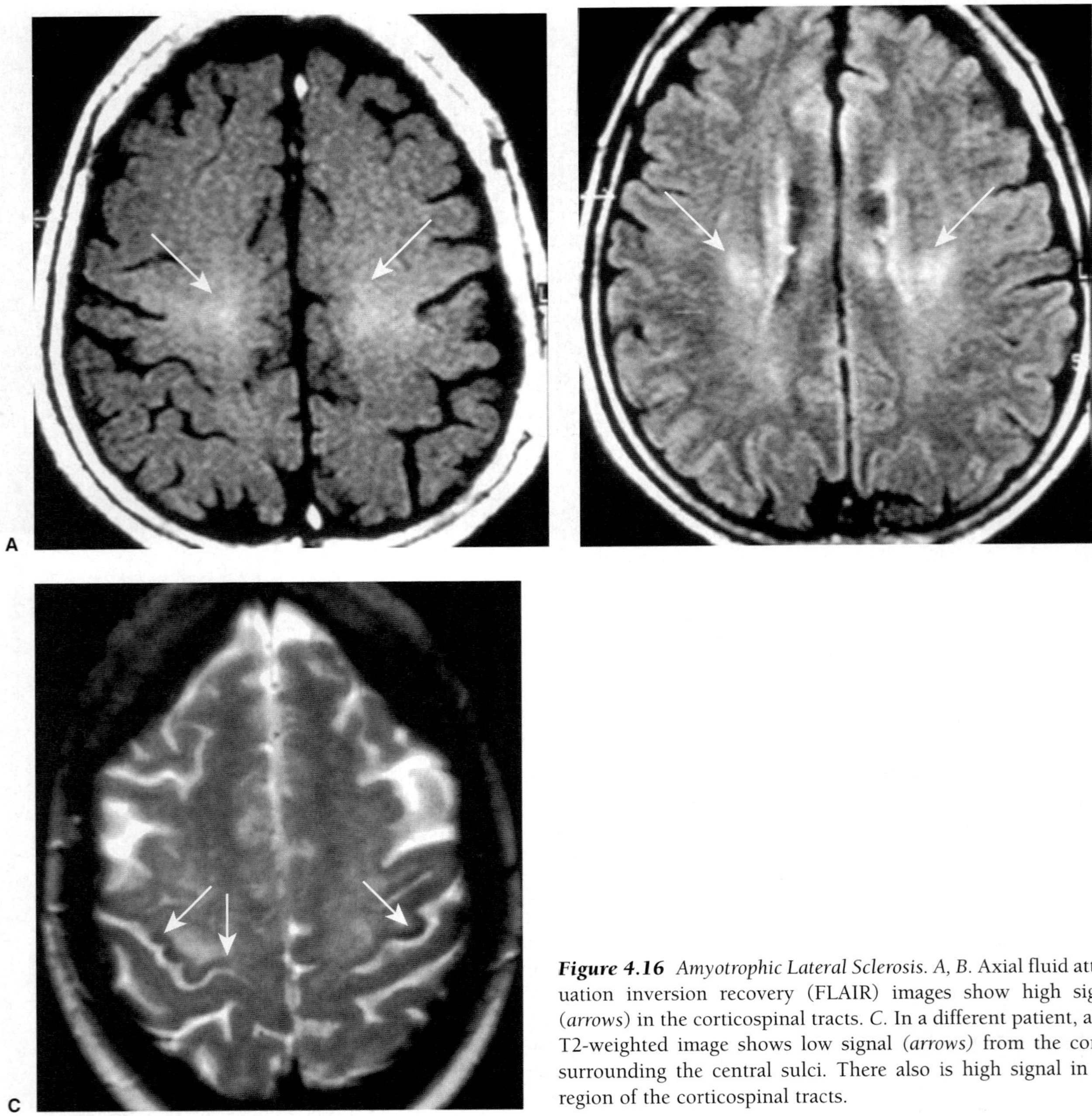

Figure 4.16 *Amyotrophic Lateral Sclerosis. A, B.* Axial fluid attenuation inversion recovery (FLAIR) images show high signal (*arrows*) in the corticospinal tracts. *C.* In a different patient, axial T2-weighted image shows low signal *(arrows)* from the cortex surrounding the central sulci. There also is high signal in the region of the corticospinal tracts.

Alzheimer's Disease

On perfusion MRI, the temporoparietal relative cerebral blood flow is reduced in patients with Alzheimer's disease.

Alzheimer's disease (AD) is the most common type of dementia in the United States (74). Most patients are diagnosed at 50 to 65 years of age, but it may occur in younger or older individuals. AD leads to death usually from 7 to 10 years after the diagnosis. The clinical diagnosis of AD is very difficult. The basic abnormalities in AD are the presence of neurofibrillary tangles and senile plaques. The neurofibrillary tangles represent protein (tau) filaments inside the axons. They probably are involved in preventing normal axonal transport. The senile plaques are accumulations of extracellular amyloid (amyloid beta protein). These plaques also occur with normal aging, but their concentration is markedly increased in AD. The origin of these plaques is debatable. The loss of neurons and the presence of senile plaques result in an inflammatory reaction. These

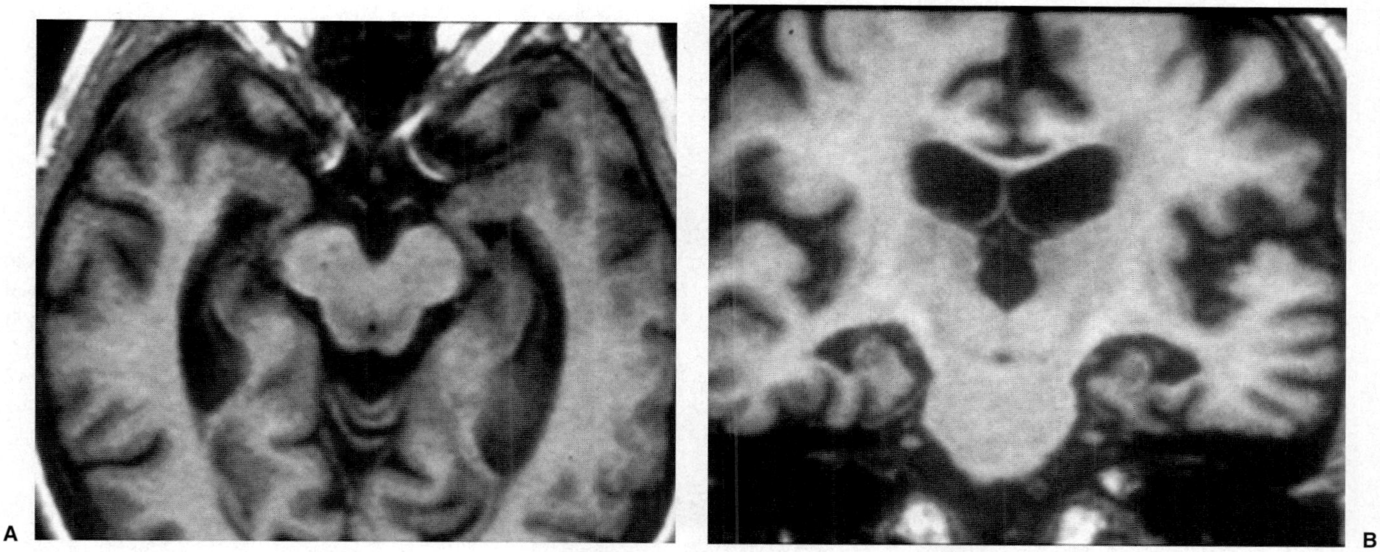

Figure 4.17 *Alzheimer's Disease.* Axial *A* and coronal *B* T1-weighted images show significant atrophy of the hippocampi and other structures in the mesial temporal lobes.

findings are seen throughout the brain but particularly in the frontal, parietal, and mesial temporal regions. CT and MRI have been used to map the degree and location of atrophy (75). Imaging studies most often are negative or show only nonspecific diffuse and atrophy that is disproportionately greater in the frontal, parietal, and temporal regions (particularly the hippocampi) may suggest AD in the correct clinical setting (Fig. 4.17). PET shows decreased glucose metabolism in the same regions, whereas SPECT shows decreased cerebral blood flow also in the same regions (76). Perfusion MRI confirms these findings. Proton MRS may be helpful in making the diagnosis. This study shows low NAA and elevated myoinositol. Elevation of myoinositol is not found in other dementias and may be typical of AD (77). A recent article shows that apparent diffusion coefficients in the hippocampi of patients with AD are higher than those in normal control subjects (78).

Parkinson's Disease

Parkinson's disease may be primary (idiopathic) or secondary (usually these patients have infarcts or other lesions in the head of the caudate nuclei). It is the most common subcortical degenerative brain disease. Symptoms are bradykinesia (slow movements), resting tremor, cogwheel rigidity, and postural abnormalities. Pathologically, there is loss of neurons in the substantia nigra (particularly in the pars compacta). When this loss exceeds 80%, symptoms ensue. By MRI, there is increased iron deposition in the midbrain narrowing the width of the pars compacta, although this finding is very hard to see on fast spin-echo (FSE) T2-weighted images (it requires the use of gradient-echo imaging) (79) (Fig. 4.18). As the disease progresses, there may be diffuse cerebral atrophy. Proton MRS shows low NAA not only in the basal ganglia but throughout the brain, implying that Parkinson's probably is a diffuse disease (80). By the time of imaging, the diagnosis of Parkinson's disease is well established in most patients. Imaging is helpful to distinguish between primary and secondary Parkinson's disease. Imaging also is helpful when a pallidotomy or thalamotomy is being considered (81). These images need to be obtained using thin sections that are accepted by most current computerized neuronavigation surgical systems. MRI also is performed after these procedures to evaluate for possible complications (mostly hemorrhages; Fig 4.19).

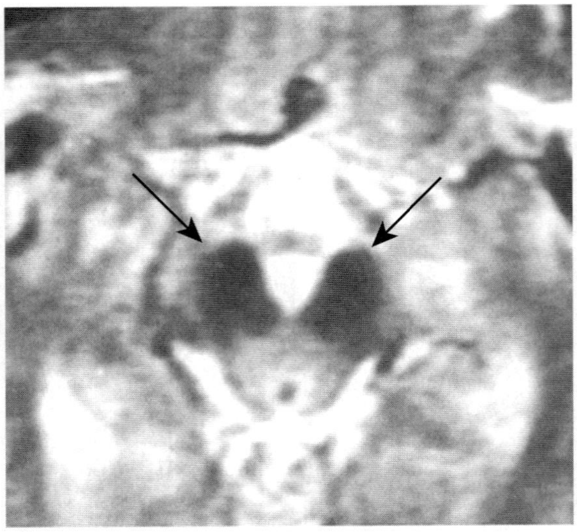

Figure 4.18 *Parkinson's Disease.* Axial T2*-weighted image shows increased iron (dark signal, *arrows*) deposition in the midbrain with complete disappearance of the normal signal intensity of the pars reticulata of the substantia nigra.

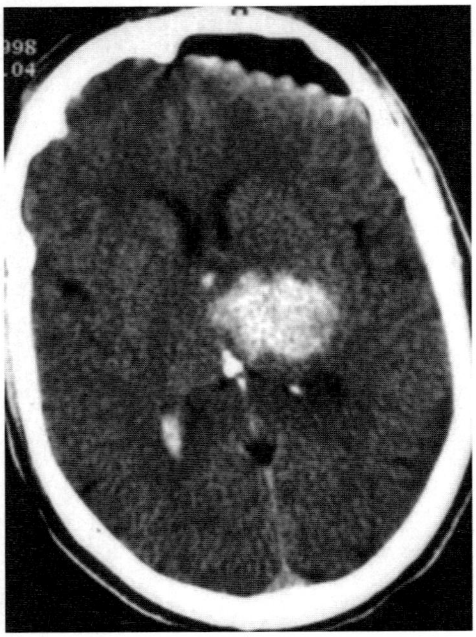

Figure 4.19 *Postthalamotomy Complication.* Axial computed tomography shows acute hemorrhage in the left thalamus.

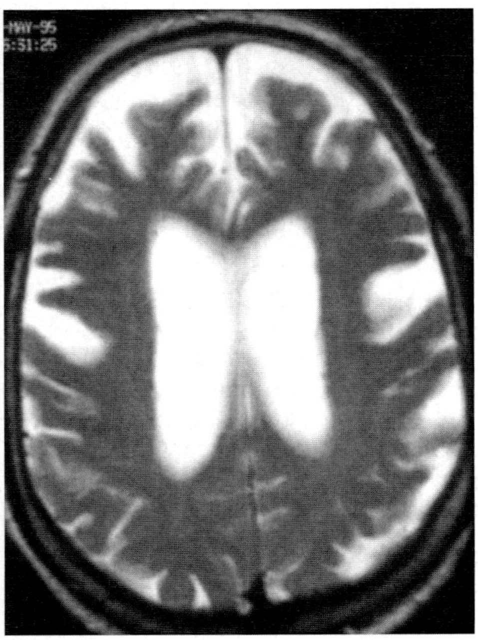

Figure 4.20 *Pick's Disease.* Axial T2-weighted image shows diffuse atrophy that is more pronounced in the frontal and temporal regions.

Pick's Disease

Differentiating between Pick's disease and Alzheimer's disease often is difficult from clinical and imaging standpoints. Pick's disease, however, is more common in female patients (82). It may be transmitted as an autosomal dominant trait. Histologically, there is neuronal loss, particularly in the frontal regions. The neurons contain cytoplasmic inclusion bodies called *Pick's bodies*. The pathology correlates well with the symptoms, and most patients exhibit abnormal behavior. MRI findings are nonspecific but show atrophy in the frontal lobes and to a lesser degree in the temporal lobes (Fig. 4.20). PET shows glucose hypometabolism in this region, and SPECT shows decreased cerebral blood flow in the frontal lobes.

Olivopontocerebellar Degeneration

Olivopontocerebellar degeneration (OPCD; also called *olivopontocerebellar atrophy*) is a part of the spectrum of multisystem atrophy syndromes. The multisystem atrophy syndromes (Parkinson's plus syndrome) are as follows:

- Olivopontocerebellar degeneration
- Shy-Drager syndrome
- Striatonigral degeneration

OPCD may be sporadic or familial (84). All 83 have clinical findings similar to those in Parkinson's disease, but are unresponsive to treatment with levodopa. The symptoms tend to be more severe and to progress rapidly. Ataxia is more common in OPCD than in the other syndromes. MRI shows significant atrophy of the brainstem, cerebellar hemispheres (reflecting a loss of Purkinje cells), and vermis that is disproportionate to the degree of supratentorial atrophy (Fig. 4.21A). Axial T2-weighted images show a typical "cross-shaped" area of increased signal intensity in the lower pons (Fig. 4.21B). These linear areas of T2 hyperintensity correspond to degeneration of the transverse pontine fibers and of the median raphe (which delimits the normal pyramidal tracts). The middle cerebellar peduncles also may be bright on T2-weighted images, but the inferior and superior cerebellar peduncles remain of normal signal intensity (although they do become atrophic). The lateral putamina occasionally also show T2 hyperintensity.

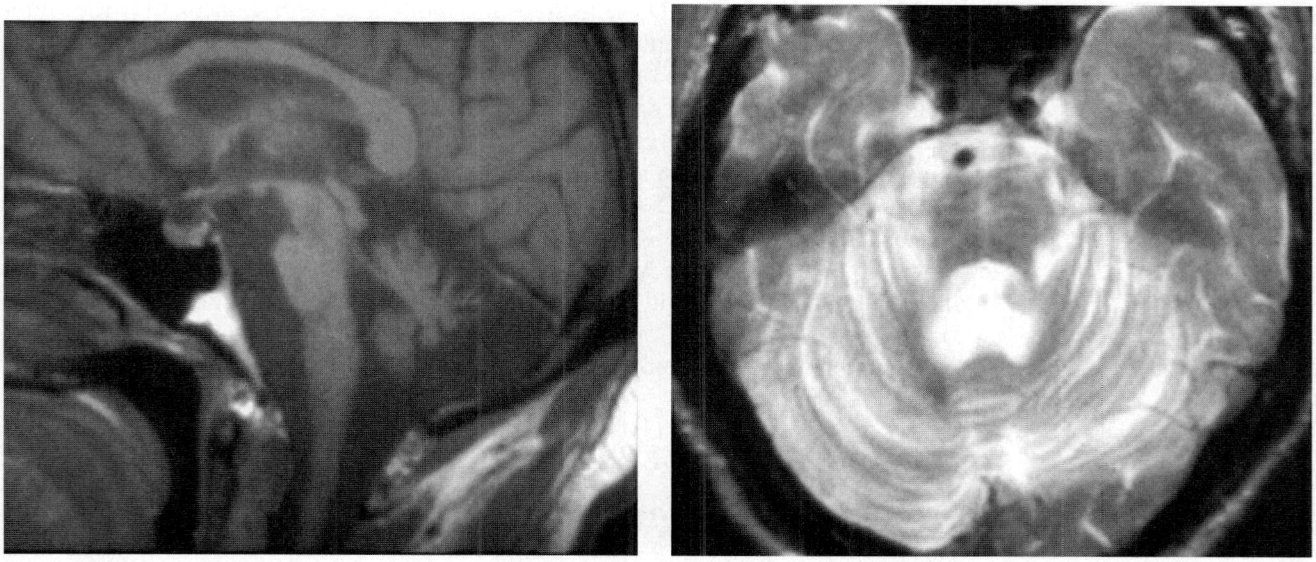

A B

Figure 4.21 *Olivopontocerebellar Degeneration.* Sagittal T1- *A* and axial T2-weighted *B* images show significant atrophy of the cerebellar hemispheres, vermis, and brainstem. On the T2-weighted image, note the increased signal in the pontine transverse fibers typical of this disease.

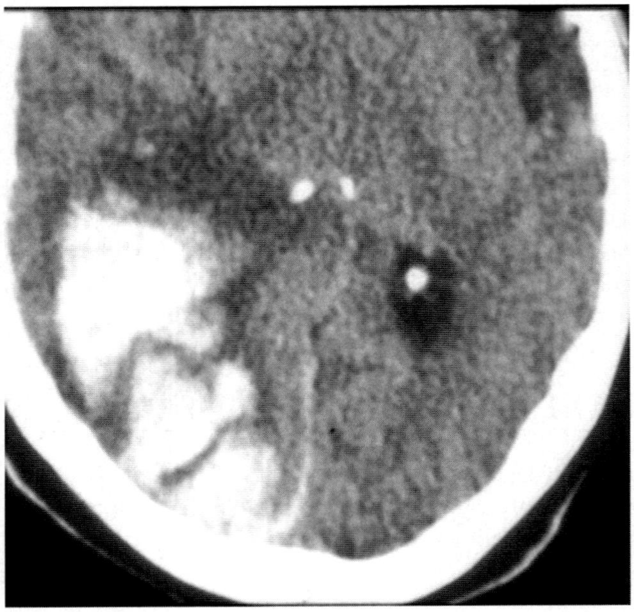

***Figure* 4.22** *Amyloid-Related Hemorrhage.* Axial computed tomography shows large right occipital acute bleed involving white and gray matter.

AMYLOIDOSIS

Amyloidosis is the underlying cause for approximately 5% to 10% of intracerebral hemorrhages in the elderly.

A detailed review of this complex entity is beyond the scope of this chapter. Amyloidosis is a group of disorders that may result in systemic or local manifestations (85,86). Amyloid is composed mostly of fibrils arranged in a cross-beta pleated fashion. These fibrils are responsible for the birefringence of amyloid under polarized light microscopy. It is an insoluble compound and is deposited in the organ that produces it. The second component that makes up amyloid (beta component) is a protein and is identical in all types of amyloid. Amyloid A is seen in inflammatory processes and in senile amyloidosis. Amyloid AL is a light chain from immunoglobulin M and commonly is found in patients with multiple myeloma. In the brain, amyloid infiltrates neurons and the media and adventitia of blood vessel walls (86). The frontal, parietal, occipital, and temporal lobes are affected. Amyloid weakens the walls of vessels and may even result in formation of microaneurysms. These features are thought to be responsible for the common brain hematomas occurring in these patients (Fig. 4.22). Senile amyloidosis is not uncommon after 80 years of life. Amyloidosis accounts for 5% to 10% of intracerebral hemorrhages in elderly people. Other cerebral manifestations of amyloidosis are recurrent transient neurologic events, rapidly progressing dementia, and masslike lesions (amyloidomas) (87). Brain amyloidomas often are isolated and not associated with systemic forms of the disease. Amyloid-related cerebral hemorrhages tend to be cortical or subcortical in location. The hematomas are large and often multifocal. The location of these hemorrhages may be mirror-like in both hemispheres. Amyloidomas may be found in the parenchyma, choroid plexuses, gasserian ganglion, spine, pituitary gland, orbits, larynx, and tongue. They manifest as nonspecific, nonenhancing masses, and the correct diagnosis requires a biopsy.

DISEASES AFFECTING THE KIDNEYS AND THE BRAIN

Patients with acute renal failure, leading to rapid accumulation of blood, commonly manifest symptoms that may lead to a coma. Symptoms of water intoxication include abnormal mentation, headache, nausea, vomiting, and muscle irritability (88). Water dilutes intracellular sodium and potassium (for a discussion of osmotic myelinolysis, see later). Brain edema is common in these patients. Uremic encephalopathy is an acute process often involving altered mental status. Other symptoms include tremor, loss of hearing and vision, choreoathetosis, and hemiballismus. Uremia affects neurotransmission, enzymes, blood vessels, membranes, and receptors. The relationship between neurologic disorders and acute and chronic renal failure is summarized in Box 4.1 (88).

Seizures, particularly status epilepticus, may result in hypertension that in turn causes areas of vasogenic and cytotoxic brain edema.

Over 40% of patients with malignant hypertension develop brain abnormalities, and approximately 20% die secondary to these lesions. Hypertension commonly results in brain edema and infarctions but also may cause thrombosis and hemorrhages. Loss of cerebral vascular autoregulation leads to the development of the so-called posterior reversible encephalopathy syndrome (PRES) (89). This syndrome is multifactorial and is characterized by fairly large and symmetric areas of increased T2 signal intensity involving the occipital and parietal regions. The abnormalities affect both gray and white matter. Using diffusion-weighted imaging, the abnormalities may be further characterized. The apparent diffusion coefficients in the zones of T2 hyperintensity seem to indicate that most of these areas are not infarctions but are related to vasogenic edema. Infarctions do, however, occur in some patients. The importance of this observation is that it may be used to establish prognosis and institute treatment, particularly in patients with cerebral infarctions. It is possible that contrast perfusion MRI also may be able to distinguish lesions representing only edema from infarctions. The clinical and imaging manifestations of PRES are identical to those found in patients receiving cyclosporine and other immunosuppressive drugs (89). It is possible that in these patients the brain abnormalities also are related to hypertension. A failure of cerebral vascular autoregulation occurs when the vasoconstrictive threshold is exceeded and perivascular edema ensues. This edema in turn compresses the microvasculature, aggravating the lesions. It also is possible that severe vasoconstriction, a mechanism initially set in motion to protect the brain, leads to compromised capillary integrity, resulting in edema, microinfarctions, and microscopic hemorrhages. This is important because hemorrhages should not be visible by MRI in PRES. Some diseases that affect both the kidneys and the brain are:

- Thrombotic thrombocytopenic purpura
- Hemolytic–uremic syndrome
- Hepatorenal syndrome
- Amyloidosis
- Metabolic disorders producing proximal tubular acidosis (cystinosis, galactosemia, glycogen storage disorders, hereditary fructose intolerance, Lowe's syndrome, pyruvate carboxylase deficiency, Sjögren's syndrome, tyrosinemia, and Wilson's disease)
- Metabolic disorders producing distal tubular acidosis (chronic active hepatitis, cryoglobulinemia, Fabry's disease, glycogen storage disease, leprosy, neuroaxonal dystrophy, primary biliary cirrhosis, hyperparathyroidism, sickle cell anemia, Sjögren's syndrome, systemic lupus erythematosus, thyroiditis, and Wilson's disease) (88)

Box 4.1: Acute and Chronic Renal Disorders that Affect the Brain

Water intoxication	Hypotension
Hyperkalemia	Hemodialysis
Uremic encephalopathy	Uremic states
Hypertensive encephalopathy	

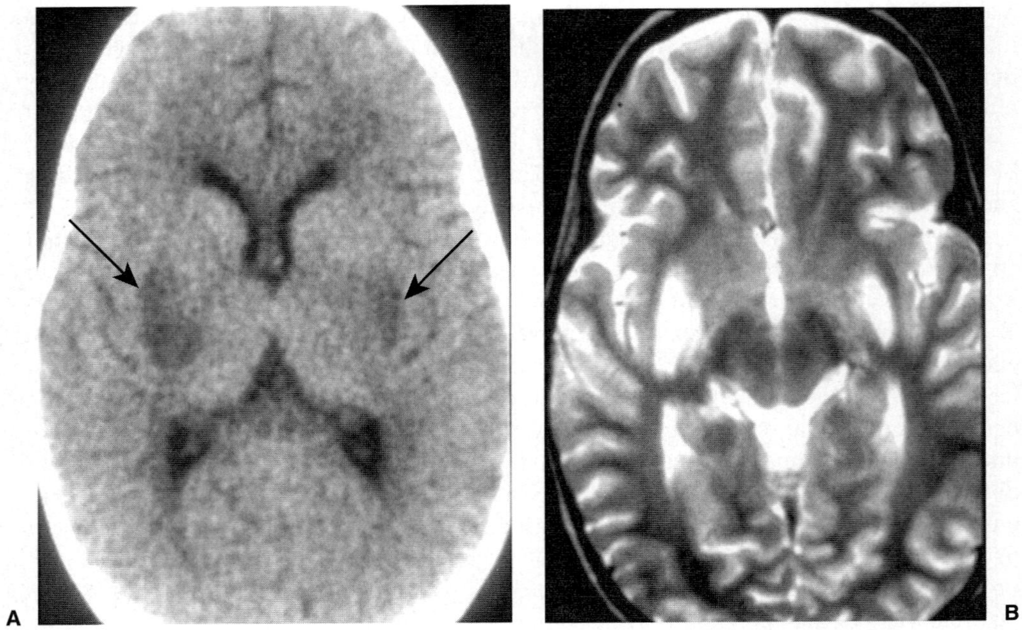

Figure 4.23 *Hemolytic–Uremic Syndrome. A.* Axial computed tomography shows low density in the putamina *(arrows). B.* Corresponding T2-weighted image shows increased signal in the same locations.

Thrombotic thrombocytopenic purpura (TTP) is a disorder characterized by thrombocytopenia, microangiopathic anemia, and neurologic symptoms (90). It results in widespread thrombosis of small vessels. It is clinically indistinguishable (and probably related) to the hemolytic–uremic syndrome (91). The neurologic symptoms are more pronounced in TTP than in hemolytic–uremic syndrome. There is an anomaly of circulating factors related to platelet adhesion in patients with TTP. Skin and mucosal purpura are typical and occur early. The neurologic symptoms are fatigue, confusion, headache, and abnormal vision and language. The imaging findings for TTP and hemolytic–uremic syndrome also are similar and often reported together. There may be small and disseminated brain hemorrhages. No large vessel occlusions are seen. Small infarctions involving the basal ganglia and thalamus occur in approximately 50% of patients (Fig. 4.23). Scattered multifocal and confluent lesions involving the cortex and underlying white matter are common. These abnormalities show high T2 signal intensity. They are similar to the lesions seen in PRES (see earlier). They may resolve or go on to become permanent infarctions, some of which show evidence of laminar necrosis. Laminar necrosis is seen as fine linear areas of increased T1 signal intensity in the deep cortex. The frontal lobes also may be involved.

Thyroid Gland Disorders Affecting the Brain

The interactions between the thyroid gland and the brain are complex. Primary thyroid gland disorders may affect the CNS, and some disorders of the brain also affect the function of this gland. Hypothyroidism may be the result of prior surgery on or around the pituitary gland or the presence of tumor in or around the pituitary gland, or it may be a sequela of prior brain irradiation. Hypothyroidism may lead to intellectual deterioration, calcium deposition in the brain, and enlargement of the pituitary gland (92). Central hypothyroidism may be an isolated defect or part of panhypopituitarism. Long-standing

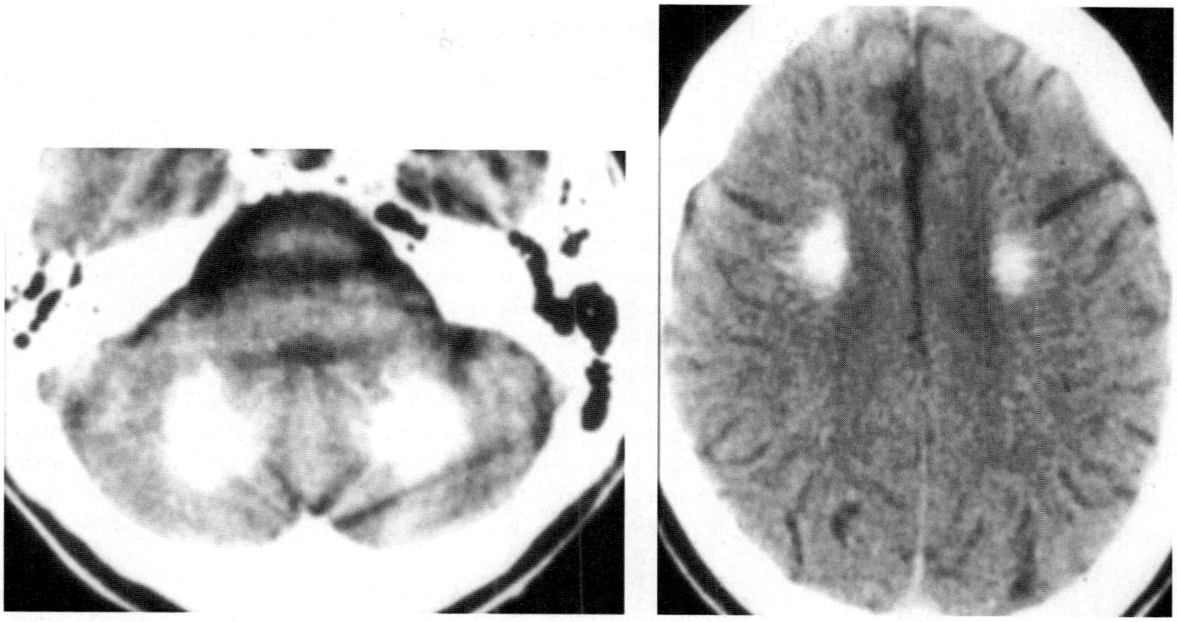

Figure 4.24 *Hypothyroidism.* Axial computed tomography scans show calcifications in the medial aspect of the cerebellar hemispheres *A* and in the white matter of the centra semiovale *B*.

untreated hypothyroidism may result in enlargement of the pituitary gland. This in turn may compress the optic chiasm and produce visual symptoms, which rarely are the presenting clinical symptoms. Circulating thyroid hormones have a negative feedback effect on the gland. If an inadequate amount of thyroid hormone is being produced by the adenohypophysis, the serum level of thyroid-stimulating hormone (produced by the hypothalamus) increases and results in hyperplasia of the thyrotropin-releasing cells (also called *thyrotrophs*). Treatment with hormone replacement results in a reduction in the size of the pituitary gland and improvement of the symptoms. In one series, hyperplasia of the pituitary gland occurred within 5 weeks of withdrawal of exogenous thyroid hormone replacement in patients with hypothyroidism. In these patients, the signal intensity of the gland remained unchanged. Hypothyroidism is said to be a rare cause of basal ganglia calcifications (93). Basal ganglia calcifications are seen in many adults and are marked in up to 2% of the population. The great majority of these individuals are normal, and thus the presence of basal ganglia calcifications cannot be used as a marker for systemic disorders. Most basal ganglia calcifications are idiopathic and of no clinical significance. Cerebellar and white matter calcifications are, however, strongly associated with hypothyroidism (93) (Fig. 4.24). Table 4.3 gives the differential diagnosis for cerebellar calcifications.

Table 4.3: Causes of Cerebellar Calcifications

Category of Disease	*Specific Conditions*
Metabolic	Hypothyroidism, hypoparathyroidism, hyperparathyroidism
Inherited	Fahr's disease, Cockayne's syndrome, tuberous sclerosis
Toxic	Lead poisoning, chemotherapy-induced microangiopathy, postirradiation
Infections	Acquired immunodeficiency syndrome in newborns

Effects of Miscellaneous Systemic Disorders on the Brain

Anorexia Nervosa

Cerebral abnormalities in patients with anorexia nervosa (AN) have been documented. In these patients, the CSF-containing spaces are wide, implying a degree of underlying cerebral atrophy (94). This atrophy may be at least partially reversible. There is a correlation between the severity and duration of the disorder, the amount of weight loss, and the degree of brain atrophy (95). The ventricles, particularly the lateral ones, also are prominent. The loss of cerebral volume may reflect an abnormal water content, abnormal glucose metabolism, or loss of cellular proteins. Patients with AN have a high level of cortisol, and this also may contribute to the development of cerebral atrophy. Patients with significant brain atrophy may show neuropsychological impairments. Patients with AN have shown significant cortical atrophy in brain volumetric studies, and this may correlate with the severity of the neuropsychological deficits.

Chronic Fatigue Syndrome

Chronic fatigue syndrome (CFS), also known as *myalgic encephalomyelitis*, is characterized by cognitive difficulties, exercise-induced fatigue, and immunologic dysfunction. The diagnosis of CFS is difficult to establish because there are no characteristic clinical or laboratory findings. It is seen most often in young women. MRI has been used to examine the brain of patients with CFS, but unfortunately most findings are nonspecific (96). Approximately 15% to 50% of patients with CFS show focal areas of increased T2 signal intensity in the white matter. There is no preferential location for these lesions, and they do not enhance after contrast administration. SPECT detects a greater number of abnormalities in the brain than MRI (97). Patients with CFS show multiple perfusion defects in the cerebral cortex and the basal ganglia. In one series, 81% of patients with CFS showed perfusion abnormalities on SPECT studies (97). It is thus possible that SPECT may be used to follow the progression of CFS and the effects of treatment. In a different report, patients with CFS were compared with those with AIDS-related dementia complex and major unipolar depression. Patients with CFS and depression had similar findings on SPECT perfusion studies, whereas control subjects and patients with AIDS dementia complex had fewer abnormalities. These authors concluded that CFS may be due to chronic viral encephalitis and that the clinical similarities between CFS and depression may be due to a similar distribution and number of defects found in the two disorders.

Porphyria

Mary, Queen of Scots and King George III suffered from porphyria. A film that convincingly portrays the devastating neurologic effects of porphyria is "The Madness of King George."

Porphyria actually is a group of disorders involving specific enzymatic defects in the biosynthesis of heme. The production of intermediate compounds, called *porphyrins*, results in clinical symptoms of abdominal pain, limb weakness, constipation, vomiting, tachycardia, photosensitive skin reactions, and porphyric encephalopathy (98). Porphyric encephalopathy is characterized by hysteria, depression, and psychosis. It is thought that these cerebral abnormalities are induced by transient ischemic attacks. Histologically, the affected parts of the brain show diffuse neuronal loss, eosinophilic changes, gliosis, a lack of inflammation, and myelin pallor, all believed to reflect ischemia. The most common type of porphyria is the cutanea tarda form due to accumulation of uroporphyrin. This type of porphyria may be sporadic or familial. MRI may demonstrate acute and chronic changes (98). Diffuse cortical infarctions with subsequent development of high T2 signal intensity in the underlying white matter have been described. Focal areas of T2 hyperintensity in the posterior parietal regions (similar to those seen in PRES) have been reported. In porphyria, these abnormalities do show contrast enhancement, suggesting that they are true infarctions. In addition, cerebral angiography may show vasospasm, which may be reversible (99). MRI may show atrophy of the frontal cortex and areas of increased intensity on T1- and T2-weighted sequences, probably related to laminar necrosis and infarction (100). CT shows atrophy of the frontal cortex and the presence of calcification, presumably due to dystrophic postischemic changes.

Hippocampal Sclerosis

One to 2% of the population has seizures, and most can be controlled with medication (101). Approximately 100,000 patients need surgery for intractable epilepsy every year. The most common sites of the epileptogenic foci in these patients are the temporal lobe (80%), frontal lobe (15%), and parietal lobe (5%) (102). The most common type of temporal lobe seizure is the complex partial seizure. Clinicians are able to lateralize the site of origin of seizures in only a small percentage of patients. Determining that only one temporal lobe produces the seizures is important because surgical (or any other invasive therapy) is indicated only in those with a unilateral focus and if the contralateral side can support memory. Imaging is used to help lateralize the seizure focus and to identify specific underlying lesions. The applications of imaging in patients with partial complex seizures are presurgical, invasive or surgical, and postsurgical.

Patients with acute generalized tonic-clonic seizures and status epilepticus may show high signal in the hippocampi on diffusion-weighted MRI and low apparent diffusion coefficient values. Most abnormalities resolve, but some are permanent.

The specific roles of neuroimaging in patients with partial complex seizures are lateralization, identification of lesions, establishing the relationship between a seizure focus and eloquent cortex, and follow-up after surgery.

MRI probably is the single most important test in the evaluation of the patient with partial complex seizures. Our imaging protocol is as follows:

1. Entire brain: conventional sagittal T1-weighted images and coronal 1.5-mm thick contiguous three-dimensional gradient-echo images [TR, 35 milliseconds; TE, 6 milliseconds; flip angle (FA), 35 degrees (total of 128 images)]. These allow for identification of cortical dysplasias, reformation of the images in different planes, and for volumetrics.
2. Hippocampi: coronal FSE T2-weighted 3-mm thick images. These high-resolution images allow for identification of increased T2 signal intensity. Coronal FLAIR images allow for the identification of subtle signal intensity alterations and additional lesions (103). The hippocampi normally are slightly brighter that other parts of the cortex on these images.

On diffusion-weighted MRI, foci of seizures demonstrate high signal intensity (i.e., restricted water diffusion). These zones correspond to those showing increased perfusion. These abnormalities tend to be transient and most disappear within 1 week. Seizures change the polarity of the cell membranes and affect the sodium–potassium pump, leading to influx of water into the intracellular compartment. This mechanism decreases the volume of extracellular water and leads to cell swelling, which eventually results in neuronal necrosis. With cell necrosis, water becomes extracellular again and the diffusion parameters normalize.

Functional imaging studies help to confirm lateralization or lesion location, particularly when MRI is negative or inconclusive, or the imaging abnormalities are bilateral. PET (using fluorodeoxyglucose [FDG]) is used between seizures episodes (interictal) and measures regional cerebral metabolism. The abnormal side/lesion therefore is seen as an area of decreased uptake of the tracer. It is said to have the highest sensitivity/specificity in lateralization. Similar information from FDG may be obtained using a coincidence scanner. With SPECT using hexamethylpropylene amine oxime (HM-PAO), the tracer is lipophilic and crosses the intact blood–brain barrier at the time of injection. The tracer is injected during the seizure (intraictal or ictal) and images are obtained 30 to 60 minutes postictal. The abnormal side/lesion is seen as an area of increased tracer uptake. Injection of the tracer sometimes is done during the Wada test to map the distribution of the Amytal/radiotracer in the brain. Functional MRI (blood oxygenation level–dependent technique) is used to identify seizure foci, lateralize memory and speech, and map functional cortex neighboring a lesion. For practical purposes, this technique currently is used only for speech lateralization, and does not yet replace the Wada test. Evaluation of memory is complex and cannot be assessed yet with this technique.

Proton MRS is done with single or angled multivolume (two-dimensional) techniques (103). At our institution, most hippocampi are now studied with two-dimensional techniques (multiple volumes), and this may help in the identification of extra-hippocampal lesions and the extent of hippocampal involvement. The abnormal hippocampus shows low NAA and, at times, lactate (particularly if obtained a short time after seizures). Correct lateralization may be achieved in 90% to 100% of patients, and contralateral abnormalities are identified in 10% to 20% of cases (104). The amount of NAA varies throughout the hippocampus and normally is lower in the head than in the body and tail of this structure.

The most common predisposing factor for the development of hippocampal sclerosis is febrile seizures.

Volumetric techniques are used to detect subtle differences in the size of the hippocampi and in cases of bilateral abnormalities that are difficult to judge visually. They are needed overall in less than 10% of patients. The normal volume of the hippocampus varies from 2.3 cc to 2.8 cc according to the technique used (border tracing versus grid). There are minimal volume differences between the sexes. It is important that only one trained person do all measurements. Because some anatomic landmarks are subjective (separation of the head of the hippocampus from the amygdala), some operators include the entire set of structures (including the subiculum) in their measurements (105). Although we measure the entire hippocampus, some authors suggest that measuring only one portion of this structure suffices because this reflects the diffuse changes (this is based on the premise that hippocampal atrophy is a diffuse process and not a segmental one). Our use of volumetry has decreased considerably, and we perform this test only in very few patients. Although some authors believe segmental hippocampal sclerosis occurs, others do not. Some believe that the entire hippocampus is affected at once.

The purpose of the Wada test is to determine if language resides on the side of surgery and if the contralateral temporal lobe can support memory (106). We begin by performing selective digital subtraction angiograms of both internal carotid arteries. The purpose of the angiogram is to detect primitive carotid–basilar communications (testing is contraindicated in these patients) and to assess the presence of a fetal posterior cerebral artery origin and degree of cross-filling. The study is done by injecting 100 to 125 mg of Amytal intraarterially over a 4-second period. Unilateral electroencephalographic slowing and contralateral loss of strength indicate adequate sedation. Aphasia and amnesia on the side of seizures (which always is studied first) indicates that the patient will not tolerate surgery. However, passing the Wada test provides no guarantee that there will be no major complications.

Imaging studies also are obtained before and after placement of depth electrodes and subdural grids. These procedures are used in patients in whom all other attempts to lateralize and locate a seizure focus have failed. These instruments are made of stainless steel, platinum alloys, and, more recently, nickel chromium. They result in far more artifact when imaged with CT than with MRI. Depth electrodes may enter the skull through occipital burr holes and travel into the amygdalae in a course parallel to the hippocampi. Orthogonal electrodes enter through temporal burr holes and travel perpendicular to the hippocampi. These are used in patients with suspected extra-hippocampal seizures. Grids usually contain 32 electrodes. The bone flap usually is replaced during the placement of the grids for protection of the brain. Complications of these procedures occur in 1% to 4% of patients and include hemorrhage, infection, edema, infarction, and gliosis.

In patients with vagal nerve stimulators, no specific imaging is required after the placement of these devices. The power source and the course of the electrode are readily identified on conventional chest and neck plain radiographs. These devices desynchronize electrical brain activity through activation of the vagal nerve nuclei, the solitary tracts, and deep brain structures in the temporal lobes. Patients with vagal stimulators may be placed in the MRI unit as long as the unit has been previously disabled.

After temporal lobe surgery, 60% to 80% of patients are seizure free and 20% to 30% experience a decrease in seizures that makes them easier to treat medically. There is an excellent correlation between the extent of resection and the outcome (the more extensive the resection, the better the prognosis). Unfortunately, extensive resections result in higher rates of complications. Imaging also is important because the actual extent of resection may vary from that estimated during surgery. Techniques used for seizure surgery are:

1. Standard temporal lobectomy: includes the anterior 5 cm of a temporal lobe, amygdala, and a part of that hippocampus
2. Selective temporal lobectomy: amygdala or hippocampus, or both
3. Lesionectomy

Complications of temporal lobectomy include memory loss (40%), visual loss (10% to 20%), hemiplegia (1% to 3%), and death (<1%). There are several semiquantitative methods for grading the degree of resection. In the compartmental methods, the temporal lobe is divided into four coronal and four axial compartments. With larger resections, there will be fewer seizures but less retention of verbal material and memory, and more visual deficits. Patients in whom the resected hippocampus demonstrates gliosis on histology will have fewer memory deficits than those in whom it does not. This probably is related to some degree of brain plasticity. A poor prognosis may be expected when one or more of the following structures is not resected: parahippocampal gyrus, hippocampus, amygdala, and uncus.

The following is a summary of the most common pathologic processes affecting the hippocampi:

1. Hippocampal sclerosis (mesial temporal sclerosis): this lesion is characterized by loss of neurons and gliosis (107). The most commonly affected regions are CA1 and CA4. Although some investigators believe segmental hippocampal sclerosis can occur, most consider it a diffuse process. By MRI, the most common finding is that of decreased volume (108) (Fig. 4.25A). This diagnosis may be made by visual inspection in approximately 90% of cases. Loss of internal characteristics and of the undulations of the pes hippocampus also is fairly common. Increased T2 signal intensity (probably reflecting gliosis) is present in approximately 65% of cases. Routine administration of gadolinium is not indicated in these patients. Ancillary findings that support the diagnosis of hippocampal sclerosis include decreased size of the ipsilateral column of the fornix and mamillary body, decreased size of the white matter in the same temporal lobe, and decreased size of the ipsilateral hemisphere (109). An enlarged temporal horn of the lateral ventricle is the least specific finding in hippocampal sclerosis. The presence of hippocampal sclerosis (as discussed previously) may be confirmed by proton MRS (Fig. 4.25B and C).
2. Developmental anomalies (cortical dysplasia, heterotopia): these anomalies account for approximately 5% to 10% of lesions resulting in temporal lobe epilepsy (110). Gray matter heterotopias are variable in size and usually abut the walls of the temporal horn of the lateral ventricle. Cortical dysplasias may be seen as areas of increased gray matter thickness with intrinsic and underlying white matter increased T2 signal intensity (Fig. 4.26). These cortical dysplasias may be impossible to distinguish from cortical-based tumors such as dysembryoplastic neuroepithelial tumor (DNET; Fig. 4.27). Recently, so-called cortical dysplasia of Taylor has received some attention in the literature. In these instances, MRI shows cortical thickening and a linear signal intensity abnormality extending into the closest ventricle. Temporal lobe encephaloceles also may result in partial complex seizures.
3. Tumors: these account for approximately 10% of lesions resulting in temporal lobe seizures. Most are low-grade astrocytomas and oligodendrogliomas. These have no specific imaging features. Ganglion cell tumors also are relatively common in the temporal lobes; they also have no specific imaging features. DNETs are cortical-based tumors with occasional cysts and calcifications and show no prominent enhancement (Fig. 4.27). They may cause scalloping of the overlying bone, and are difficult to differentiate from cortical dysplasias. In adults, infarctions and metastasis also may result in new-onset partial complex seizures.

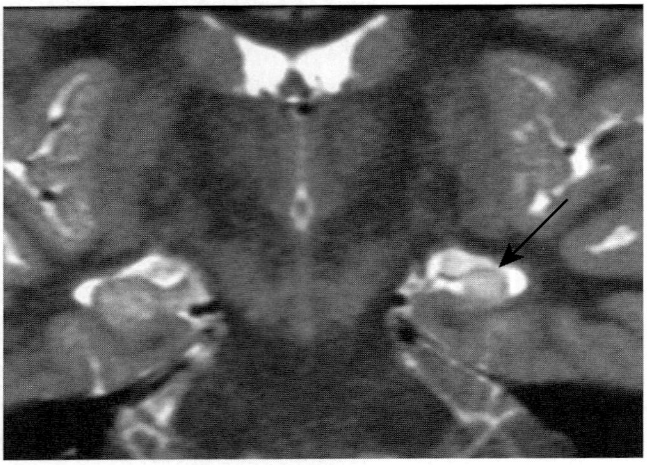

A

Figure 4.25 *Hippocampal Sclerosis.* Coronal T2-weighted image *A* shows small, bright left hippocampus *(arrow)*. In a different patient, proton magnetic resonance spectroscopy shows low *N*-acetyl aspartate (NAA) in posterior left hippocampus *B* compared with the right one *C*.

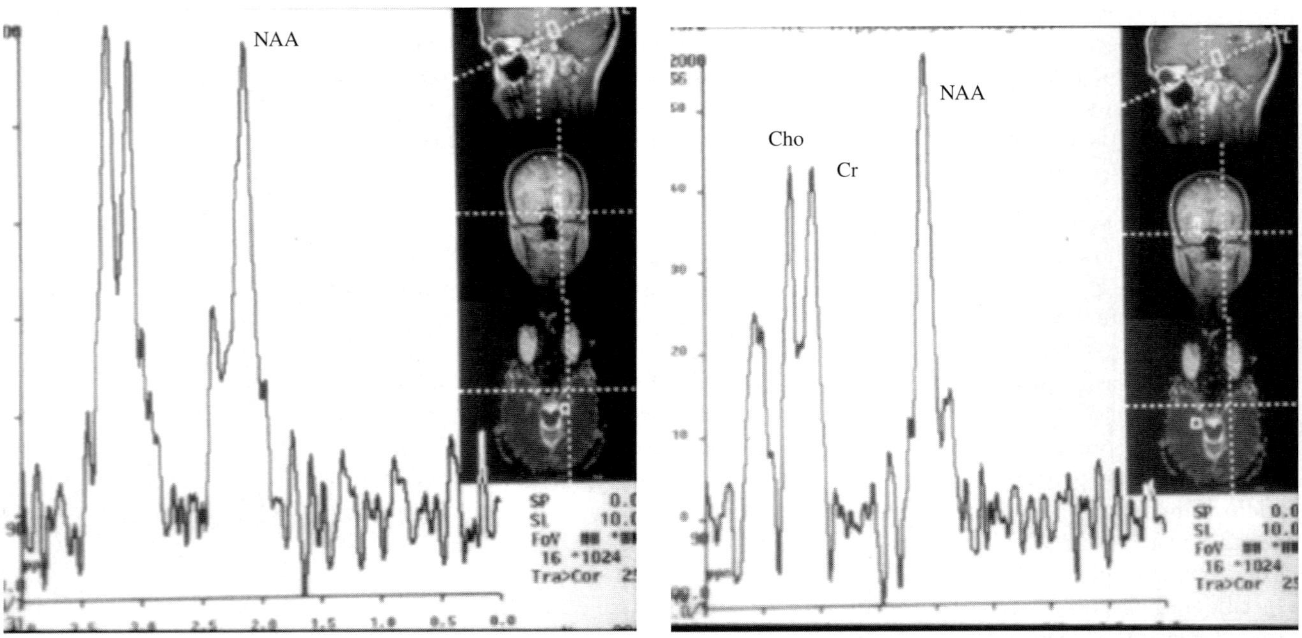

B

C

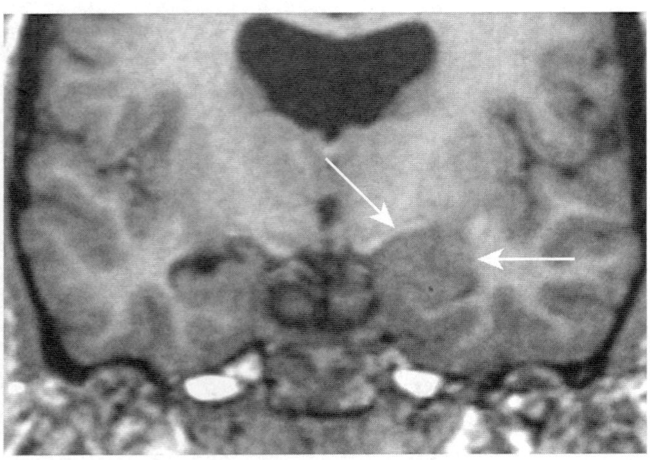

Figure 4.26 *Hippocampal Developmental Anomaly.* Coronal T1-weighted image shows large gray matter dysplasia (*arrows*) in the region of the left hippocampal head and amygdala.

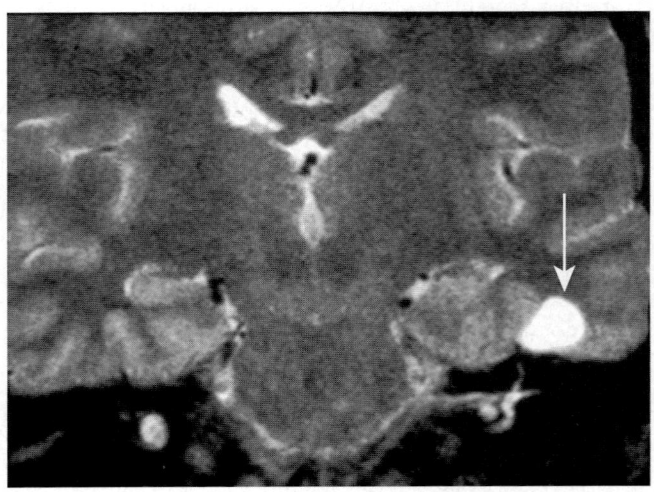

Figure 4.27 *Dysembryoplastic Neuroepithelial Tumor (DNET) of the Temporal Lobe.* Coronal T2-weighted image shows well defined high-intensity mass (*arrow*) located mostly in the cortex of the left inferior temporal gyrus.

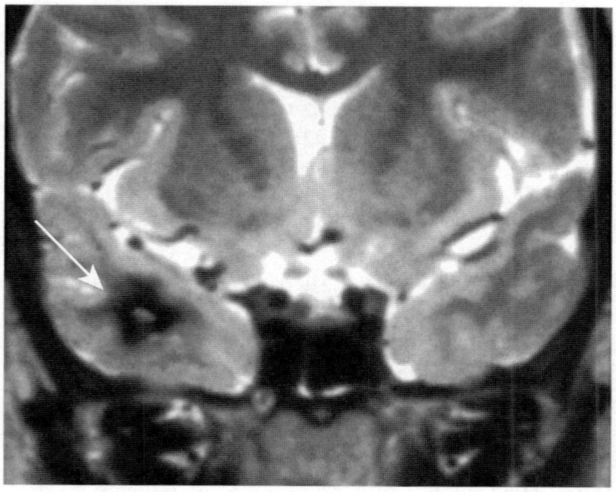

Figure 4.28 *Cavernous Angioma.* Coronal T2-weighted image shows typical cavernous angioma *(arrow)* in the white matter of the anterior pole of the right temporal lobe. The lesion is centrally bright and is surrounded by a hypointense rim due to deposition of chronic blood products.

4. Vascular malformations: these account for approximately 1% to 2% of lesions producing partial complex seizures. Both high-flow malformations (arteriovenous malformations) and cryptic malformations (mainly cavernous angiomas) occur with equal frequency in this location. MRI identifies dual abnormalities in approximately 10% of all patients with partial complex seizures (Fig. 4.28).
5. Others: pathologic processes that also may result in temporal lobe epilepsy include gliosis and atrophy on a posttraumatic basis, ischemia, inflammation (Rasmussen's encephalitis), infection (cysticercosis), and the sequelae of surgery (gliosis after depth electrode placement). Limbic encephalitis is a rare paraneoplastic process in which an immunologic reaction results in the formation of anti-neuronal antibodies (111–113). Patients present with memory problems, seizures, and irritability. The most common primary tumors to produce it arise in the lung, testicle, and breast. On T2 and FLAIR images, the mesial temporal lobes are swollen and bright and may enhance after administration of gadolinium (Fig. 4.29). In my experience, proton MRS shows low NAA, but the absence of elevated choline excludes the presence of metastases.

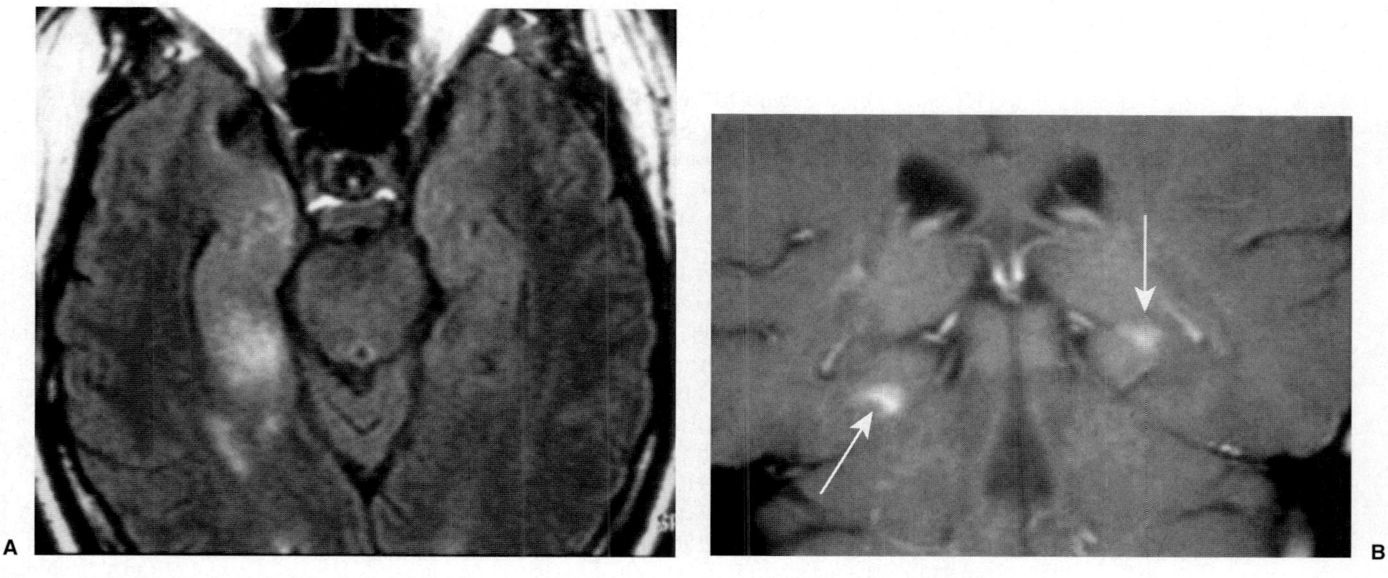

Figure 4.29 *Limbic Encephalitis. A.* Axial fluid attenuation inversion recovery (FLAIR) image shows increased signal in both mesial temporal lobes (right greater than left). *B.* After gadolinium administration, coronal T2-weighted image shows areas of enhancement *(arrows)* in both mesial temporal lobes.

References

1. Etsuo I, Shinichi H, Narumi Y, et al. Portal-systemic encephalopathy: presence of basal ganglia lesions with high signal intensity on MR images. Radiology 1991;179:551–555.
2. Ho VB, Fitz CR, Chuang SH, et al. Bilateral basal ganglia lesions: pediatric differential considerations. Radiographics 1993;13:269–292.
3. Pomier-Layrargues G, Spahr L, Butterworth RF. Increased manganese concentrations in pallidum of cirrhotic patients. Lancet 1995;345:735.
4. Krieger D, Krieger S, Jansen O, et al. Manganese and chronic hepatic encephalopathy. Lancet 1995;346:270–274.
5. Mirowitz SA, Westrich TJ. Basal ganglial signal intensity alterations: reversal after discontinuation of parenteral manganese administration. Radiology 1992;185:535–536.
6. Iwasa M, Kinosada Y, Nakatsuka A, et al. Magnetization transfer contrast of various regions of the brain in liver cirrhosis. AJNR Am J Neuroradiol 1999;20:652–654.
7. Ross BD, Jacobson S, Villamil F, et al. Subclinical hepatic encephalopathy: proton MR spectroscopic abnormalities. Radiology 1994;193:457–463.
8. van den Heuvel AG, van der Grond J, van Rooij LG, et al. Differentiation between portal-systemic encephalopathy and neurodegenerative disorders in patients with Wilson disease: H-1 MR spectroscopy. Radiology 1997;203:539–543.
9. Haseler LJ, Sibbitt WL Jr, Mojtahedzadeh HN, et al. Proton MR spectroscopic measurement of neurometabolites in hepatic encephalopathy during oral lactulose therapy. AJNR Am J Neuroradiol 1998;19:1681–1686.
10. Smith JK, Mah JK, Castillo M. Brain MR imaging findings in two patients with Alper's syndrome. Clin Imaging 1996;20:235–237.
11. Erbetta A, Ciceri E, Chiapparini L, et al. Magnetic resonance imaging findings in bilirubin encephalopathy. Int J Neuroradiol 1998;4:161–164.
12. Castillo M, Kwock, Green C. MELAS syndrome: imaging and proton MR spectroscopic findings. AJNR Am J Neuroradiol 1995;16:233–239.
13. Allard JC, Tilak S, Carter AP. CT and MR of MELAS syndrome. AJNR Am J Neuroradiol 1988;9:1234–1238.
14. Kim IO, Kim JH, Kim WS, et al. Mitochondrial myopathy-encephalopathy-lactic acidosis and strokelike episodes (MELAS) syndrome: CT and MR findings in seven children. AJR Am J Radiol 1996;166:641–645.
15. Medina L, Chi TL, DeVivo DC, et al. MR findings in patients with subacute necrotizing encephalomyelopathy (Leigh syndrome): correlation with biochemical defect. AJNR Am J Neuroradiol 1990;11:379–384.
16. Paltiel HJ, O'Gorman AM, Meagher-Villemure K, et al. Subacute necrotizing encephalomyelopathy (Leigh disease): CT study. Radiology 1987;162:115–118.
17. Demange P, Pham Gia H, et al. MR of Kearns-Sayre syndrome. AJNR Am J Neuroradiol 1989;S91.
18. Shaw DW, Maravilla KR, Weinberger E, et al. MR imaging of phenylketonuria. AJNR Am J Neuroradiol 1991;12:403–406.
19. Brismar J, Aqueel A, Brismar G, et al. Maple syrup urine disease: findings on CT and MR scans of the brain in 10 infants. AJNR Am J Neuroradiol 1990;11:1219–1228.
20. Ruano MM, Castillo M, Thompson JE. MR imaging in a patient with homocystinuria. AJR Am J Radiol 1998;171:1147–1149.
21. Brismar J, Ozand PT. CT and MR of the brain in glutaric acidemia type I: a review of 59 published cases and a report of 5 new patients. AJNR Am J Neuroradiol 1995;16:675–683.
22. Hald JK, Nakstad PH, Skjeldal, et al. Bilateral arachnoid cysts of the temporal fossa in four children with glutaric aciduria type I. AJNR Am J Neuroradiol 1991;12:407–409.
23. Gebarski SS, Gabrielsen TO, Knake JE, et al. Cerebral CT findings in methylmalonic acid propionic acidemas. AJNR Am J Neuroradiol 1983;4:955–957.
24. Andreula CF, De Blasi R, Carella A. CT and MR studies of methylmalonic acidemia. AJNR Am J Neuroradiol 1991;12:410–412.
25. King AD, Walshe JM, Kendall BE, et al. Cranial MR imaging in Wilson's disease. AJR Am J Radiol 1996;167:1579–1584.
26. van Wassenaer-van Hall HN, van den Heuvel AG, Jansen GH, et al. Cranial MR in Wilson disease: abnormal white matter in extrapyramidal and pyramidal tracts. AJNR Am J Neuroradiol 1995;16:2021–2027.

27. van Wassenaer-van Hall HN, van den Heuvel AG, Algra A, et al. Wilson disease: findings at MR imaging and CT of the brain with clinical correlation. Radiology 1996;198:531–536.
28. Kuwert T, Hefter H, Scholz D, et al. Regional cerebral glucose consumption measured by positron emission tomography in patients with Wilson's disease. Eur J Nucl Med 1992;19: 96–101.
29. Houston CS, Harding SR. Menkes kinky hair syndrome. AJNR Am J Neuroradiol 1993;14:785.
30. Faerber EN, Grover WD, DeFilipp GJ, et al. Cerebral MR of Menkes kinky-hair disease. AJNR Am J Neuroradiol 1989;10:190–192.
31. Jacobs DS, Smith AS, Finelli DA, et al. Menkes kinky hair disease: characteristic MR angiographic findings. AJNR Am J Neuroradiol 1993;14:1160–1163.
32. Andrews NC. Medical progress: disorders or iron metabolism. N Engl J Med 1999;341: 1986–1995.
33. Geremia GK, McClunney K, Adler S, et al. The magnetic-resonance hypointense spine of AIDS. AJNR Am J Neuroradiol 1989;10:880–881.
34. Sparacia G, Midiri M, D'Angelo P, et al. Magnetic resonance imaging of the pituitary gland in patients with secondary hypogonadism due to transfusional hemochromatosis. MAGMA 1999;8:87–90.
35. Berg D, Hoggenmuller U, Hofmann E, et al. The basal ganglia in haemochromatosis. Neuroradiology 2000;42:9–13.
36. Savoiardo M, Halliday WC, Nardocci N, et al. Hallervorden-Spatz disease: MR and pathologic findings. AJNR Am J Neuroradiol 1993;14:155–162.
37. Ramos A, Quintana F, Díez C, et al. CT findings in spinocerebellar degeneration. AJNR Am J Neuroradiol 1987;8:635–640.
38. Barkovich AJ, Ali FA, Rowley HA, et al. Imaging patterns of neonatal hypoglycemia. AJNR Am J Neuroradiol 1998;19:523–528.
39. Richardson ML, Kinard RE, Gray MB. CT of generalized gray matter infarction due to hypoglycemia. AJNR Am J Neuroradiol 1981;2:366–367.
40. Spar JA, Lewine JD, Orrison WW Jr. Neonatal hypoglycemia: CT and MR findings. AJNR Am J Neuroradiol 1994;15:1477–1478.
41. Harper C, Bitterworth R. Nutritional and metabolic disorders. In: Graham DI, Lantos PL, eds. Greenfield's neuropathology, 6th ed. London: Arnold, 1997:613–615.
42. Doraiswamy PM, Massey EW, Enright K, et al. Wernicke-Korsakoff syndrome caused by psychogenic food refusal: MR findings. AJNR Am J Neuroradiol 1994;15:594–596.
43. Galluzzi M, Bozzao A, Splendiani A, et al. Wernicke encephalopathy: MR findings in five patients. AJNR Am J Neuroradiol 1990;11:887–892.
44. Shogry ME, Curnes JT. Mamillary body enhancement on MR as the only sign of acute Wernicke encephalopathy. AJNR Am J Neuroradiol 1994;15:172–174.
45. Harter SB, Nokes SR. Gadolinium-enhanced MR findings in a pediatric case of Wernicke encephalopathy. AJNR Am J Neuroradiol 1995;16:700–702.
46. d'Aprile P, Gentile MA, Carella A. Enhance MR in the acute phase of Wernicke encephalopathy. AJNR Am J Neuroradiol 1994;15:591–593.
47. Kamaki M, Kawamura M, Moriya H, et al. "Crossed homonymous hemianopia" and "crossed left hemispatial neglect" in a case of Marchiafava-Bignami disease. J Neurol Neurosurg Psychiatry 1993;56:1027–1032.
48. Lechevalier B, Andersson JC, Morin P. Hemispheric disconnection syndrome with a "crossed avoiding" reaction in a case of Marchiafava-Bignami disease. J Neurol Neurosurg Psychiatry 1977;40:483–497.
49. Thackray HM, Tifft C. Fetal alcohol syndrome. Pediatr Rev 2001;22:45–47.
50. Silverman CS, Brenner J, Murtagh FR. Hemorrhagic necrosis and vascular injury in carbon monoxide poisoning: MR demonstration. AJNR Am J Neuroradiol 1993;14:168–170.
51. Miura T, Mitomo M, Kawai R, et al. CT of the brain in acute carbon monoxide intoxication: characteristic features and prognosis. AJNR Am J Neuroradiol 1985;6:739–742.
52. Taylor R, Holgate RC. Carbon monoxide poisoning: asymmetric and unilateral changes on CT. AJNR Am J Neuroradiol 1988;9:975–977.
53. Nau T, Seitz H, Kapral S, et al. Ethylene glycol poisoning and brain injury: a dangerous combination. Anasthesiologie 1999;34:318–320.
54. Teo JGC, Goh KYC, Ahuja A, et al. Intracranial vascular calcifications, glioblastoma multiforme, and lead poisoning. AJNR Am J Neuroradiol 1997;18:576–579.
55. López-Villegas D, Lenkinski RE. Magnetic resonance imaging and spectroscopy of regional brain structure in a 10-year-old boy with elevated blood lead levels. Pediatrics 1998;101:7.

56. Tayfun C, Kurtaran HK, Bulakbasi N, et al. Cerebral and orbital magnetic resonance imaging findings in methyl alcohol intoxication. Int J Neuroradiol 1999;5:145–150.
57. Rubinstein D, Escott E, Kelly JP. Methanol intoxication with putaminal and white matter necrosis: MC and CT findings. AJNR Am J Neuroradiol 1995;16:1492–1494.
58. Gaul HP, Wallace CJ, Auer RN, et al. MR findings in methanol intoxication. AJNR Am J Neuroradiol 1995;16:1783–1786.
59. Nierenberg DW, Nordgren RE, Change MB, et al. Delayed cerebellar disease and death after accidental exposure to dimethylmercury. N Engl J Med 1998;338:1672–1676.
60. Korogi Y, Takahasi M, Okajima T, et al. MR findings of Minamata disease: organic mercury poisoning. J Magn Reson Imaging 1998;8:308–316.
61. Committee on Substance Abuse and Committee on Native American Child Health. Inhalant abuse. Pediatrics 1996;97:420–423.
62. Unger E, Alexander A, Fritz T, et al. Toluene abuse: physical basis for hypointensity of the basal ganglia on T2-weighted MR images. Radiology 1994;193:473–476.
63. Xiong L, Matthes JD, Li J, et al. MR imaging of "spray heads:" toluene abuse via aerosol paint inhalation. AJNR Am J Neuroradiol 1993;14:1195–1199.
64. Ashina M, Bendtsen L, Jensen R, et al. Nitric oxide-induced headache in patients with chronic tension-type headache. Brain 2000;123:1830–1837.
65. Simmons JT, Pastakia B, Chase TN, et al. Magnetic resonance imaging in Huntington disease. AJNR Am J Neuroradiol 1986;7:25–28.
66. Ho VB, Chuang HS, Rovira MJ, et al. Juvenile Huntington disease: CT and MR features. AJNR Am J Neuroradiol 1995;16:1405–1412.
67. Chew W, Kucharczyk J, Moseley M, et al. Hyperglycemia augments ischemic brain injury: in vivo MR imaging/spectroscopic study with nicardipine in cats with occluded middle cerebral arteries. AJNR Am J Neuroradiol 1991;12:603–609.
68. Lai PH, Tien RD, Chang MH, et al. Chorea-ballismus with nonketotic hyperglycemia in primary diabetes mellitus. AJNR Am J Neuroradiol 1996;17:1057–1064.
69. Nagai C, Kato T, Katagiri T, et al. Hyperintense putamen on T1-weighted MR images in a case of chorea with hyperglycemia. AJNR Am J Neuroradiol 1995;16:1243–1246.
70. Shan DE, Ho DM, Chang C, et al. Hemichorea-hemiballism: an explanation for MR signal changes. AJNR Am J Neuroradiol 1998;19:863–870.
71. Cheung G, Gawal MJ, Cooper PW, et al. Amyotrophic lateral sclerosis: correlation of clinical and MR imaging findings. Radiology 1995;194:263–270.
72. Oba H, Araki T, Ohtomo K, et al. Amyotrophic lateral sclerosis: T2 shortening in motor cortex at MR imaging. Radiology 1993;189:843–846.
73. Kato Y, Matsumura K, Kinosada Y, et al. Detection of pyramidal tract lesions in amyotrophic lateral sclerosis with magnetization-transfer measurements. AJNR Am J Neuroradiol 1997;18:1541–1547.
74. Tien RD, Felsberg GJ, Ferris NJ, et al. The dementias: correlation of clinical features, pathophysiology, and neuroradiology. AJR Am J Radiol 1993;161:245–255.
75. Rusinek H, de Leon MJ, George AE, et al. Alzheimer disease: measuring loss of cerebral gray matter with MR imaging. Radiology 1991;178:109–114.
76. Bonte FJ, Tintner R, Weiner MF, et al. Brain blood flow in the dementias: SPECT with histopathologic correlation. Radiology 1993;186:361–365.
77. Ernst T, Chang L, Melchor R, et al. Frontotemporal dementia and early Alzheimer disease: differentiation with frontal lobe H-1 MR spectroscopy. Radiology 1997;203:829–836.
78. Kantarci K, Jack CR, Campeau NC, et al. Mild cognitive impairment and Alzheimer disease: regional diffusivity of water. Radiology 2001;219:101–107.
79. Chen JC, Hardy PA, Kucharczyk W, et al. MR of human postmortem brain tissue: correlative study between T2 and assays of iron and ferritin in Parkinson and Huntington disease. AJNR Am J Neuroradiol 1993;14:275–281.
80. Bowen BC, Block RE, Sánchez-Ramos J, et al. Proton MR spectroscopy of the brain in 14 patients with Parkinson disease. AJNR Am J Neuroradiol 1995;16:61–68.
81. Cohn MC, Hudgins PA, Sheppard SK, et al. Pre- and postoperative MR evaluation of stereotactic pallidotomy. AJNR Am J Neuroradiol 1998;19:1075–1080.
82. Groen JJ, Endtz LJ. Hereditary Pick's disease: second re-examination of the large family and discussion of other hereditary cases, with particular reference to electroencephalography, and computerized tomography. Brain 1982;105:443–459.

83. Drayer BP, Olanow W, Burger P, et al. Parkinson Plus syndrome: diagnosis using high field MR imaging of brain iron. Radiology 1986;159:493–498.
84. Savoiardo M, Strada L, Girotti F, et al. Olivopontocerebellar atrophy: MR diagnosis and relationship to multisystem atrophy. Radiology 1990;174:693–696.
85. Ortiz O, Reed L. Cerebral amyloid angiopathy presenting as a nonhemorrhagic, infiltrating mass. Neuroradiology 1996;38:449–452.
86. Wagle WA, Smith TW, Weiner M. Intracerebral hemorrhage caused by cerebral amyloid angiopathy: radiographic-pathologic correlation. AJNR Am J Neuroradiol 1984;5:171–176.
87. Lee J, Krol G, Rosenblum M. Primary amyloidoma of the brain: CT and MR presentation. AJNR Am J Neuroradiol 1995;16:712–714.
88. Rust RS, Chun RWM. Interrelationships between renal and neurologic diseases and therapies. In: Swaiman KF, Ashwal S, eds. Pediatric neurology: principles and practice, 3rd ed. St. Louis: Mosby, 1999:1403–1437.
89. Schwartz RB, Bravo SM, Klufas RA, et al. Cyclosporine neurotoxicity and its relationship to hypertensive encephalopathy: CT and MR findings in 16 cases. AJR Am J Radiol 1995; 165:627–631.
90. Moore KR, Osborn AG, Townsend JJ, et al. The imaging and pathologic spectrum of hemolytic-uremic syndrome-thrombotic thrombocytopenic purpura (HUS-TTP syndrome). Int J Neuroradiol 1997;3:147–159.
91. Okada J, Yoshikawa K, Matsuo H, et al. Reversible MRI and CT findings in uremic encephalopathy. Neuroradiology 1991;33:524–526.
92. Shimono T, Hatabu H, Kasagi K, et al. Rapid progression of pituitary hyperplasia in humans with primary hypothyroidism: demonstration with MR imaging. Radiology 1999;213:383–388.
93. Burke JW, Williamson BRJ, Hurst RW. "Idiopathic" cerebellar calcifications: association with hypothyroidism. Radiology 1998;167:533–536.
94. Kornreich L, Shapira A, Horev G, et al. CT and MR evaluation of the brain in patients with anorexia nervosa. AJNR Am J Neuroradiol 1991;12:1213–1216.
95. Lambe EK, Katzman DK, Mikulis DJ, et al. Cerebral gray matter volume deficits after weight recovery from anorexia nervosa. Arch Gen Psychiatry 1997;54:537–542.
96. Greco A, Tannock C, Brotsoff J, et al. Brain MR in chronic fatigue syndrome. AJNR Am J Neuroradiol 1997;18:1265–1269.
97. Schwartz RB, Garada BM, Komaroff AL, et al. Detection of intracranial abnormalities in patients with chronic fatigue syndrome: comparison of MR imaging and SPECT. AJT 1994;162: 935–941.
98. Aggarwal A, Quint DJ, Lynch JP III. MR imaging of porphyric encephalopathy. AJR Am J Radiol 1994;162:1218–1220.
99. Black KS, Mirsky P, Kalina P, et al. Angiographic demonstration of reversible cerebral vasospasm in porphyric encephalopathy. AJNR Am J Neuroradiol 1995;16:1650–1652.
100. Berenguer J, Blasco J, Cardenal C, et al. Hepatoerythropoietic porphyria: neuroimaging findings. AJNR Am J Neuroradiol 1997;18:1557–1560.
101. Fischer RS, et al. Epilepsy for the Neuroradiologist. AJNR Am J Neuroradiol 1997;18:851.
102. Bronen RA, et al. A systematic approach for interpreting MR images of the seizure patient. AJR Am J Radiol 1997;169:241.
103. Thompson JE, Castillo M, Kwock L, et al. Usefulness of proton MR spectroscopy in the evaluation of temporal lobe epilepsy. AJR Am J Radiol 1998;170:771–776.
104. Achten E, et al. Value of single voxel proton MR spectroscopy in temporal lobe epilepsy. AJNR Am J Neuroradiol 1997;18:1131.
105. Kim JH, et al. MR measurement of the hippocampus for lateralization of temporal lobe epilepsy: value of measurements of the body vs. the whole structure. AJR Am J Radiol 1994; 163:1453.
106. Castillo M, Mukherji SK, McCartney WH. Cerebral amobarbital sodium distribution during Wada testing: utility of digital subtraction angiography and single-photon emission tomography. Neuroradiology 2000;42:814–817.
107. Tien RD, et al. Complex partial seizures and mesial temporal sclerosis, evaluation with fast spin echo MR imaging. Radiology 1993;189:835.
108. Grattan-Smith JD, Harvey AS, Desmond PM, et al. Hippocampal sclerosis in children with intractable temporal lobe epilepsy: detection with MR imaging. AJR Am J Radiol 1993;161: 1045–1048.

109. Baldwin GN, Tsuruda JS, Maravilla KR, et al. The fornix in patients with seizures caused by unilateral hippocampal sclerosis: detection of unilateral volume loss on MR images. AJR Am J Radiol 1994;162:1185–1189.
110. Barkovich AJ, Rowley HA, Andermann F. MR in partial epilepsy: value of high-resolution volumetric techniques. AJNR Am J Neuroradiol 1995;16:339–343.
111. Gultekin SH, Rosenfeld MR, Voltz R, et al. Paraneoplastic limbic encephalitis: neurological symptoms, immunological findings, and tumour association in 50 patients. Brain 2000;123: 1481–1494.
112. Provenzale JM, Barboriak DP, Coleman RE. Limbic encephalitis: comparison of FDG PET and MR imaging findings. AJR Am J Radiol 1998;170:1659–1660.
113. Kodama T, Numaguchi Y, Gellad FE, et al. Magnetic resonance imaging of limbic encephalitis. Neuroradiology 1991;33:520–523.

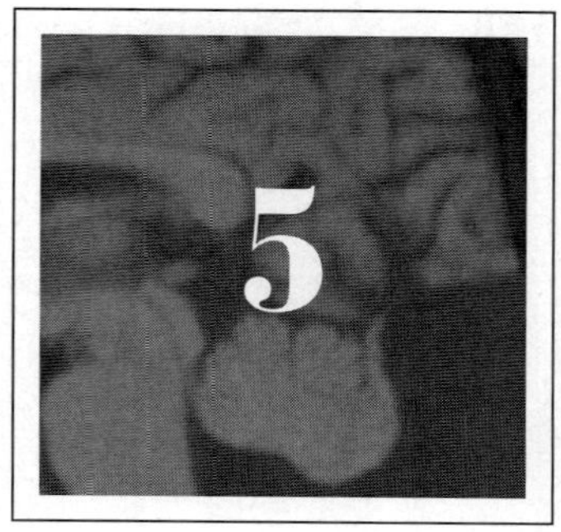

Disorders of Cerebral Spinal Fluid Flow

- Pathophysiology
- Noncommunicating Hydrocephalus
- Communicating Hydrocephalus
- Benign External Hydrocephalus (Benign Enlargement of the Subarachnoid Spaces)
- Slit Ventricle Syndrome
- Intracranial Hypotension
- Complications of Ventricular Shunts
- Trapped Ventricles
- Endoscopic Ventriculostomies

Pathophysiology

Traditionally, hydrocephalus has been divided into obstructive and nonobstructive types (1). However, all hydrocephalus is fundamentally obstructive, and thus it is better to classify it as communicating and noncommunicating. Even in noncommunicating hydrocephalus, there is some absorption of cerebrospinal fluid (CSF). CSF is a filtrate mostly produced by the choroid plexus, but it also is produced by the brain and the spinal cord. Approximately 0.4 mL of CSF is produced every minute (approximately 500 mL in 1 day) (1). CSF flows from the ventricles into the subarachnoid space aided by contraction and expansion of the brain parenchyma in response to arterial systole and diastole, respectively. As the ventricular CSF exits through the outlet foramina of the fourth ventricle, some of it continues down into the spinal canal while another part is directed toward the convexities. Even the CSF that travels into the spinal canal eventually is directed toward the cerebral convexities. This pulsatile motion of CSF is called *bulk flow*. Bulk flow was believed to explain the motion of CSF, but this concept recently has been challenged (2). The major causes of hydrocephalus are shown in Table 5.1.

The mechanism for absorption of CSF is complex and poorly understood. It was thought that the pacchionian (arachnoid) granulations played an important role, but this now is considered questionable. The pacchionian granulations are invaginations of arachnoid into the venous sinuses. These protuberances contain fibrous connective tissue, arachnoid cells, and small vessels (3). It was thought that most CSF absorption occurred because these arachnoid granulations channeled CSF into the venous sinuses. The exact role (if any) that pacchionian granulations play in the absorption of CSF is uncertain. The pacchionian granulations are clearly seen on imaging studies as defects protruding most often into the transverse sinuses, the venous torcular, or the superior sagittal sinus (3,4) (Fig. 5.1). Most measure approximately 2 to 3 mm and may show some contrast enhancement. Occasionally, they can be very large (giant pacchionian granulation).

Pacchionian (arachnoid) granulations commonly are seen in the regions of the transverse and superior sagittal sinuses. Occasionally, they may be very large.

A new explanation attempting to clarify the mechanism by which CSF is absorbed states that the pacchionian granulations and villi play a small or no role in this event (2,5). CSF instead is absorbed by the capillaries (including their surrounding Virchow-Robin

In skull base dysplasias, such as achondroplasia, a restriction of the venous outflow may account for the development of communicating hydrocephalus.

Table 5.1: Etiologies of Hydrocephalus

Noncommunicating Hydrocephalus	*Communicating Hydrocephalus*
Intraventricular obstruction(s)	Extraventricular (subarachnoid space) obstruction(s) Overproduction of cerebrospinal fluid Normal-pressure hydrocephalus Immaturity of resorption (so-called benign external hydrocephalus of childhood) Increased intracranial venous pressure

spaces). The CSF pulsations cause the postcapillary veins to become slightly reduced in caliber and have increased pressure (5). This pressure is transmitted to the capillary bed, where the vessels remain open and participate in the resorption of CSF. If the arterial pulsations are diminished, the veins are not compressed and the capillaries remain narrowed. This has been termed *reduced arterial pulsation hydrocephalus* (communicating hydrocephalus). The relatively low pressure in the subarachnoid space is at odds with the relatively increased intraventricular pressure, resulting in dilatation of the ventricles. In addition, because the capillaries are somewhat collapsed, oxygen transport to neighboring tissues is decreased, resulting in symptoms. The opposite also happens. If the ventricles become obstructed, the parenchyma narrows the subarachnoid space and compresses the veins. As a result, venous congestion increases the intracranial pressure. The imaging appearance of hydrocephalus is summarized in the Table 5.2.

The development of periventricular edema deserves special mention because many neurosurgeons use it as an indicator for the need for shunting. It is known that periventricular lucency represents an attempt by the brain to absorb CSF. When present, the edema initially is located around the frontal and occipital horns of the lateral ventricles (Fig. 5.2). Although this edema may progress and completely surround the lateral ventricles, it always is more prominent in the frontal and occipital regions. With normal aging, the brain parenchyma immediately anterior to the frontal horns of the lateral ventricles may develop thin and fairly symmetric areas of high T2 signal intensity. These are presumed to represent denudation of the ependyma and adjacent gliosis ("ependymosa granularis") and are normal and not to be confused with early transependymal CSF absorption. As the ventricles enlarge, they may develop diverticula at their weak points (Fig. 5.3). Table 5.3 describes the most common locations of ventricular diverticula resulting from hydrocephalus (6).

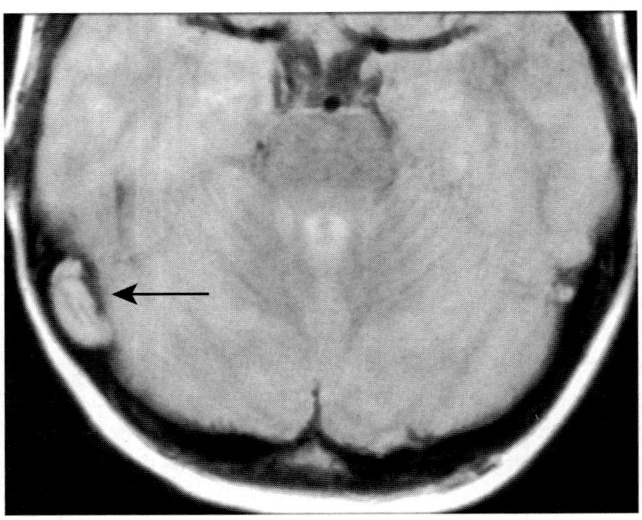

Figure 5.1 *Arachnoid Granulation.* Axial proton-density image shows arachnoid granulation *(arrow)* protruding into the right transverse sinus. This and along the superior sagittal sinus are their most common locations.

Table 5.2: Features of Hydrocephalus on Imaging Studies

Most Reliable	*Least Reliable*
Dilatation and rounding of the anterior and posterior aspects of the third ventricle	Rounding of the anterior border of the frontal horns of the lateral ventricles
Dilatation of the temporal horns with dilatation of the lateral ventricles	Narrowed angle between frontal horns of the lateral ventricles
Effacement of cortical sulci and cisterns	Isolated dilatation of the temporal horns of the lateral ventricles
Periventricular edema	
Narrowed mamillopontine angle	

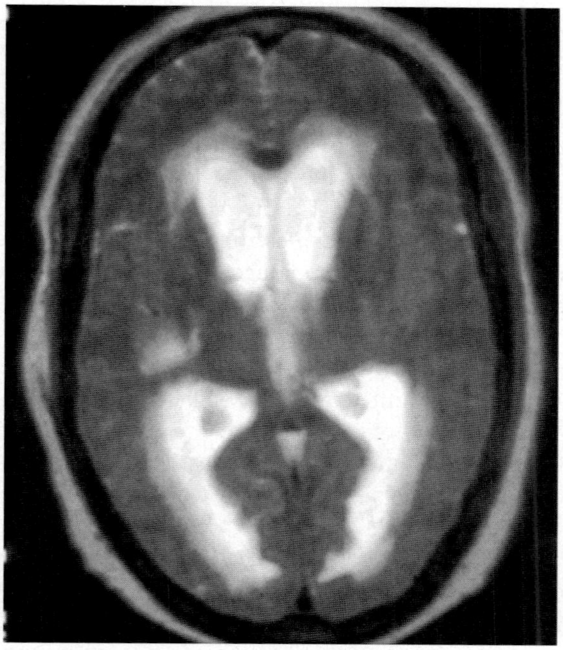

Figure 5.2 *Acute Noncommunicating Hydrocephalus.* Axial T2-weighted image shows dilated lateral ventricles with a halo of increased intensity (edema) in the periventricular white matter.

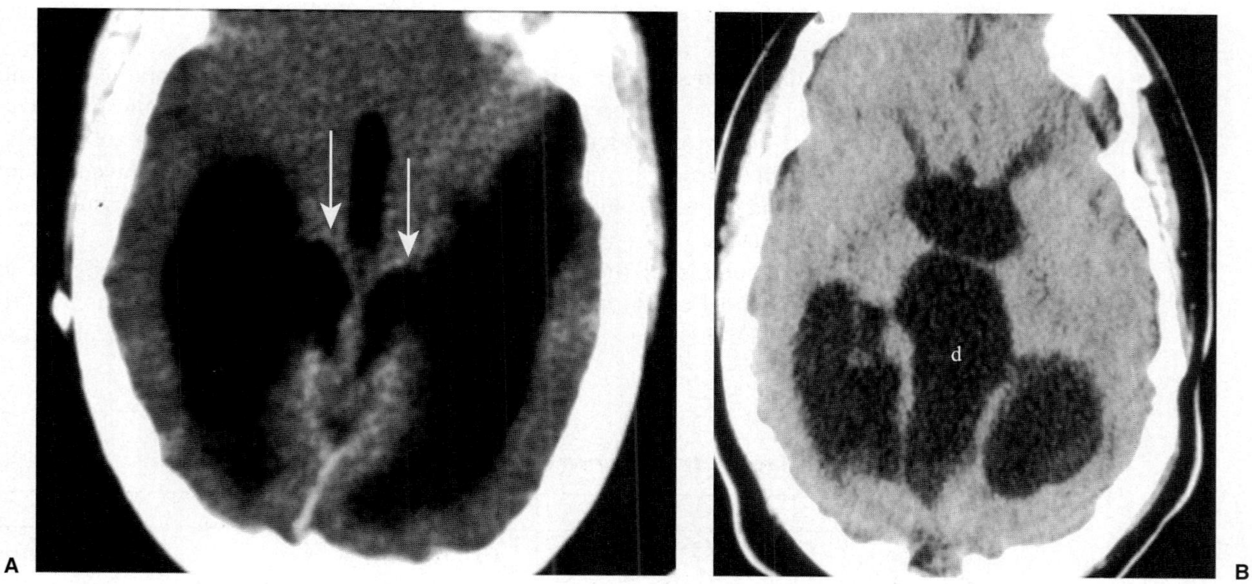

Figure 5.3 *Ventricular Diverticula in Hydrocephalus. A.* Axial computed tomography (CT) shows markedly dilated lateral ventricles and diverticula *(arrows)* arising from the medial aspects of the atria. *B.* Axial CT shows large diverticulum *(d)* arising from the posterior aspect of the third ventricle.

Table 5.3: Ventricular Diverticula Resulting from Hyrdrocephalus

Common Sites	*Uncommon Sites*
Suprachiasmatic and infundibular recesses of the third ventricle Posterior third ventricle (pineal recess)	Medial atria of the lateral ventricles (may remain supratentorial or be infratentorial) Medial temporal horns (through the choroidal fissures)

Noncommunicating Hydrocephalus

Aqueductal stenosis first may become clinically evident at birth, during infancy, and even during adulthood.

The major causes of noncommunicating hydrocephalus are listed in Table 5.4.

The most common cause of congenital noncommunicating hydrocephalus is aqueductal stenosis (7). It accounts for over 20% of patients with hydrocephalus. Its onset may be acute or insidious, in childhood or during adulthood. Many patients have a history of neonatal intracranial hemorrhage or meningitis, and presumably this leads to scarring and formation of webs in the aqueduct (this process is sometimes called *aqueductal gliosis*). Some webs are believed to be truly developmental in origin (Fig. 5.4A). Congenital deformities of the aqueduct, such as forking, also may result in its obstruction (1) (Fig. 5.4B). Thin sagittal T1-weighted images show the anatomy of the aqueduct, but sagittal T2-weighted images are needed to assess the tectum. High T2 signal in the tectum should rise the suspicion of an intrinsic lesion producing the hydrocephalus. Flow-sensitive gradient-echo imaging also may be useful in the evaluation of the aqueductal patency (8). These images need to be obtained in a plane that is perpendicular to the long axis of the aqueduct to maximize their sensitivity. High signal intensity in the aqueduct signifies patency. Cardiac-gated (prospective or retrospective) phase-contrast imaging also is useful. Aqueductal stenosis also is seen in congenital anomalies such as Chiari 2 and the Dandy-Walker spectrum of malformations (Chapter 1).

Intraventricular blood may be due to germinal matrix hemorrhage, dissection into the ventricles from an intraaxial hematoma (usually due to hypertension), rupture of subependymal veins (usually secondary to trauma), intraventricular arteriovenous malformations, intraventricular tumors, or the reflux from subarachnoid hemorrhage. In these patients, the clot and hydrocephalus are clearly visible on computed tomography (CT) or magnetic resonance imaging (MRI), but contrast-enhanced MRI is needed if a mass is suspected.

Intraventricular tumors resulting in hydrocephalus are not very common. Choroid plexus papillomas produce hydrocephalus due to overproduction of CSF and other reasons (see later). Other intraventricular tumors that result in hydrocephalus are ependymomas of the fourth ventricle in children and less commonly in adults, intraventricular astrocytomas, ependymomas, subependymomas, central neurocytoma, lymphoma, leukemia, and metastases.

Masses arising outside of the ventricular system may compress it and result in hydrocephalus. The most common intraaxial masses to produce hydrocephalus in children are cerebellar astrocytomas, medulloblastomas, tectal astrocytomas, pineal region

Table 5.4: Etiologies of Noncommunicating Hyrdrocephalus

Common	*Uncommon*
Congenital Intraventricular hemorrhage Intraventricular tumors	Extraventricular masses

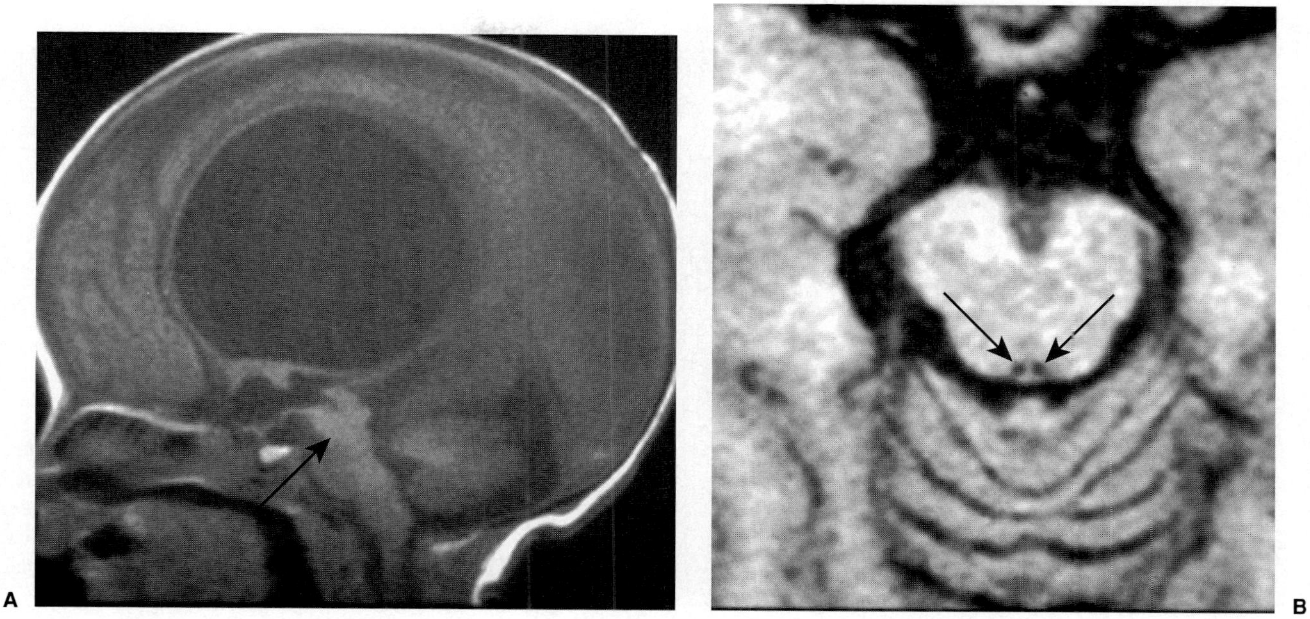

Figure 5.4 *Aqueductal Anomalies. A.* Sagittal T1-weighted image shows marked stenosis or atresia of the distal aqueduct *(arrow)* and massive hydrocephalus. *B.* In a different patient, axial T1-weighted image shows forking *(arrows)* of the aqueduct.

masses (germ cell tumors), giant cell astrocytomas (in patients with tuberous sclerosis), optic chiasm gliomas, and arachnoid cysts. All of these entities are discussed in detail in Chapter 6.

Communicating Hydrocephalus

The passage of CSF through the subarachnoid space may be affected by the presence of tumor, hemorrhage, or infection. The most common tumors to cause this in children are primitive neuroectodermal tumors, germ cells tumors, and leukemia. In adults, common tumors that obstruct the subarachnoid space are metastases, leukemia, and lymphoma. The most common infections/inflammations to result in communicating hydrocephalus are bacterial infections, tuberculosis, and sarcoidosis.

Overproduction of CSF is the result of an abnormality in the choroid plexus. This abnormality may be in the form of a mass (papilloma and carcinoma) or may consist of diffuse hypertrophy of the choroid plexus (1). In reality, the hydrocephalus resulting from choroid plexus tumors is due to a combination of overproduction of CSF, increased proteins in the CSF, hemorrhage, desquamated tumor cells, and metastatic seeding.

Normal-pressure hydrocephalus is an entity seen in adults (9). The typical clinical triad is gait apraxia, dementia, and incontinence. Unfortunately, most patients are difficult to diagnose (the triad is not present in all), and once the dementia has occurred very few patients show any improvement after treatment. The diagnosis of normal-pressure hydrocephalus is based on the following:

- Clinical triad of symptoms
- Imaging studies showing the lateral ventricles dilated out of proportion to the degree of cortical sulci dilatation
- Intraventricular reflux of radiotracer into the ventricles on cisternography
- Increased velocity of CSF in the aqueduct on phase-contrast MRI or pronounced flow void on T2-weighted images

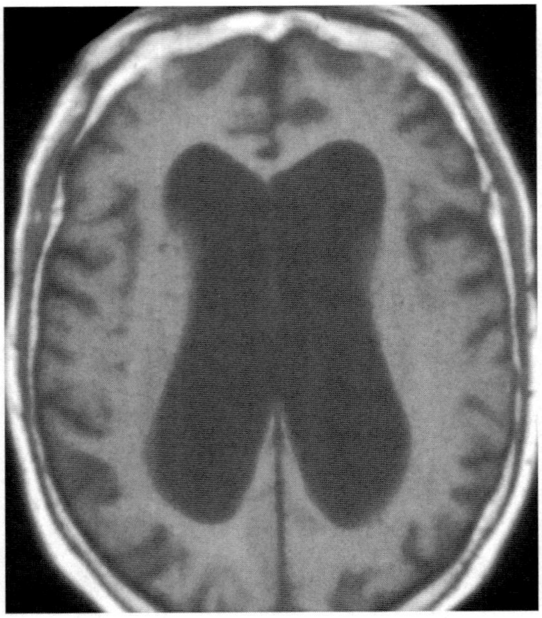

Figure 5.5 *Normal-Pressure Hydrocephalus.* Axial T1-weighted image shows dilated lateral ventricles that are out of proportion to the degree of dilatation of the cortical sulci. Note absence of periventricular edema.

The dilated ventricles presumably expand the brain outward and narrow the subarachnoid spaces (Fig. 5.5). As the brain responds to arterial systole, most of its force is directed to the widely patent ventricles and transmitted to the CSF, resulting in increasing velocity of the fluid in the aqueduct. Patients with increased aqueductal CSF velocity are believed to respond better to shunting. Unfortunately, despite shunting, many patients with normal-pressure hydrocephalus fare poorly. The dilated ventricles result in impingement of the corpus callosum against the falx, and this also may contribute to their symptoms (10).

Increased venous pressure may be due to occlusion or narrowing of the venous sinuses (11). The occlusion may be acute (thrombosis) or chronic (narrowing of the sinuses at the base of the skull). In the presence of venous flow restriction, hydrocephalus is more common in children, whereas increased intracranial pressure ("pseudotumor") is more common in adults. Abnormalities in the base of the skull may narrow the region of the sigmoid sinuses and the jugular foramina, resulting in diminished venous outflow. The osseous abnormalities are seen primarily in achondroplasia or in patients with syndromes resulting in craniosynostosis and skull base deformities (e.g., Apert's, Carpenter's, Crouzon's) (1). The restriction of venous outflow creates backup pressure on the pacchionian (arachnoid) granulations, presumably leading to decreased CSF resorption.

Benign External Hydrocephalus (Benign Enlargement of the Subarachnoid Spaces)

Benign external hydrocephalus (benign extraaxial fluid collections of infancy) is a diagnosis of exclusion.

This is a relatively common entity in children, and hence I address it separately. These are children in whom the head circumference is increased (1,6). They are asymptomatic. The macrocephaly becomes obvious during the first year of life, then plateaus around 1.5 years of age, and normalizes usually by 3 years of age. The findings presumably are due to an immaturity of the pacchionian granulations, although this has not been proven to be the actual etiology. CT usually is obtained in these patients, and it shows enlargement of the subarachnoid spaces, particularly in the frontal regions and along the anterior aspect of the interhemispheric fissure (12) (Fig. 5.6). The lateral ventricles usually are mildly

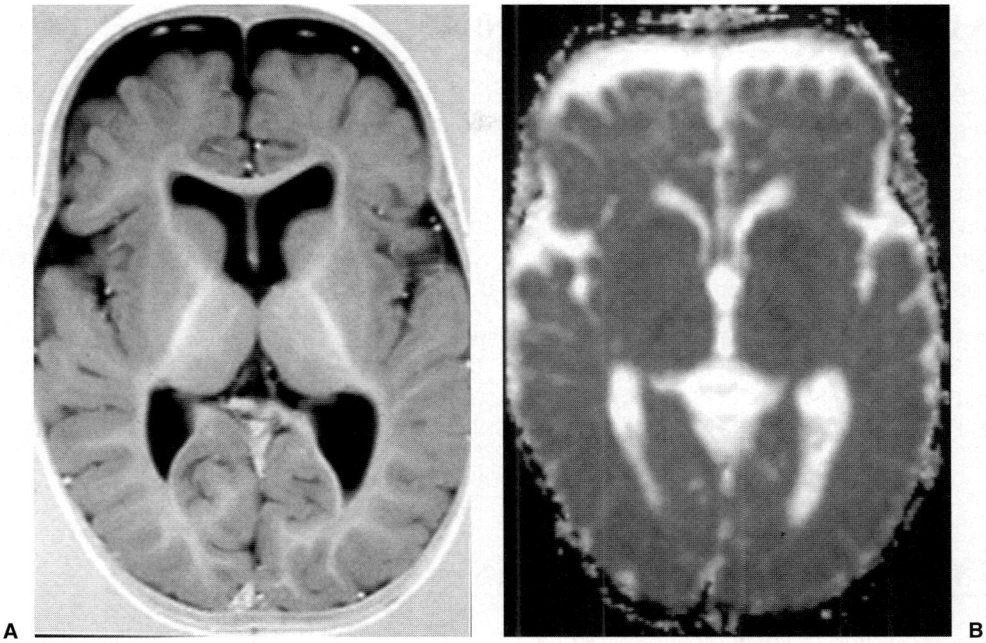

Figure 5.6 *Benign External Hydrocephalus. A.* T1-weighted axial inversion recovery image shows enlarged cerebrospinal fluid (CSF)–containing spaces, particularly in the frontal regions. The lateral ventricles also are somewhat prominent. *B.* Corresponding apparent diffusion coefficient map shows that the contents of the subarachnoid spaces behave similar to the intraventricular CSF, thus excluding the presence of chronic subdural hematomas or effusions (which would have different signal intensity). In this patient with progressive macrocephaly, the presumptive diagnosis of benign external hydrocephalus was made.

prominent, especially their frontal horns. The basilar cisterns also are prominent. The differential diagnosis for enlarged subarachnoid spaces in children is as follows (1):

- Benign external hydrocephalus
- Current or prior meningitis
- Current or prior trauma
- Malnutrition
- Dehydration
- Atrophy
- Steroids
- Chronic illnesses

The most important aspect in these children is to differentiate benign external hydrocephalus from subdural collections such as seen in trauma or meningitis. Subdural collections tend to be asymmetric, whereas dilatation of the subarachnoid spaces is fairly symmetric. In the presence of enlarged subarachnoid spaces, most of the superficial veins remain close to the inner table of the skull and the bridging veins (about the region of the superior sagittal sinus) are visualized crossing the CSF-filled space With subdural collections, the superficial veins are inwardly displaced and lay on the brain cortex, and the bridging veins are not seen. In addition, subdural collections may show different signal intensity compared with CSF, particularly on proton-density and fluid attenuation inversion recovery (FLAIR) images. We usually recommend a repeat imaging study between 3 and 5 years of age to document the resolution of benign subdural collections (many neuroradiologists do not recommend a follow-up imaging study if the head circumference normalizes). If the head circumference continues to increase or clinical symptoms ensue, then prompt imaging is needed.

Slit Ventricle Syndrome

This rare entity is more familiar to neurosurgeons than to radiologists. Patients with the slit ventricle syndrome are those who have been previously shunted and present with signs and symptoms of increased intracranial pressure (shunt failure) but show normal or reduced size of lateral ventricles on imaging studies (1,6). Conversely, the ventricles also may be small when too much CSF is being drained. Intermittent shunt obstruction may produce symptoms, but when these patients are imaged, the patency of the shunt may have been reestablished and the ventricles appear normal. The causes of the small ventricles are:

- Inability of the brain parenchyma to be displaced (noncompliance)
- Intraventricular (ependymal) scars
- Overdrainage of CSF (intracranial hypotension)
- "Pseudotumor" cerebri

In reality, slit ventricle syndrome is very rare. It is mainly a clinical diagnosis.

Intracranial Hypotension

Thickened and enhancing dura and engorged veins in either the intracranial or intraspinal compartments should raise the suspicion of intracranial hypotension due to loss of CSF.

The syndrome of spontaneous intracranial hypotension (SIH) has received considerable attention (13). Before MRI, this syndrome was not well known and its imaging manifestations were not appreciable. Many years ago SIH was described, from a clinical standpoint, in patients presenting with chronic headaches in the absence of a history of trauma, surgery, or a lumbar puncture. The etiology of this rare entity is an occult leak of CSF (often in the spine) that results in decreased intracranial fluid volume and hence pressure. Symptoms are postural headache, stiff neck, nausea, vomiting, cranial nerve palsies, vertigo, tinnitus, and photophobia (13,14). The CSF usually is normal but may show increased proteins. The CSF pressure usually is less than 6 cm H_2O. Most patients can be treated symptomatically because the leaks most likely will resolve spontaneously. In patients with chronic symptoms, imaging is indicated. On brain MRI, there may be widening of the subarachnoid convexity spaces, small ventricular size, and downward sagging of the midline structures (cerebellar tonsils and floor of the third ventricle; Fig. 5.7). The venous sinuses (particularly the superior sagittal sinus) may be prominent. After contrast administration, there is significant enhancement of thick dura with sparing of the leptomeninges and of the venous sinuses. In the spine, the epidural space is thick, enhances, and may contain dilated epidural veins (14,15). All of these findings may lead to com-

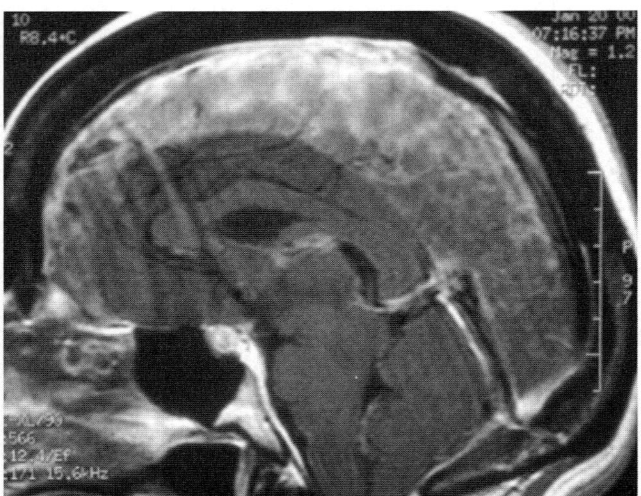

Figure 5.7 *Intracranial Hypotension.* Sagittal postcontrast T1-weighted image of a "sagging" third ventricle, poorly visualized suprasellar cistern, low-lying cerebellar tonsils, prominent venous sinuses, and marked enhancement of falx cerebri. Note that the venous plexus on the dorsal surface of the clivus also is prominent.

pression of the spinal cord. If the site of leak needs to be documented for treatment purposes, we usually use a combination of iodinated contrast and radionuclide cisternography. I prefer to use a radionuclide with a long half-life and image the patient on several consecutive days because the CSF leak may be intermittent. If the leak is found on immediate studies, then the anatomic details of that site may be evaluated with postmyelography CT while there is still an adequate amount of iodinated contrast in the thecal sac. An indirect sign of a CSF leak on nuclear medicine studies is premature visualization of the urinary system. It is believed that Tarlov (perineurial) cysts may play a role in the development of SIH. These cysts may result in tiny dural tears leading to the escape of CSF. Occasionally, an intraspinal fluid-filled cyst is found at the site of the tear.

Complications of Ventricular Shunts

The most common complication of shunt is its failure to function properly (1,6). Shunt malfunction occurs in 25% to 70% of patients. These patients unfortunately present with nonspecific clinical signs, including headaches, lethargy, and altered mental status (6). In many children, these are similar to the symptoms that occur with most viral illnesses, and therefore many of them receive frequent imaging studies. The only reliable way to make the diagnosis of shunt malfunction is by comparison with previous imaging studies. Most shunts are inserted through frontal or occipital burr holes. The goal is to position the tip of the shunt away from choroid plexus, usually in the frontal horns of the lateral ventricles (choroid plexus stops at the level of the foramina of Monro). The shunt commonly perforates the septum pellucidum and crosses into the contralateral ventricle. If the tip of the shunt is close to the choroid plexus, this organ may grow around it and occlude it. The presence of periventricular edema (transependymal CSF resorption) usually indicates acute hydrocephalus, but this is not always present in patients in whom hydrocephalus has occurred many times owing to shunt malfunction (Fig. 5.8A). Table 5.5 lists the possible complications from a shunt (16).

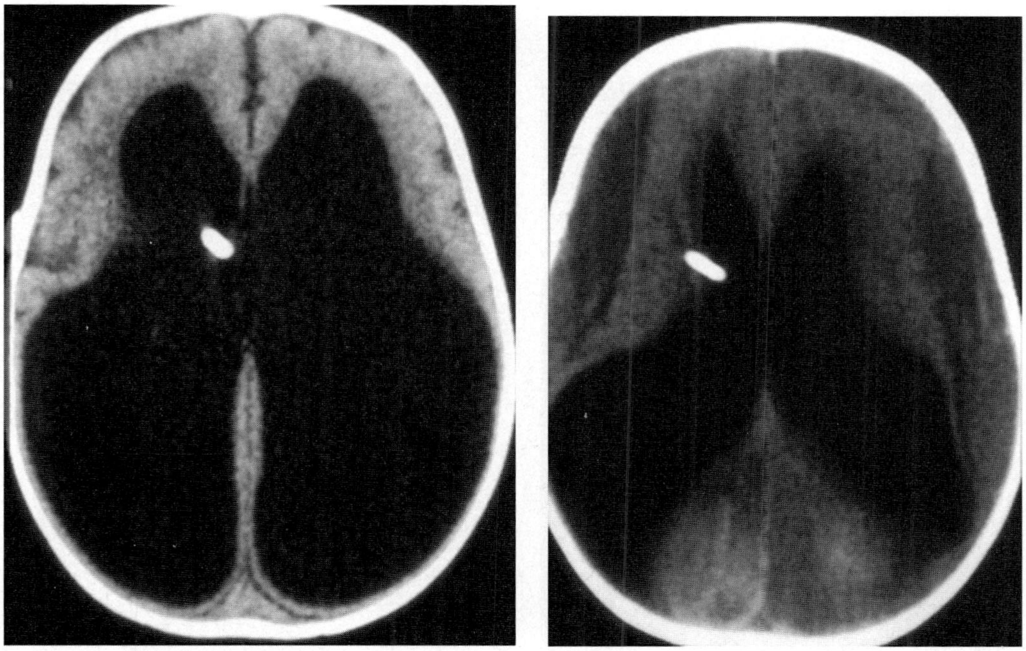

A B

Figure 5.8 *Shunt Malfunction and Subdural Collections Postshunting. A.* Axial computed tomography shows massive dilatation of the lateral ventricles secondary to shunt malfunction. *B.* After shunt revision in the same patient, the lateral ventricles are smaller but bilateral subdural fluid collections have developed.

Table 5.5: Shunt Complications

Common	Uncommon
Shunt failure and hydrocephalus	Slit ventricle syndrome
Meningeal fibrosis	Perishunt edema and cyst formation
Subdural hematomas	Scalp CSF cysts about catheter and reservoir
Infection	Intraperitoneal CSF cyst formation
	Intraabdominal tumor or choroid plexus seeding
	Intestinal obstruction
	Ascites
	Perforation of abdominal viscera
	Peritonitis
	Catheter degradation (seen as calcifications)

CSF, cerebrospinal fluid.

The tip of an intraventricular shunt needs to be in the frontal horns, in which there is no choroid plexus.

Subdural hematomas occur after rapid shunting or overdrainage of CSF, as may happen with low-pressure valves (most shunts today have medium-pressure valves). Rapid decompression of the lateral ventricles leads to collapse of the brain parenchyma with stretching and tearing of the bridging veins and development of subdural hematomas or hygromas (Fig. 5.8B). These hematomas are more common in older persons (but also are seen in children), particularly those shunted for normal-pressure hydrocephalus. Postshunt subdural hematomas are less common in patients younger than 3 years of age.

Meningeal fibrosis is a common occurrence after shunt placement (17). This fibrosis usually involves the dura and spares the leptomeninges. The pachymeninges become thick and show prominent contrast enhancement. By MRI, they are of low signal intensity on T1-weighted images and bright on proton-density and T2 sequences (18). They may be mistaken for postshunt subdural hematomas, but fibrosis enhances after gadolinium is given (19) (Fig. 5.9). I have seen fibrosis as early as 5 to 7 days after shunting.

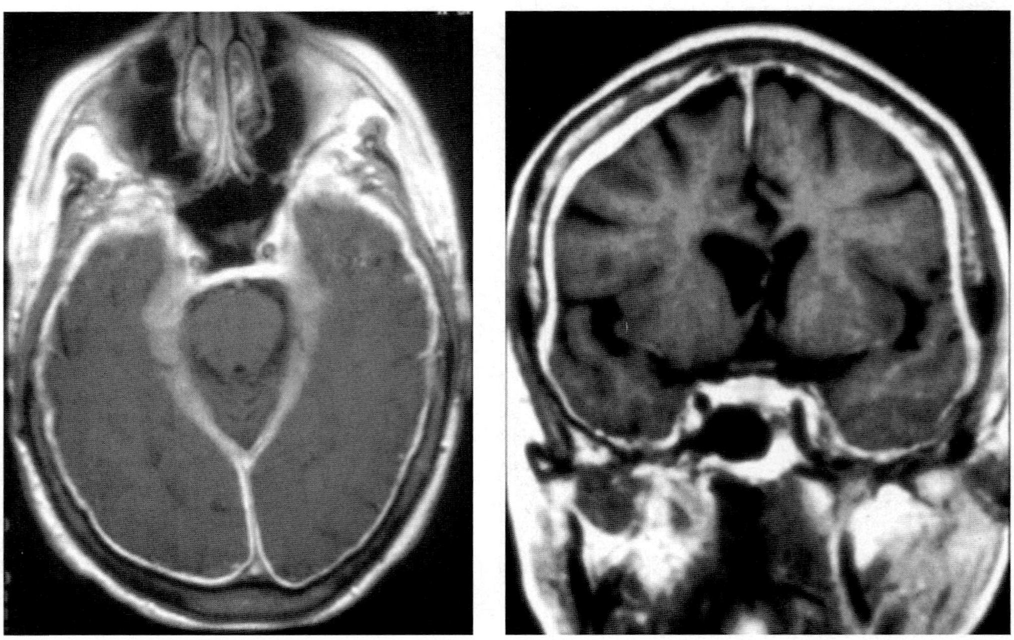

Figure 5.9 *Postventricular Shunting Dural Fibrosis.* Axial *(A)* and coronal *(B)* postcontrast T1-weighted images show thick enhancing dura.

Symptoms of shunt-related infections are intermittent low-grade fever, meningismus, anemia, dehydration, and hepatosplenomegaly (1,6). Shunt infections occur in approximately 1% to 5% of patients. Signs of infections on the skin overlying the shunt course or the reservoir may be present. The infection may extend into the ventricles or the abdomen. Contrast-enhanced studies are needed to document the presence of ventriculitis (ependymitis). Chronically or previously infected ventricles may contain septations. If a shunt is infected, it usually is removed and a temporary ventriculostomy is placed while the patient receives antibiotics.

Degeneration of a shunt leads to its calcification. Calcification of a shunt anywhere along its course correlates with shunt failure.

Perishunt cysts, fluid-filled tracts, and edema are rare imaging findings of shunt malfunction (6) (Fig. 5.10). At times, choroid plexus is clearly seen encasing the distal end of the intracranial shunt. Rarely, a fibrotic mass (enhancing just like the choroid plexus) may form about the intraventricular tip of the catheter and result in its obstruction. This mass may become a combination of fibrosis and granulation, and may even calcify (Fig. 5.11A). Calcifications of shunt catheters correlate closely with shunt malfunction. These calcifications may occur in the tip of the intraventricular portion of the shunt or anywhere along its course (Fig. 5.11B). Last, skull changes may occur in chronically shunted patients (1) (Fig. 5.12). The skull becomes thick with a prominent diploic bone marrow space. The paranasal sinuses and mastoid air cells may grow inward to compensate for lack of brain growth. Intraabdominal complications are rare and necessitate imaging with CT or sonography. Intraperitoneal tumor seeding is uncommon and better evaluated by CT. Intraperitoneal tumor seeding is indistinguishable from benign choroid plexus hyperplasia extending into the abdomen. This is seen particularly if shunting was started when the patient was a child. Large CSF cysts ("CSF-omas") may form around the distal end of the intraperitoneal portion of a shunt (Fig. 5.10B).

Rarely, the neurosurgeon may not be able to assess the functioning of the shunt's proximal limb. This usually is accomplished by tapping the reservoir or documenting its filling after manual compression. In some cases, instillation of iodinated contrast material may be needed. In these patients, we usually provide fluoroscopic guidance to confirm that the drainage of contrast is intraventricular. We usually use 2 to 5 mL of nonionic contrast at concentrations of 180 or 200 mg/mL of iodine. This procedure also is useful to

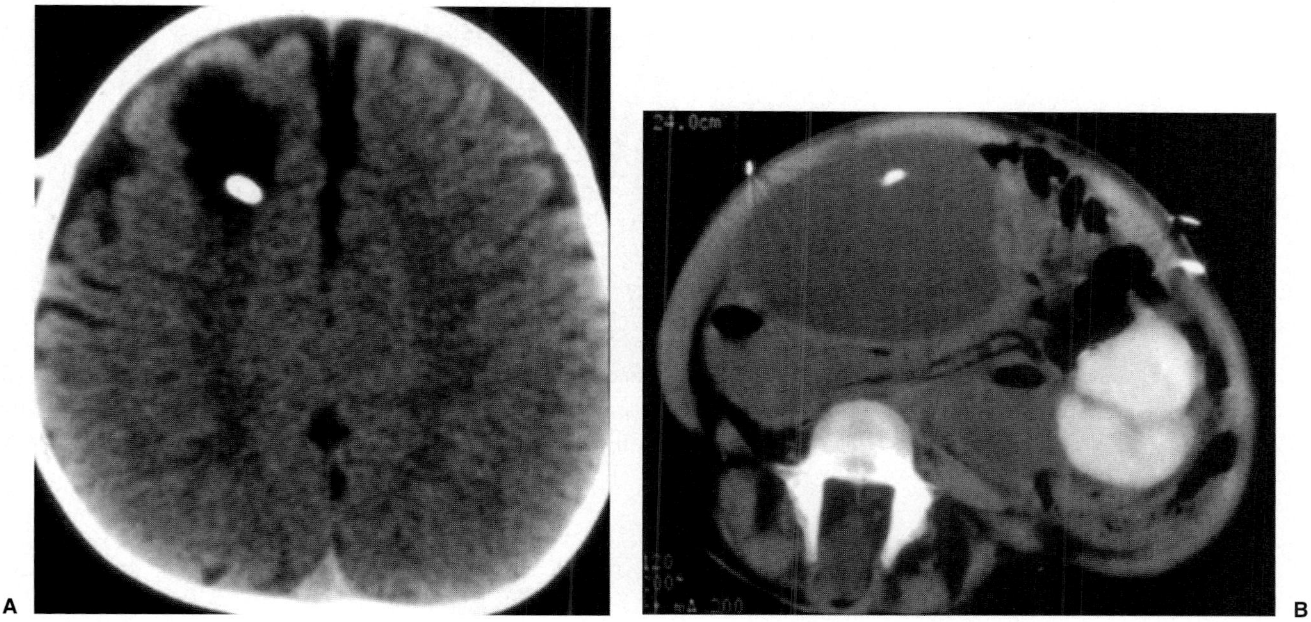

Figure 5.10 *Perishunt Cyst. A.* Axial computed tomography (CT) in a patient with shunt failure shows formation of a cerebrospinal fluid (CSF)–filled cyst around the catheter. *B.* Axial CT of the abdomen shows large CSF cyst surrounding the distal limb of the shunt catheter.

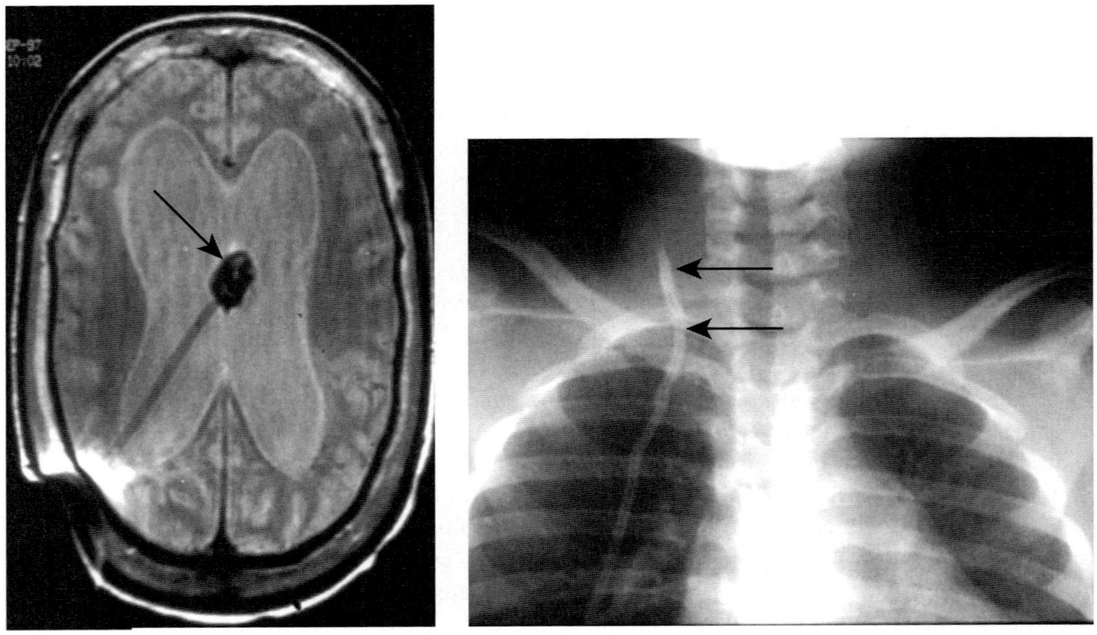

Figure 5.11 *Degeneration of Shunt Catheters. A.* Axial proton-density image shows masslike thickening *(arrow)* of the tip of the ventricular catheter that represents a granulomatous reaction. *B.* Frontal chest radiograph shows calcification *(arrows)* of the distal limb of a shunt catheter. The superior aspect of the catheter is not visualized.

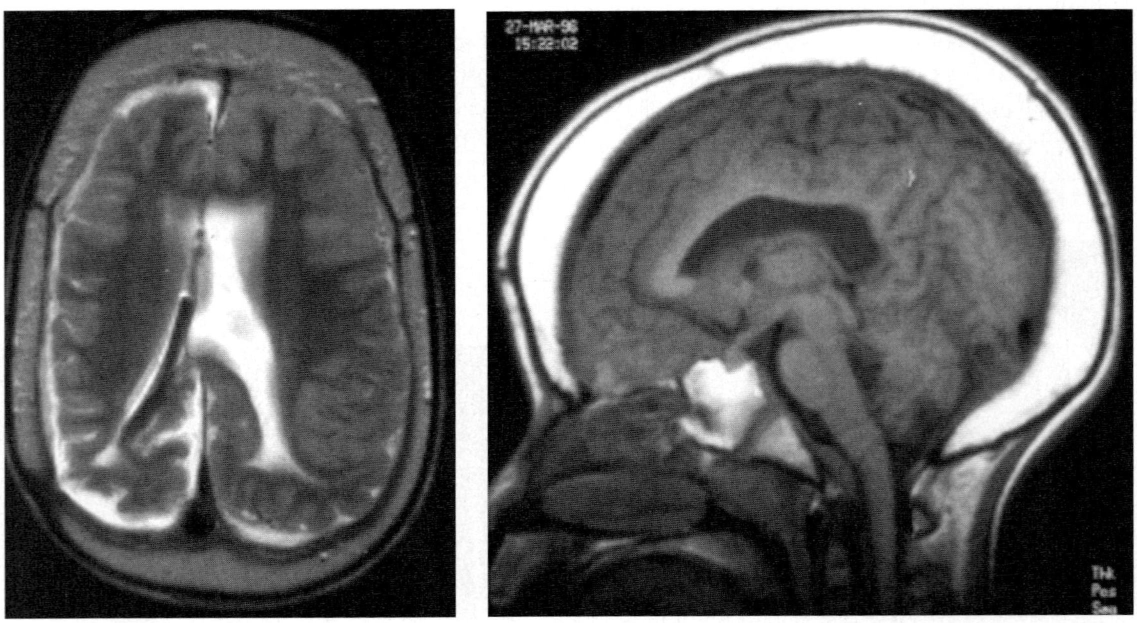

Figure 5.12 *Skull Changes after Ventricular Shunting.* Axial T2- *(A)* and sagittal T1-weighted *(B)* images show marked thickening of the diploic space of the calvarium in a patient who has been shunted for many years.

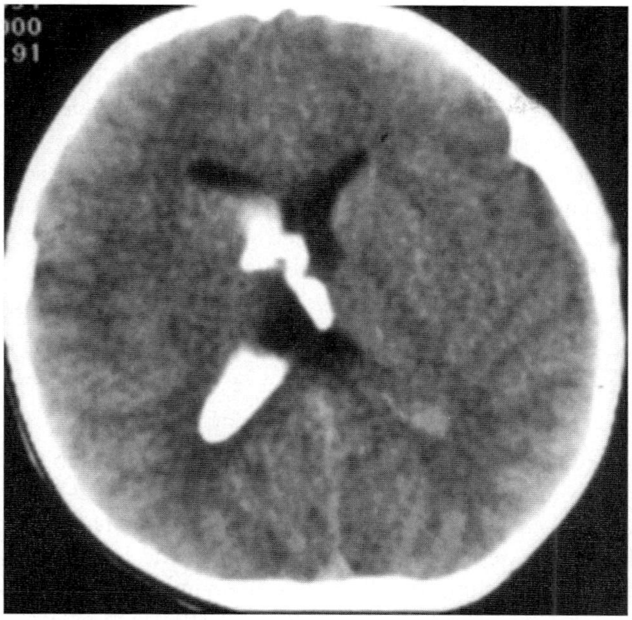

Figure 5.13 *Multiple Intraventricular Septations Secondary to Prior Infection.* Computed tomography obtained after introduction of contrast material into the proximal limb of a shunt catheter shows that the lateral ventricles contain many compartments not communicating with others.

evaluate the presence or absence of communications among the different compartments in patients with intraventricular scars (Fig. 5.13).

TRAPPED VENTRICLES

A trapped ventricle, as it name implies, is one in which lack of egress of CSF causes it to enlarge. The most common trapped ventricle is the fourth. The fourth ventricle becomes trapped when its outlet foramina and the aqueduct of Sylvius are blocked (Fig. 5.14). The choroid plexus produces CSF that is unable to escape, leading to ventricular dilatation. A

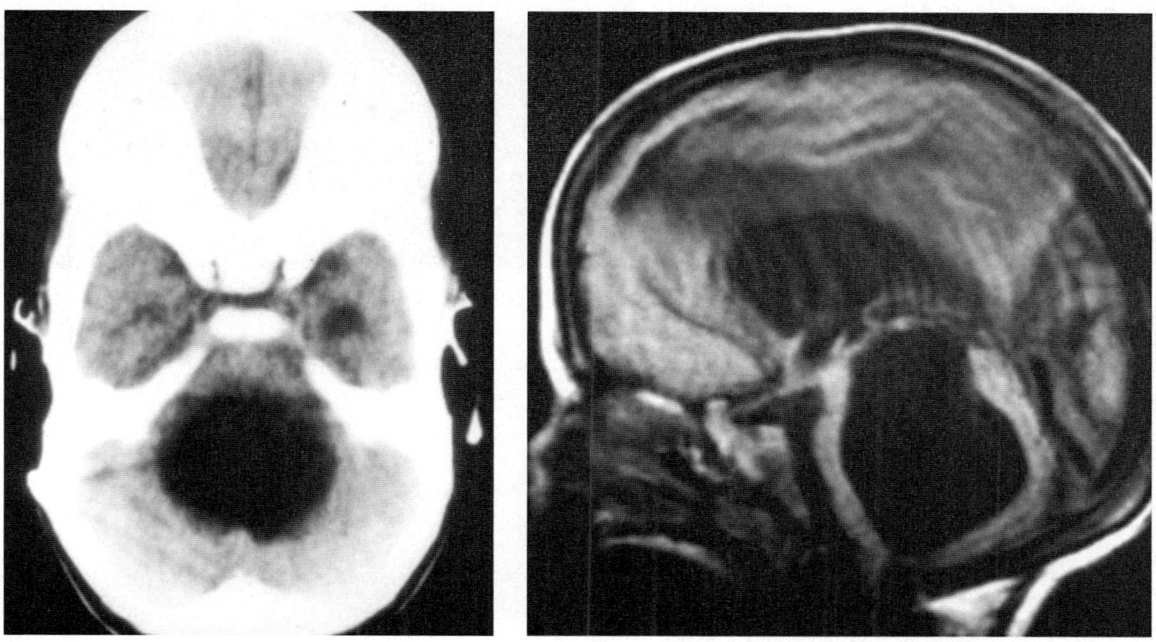

A B

Figure 5.14 *Trapped Ventricle.* Axial computed tomography *A* and sagittal T1-weighted image *B* show markedly dilated fourth ventricles (different patients) due to entrapment.

ball-valve mechanism allowing CSF to enter the ventricle also may be responsible for the findings. A lateral ventricle may become trapped by two mechanisms. A mass or lesion (such as scar) may obstruct the foramen of Monro, or displacement (midline shift) of the ventricle may result in obstruction of its foramen. A portion of a lateral ventricle may become trapped by an intraparenchymal mass, obstructing its communication with the rest of the ventricle, or an intraventricular mass or scar can isolate a region of a ventricle. Trapped ventricles are common in patients with a history of previous shunt infection. Regardless of its etiology, the trapped portion needs to be shunted and will behave exactly (including all of the aforementioned complications) as a shunted ventricle.

Endoscopic Ventriculostomies

After endoscopic third ventriculostomies, the hydrocephalus resolves slowly and a significant change in size of the ventricles may not be evident acutely.

Because shunt failure is so common, endoscopic ventriculostomies represent an attractive therapy. This, coupled with improvements in endoscope technology (smaller, capable of making acute turns) has led to the common use of endoscopic ventriculostomies (20). Endoscopic ventriculostomies may be used to relieve the pressure from one dilated lateral ventricle by creating a fenestration in the septum pellucidum. Scars at the level of the foramina of Monro may be treated, thus avoiding the placement of a shunt catheter. The most common type of ventriculostomy involves the third ventricle. The hypothalamus between the mamillary bodies and pituitary stalk is fenestrated, creating a communication between the third ventricle and the suprasellar cistern. Unlike in catheter shunting, an immediate decrease in the size of the ventricles is not evident. Rather, there is a progressive diminution of ventricular size in the weeks that follow the ventriculostomy (therefore, this is a more physiologic treatment). Not all third ventriculostomies are successful; over 50% of them fail owing to closure of the perforation. Occasionally, spontaneous third ven-

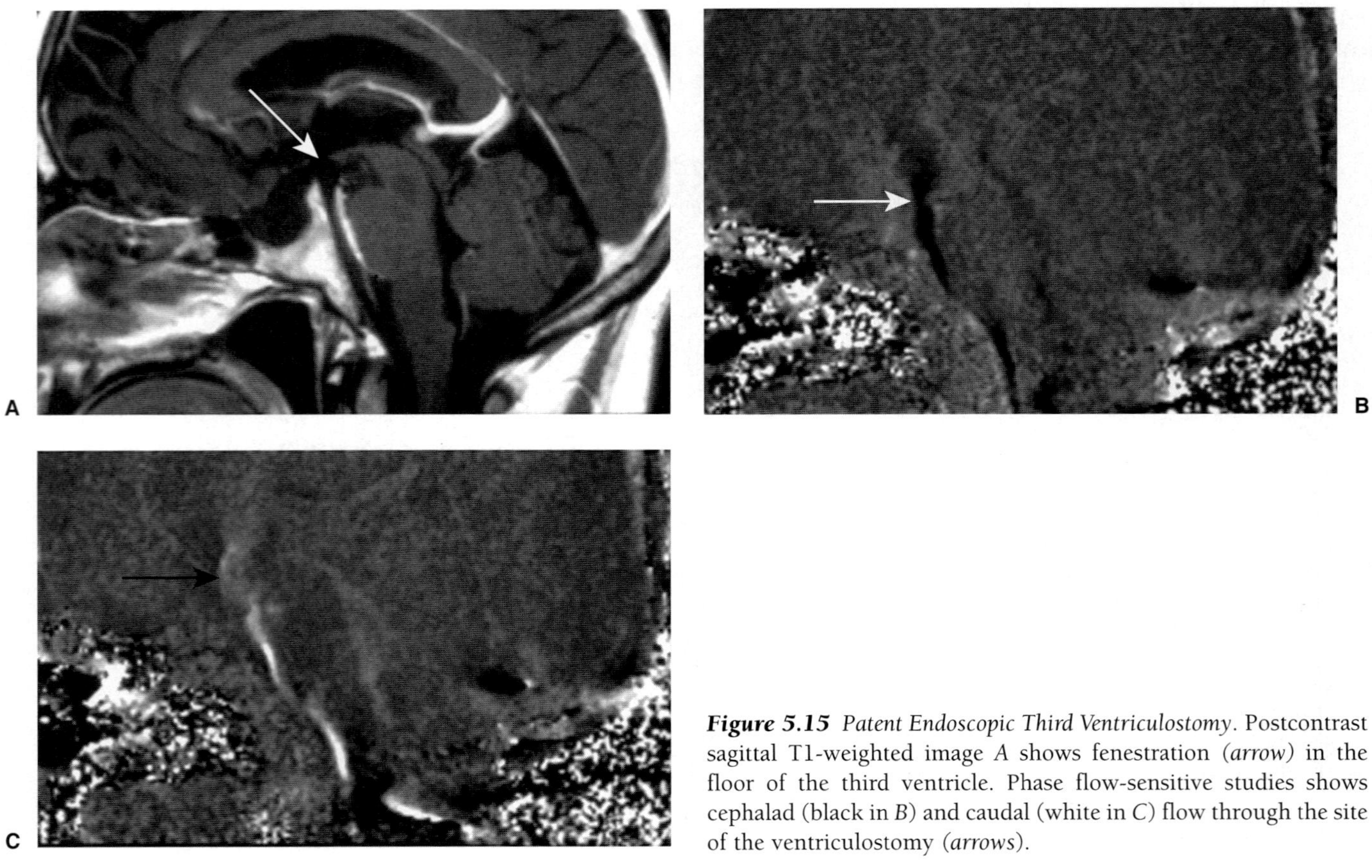

Figure 5.15 *Patent Endoscopic Third Ventriculostomy*. Postcontrast sagittal T1-weighted image *A* shows fenestration *(arrow)* in the floor of the third ventricle. Phase flow-sensitive studies shows cephalad (black in *B*) and caudal (white in *C*) flow through the site of the ventriculostomy *(arrows)*.

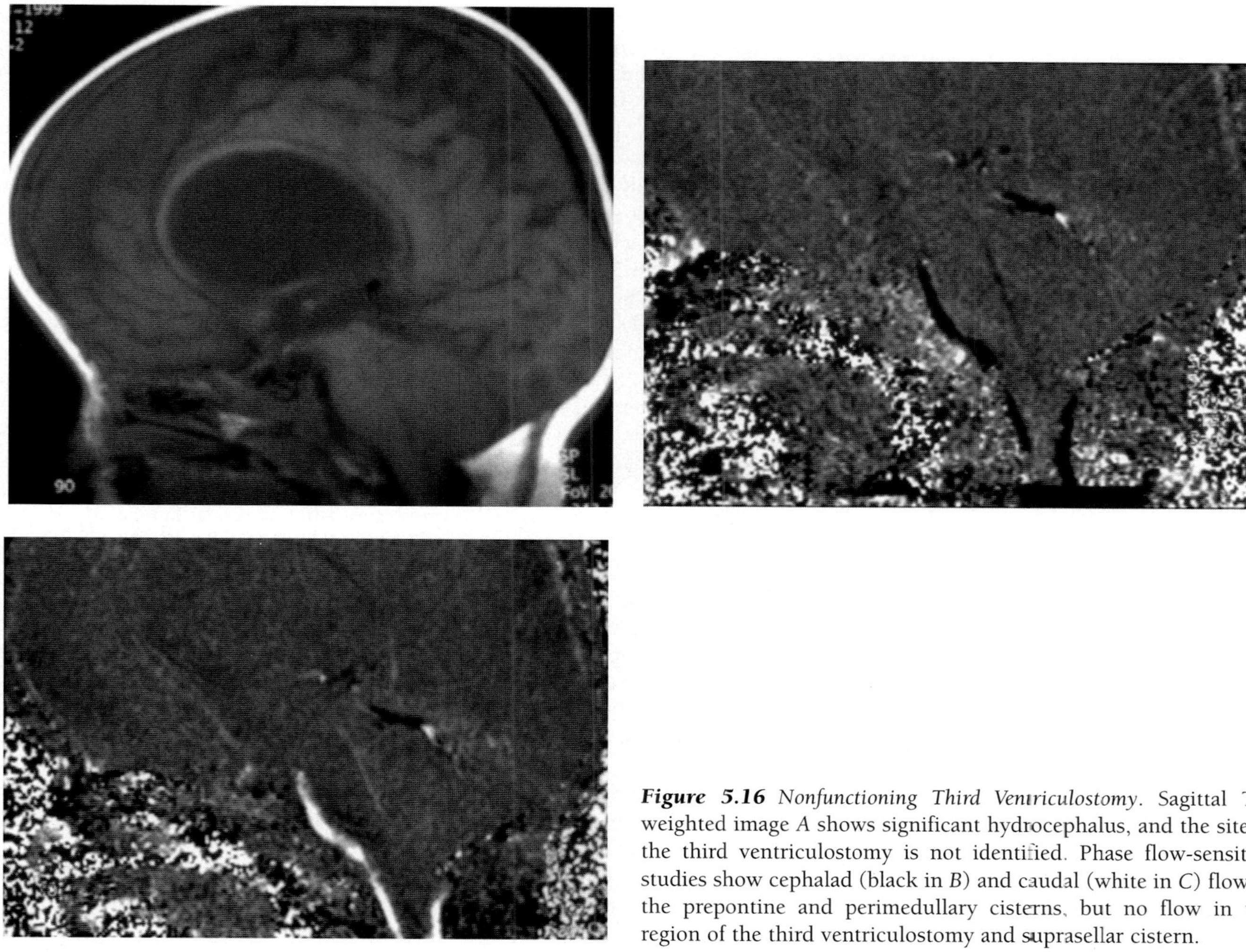

A B C

Figure 5.16 *Nonfunctioning Third Ventriculostomy.* Sagittal T1-weighted image *A* shows significant hydrocephalus, and the site of the third ventriculostomy is not identified. Phase flow-sensitive studies show cephalad (black in *B*) and caudal (white in *C*) flow in the prepontine and perimedullary cisterns, but no flow in the region of the third ventriculostomy and suprasellar cistern.

triculostomies may develop in patients with massive hydrocephalus (21). The patency of third ventriculostomies may be evaluated with MRI. Thin (3-mm) sagittal T1- and T2-weighted images may be used to visualize the fenestration. Flow-sensitive phase-contrast (ideally using retrospective cardiac gating) MRI identifies the presence of synchronous flow at the ventriculostomy site compared with the CSF flow in the third ventricle and suprasellar cistern (Figs. 5.15 and 5.16).

References

1. Barkovich AJ. Pediatric neuroimaging, 3rd ed. Philadelphia: Lippincott Williams & Wilkins, 2000:581–620.
2. Greitz D, Greitz T. The pathogenesis and hemodynamics of hydrocephalus: proposal for a new understanding. Int J Neuroradiol 1997;3:367–375.
3. Leach JL, Jones BV, Tomsick TA, et al. Normal appearance of arachnoid granulations on contrast-enhanced CT and MR of the brain: differentiation from dural sinus disease. AJNR Am J Neuroradiol 1996;17:1523–1532.
4. Roche J, Warner D. Arachnoid granulations in the transverse and sigmoid sinuses: CT, MR and MR angiographic appearance of a normal anatomic variation. AJNR Am J Neuroradiol 1996;17: 677–683.
5. Greitz D, Hannerz J. A proposed model of cerebrospinal fluid circulation: observations with radionuclide cisternography. AJNR Am J Neuroradiol 1996;17:431–438.
6. Castillo M, Mukherji SK. Imaging of the pediatric head, neck, and spine. Philadelphia: Lippincott–Raven, 1996:319–326.

7. Barkovich AJ, Newton TH. MR of aqueductal stenosis: evidence of a broad spectrum of tectal distortion. AJNR Am J Neuroradiol 1989;10:471–476.
8. Atlas SW, Mark AS, Fram EK. Aqueductal stenosis: evaluation with gradient-echo rapid MR imaging. Radiology 1988;169:449–453.
9. Bradley WG Jr, Scalzo D, Queralt J, et al. Normal-pressure hydrocephalus: evaluation with cerebrospinal fluid flow measurements at MR imaging. Radiology 1996;198:523–529.
10. Jinkins JR. Clinical manifestations of hydrocephalus caused by impingement of the corpus callosum on the falx: an MR study in 40 patients. AJNR Am J Neuroradiol 1991;12:331–340.
11. Mueller SM, Bell W, Cornell S, et al. Achondroplasia and hydrocephalus: a computerized tomographic, roentgenographic, and psycho-metric study. Neurology 1977;27:430–434.
12. Wilms G, Vanderschueren G, Demaerel PH, et al. CT and MR in infants with pericerebral collections and macrocephaly: benign enlargement of the subarachnoid spaces versus subdural collections. AJNR Am J Neuroradiol 1993;14:855–860.
13. Dillon WP, Fishman RA. Some lessons learned about the diagnosis and treatment of spontaneous intracranial hypotension. AJNR Am J Neuroradiol 1998;19:1001b–1002b.
14. Rabin BM, Roychowdhury S, Meyer JR, et al. Spontaneous intracranial hypotension: spinal MR findings. AJNR Am J Neuroradiol 1998;19:1034–1039.
15. Yousry I, Forderreuther S, Moriggl B, et al. Cervical MR imaging in postural headache: MR signs and pathophysiological implications. AJNR Am J Neuroradiol 2001;22:1239–1250.
16. Murtagh FR, Quencer RM, Poole CA. Cerebrospinal fluid shunt function and hydrocephalus in the pediatric age group: a radiographic/clinical correlation. Radiology 1979;132:385–388.
17. Martin DS, Awwad EE, Pittman T. Meningeal fibrosis appearing shortly after ventricular shunting. AJNR Am J Neuroradiol 1990;11:617–618.
18. Destian S, Heier LA, Zimmerman RD, et al. Differentiation between meningeal fibrosis and chronic subdural hematoma after ventricular shunting: value of enhanced CT and MR scans. AJNR Am J Neuroradiol 1989;10:1021–1026.
19. Hudgins PA, Davis PC, Hoffman JC Jr. Gadopentetate dimeglumine-enhanced MR imaging in children following surgery for brain tumor: spectrum of meningeal findings. AJNR Am J Neuroradiol 1991;12:301–307.
20. Jack CR Jr, Kelly PJ. Stereotactic third ventriculostomy: assessment of patency with MR imaging. AJNR Am J Neuroradiol 1989;10:515–522.
21. Rovira A, Capellades J, Grivé E, et al. Spontaneous ventriculostomy: report of three cases revealed by flow-sensitive phase-contrast cine MR imaging. AJNR Am J Neuroradiol 1999;20:1647–1652.

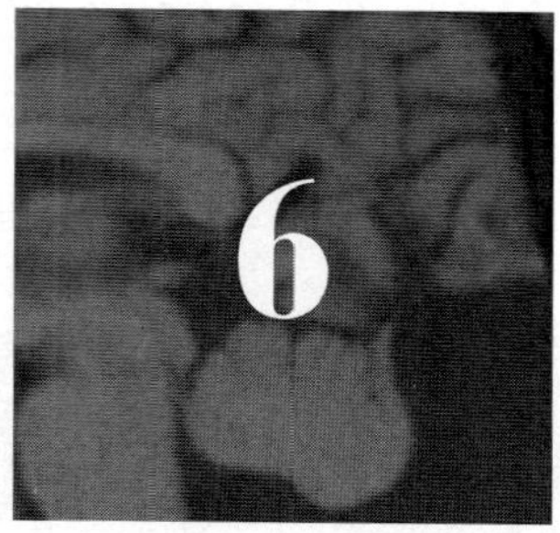

INTRACRANIAL TUMORS

- Childhood Tumors
- Adult Tumors

CHILDHOOD TUMORS

INFRATENTORIAL TUMORS

Pilocytic Astrocytoma (Juvenile Pilocytic Astrocytoma)

Juvenile pilocytic astrocytoma (JPA) is the second most common primary cerebellar tumor after medulloblastoma occurring in children. JPAs are more common in boys and usually are found between 5 and 10 years of age (1). JPA accounts for over 30% of all brain tumors in children, but occasionally may be found in adults. Most JPAs arise in the cerebellar hemispheres, slightly off midline, or in the vermis. The typical clinical findings are related mostly to increased intracranial pressure due to hydrocephalus and cerebellar or brainstem symptoms due to compression. Hydrocephalus occurs relatively early in the course of the disease, and ventricular shunting markedly improves the symptoms. The name of these tumors is derived from the fact that the neoplastic astrocytes are elongated ("piloid" or hairlike) and are arranged in parallel rows. JPAs are well defined tumors. According to the World Health Organization (WHO) classification, JPAs are grade I astrocytomas. Other well defined (localized) intracranial astrocytomas include giant cell astrocytoma (in tuberous sclerosis) and pleomorphic xanthoastrocytoma (2).

The importance of dividing astrocytomas into those that are localized and those that are diffuse is that the localized ones have a much better prognosis because they are amenable to surgical resection. As such, the 20-year survival rate is nearly 80% to 90% for patients with JPAs, and many of them are considered cured if the resection is total. Conversely, approximately 20% of JPAs recur, some of them aggressively with subarachnoid tumor spread. Tumor spread into the adjacent leptomeninges is a not uncommon finding at histologic studies, but it tends to be limited (2).

The imaging appearance of JPA is fairly typical (3). Most tumors are 2 to 4 cm in diameter and present as well demarcated masses slightly off the midline in the cerebellum. They are of intermediate T1 signal and hyperintense on T2-weighted and fluid attenuation inversion recovery (FLAIR) images. They usually have no surrounding edema. Approximately 80% of these tumors contain one (50%) or multiple cysts (30%) (Fig. 6.1A and B). The wall of the cyst(s) usually consists of compressed cerebellum and gliosis, and not tumor. Occasionally, the wall may be lined with tumor. Tumoral calcifications are rare (<10%). After contrast administration, there is intense enhancement of one or more tumor nodules. Approximately 20% to 30% of JPAs are completely solid (Fig. 6.1C). Despite their benign histology, these tumors have several unique imaging findings. Their intense enhancement does not correlate with a higher grade of malignancy. On positron emission

Approximately 80% of cerebellar juvenile pilocytic astrocytomas are cystic, whereas approximately 20% of them are solid.

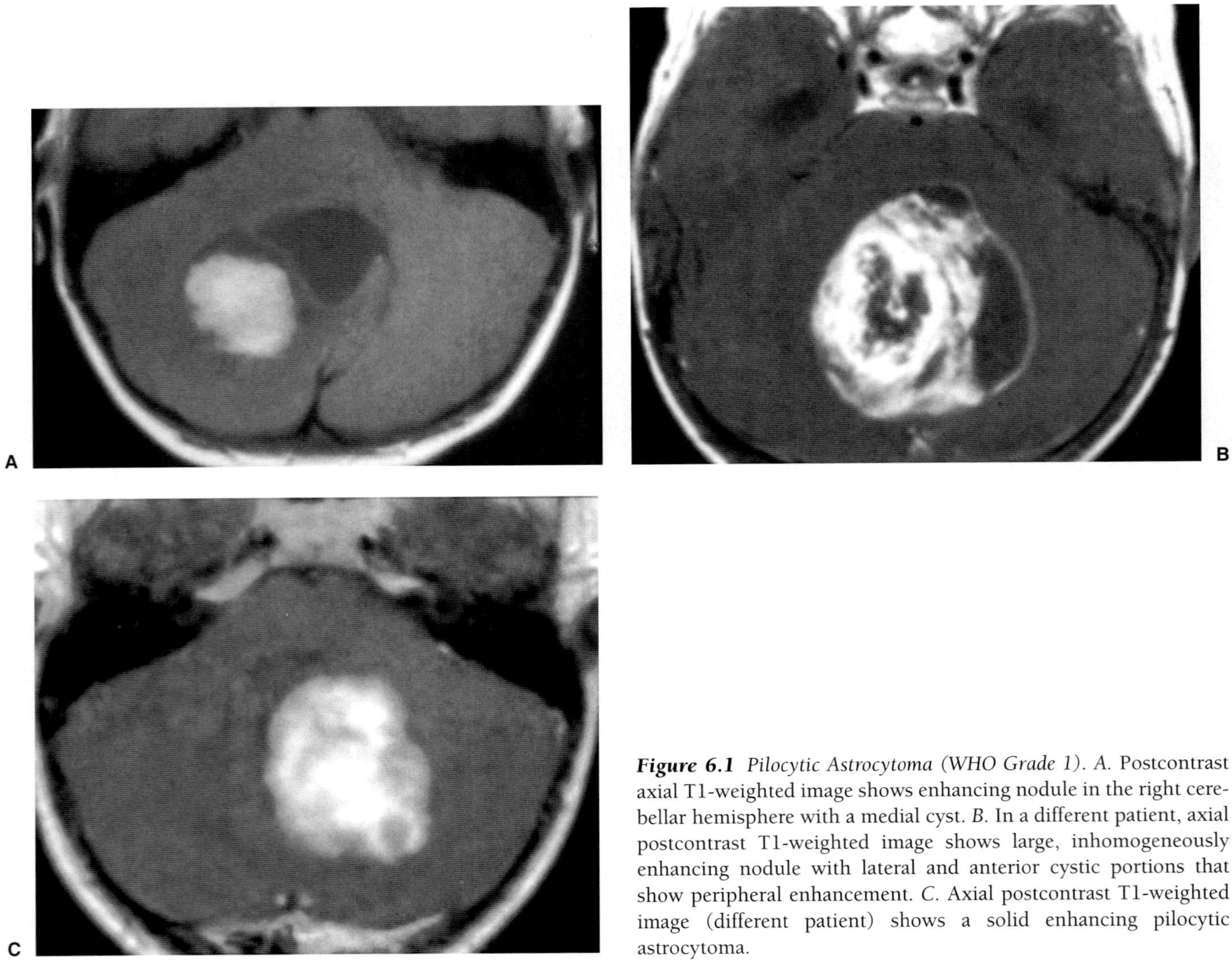

Figure 6.1 *Pilocytic Astrocytoma (WHO Grade 1). A.* Postcontrast axial T1-weighted image shows enhancing nodule in the right cerebellar hemisphere with a medial cyst. *B.* In a different patient, axial postcontrast T1-weighted image shows large, inhomogeneously enhancing nodule with lateral and anterior cystic portions that show peripheral enhancement. *C.* Axial postcontrast T1-weighted image (different patient) shows a solid enhancing pilocytic astrocytoma.

tomography, they show avid uptake of glucose tracers (similar to more malignant tumors) (1). On proton magnetic resonance (MR) spectroscopy they show significant elevation of choline and presence of lactate (because of their glycolytic nature), as well as high levels of myoinositol.

Brainstem Astrocytomas

These are relatively common lesions probably accounting for approximately one-fourth of posterior fossa tumors. If brainstem and cerebellar astrocytomas are grouped together, they comprise the most common tumors in the posterior fossa of children (2). Brainstem astrocytomas are more common in boys and usually are found in patients younger than 10 years of age. There is an association between brainstem gliomas and neurofibromatosis type 1 (NF-1) (2). Approximately 50% of brainstem gliomas are of the pilocytic type, and the remainder are infiltrative fibrillary astrocytomas that have a tendency to degenerate into higher malignant grades. The tumor may be isolated to the pons, involve both the pons and the medulla (50%) or midbrain, and may extend into the thalami (4). Approximately 60% of these tumors show an exophytic component protruding into one of the adjacent cisterns. Brainstem astrocytomas projecting into the fourth ventricle tend to be of the pilocytic type and thus may have a better prognosis. Despite their low histologic grade, brainstem gliomas have a poor prognosis, with most patients dying approximately 2 years after the diagnosis.

Many patients have very few clinical symptoms until the terminal phase of the disease. Unlike cerebellar JPAs, brainstem gliomas result in hydrocephalus only late in the course of the disease. This presumably is due to a gradual posterior bowing of the fourth ventricle and aqueduct that allows for flow of CSF. Brainstem gliomas often are of low T1 signal intensity and bright on T2 and FLAIR images (4) (Fig. 6.2A). Their enhancement is extremely variable (diffuse, nodular, or absent; Fig. 6.2B). Ringlike enhancement may suggest degeneration into higher malignant grades. When a JPA occurs in the brainstem, its imaging characteristics are similar to those of tumors arising in the cerebellum, but they may lack cysts. JPAs in the brainstem tend to protrude posteriorly into the fourth ventricle and have variable enhancement (Fig. 6.2C and D). Calcifications and hemorrhage are rare in brainstem

Unlike with cerebellar juvenile pilocytic astrocytomas, hydrocephalus is a late complication with brainstem astrocytomas.

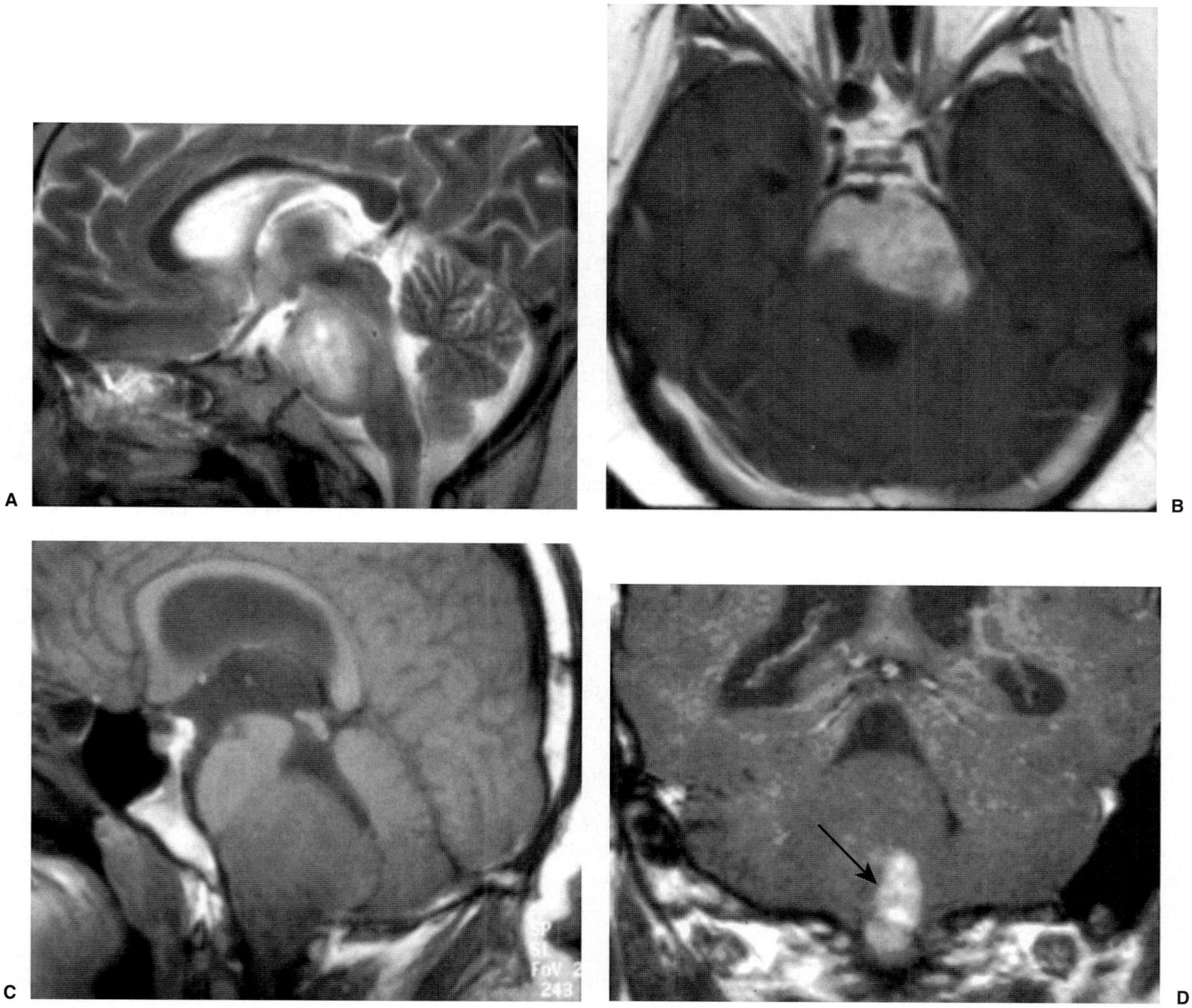

Figure 6.2 *Brainstem Astrocytoma. A.* Sagittal T2-weighted image shows high signal and expansion of the pons without significant hydrocephalus. *B.* In the same patient, there is contrast enhancement of the ventral portion of this diffuse astrocytoma (WHO grade 2). *C.* In a different patient, axial T1-weighted image shows large, dorsally exophytic pilocytic astrocytoma (WHO grade 1) involving the pons, medulla, and fourth ventricle. These tumors often are adherent to the brainstem, and unlike other pilocytic gliomas cannot be totally resected. *D.* In the same patient, the tumor shows some contrast enhancement *(arrow)*.

gliomas. Brainstem gliomas need to be differentiated from viral pontomesencephalitis. We have found proton MR spectroscopy to be helpful in this regard.

Midbrain (mesencephalic) gliomas deserve special mention because this is the second most common site for brainstem tumors (2). Most of these midbrain tumors are localized and present early with hydrocephalus. Some are diffuse and tend to infiltrate the brainstem and present with cranial neuropathies. They are associated with NF-1. The symptoms of midbrain gliomas are as follows:

- Increased intracranial pressure (hydrocephalus)
- Parinaud's syndrome (paralysis of upward gaze)
- Blurred or double vision
- Motor weakness

Most midbrain gliomas show low T1 signal and variable contrast enhancement. Approximately 25% of them show hemorrhage or cyst. They always are bright on T2-weighted sequences. Not uncommonly, they extend to the thalami. In reality, many thalamic astrocytomas begin as midbrain tumors.

Tumors of Primitive Cells

Atypical teratoid rhabdoid tumor of the cerebellum appears identical to cerebellar medulloblastoma in imaging studies, but has a worse prognosis.

Medulloblastoma. Under "Tumors of Primitive Cells," I include medulloblastoma and atypical teratoid rhabdoid tumor (ATRT). Medulloblastoma belongs to the primitive neuroectodermal tumors (PNET) (2). Because medulloblastoma has been well studied, its imaging features are well known, and its treatment and prognosis are well established, it often is discussed as one specific entity. Medulloblastomas are the most common tumors originating in the cerebellum of children (5). They are more common in boys, and approximately 50% are discovered during the first 5 years of life and 40% before 12 years of age. Only 10% of medulloblastomas are found in older individuals (lateral cerebellar medulloblastomas, usually of the "desmoplastic" subtype) (5). In children, most medulloblastomas arise in the midline vermis at the level of the superior or inferior medullary veli. They may protrude into the fourth ventricle and may be indistinguishable from other intraventricular tumors. The symptoms usually are due to hydrocephalus. By the time of diagnosis, all children are considered to have CSF spread. The "rules of 90" for medulloblastoma are listed in Table 6.1.

Medulloblastomas are hypercellular, resulting in high density on computed tomography (CT) and low T2 signal intensity (5) (Fig. 6.3A–D). Most show contrast enhance-

Table 6.1: Rule of 90s for Medulloblastoma

Finding	*Percentage*
Found in children <10 yr of age	90%
Solid and enhancing	90%
Cerebrospinal fluid spread at diagnosis	90%
Absence of cysts/calcifications	90%
Hydrocephalus at presentation	90%

Figure 6.3 *Medulloblastoma (WHO Grade 4). A.* Sagittal T2-weighted image shows mass (M) arising from the superior medullary velum and compressing the aqueduct, resulting in hydrocephalus. *B.* In a different patient, postcontrast sagittal T1-weighted image shows inhomogeneously enhancing tumor arising from the superior medullary velum and herniating cephalad through the tentorial incisura. There is hydrocephalus. *C.* Axial T2-weighted image (different patient) shows a medulloblastoma inside the fourth ventricle. Note that the tumor is somewhat hypointense. *D.* In the same patient, postcontrast T1-weighted image shows that the tumor is definitively inside the fourth ventricle and enhances homogeneously. Hydrocephalus is present. *E.* In a different patient, there is enhancement of the subarachnoid space because of metastases from medulloblastoma. *F.* In the same patient, there also is metastatic seeding (arrows) from medulloblastoma on the dorsal surface of the cervicothoracic spinal cord.

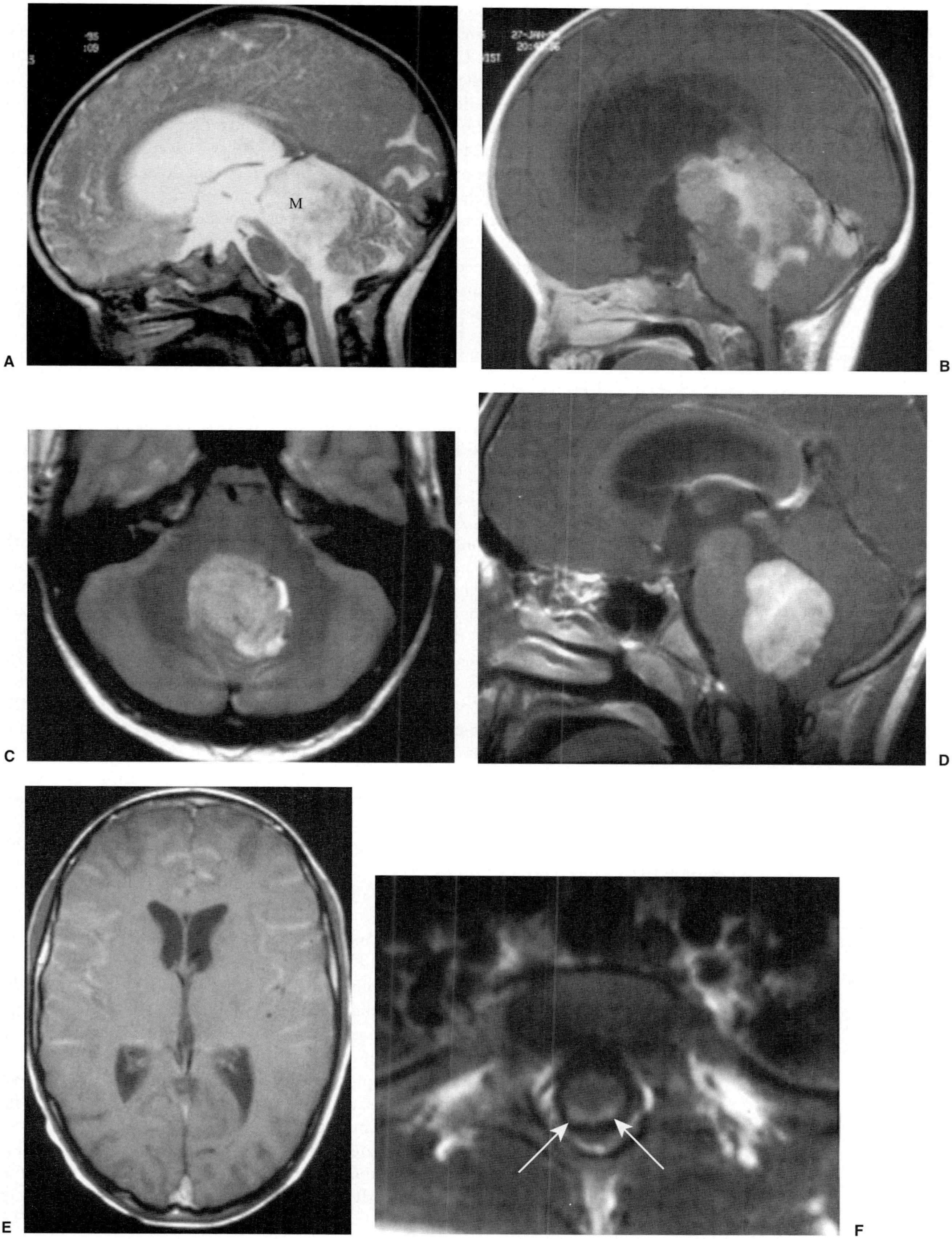
M
A
B
C
D
E
F

ment, which may be variable and patchy or homogeneous and solid (Fig. 6.3A–D). Proton MR spectroscopy shows significant elevation of choline and lipids/lactate, and in some patients the presence of taurine (7). The level of *N*-acetyl aspartate (NAA) is very low. Leptomeningeal tumor spread in the head and spine is not uncommon and is best evaluated with contrast-enhanced magnetic resonance imaging (MRI; Fig. 6.3E and F). Imaging of the spine needs to be obtained before surgery and shows enhancing lesions in more than 50% of patients (8,9). If spinal imaging is obtained after surgery, I recommend waiting 3 to 4 weeks to allow for postoperative inflammation-induced changes to resolve (these may mimic metastases!). Medulloblastoma may be a part of Gorlin's syndrome (basal cell nevus) and of ataxia–telangiectasia. With a combination of chemotherapy and irradiation, the 5-year survival rate is approximately 50% for patients with medulloblastoma. Postoperative imaging is needed for surveillance. Dural enhancement is nonspecific, but pial enhancement and focal nodular enhancement are highly suspect for tumor (10). Proton MR spectroscopy is very helpful in this situation and adds confidence to the diagnosis of recurrent/residual tumor.

Although most childhood cerebellar medulloblastomas arise in the midline, most adult cerebellar medulloblastomas are peripheral (lateral) in location.

Lateral cerebellar medulloblastomas deserve special mention. These tumors are found mostly in adults (2,6). They are located in the lateral aspect of one cerebellar hemisphere, often extending to the meninges. They result in an intense inflammatory and desmoplastic reaction of the adjacent meninges, and thus are called *desmoplastic* medulloblastomas. Because of their location, they may resemble meningiomas on imaging studies. They are hypointense on T1- and bright on T2-weighted images (6). Their pattern of enhancement is variable, and most show a "dural tail" of enhancement.

Atypical Teratoid Rhabdoid Tumor. ATRTs are rare but now are being recognized with increasing frequency by both neuroradiologists and neuropathologists. They are more common in boys and occur at a younger age than medulloblastomas and pilocytic astrocytomas. ATRTs are highly malignant and aggressive. Histologically, these tumors contain undifferentiated primitive cells, rhabdoid cells, malignant glial cells, and regions of malignant epithelial and mesenchymal degeneration (11). Mitosis and necrosis are common. Despite aggressive therapy, most patients die within 1 year (many of the so-called aggressive medulloblastomas of the past were probably ATRTs). They have nonspecific MRI appearances (they occasionally show no enhancement), and in children they are indistinguishable from medulloblastomas (11) (Fig. 6.4). Because of their rhabdoid components, a primary rhabdoid tumor in the kidneys must be ruled out before the diagnosis of primary intracranial ATRT is made. Although most ATRTs are found in the posterior fossa, they also occur in the cerebral hemispheres, pineal gland region, and hypothalamus. Proton MR spectroscopy is nonspecific and shows markedly high choline and lipids/lactate with low NAA.

Ependymoma

The differential diagnosis of a tumor arising in the fourth ventricle and extending into the adjacent cisterns primarily includes ependymoma and choroid plexus papilloma.

Ependymomas are the third most common infratentorial tumor in children, and most are found in boys approximately 5 years of age (2). They also are found in adults (peak age: 40 years). When they occur in children, more than 70% of them are located in the fourth ventricle (Fig. 6.5). In adults (and some children), another common location is the cerebral hemispheres (frontal and parietal lobes). The clinical symptoms are similar to those found in other posterior fossa tumors—that is, most symptoms are due to early onset of hydrocephalus with increased intracranial pressure. On CT, approximately 50% of these tumors show calcifications, 50% have cysts, and 50% have surrounding edema (2). The cysts tend to be small. MRI shows varied patterns of enhancement (12). Areas of hemorrhage may be observed in up to 10% of ependymomas. The tumor is soft and at times it may extend out of the fourth ventricle into the cerebellopontine angle cisterns through the foramina of Luschka. This appearance is fairly typical for an ependymoma. Approximately 10% of patients show leptomeningeal spread of tumor at the time of diagnosis, and the entire neuraxis needs to be imaged when this is a consideration. Despite their low malignant potential, the overall 5-year survival rate is only 50%.

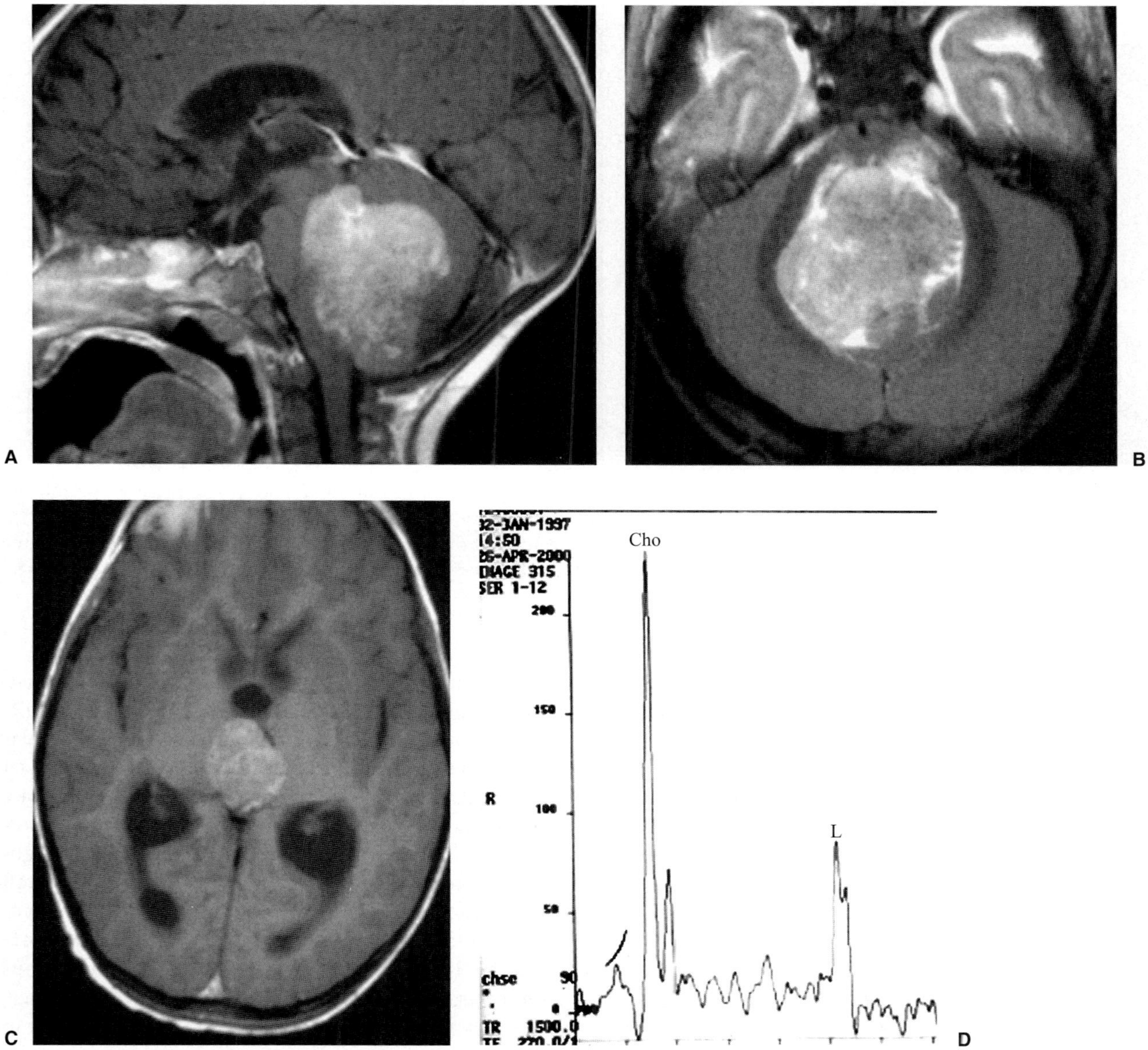

Figure 6.4 *Atypical Teratoid Rhabdoid Tumor (WHO Grade 4). A.* Postcontrast sagittal T1-weighted image shows large and mostly enhancing tumor in the fourth ventricle. *B.* On an axial T2-weighted image (same patient), the tumor is relatively hypointense, a feature seen in many highly malignant brain tumors. *C.* In a different case, a postcontrast axial T1-weighted image shows an enhancing tumor in the pineal gland region. *D.* Long–echo-time proton magnetic resonance spectroscopy in a different atypical teratoid rhabdoid tumor shows markedly elevated choline *(Cho)*, absent *N*-acetyl aspartate, and presence of lactate *(L)*.

A variant of ependymoma that has received attention lately is the subependymoma. Most of these tumors are asymptomatic and are found only at autopsy (2). They are found in adults in the third and fourth decades of life. Most subependymomas are found in the lateral and fourth ventricles (13). The third ventricle, septum pellucidum, aqueduct, and spinal central canal also may be involved. Subependymomas are histologically benign. They show low T1 and high T2 signal intensity and solid or heterogeneous enhancement (14). Intratumoral calcifications are typical. Subependymomas usually are devoid of surrounding edema.

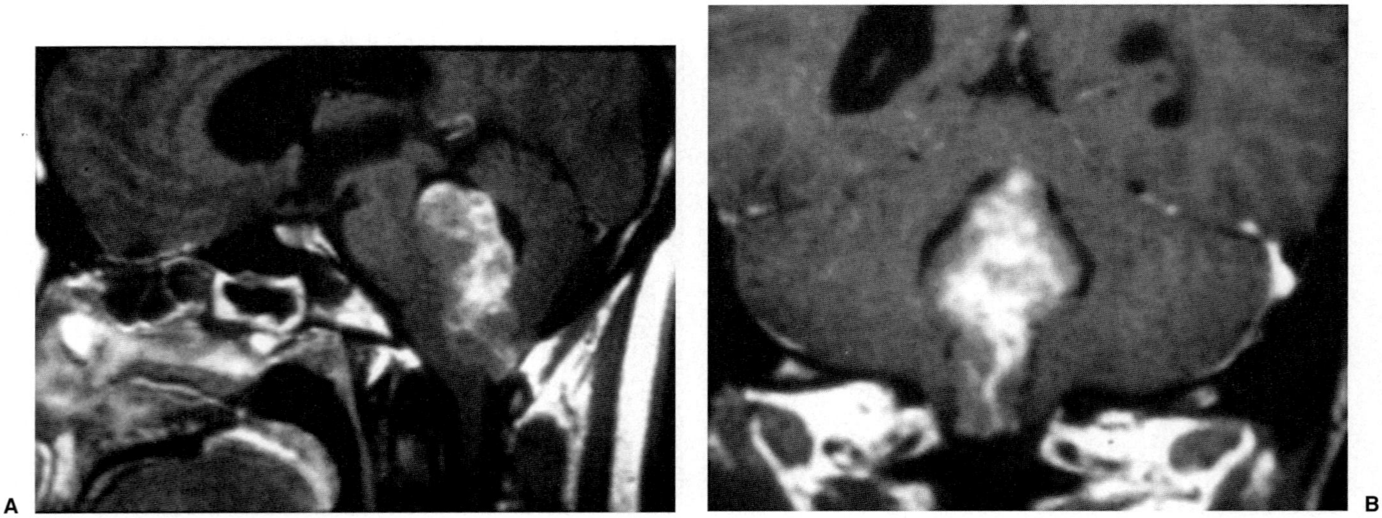

Figure 6.5 *Ependymoma (WHO Grade 2). A.* Sagittal postcontrast T1-weighted image shows enhancing mass in the fourth ventricle protruding inferiorly through the foramen of Magendie, a feature typical of ependymoma. *B.* In the same patient, the enhancing tumor is seen to be surrounded by the fourth ventricle (and thus is intraventricular) and projecting inferiorly through the midline foramen.

Ganglion Cell Tumors

These tumors are, in order of frequency, ganglioglioma, gangliocytoma, and ganglioneuroma. Gangliogliomas account for approximately 1% of all primary brain tumors in adults and approximately 4% in children (15). Most ganglion cell tumors are found in males younger than 30 years of age. The relatively young age at presentation is due to the fact that these tumors often cause intractable seizures (16). Although most gangliogliomas are histologically benign, some are malignant *de novo* and some undergo malignant degeneration. Complete resection however, most often provides a permanent cure. Most gangliogliomas are found in the cerebellum, the mesial temporal lobes (where they may result in partial complex seizures), and frontal and parietal regions (Fig. 6.6). Spinal cord gangliogliomas are rare, extensive (holocord), and usually indistinguishable from the more common cord astrocytoma (17). In the brain, gangliogliomas have a heterogeneous appearance; approximately 50% have cysts, 50% have calcifications, and 50% enhance. Surrounding edema, however, is rare. They tend to involve the cortex (and thus result in seizures) and may even scallop the inner table of the skull.

Remember the rule of 50s for intracranial gangliogliomas: 50% are in the cerebellum, 50% enhance, 50% have cysts, 50% have calcifications.

Gangliocytomas are very rare. They are tumors of children and usually produce seizures that are refractory to medical treatment. By CT they are hyperdense and show little or no contrast enhancement (18). Their signal characteristics on MRI are nonspecific. They produce little mass effect and show no surrounding edema.

Desmoplastic infantile gangliocytomas/gangliogliomas are rare tumors but have a fairly typical appearance on imaging studies (19,20). They are found before 2 years of age, predominantly in boys. Most are supratentorial and very large (>60% involve an entire cerebral hemisphere; Fig. 6.7). The most common locations are frontal, parietal, and occipital lobes. They are large, predominantly cystic masses that contain a nodule or nodules of enhancing tumor. These nodules usually involve the gray matter and are subpial in location.

Lhermitte-Duclos disease is so rare that when found, patients may need to be evaluated for the possibility of underlying Cowden's disease.

Dysplastic gangliocytomas of the cerebellum are a specific entity also known as *Lhermitte-Duclos disease* (LDD) (21). They are very rare but also have a fairly typical appearance on imaging studies. Most are found in men in the third and fourth decades of life. The symptoms usually are mild and slowly progressive and consist mostly of increased intracranial pressure and ataxia. The lesions result in a mass effect on the fourth ventricle and grow very slowly. LDD is associated with the multiple hamartoma syndrome (Cowden's disease). LDD is so rare that some authors suggest that all patients harboring this lesion should be evaluated for the possibility of Cowden's disease (22). Histologically, LDD

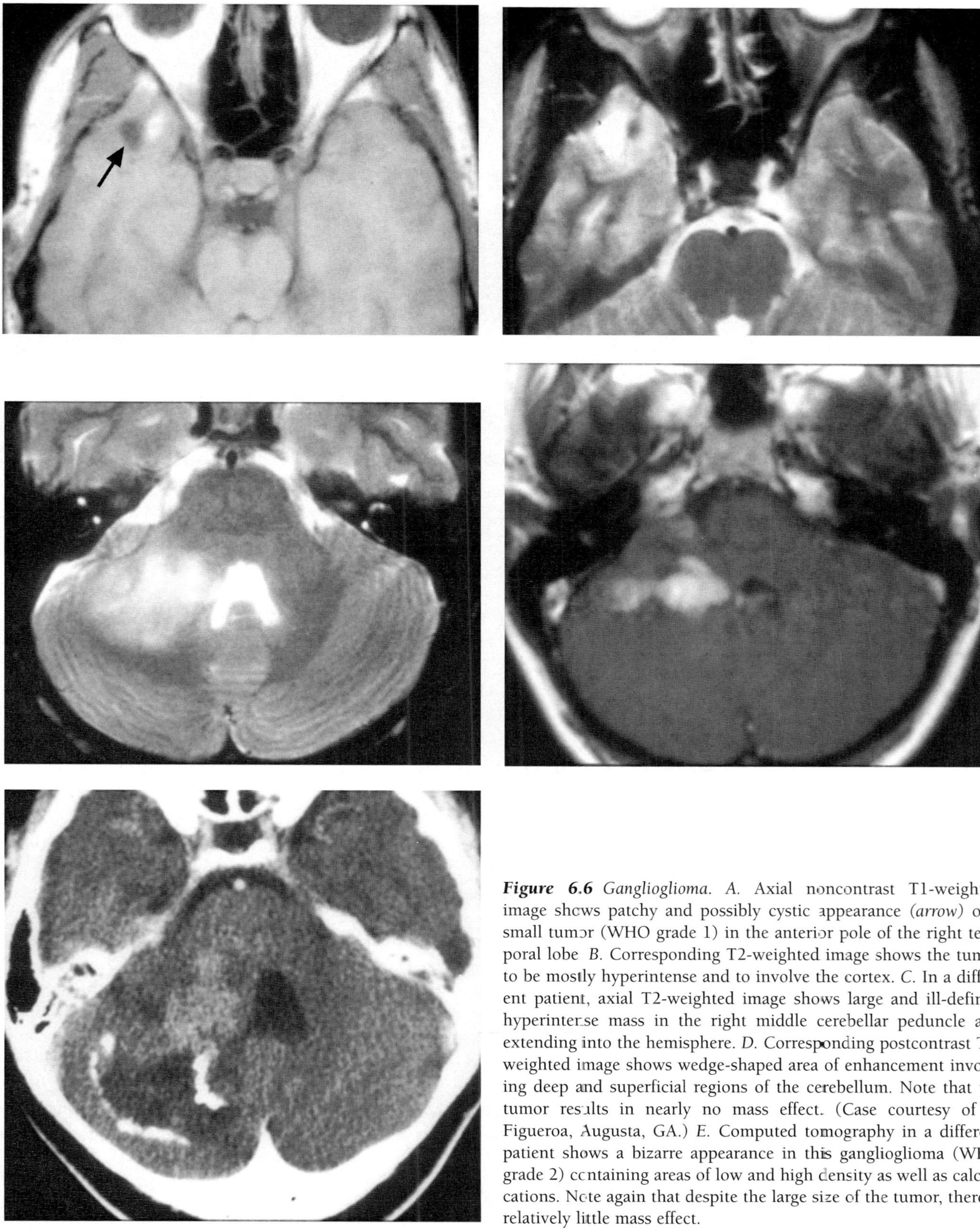

Figure 6.6 *Ganglioglioma. A.* Axial noncontrast T1-weighted image shows patchy and possibly cystic appearance *(arrow)* of a small tumor (WHO grade 1) in the anterior pole of the right temporal lobe *B.* Corresponding T2-weighted image shows the tumor to be mostly hyperintense and to involve the cortex. *C.* In a different patient, axial T2-weighted image shows large and ill-defined hyperintense mass in the right middle cerebellar peduncle and extending into the hemisphere. *D.* Corresponding postcontrast T1-weighted image shows wedge-shaped area of enhancement involving deep and superficial regions of the cerebellum. Note that the tumor results in nearly no mass effect. (Case courtesy of R. Figueroa, Augusta, GA.) *E.* Computed tomography in a different patient shows a bizarre appearance in this ganglioglioma (WHO grade 2) containing areas of low and high density as well as calcifications. Note again that despite the large size of the tumor, there is relatively little mass effect.

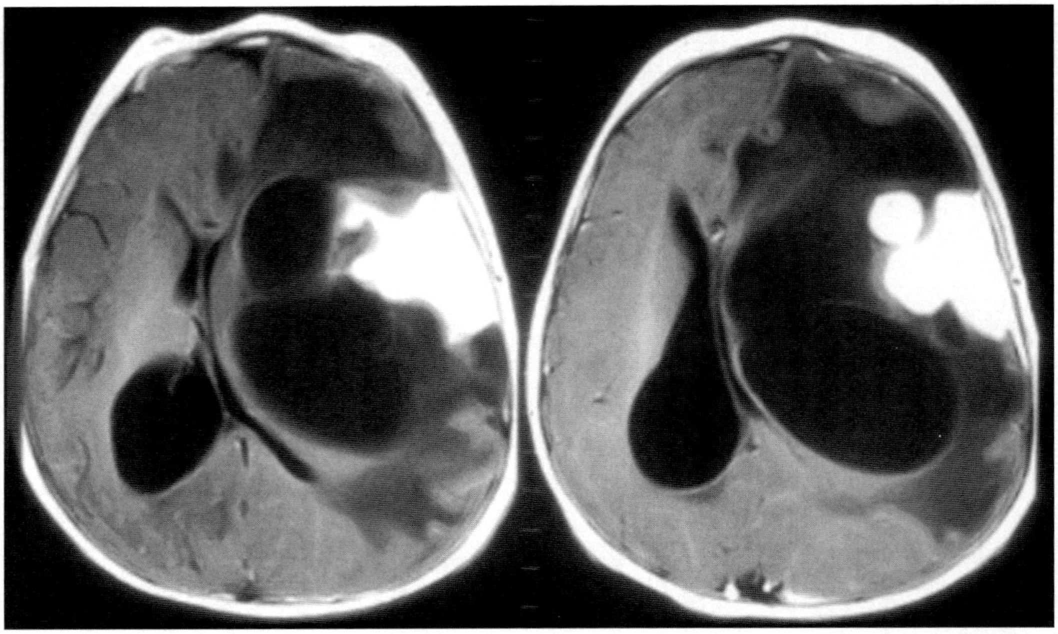

Figure 6.7 *Desmoplastic Infantile Gangliocytoma (WHO Grade 1).* Sequential axial postcontrast T1-weighted images shows large, left-sided cystic mass with a peripherally located and enhancing nodule. There is significant mass effect and dilatation of the right lateral ventricle. (Courtesy of P. Tortori, Genova, Italy.)

consists of hypertrophy of the granular and molecular layers of the cerebellar cortex with a thin Purkinje cell layer. This results in thick folia. The imaging features are better seen on MRI. The lesion, which usually does not enhance, shows a striated (corduroy) appearance owing to the thick folia and is most often located in one cerebellar hemisphere. Contrast enhancement does occur but is considered atypical (23).

Supratentorial Tumors

Craniopharyngioma

In the suprasellar region, the most common childhood tumors are craniopharyngioma and astrocytoma. Craniopharyngiomas are histologically benign epithelial tumors, but they are difficult to resect and recurrences are common. The locations for craniopharyngiomas are listed in Table 6.2 (2).

In children, the most common suprasellar tumors are craniopharyngioma and optic chiasm/hypothalamic astrocytoma.

Most craniopharyngiomas are found in children (peak age, 5 years), but they also may be seen in adults (peak age, 45 years). There are two histologic types: adamantinomatous (mostly seen in children) and papillary (seen almost exclusively in adults). Craniopharyngiomas represent approximately 5% of all intracranial tumors. They are thought to arise from remnants of Rathke's pouch, although this has not been proved. The common symptoms at presentation are shown in Table 6.3. Table 6.4 describes the "rules of 80%" for craniopharyngiomas.

By CT, craniopharyngiomas contain calcifications, cysts, and solid enhancing tissues (Fig. 6.8A). Most of the tumor cysts are of low T1 and T2 signal intensity (24). However,

Table 6.2: *Location of Craniopharyngioma*

Location	*Incidence*
Suprasellar/sellar	75%
Purely suprasellar	20%
Purely intrasellar	5%

Table 6.3: Symptoms Produced by Craniopharyngioma

Category of Symptoms	*Specific Symptoms*
Compression of optic chiasm	Bitemporal hemianopsia
Endocrine dysfunction	Growth retardation, delayed or precocious puberty, diabetes insipidus
Increased intracranial pressure	Hydrocephalus

Table 6.4: Imaging Features of Craniopharyngioma in Children

Imaging Characteristics	*Incidence*
Cysts	80%
Size from 2–6 cm	80%
Calcifications	80%
Contrast enhancement	80%

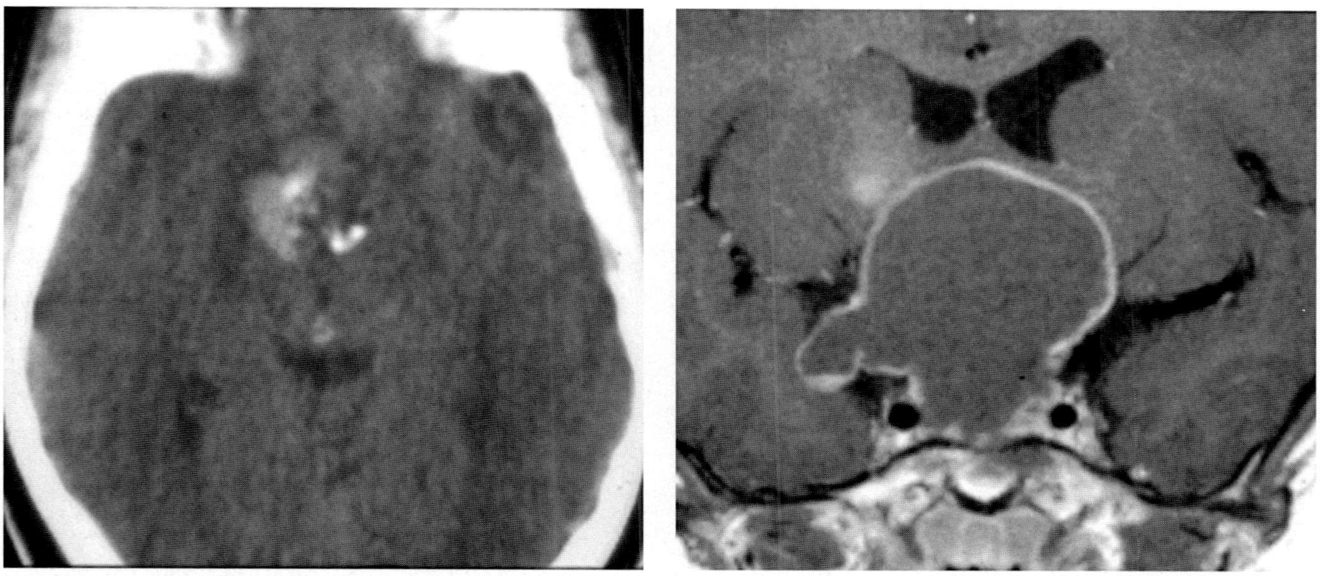

A B

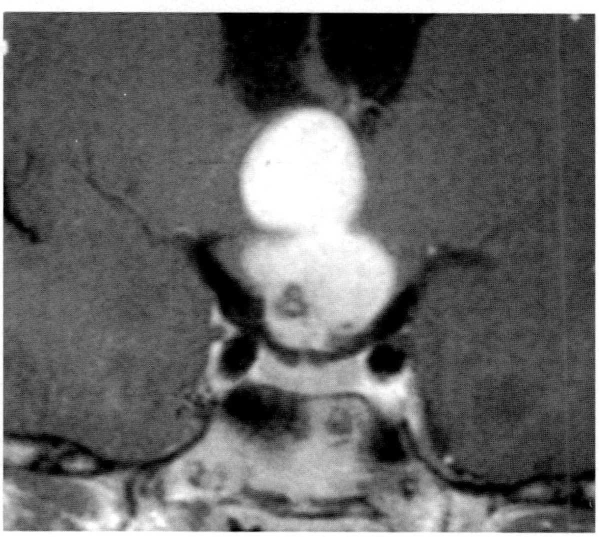

C

Figure 6.8 *Craniopharyngioma. A.* Axial computed tomography shows suprasellar mass containing calcifications and zones of high density. *B.* Coronal postcontrast T1-weighted image shows a large suprasellar and intrasellar, mostly cystic craniopharyngioma with peripheral enhancement. There is extension into the right middle cranial fossa. *C.* In a different patient, postcontrast coronal T1-weighted image shows enhancing mass with a suprasellar component and another component in the region of the third ventricle. Note the "waist" of the tumor where it crosses the sellar diaphragm. There is hydrocephalus.

occasionally the cysts are bright on T1-weighted images, reflecting hemorrhage or liquid cholesterol (this typically is referred to as *crank-case oil* by neurosurgeons). All cystic craniopharyngiomas have areas of enhancement (Fig. 6.8B). These solid and enhancing regions have variable appearances (Fig. 6.8C). Craniopharyngiomas are large and multilobulated at presentation (so-called "giant" craniopharyngiomas account for 25% of these tumors). Craniopharyngiomas tend to extend into several intracranial compartments and cisterns. The sella is enlarged and may be eroded. Proton MR spectroscopy shows that they contain abundant lipids (peaks at 1 to 2 parts per million [ppm]).

Unlike childhood craniopharyngiomas, adult craniopharyngiomas usually involve the third ventricle (2). They lack cysts, cholesterol, and keratin. They are solid and richly vascularized, and they are easier to remove than the adamantinomatous type. By MRI, their features are nonspecific and the differential diagnosis is based on the age of the patient and the location of the tumor.

Astrocytoma

Suprasellar Astrocytomas. Astrocytomas may occur in the optic chiasm, hypothalamus, and cerebral hemispheres. Many suprasellar gliomas are so large at the time of diagnosis that determining their site of origin is not possible, and thus the term *chiasmatic* or *hypothalamic* astrocytoma is better avoided (25) (Fig. 6.9). Regardless of the site of origin, the histology and treatment are similar. Suprasellar gliomas comprise approximately 15% of all intracranial tumors in children (2). When they originate in the hypothalamus, they produce endocrine abnormalities and tend to present earlier. When they originate in the optic chiasm, the visual deficits may be difficult to assess, and they present later. Fortu-

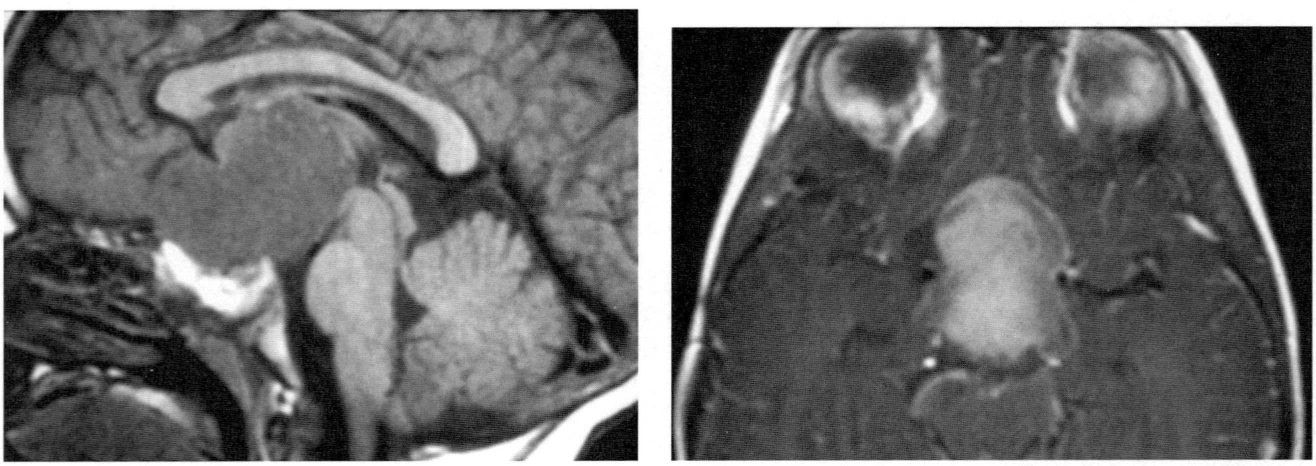

A B

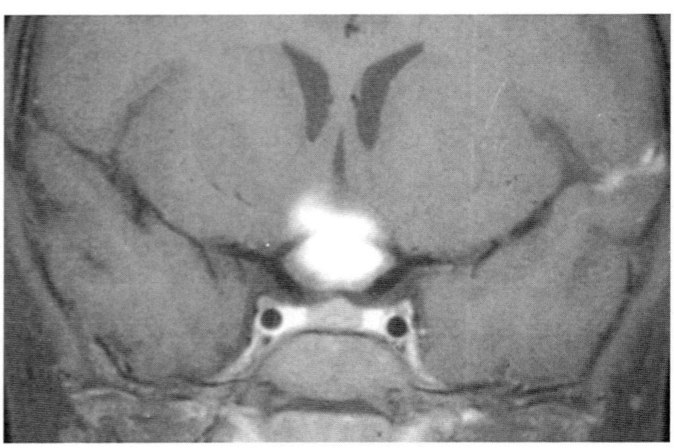

C

Figure 6.9 *Suprasellar Astrocytoma. A.* Noncontrast sagittal T1-weighted image shows very large suprasellar tumor with inferior extension into an expanded sella turcica. It is not possible to determine the site of origin of the lesion. *B.* Axial postcontrast T1-weighted image (different patient) shows diffuse enhancement in this presumed optic chiasm astrocytoma. *C.* In a patient with neurofibromatosis type 1, there is an enhancing optic chiasm glioma superiorly extending into the hypothalamus.

Table 6.5: Symptoms Produced by Suprasellar Astrocytomas

Symptom	Incidence
Visual deficits	50%
Hydrocephalus	50%
Endocrine dysfunction	20%
Diencephalic syndrome	<10%

nately, most patients have very few symptoms until the terminal phase of the disease. The symptoms due to these tumors are listed in Table 6.5.

Histologically, most suprasellar astrocytomas are of the pilocytic type (2). Despite their low malignancy, they may be infiltrative (Fig. 6.9C). Some chiasmatic astrocytomas seen in patients with NF-1 show benign behavior, even regressing in size, and are believed to be more akin to a hamartoma than to a glioma. Approximately 20% to 50% of patients with chiasmatic gliomas also have NF-1. In NF-1, the gliomas tend to originate in the optic nerves and commonly are multicentric. In the absence of NF-1, these gliomas tend to arise in the chiasm as a unifocal mass. Regardless of whether NF-1 is present, all chiasmatic gliomas may extend posteriorly along the optic radiations and may seed the subarachnoid spaces. By MRI, suprasellar gliomas are hypointense on T1- and bright on T2 weighted images (25). They usually are bulky and lobulated and may expand the sella turcica. Cysts may be present and the solid portions of the tumor may or may not enhance. There is no correlation between enhancement and histologic grade of the tumor. Enhancement may disappear with time regardless of treatment.

Hemispheric Astrocytomas. Hemispheric astrocytomas in children usually are malignant (2). Hemispheric gliomas comprise approximately 30% to 50% of all supratentorial primary tumors in children (26). The most common symptoms at presentation are seizures and increased intracranial pressure due to hydrocephalus. Most are found before 10 years of age. Unlike the localized gliomas, most hemispheric astrocytomas are diffuse, but they may have a better prognosis than those seen in adults despite many of them being of high histologic grade. Their imaging features are nonspecific and similar to those seen for adult astrocytomas (see below; Fig. 6.10A).

Regardless of their exact origin and histology, suprasellar astrocytomas are diffusely infiltrating, nonsurgical lesions. Contrary to those in adults, highly malignant cerebral astrocytomas in children are well demarcated and have a better prognosis.

A specific type of glioma occurring in the cerebral hemispheres is the giant cell astrocytoma (GCA), which is seen almost exclusively in the setting of tuberous sclerosis (Chapter 2). They are so rare in the absence of tuberous sclerosis that, if found, a search for that phakomatosis is indicated (2). Most GCAs are found in patients 5 to 10 years of age. They usually are located at the level of the foramina of Monro (27) (Fig. 6.10B and C). They tend to arise from subependymal nodules of tuberous sclerosis and nearly always are benign, although malignant degeneration may occur. All GCAs enhance by MRI and show progressive growth on serial studies. They result in unilateral or bilateral dilated lateral ventricles. Because most patients are devastated by the underlying disease, many surgeons opt to treat the patients conservatively by placing a ventricular shunt for the relief of hydrocephalus. In patients with less severe symptoms (or if the parents/guardians desire), the tumors may be resected.

Choroid Plexus Tumors

Choroid plexus tumors are rare and represent less than 1% of intracranial tumors in adults and approximately 1% to 4% of childhood intracranial tumors (2). Most childhood choroid plexus tumors are found before 5 years of age (28,29). The great majority of these tumors are choroid plexus papillomas (CPP). Most childhood CPPs arise in the atria of the lateral ventricles, whereas most of the adult ones are found in the fourth ventricle. CPP produce hydrocephalus by virtue of increased CSF filtration, hemorrhage, and desqua-

Frank invasion of the adjacent brain parenchyma is the best way to differentiate a choroid plexus papilloma from a choroid plexus carcinoma.

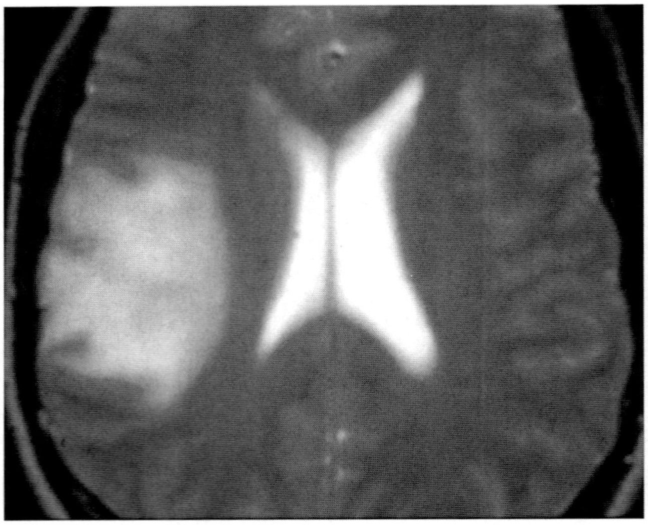
A

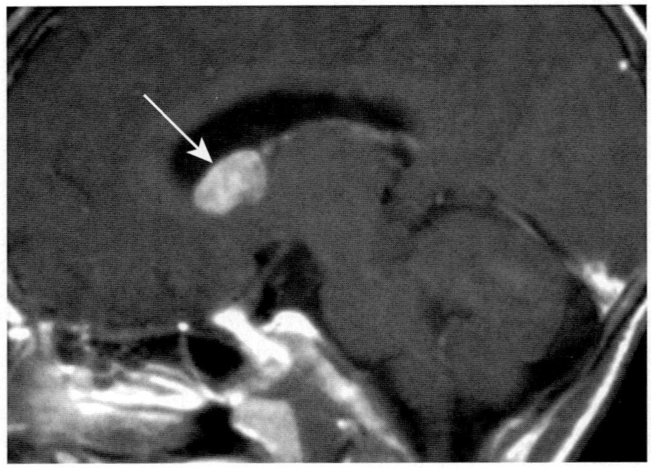
B

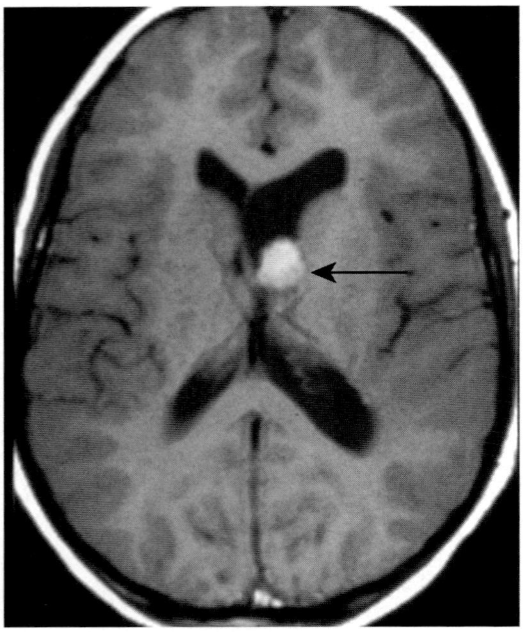
C

Figure 6.10 *Supratentorial Astrocytomas in Children. A.* Axial T2-weighted image in a young adolescent patient shows a nonspecific-appearing, hyperintense anaplastic astrocytoma (WHO grade 3) in the right temporal lobe. *B.* Parasagittal postcontrast T1-weighted image in a patient with tuberous sclerosis shows enhancing giant cell astrocytoma (*arrow*, WHO grade 1) in the region of the foramen on Monro. *C.* In a different patient with tuberous sclerosis, axial postcontrast T1-weighted image shows enhancing mass (*arrow*) in the region of the left foramen of Monro and mild dilatation of the corresponding lateral ventricle.

mated debris (Chapter 5). These tumors are histologically benign but may seed the leptomeninges and even the peritoneal cavity if a ventricular shunt has been previously placed. By CT, most CPPs are large, hyperdense, and show contrast enhancement (30). Approximately 20% of them contain calcifications. On MRI, they are of low T1 and intermediate to low T2 signal intensity (Fig. 6.11A). They may contain foci of hemorrhage. Flow voids representing large vessels may be present (some patients may benefit from preoperative embolization to decrease bleeding at resection). All CPPs show marked contrast enhancement and most have surrounding edema (Fig. 6.11B). CPPs arising in the fourth ventricle are smaller at presentation because they produce obstructive hydrocephalus early in the course of the disease. If they are large, they may protrude into the cerebellopontine angle cisterns by extending through the foramina of Luschka. CPPs in the fourth ventricle have a nonspecific imaging appearance, but all show contrast enhancement. The differential diagnosis for lesions arising in the choroid plexus is shown in Table 6.6.

The counterparts of CPP are the choroid plexus carcinomas (2). These malignant tumors represent approximately 10% to 20% of all choroid plexus tumors and are found mostly in children. They are large and multilobulated, show prominent contrast enhance-

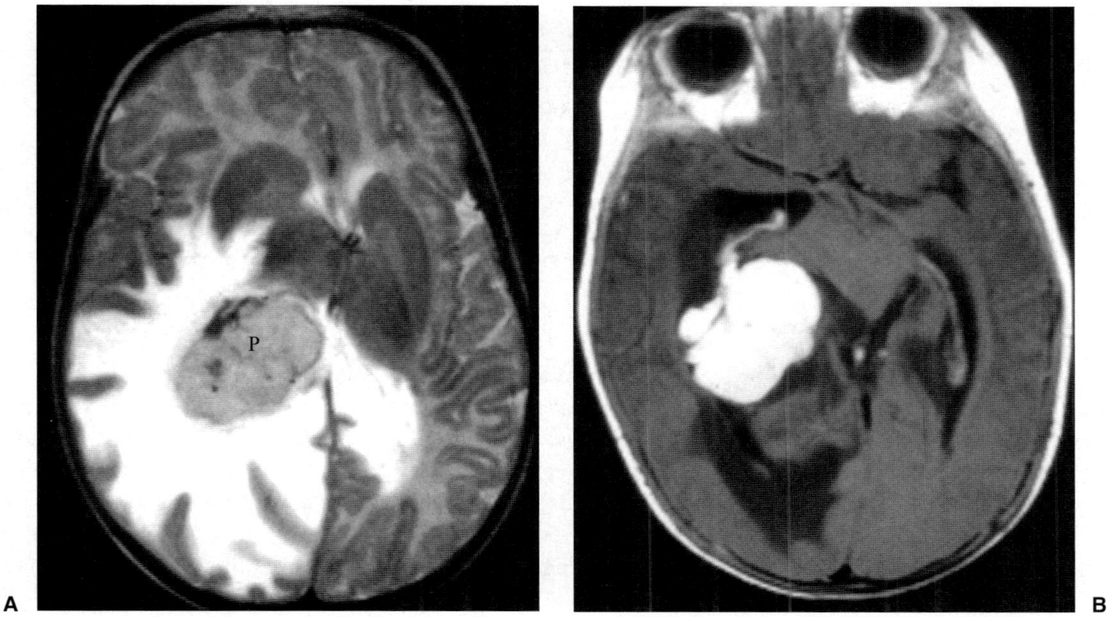

Figure 6.11 *Choroid Plexus Papilloma (WHO Grade 1). A.* Axial T2-weighted image shows hypointense mass *(P)* containing some areas of flow void due to the presence of large vessels and considerable surrounding edema despite the benign histology of the lesion. *B.* Corresponding post-contrast T1-weighted image shows marked and homogeneous enhancement in the tumor. There is entrapment and dilatation of the temporal horn of the right lateral ventricle.

ment, and have surrounding edema. Only frank invasion of the brain may be used to distinguish them from CPP.

Dysembryoplastic Neuroepithelial Tumors

Dysembryoplastic neuroepithelial tumors (DNET) have received considerable attention lately, although they are very rare (<1% of intracranial tumors) (2). However, they are a not uncommon cause of medically refractory seizures (usually of the partial complex type). Most DNETs are found in the temporal and frontal lobes. They are histologically benign and their features include the presence of microcysts underlying an area of cortical dysplasia. Neurons are found amid the microcyst matrix. These tumors grow very slowly. Because the cortex is nearly always involved, scalloping of adjacent bones is common. By MRI, DNETs usually are small, cortically based, and have low T1 and high T2 signal intensity (31). Cysts and calcifications are identified in 30% to 40% of these tumors. Contrast enhancement is present in approximately one-half of DNETs.

Table 6.6: Diagnostic Considerations in Choroid Plexus Masses

Tumor or Mass	*Age Group*
Papilloma	Children
Carcinoma	Children
Meningioma	Adults
Metastases	Adults
Lymphoma	Adults
Cysts	Adults
Xanthogranulomas	Adults
Lipoma	Any
Cryptococcus	Adults (especially those with acquired immunodeficiency syndrome)

Table 6.7: The Histiocytoses

Name	*Type of Disease*	*Predominant Age (yr)*
Letterer-Siwe disease	Acute disseminated	<1
Hand-Schüller-Christian disease	Bone involvement, exophthalmos, diabetes insipidus	1–10
Eosinophilic granuloma	One or few bone lesions	10–30

Histiocytoses

The Langerhans cell histiocytoses include the disorders listed in Table 6.7 (2).

Many calvarial eosinophilic granulomas heal spontaneously or after biopsy with or without the intralesional instillation of steroids.

Only eosinophilic granuloma and Hand-Schüller-Christian disease are discussed here because they are the ones affecting the brain. Histologically, all lesions contain macrophage-like cells (Langerhans cells) admixed with eosinophils, plasma cells, macrophages, and multinucleated giant cells (32). Necrosis and fibrosis also commonly are found. The most common site for eosinophilic granuloma is the calvarium, where it results in lesions that show different degrees of involvement of the inner and outer tables ("beveled edge" sign; Fig. 6.12A). These lesions are of low T1 and high T2 signal and all enhance to some degree after contrast administration (Fig. 6.12B). The enhancement may

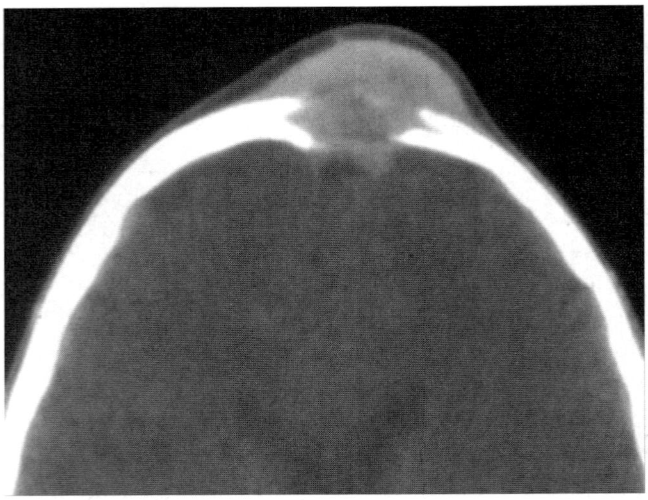

A

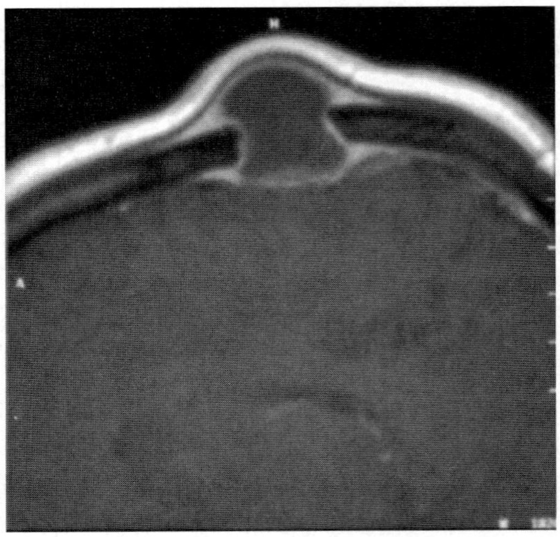

B

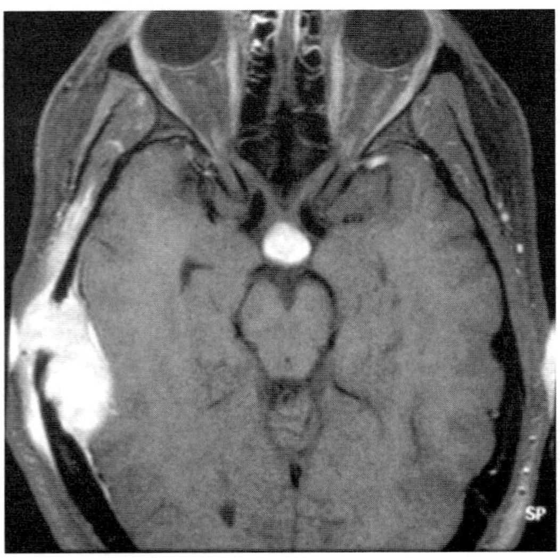

C

Figure 6.12 *Eosinophilic Granuloma. A.* Axial postcontrast computed tomography shows enhancing soft tissue mass destroying the frontal bones. Note asymmetric erosion of the outer and inner tables of the skull. *B.* In a different patient, parasagittal postcontrast T1-weighted image shows a mostly nonenhancing mass destroying the skull. *C.* Axial postcontrast fat-suppressed T1-weighted image shows eosinophilic granuloma destroying the right temporal bone squama with intracranial extension. Also note enhancing mass in the suprasellar region.

extend to the overlying soft tissues and into the dura. The temporal bone is not uncommonly affected (Fig. 6.12C). In Hand-Schüller-Christian disease, the bone (and even the soft tissues) of the orbits may be involved, leading to exophthalmos. The lateral wall of the orbits commonly is involved, and the lesion nearly always destroys the greater wing of the sphenoid and may extend into the cavernous sinus (33). MRI of the sella usually shows an enhancing lesion involving the pituitary, the stalk, and the hypothalamus (34,35) (Fig. 6.12C).

Adult Tumors

Infratentorial Tumors

Hemangioblastoma

Hemangioblastomas are rare lesions accounting for less than 2% of all intracranial tumors (36). They are the most common primary tumor of the cerebellum in adults, and most are discovered in patients 30 to 50 years of age (37). Hemangioblastomas are more common in men. Approximately 20% of patients with hemangioblastoma have von Hippel-Lindau disease (VHL) (Chapter 2). The solid portion of the tumor nodule is composed of a hypervascular capillary network embedded in a stroma of polygonal cells without evidence of mitosis. The exact cell of origin for hemangioblastoma is not certain. Approximately 60% of hemangioblastomas have accompanying cysts. The wall of the cyst is devoid of tumor and consists of compressed brain tissue that becomes gliotic. The fluid content of the cyst is probably an exudate or a filtrate, but its etiology (and why only some hemangioblastomas have cysts) is unknown. The fluid may contain evidence of acute or prior hemorrhage. Despite their benign histology, approximately 25% of hemangioblastomas recur after resection. Hemangioblastomas are hypervascular tumors that may benefit from preoperative embolization (38). Some patients are said to be polycythemic because of production of erythropoietin by the tumor, but this is very rare. Multiple hemangioblastomas are found in 5% to 20% of patients, most of whom have VHL (Chapter 2).

Patients with Von Hippel-Lindau disease may have cerebral, cerebellar and spinal cord hemangioblastomas as well as endolymphatic sac tumors.

Approximately 60% of hemangioblastomas are cystic masses (Fig. 6.13A). The cyst is always isointense or slightly hyperintense with respect to CSF on both T1- and T2-weighted images. This is believed to be due to the presence of blood, increased proteins,

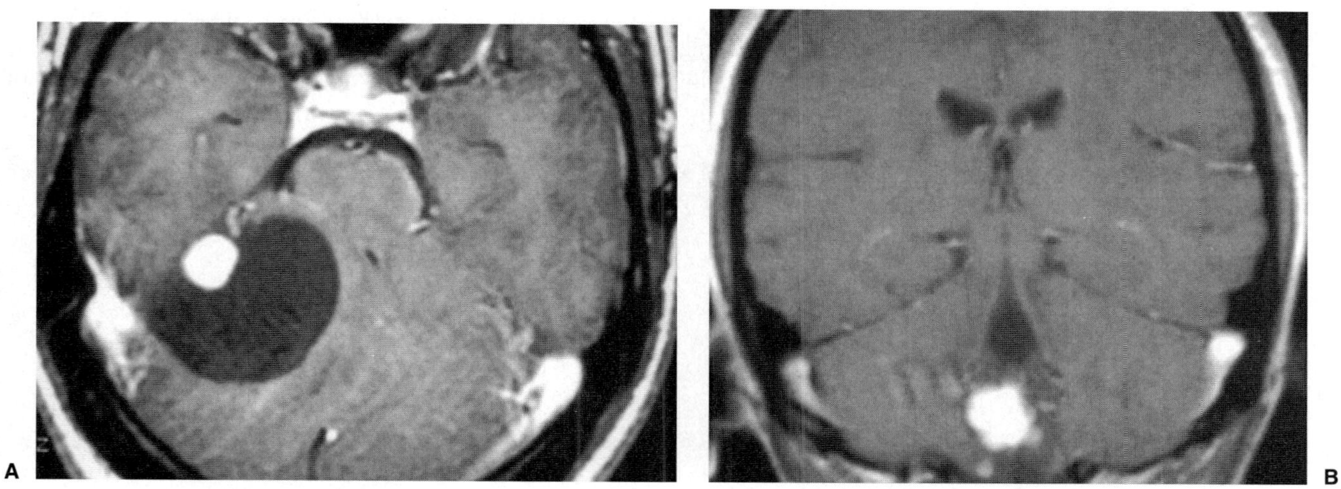

Figure 6.13 *Hemangioblastoma (WHO Grade 1). A.* Axial postcontrast T1-weighted image shows mass in the right cerebellum containing a laterally (subpial) enhancing nodule and a large cyst medially. *B.* In a different patient, coronal postcontrast T1-weighted image shows a solid and enhancing hemangioblastoma inferior to the fourth ventricle.

or decreased motion and pulsatility of the fluid. The tumor nodule is hypointense on T1- and bright on T2-weighted images (37). The nodule shows marked contrast enhancement and always is in a subpial location. Often, large flow voids from hypertrophied feeding arteries and draining veins may be appreciated in the tumor nodule. Hemangioblastomas may be completely solid, particularly when multiple and secondary to VHL (Fig. 6.13B).

Schwannoma

Schwannomas are the most common posterior fossa tumor in adults and the second most common intracranial extraaxial tumor after meningioma in adults (39). Approximately 75% to 80% of masses in the cerebellopontine angle cistern are vestibular schwannomas. Box 6.1 lists the differential diagnosis of masses in this location is (40,41).

Vestibular schwannomas are encountered in only approximately 2% of adult patients imaged for hearing loss.

Vestibular schwannomas arise from Scarpa's ganglion (glial–Schwann cell junction) in the superior division of the vestibular nerve. They are found most commonly in women 40 to 60 years of age. The most common symptoms include sensorineural hearing loss, tinnitus, headache, and disequilibrium (39). Facial nerve palsy is uncommon because the seventh cranial nerve is fairly resistant to pressure caused by the vestibular schwannoma. Bilateral eighth nerve schwannomas are pathognomonic for NF-2 (Chapter 2). By MRI, vestibular schwannomas tend to enhance, but always in a heterogeneous fashion (42). The term *intracanalicular* is used when the tumor resides inside the internal auditory canal (Fig. 6.14A). More often, the schwannoma has an "ice cream cone" appearance with an intracanalicular portion and another masslike portion in the cerebellopontine angle cistern (Fig. 6.14B). Occasionally, vestibular schwannomas show extension into the cochlea and "dural tails" of enhancement. Approximately 5% to 22% of vestibular schwannomas have atypical imaging features and may have associated arachnoid cysts or central necrosis, or be partially or completely cystic (Fig. 6.14C). Initial screening of patients suspected of having vestibular schwannoma may be done with constructive interference in the steady state (CISS) images; after surgery, contrast-enhanced MRI is needed. After surgery, linear or somewhat nodular enhancement in the internal auditory canal may be seen. Linear enhancement does not indicate tumor, but nodular enhancement is suspect for tumor and needs to be followed with MRI. In consecutive MRI studies (on a yearly basis), this nodular enhancement is seen to disappear in most patients. Because vestibular schwannomas grow very slowly, studies can be obtained on a yearly basis. Recently, many of these schwannomas are being treated with stereotactic radiation. Previously irradiated schwannomas shrink very slowly. They do, however, enhance less and develop central areas of presumed necrosis or cystic changes.

Chordoma

Chordomas arise from notochordal remnants at the sacrum (50%; they are the most common primary sacral tumor), clivus (35%), and cervical and thoracic regions (15%) (43). Despite being histologically benign tumors, chordomas show local aggressive behavior,

Box 6.1: Most Common Masses Occurring in Adults at the Cerebellopontine Angle

Schwannoma
Meningioma
Metastasis
Glomus tumors
Epidermoid
Arachnoid cyst
Cholesterol granuloma
Ramsay-Hunt syndrome (intracanalicular)
Rare (endolymphatic sac tumor, lipoma, aneurysm, chordoma, sarcoidosis)

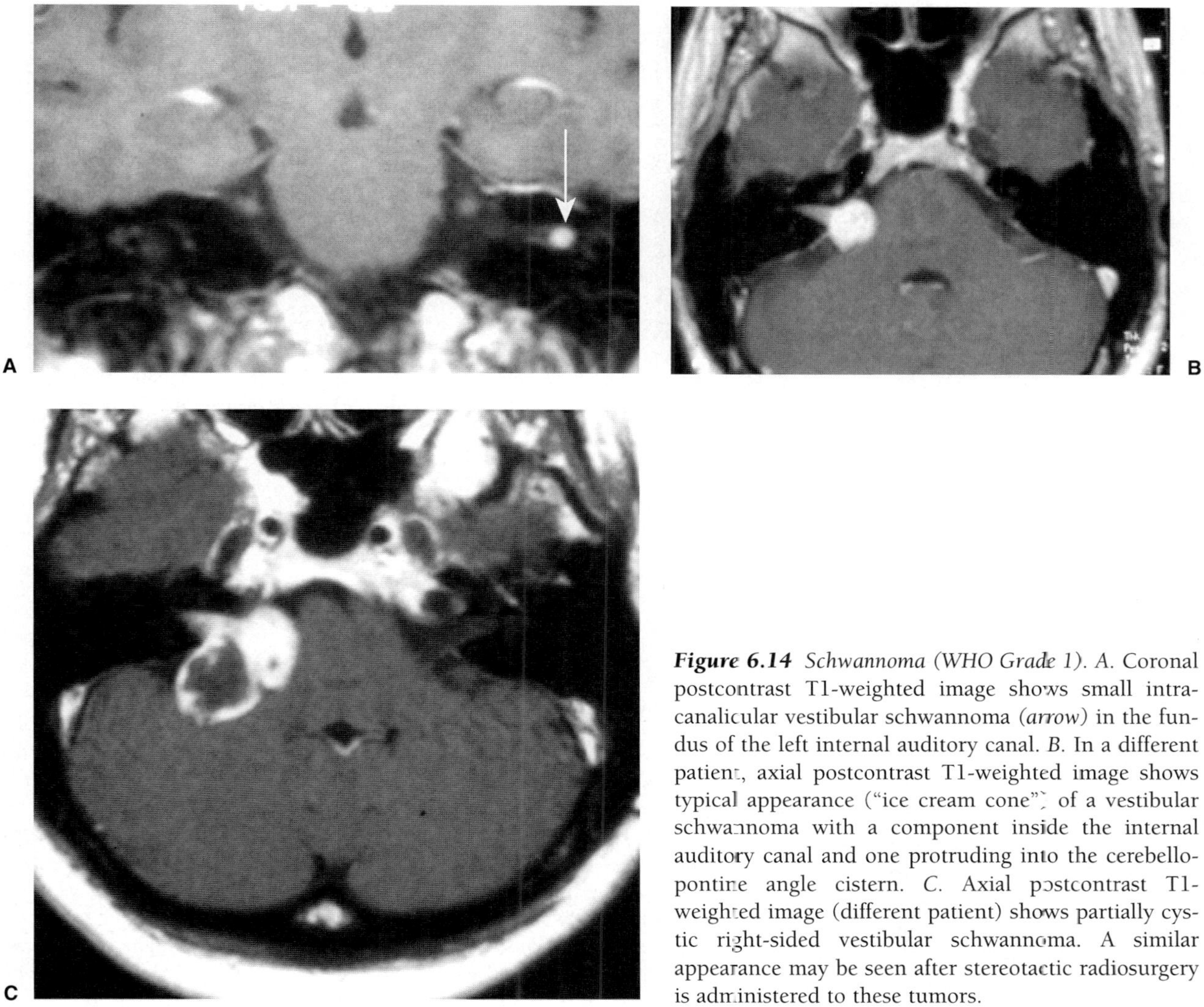

Figure 6.14 *Schwannoma (WHO Grade 1). A.* Coronal postcontrast T1-weighted image shows small intracanalicular vestibular schwannoma *(arrow)* in the fundus of the left internal auditory canal. *B.* In a different patient, axial postcontrast T1-weighted image shows typical appearance ("ice cream cone") of a vestibular schwannoma with a component inside the internal auditory canal and one protruding into the cerebellopontine angle cistern. *C.* Axial postcontrast T1-weighted image (different patient) shows partially cystic right-sided vestibular schwannoma. A similar appearance may be seen after stereotactic radiosurgery is administered to these tumors.

and distant metastases are seen in 10% to 40% of patients. Chordomas usually are found in men in the fourth to seventh decades of life, although vertebral body chordomas occur earlier. Sacral chordomas usually are lytic and destructive lesions presenting with pain, rectal dysfunction, mass, and urinary incontinence. In the head, they destroy bone and invade the adjacent sinonasal cavities, but do not invade the brain. Histologically, the most typical finding is that of cells that have abundant cytoplasm containing many bubble-like changes ("physaliphorous" cells) (2). Chordomas have no capsule. When they have significant cartilaginous, areas they are called *chondroid* chordomas; chondroid chordomas present at an earlier age and have a better prognosis than the typical chordoma.

CT shows that 30% to 70% of chordomas contain calcifications (Fig. 6.15A). On MRI, most are of relatively low T2 signal intensity, but the chondroid type may show relatively high signal intensity on T2-weighted images (Fig. 6.15B and C). All chordomas show patchy areas of enhancement and some nearly cystlike areas that do not enhance. The differential diagnosis for masses arising in the clivus in adults includes:

- Chordomas
- Metastasis
- Plasmacytoma
- Primary sarcomas
- Ecchordosis physaliphora
- Masses secondarily invading the clivus (nasopharyngeal carcinoma, meningioma)

A
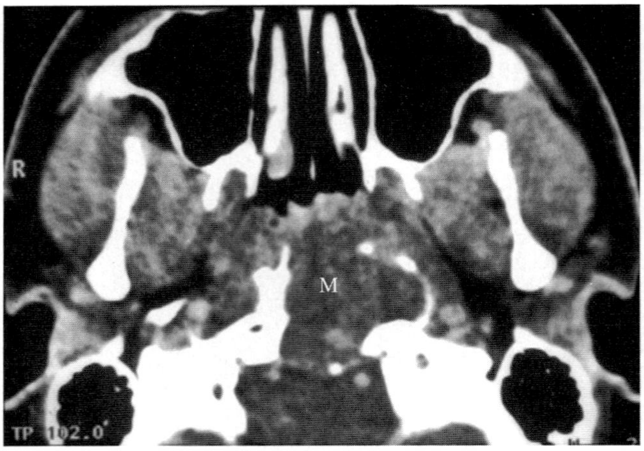

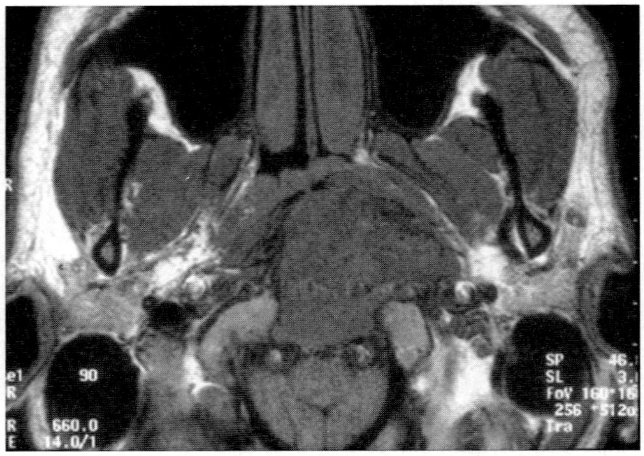

B

C
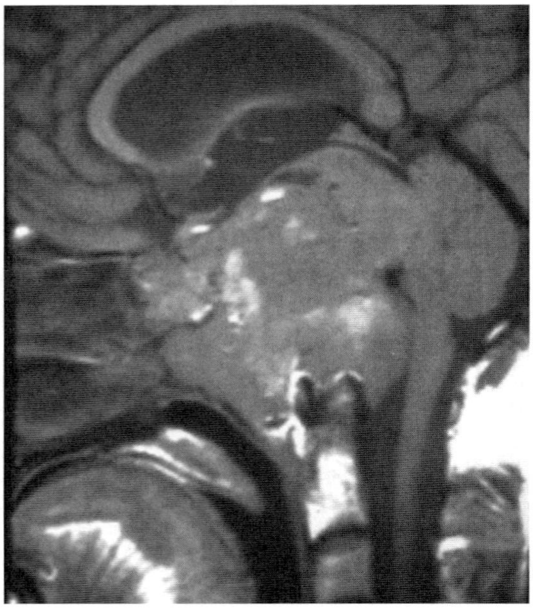

Figure 6.15 *Chordoma. A.* Axial contrast-enhanced computed tomography shows nonenhancing mass *(M)* destroying the clivus and extending anteriorly into the nasopharynx. *B.* Corresponding noncontrast T1-weighted image shows to better advantage the extension of the mass. Note extension into the anterior perimedullary cistern. *C.* In a different patient, noncontrast sagittal T1-weighted image shows a large tumor centered in the clivus with considerable intracranial extension, compression of the brainstem, and hydrocephalus. The mass also extends into the nasopharynx.

Supratentorial Tumors

Astrocytoma

Overall, glioblastoma multiforme (GBM) is the most common brain tumor in adults (more common than metastases and lymphoma). Most supratentorial astrocytomas, regardless of their histologic grade, are considered to be diffuse tumors. The diffuse cerebral astrocytomas are as follows:

- Low-grade astrocytoma
- Anaplastic astrocytoma
- GBM
- Gliomatosis cerebri
- Pontine astrocytoma
- Midbrain astrocytoma
- (Bi)thalamic astrocytoma
- Optic pathway astrocytoma

Astrocytomas are graded according to the scheme in Table 6.8, and cerebral astrocytomas may be subdivided according to their histology (2) (Table 6.9).

Table 6.8: Grading of Cerebral Astrocytomas

WHO Grade II	*WHO Grade III*	*WHO Grade IV*
Low-grade astrocytomas (Mayo grade II)	Anaplastic astrocytomas (Mayo grade III)	Glioblastoma multiforme (Mayo grade IV)

WHO, World Health Organization.

Table 6.9: Histologic Features of Cerebral Astrocytomas

Fibrillary	*Gemistocytic*	*Protoplasmic*	*Anaplastic*	*Glioblastoma Multiforme*
Most frequent variant, low to moderate cellularity	Gemistocytic astrocytes, may have a better prognosis	Rare, low cellularity and absent mitosis, mucoid degeneration and cyst formation	Increased cellularity, pleomorphism, mitotic activity, occasional necrosis and neovascularity	Highly anaplastic glial cells, mitoses, necrosis, vascular proliferation

Low-Grade Astrocytoma. Low-grade astrocytomas account for 10% to 30% of cerebral gliomas in adults (2). Histologically, they are fibrillary (diffuse), and over 80% eventually show anaplastic transformation. They usually occur in one cerebral hemisphere in patients 20 to 40 years of age. Approximately 10% to 20% of astrocytomas show calcifications by CT. All low-grade astrocytomas are hyperintense on MRI T2-weighted images, and most are hypointense on T1-weighted images (Fig. 6.16). Their borders may be well defined or ill defined. Contrast enhancement may be absent or mild; edema and hemorrhage are rare (44). By proton MR spectroscopy, most show elevation of choline and low NAA (45). When a short echo time (TE) is used, most low-grade astrocytomas show elevated myoinositol (46). Perfusion MR studies show that low-grade astrocytomas have low relative cerebral blood volume (rCBV) compared with higher-grade tumors (47). Median survival varies between 2 and 8 years for patients with low-grade cerebral astrocytomas.

In adults, malignant brain astrocytomas are more common than benign ones.

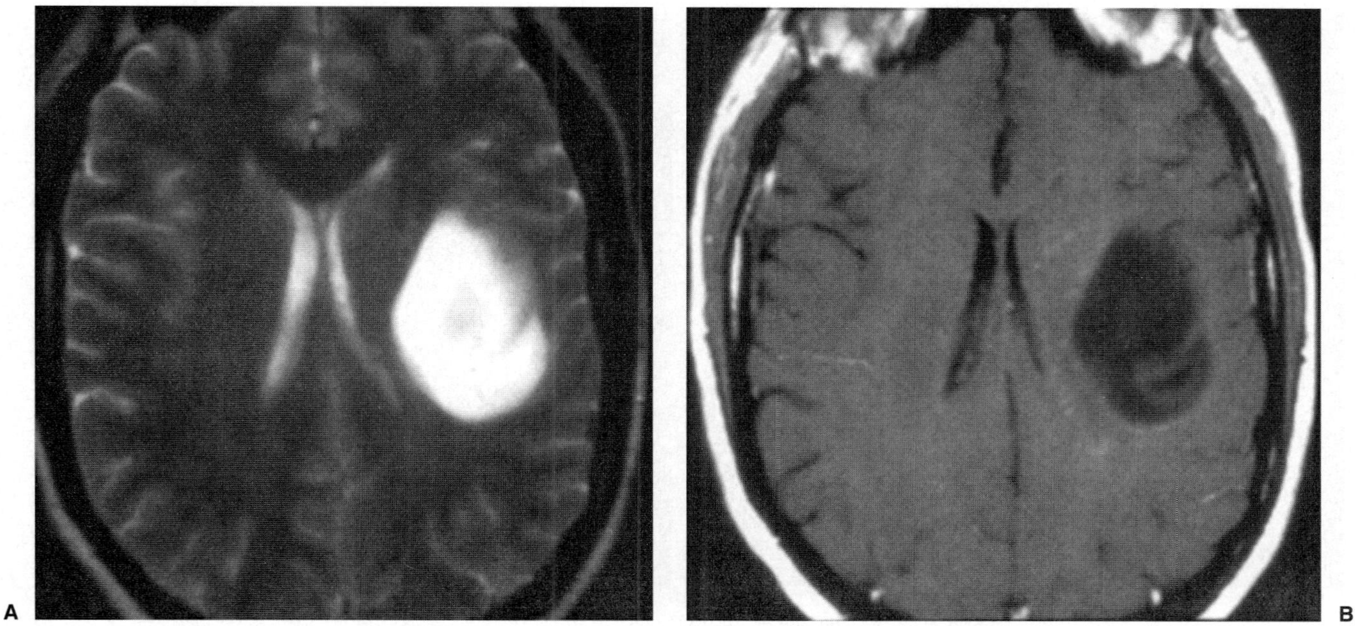

Figure 6.16 *Low-Grade Astrocytoma (WHO Grade 2). A.* Axial T2-weighted image shows well defined, hyperintense mass in the left temporal lobe. There is no associated edema. *B.* Corresponding postcontrast T1-weighted image shows no enhancement and little mass effect.

Anaplastic Astrocytoma. Anaplastic astrocytomas account for 30% of cerebral gliomas in adults and are found more frequently in patients 40 to 60 years of age (2). Dissemination through the white matter tracts, ependyma, and subarachnoid space is relatively common. Anaplastic astrocytomas tend to invade structures without destroying them, and commonly result in thickening of the white matter. They arise in the white matter of the cerebral hemispheres (frontal, parietal, temporal, and occipital). Imaging studies show an inhomogeneous mass (bright on T2 images), surrounded by edema, and sometimes peripheral or central areas of enhancement (Fig. 6.17). The borders of these tumors are ill defined. By proton MR spectroscopy, anaplastic astrocytomas show high choline and low NAA, and on short TE studies very little myoinositol (45,46). Prognosis is poor, with a median survival of 2 years.

The main differential diagnosis of a butterfly-type lesion includes GBM, lymphoma, oligodendroglioma, and demyelinating disease.

Glioblastoma Multiforme. GBM accounts for over 50% to 60% of cerebral gliomas in adults (47). Necrosis, neovascularity, and cellular pleomorphism ("multiforme") are typical histologic features. Most GBMs arise in white matter of the cerebral hemispheres (frontal, temporal, parietal, and corpus callosum) in men older than 50 years of age. Symptoms vary but usually are less than 3 months in duration. GBM is a diffuse disease for which there usually is no cure. Imaging studies often reveal these tumors to have a typical nodular rim of enhancement with a large amount of surrounding edema and mass effect (Fig. 6.18A). Hemorrhage may occur and calcifications are rare. Extension through the corpus callosum is typical and results in the "butterfly"-type GBM (26) (Fig. 6.18B). GBM commonly extends into the leptomeninges and the ventricular ependyma (2). Multifocal GBMs are of polyclonal origin, whereas multicentric ones (2%) represent extension of one primary lesion (Fig. 6.18C). Proton MR spectroscopy shows very high choline, low NAA, and the presence of lipids and lactate, reflecting necrosis (45) (Fig. 6.18D). On short TE studies, the myoinositol peak is absent or markedly reduced (46). Spectroscopy shows presence of tumor in zones of edema and even in normal-appearing areas. Thus, two-dimensional proton MR spectroscopy may be a better means to map the tumor than simple imaging studies. Perfusion studies show elevated rCBV (48,49). Perfusion MR studies have been used to differentiate tumor grades, with the highest rCBV found in GBMs. Ten percent of GBMs occur in multiple sites (2). Prognosis is very poor and most patients die

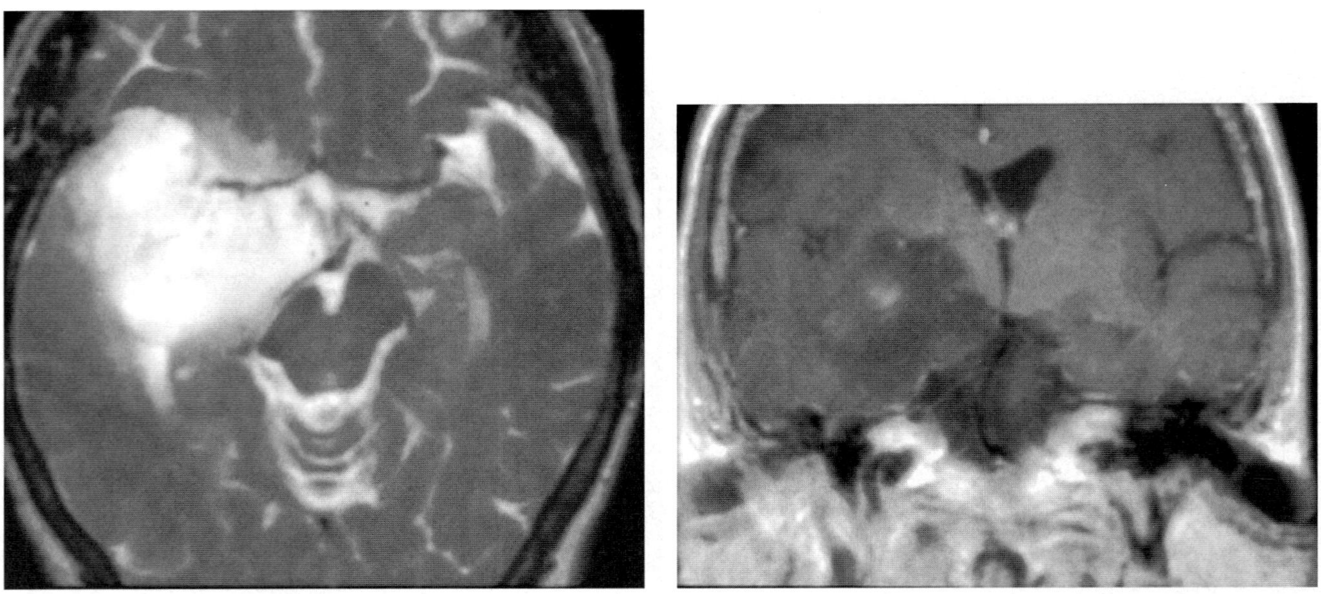

A B

Figure 6.17 *Anaplastic Astrocytoma (WHO Grade 3). A.* Axial T2-weighted image shows bright, large mass in the right temporal lobe with mass effect and somewhat indistinct margins. *B.* Coronal postcontrast T1-weighted image shows areas of patchy enhancement in the tumor without evidence of frank necrosis.

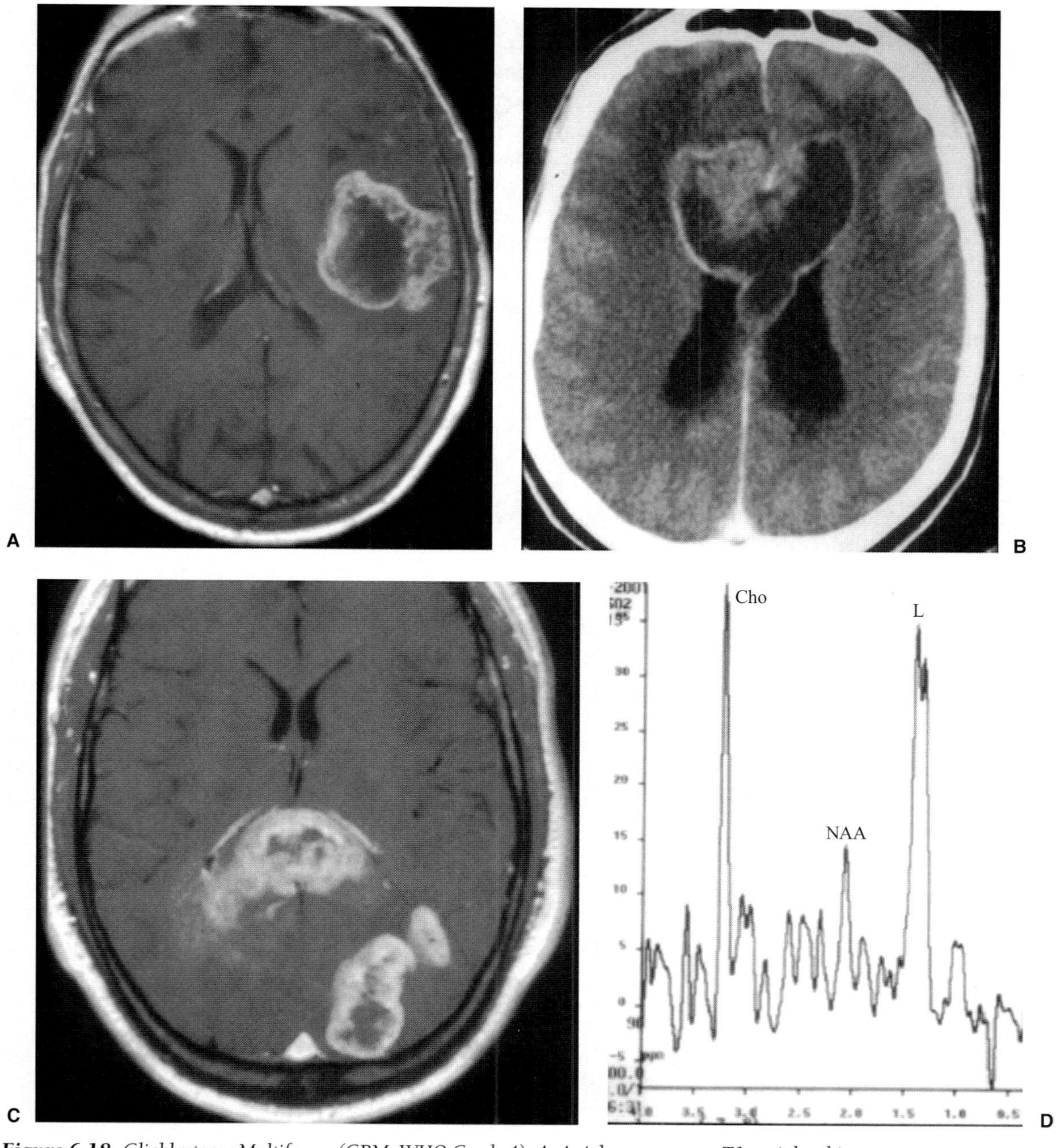

Figure 6.18 *Glioblastoma Multiforme (GBM; WHO Grade 4). A.* Axial postcontrast T1-weighted image shows a mass in the left temporal lobe. Note central nonenhancing region, presumed to be necrosis, and the irregular and thick rim of enhancement. *B.* Axial postcontrast computed tomography shows necrotic and ring-enhancing tumor in the genu of the corpus callosum (so-called butterfly glioma). *C.* Axial postcontrast T1-weighted image shows multifocal GBM with tumor in the splenium of the corpus callosum and in the left occipital lobe. *D.* Long–echo-time magnetic resonance spectroscopy in a GBM shows high choline *(Cho)*, low *N*-acetyl aspartate *(NAA)*, and presence of lactate *(L)*.

8 to 12 months after diagnosis. GBMs also may occur as a consequence of prior irradiation.

Recently, GBMs have been divided into primary or secondary types. Primary GBMs are more common in adults and arise *de novo*. Secondary GBMs are found in younger patients and represent the malignant degeneration from originally lower-grade astrocytomas. Tumors undergo a series of mutations before becoming GBMs. The formation of grade II astrocytomas involves the following (2):

Inactivation of tumor suppressor gene *p53* (located in chromosome 17q); this gene is involved in the control of apoptosis, cell cycle arrest, and angiogenesis

Activation of a platelet-derived growth factor

In 20% to 30% of tumors, loss of a tumor suppressor gene located in chromosome 22q (not the neurofibromatosis gene)

- Formation of anaplastic astrocytomas involves the following:

Inactivation of tumor suppressor genes in chromosomes 9p, 11p, 13p, and 19p, all of which encode for proteins that are crucial in cell cycle regulations.

The gene in chromosome19p is unique to glial-line tumors.

- Formation of GBMs involves the following:

Inactivation of tumor suppressor gene in chromosome 10q (this occurs in 65% to 85% of tumors).

Amplification of epidermal growth factor receptor gene in 40% of tumors (this gene facilitates tumor growth).

High tumor metabolism leads to hypoxia, which in turn results in upregulation of angiogenic factors that promote cloning of resistant cells.

Thickening of white matter tracts in more than one cerebral lobe suggests the possibility of underlying gliomatosis cerebri.

Gliomatosis Cerebri. Gliomatosis cerebri is a very rare of form of a common disease (astrocytoma) (50). It probably represents true multicentric gliomas of varying degrees of malignancy. Gliomatosis cerebri results in proliferation of malignant glial cells, destruction of the myelin sheaths, and preservation of axons and neurons. Gliomatosis extends through the white matter tracts but preserves the cortex (51). The diagnosis can be made when a glioma involves at least two or three cerebral lobes. The most common presentation of gliomatosis is seizures followed by bizarre behavior. There is no specific age for presentation, and both sexes are similarly affected. Histologically, the malignant grade of the lesion varies from grade II to III, depending on the site targeted for biopsy, but true GBM is rare (2). By imaging studies, a typical finding is that of widening of the white matter tracts (particularly the corpus callosum and posterior limb of the internal capsule) (52). Enhancement is patchy and sometimes absent (53). The lesion is difficult to appreciate on noncontrast T1-weighted images, but is always bright on T2-weighted images (Fig. 6.19). Mass effect is present, but there is no significant surrounding edema. Proton MR spectroscopy (especially using multivolume techniques) shows varying degrees of elevation of choline and myoinositol, low NAA, and at times lipids and lactate (54).

Oligodendroglioma

Oligodendrogliomas account for less than 5% of cerebral gliomas in adults and usually are found in the fifth and sixth decades of life (2). Oligodendrogliomas in children are rare (55). These tumors are more common in males. The most common symptom is seizures. Approximately 50% of oligodendrogliomas are histologically "mixed" and contain neoplastic astrocytes (called an *oligoastrocytoma*, which is identical to oligodendroglioma on imaging studies); growth is very slow. Similar to GBMs, oligodendrogliomas undergo a series of genetic mutations involving chromosomes 9, 10, and 19, leading to the upregulation of a tumor growth factor (2). Over 85% of oligodendrogliomas are supratentorial. Multiple sites of involvement are seen in 50% of patients, and bilateral tumors in 20%. Oligodendrogliomas typically involve the subcortical white matter in the frontotemporal regions, but also may occur in temporal and occipital lobes and in the corpus callosum. These tumors are slow growing, and several years may be needed to demonstrate any change in them. They are the most common intraaxial tumor to calcify (70%), and this feature is readily visible with CT (Fig. 6.20). Because of their peripheral location, they may cause scalloping of the inner table of the skull (17%). Cysts are present in 20%, hemorrhage occurs in 20%, and contrast enhancement is seen in 50% of oligodendrogliomas. The tumors usually measure 3.5 cm at discovery. They are of low T1 signal and high T2 signal intensity. MRI with contrast shows variable patterns of enhancement. The 5-year survival rate is 75% for pure oligodendroglioma and less for the mixed type. When they

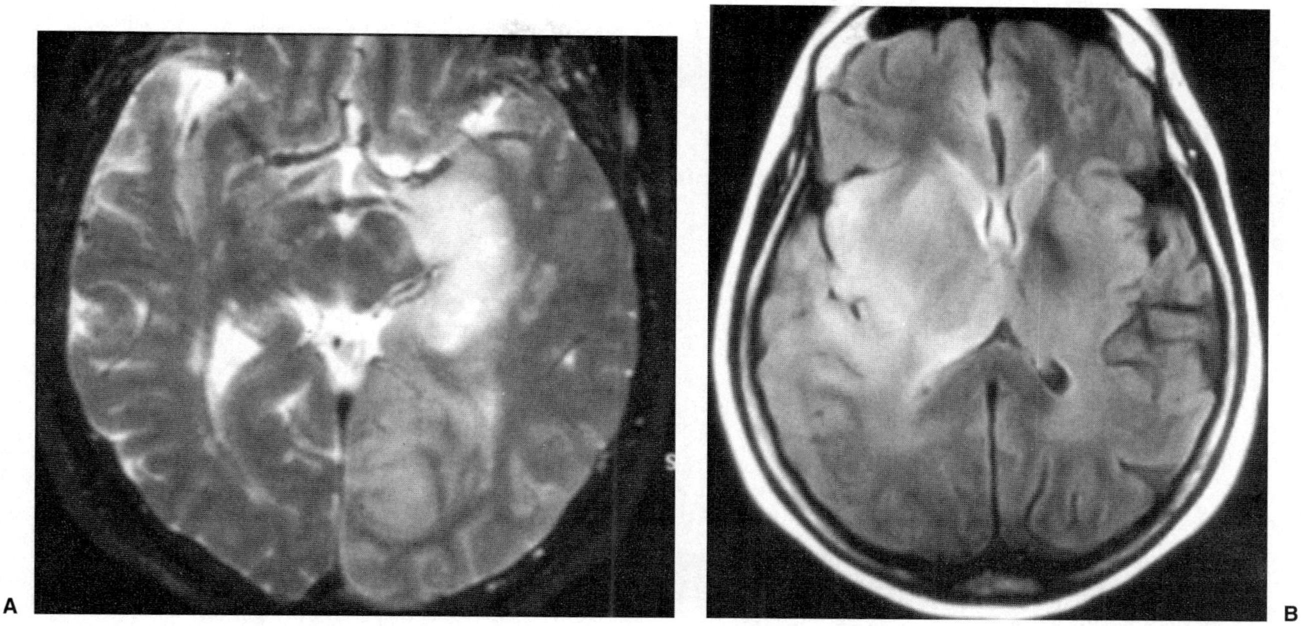

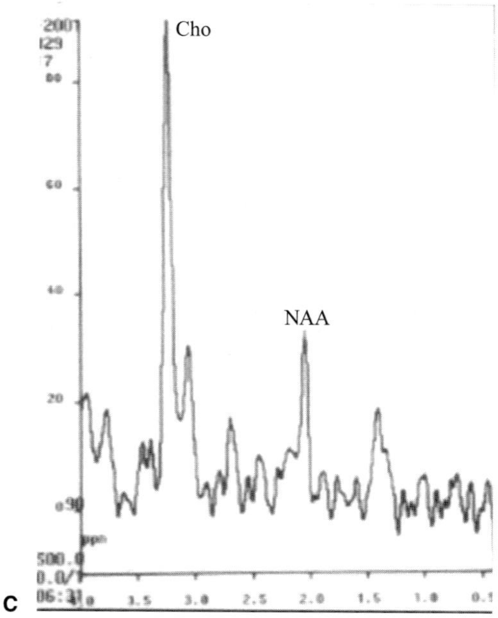

Figure 6.19 *Gliomatosis Cerebri (WHO Grade 3). A.* Axial T2-weighted image shows high signal intensity in the mesial left temporal lobe extending to the left occipital region. The white matter is slightly "expanded" and the tumor involves the cortex. *B.* Fluid attenuation inversion recovery (FLAIR) image (different patient) shows high signal of tumor diffusely involving the right temporal lobe (white matter tracts and deep gray matter nuclei). Note relatively little mass effect. (Case courtesy of J. Thompson, Gastonia, NC.) *C.* Long–echo-time magnetic resonance spectroscopy (same patient as *A*) shows high choline *(Cho)*, low *N*-acetyl aspartate *(NAA)*, but no definite lipids or lactate.

arise inside the lateral ventricles, they may be histologically confused with central neurocytoma (55).

Lymphoma

Secondary brain lymphoma most commonly presents as leptomeningeal spread, whereas primary brain lymphoma (usually non-Hodgkin's and B-cell types) presents as parenchymal masses (2). Lymphomas account for less than 1% of all primary brain tumors in adults (>60 years of age), but occur in 6% of patients with acquired immunodeficiency syndrome (AIDS) (52). It previously was thought that lymphoma would become the most common primary brain tumor because of the large AIDS population. This, however, has not occurred because treatment for patients with AIDS has improved considerably, and GBM

Most toxoplasmosis lesions show some improvement after 2 to 4 weeks of antibiotics, whereas lymphoma remains unchanged.

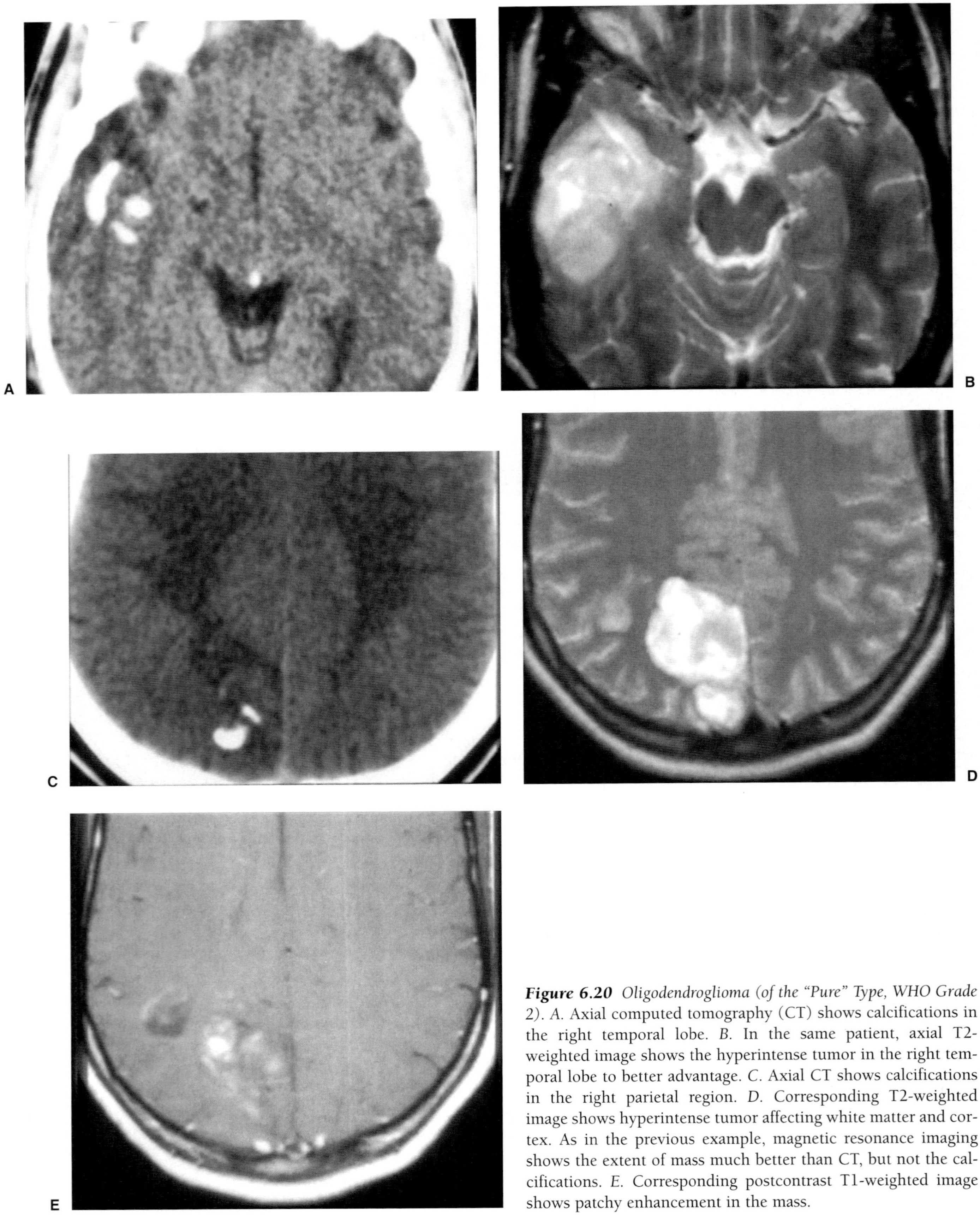

Figure 6.20 Oligodendroglioma (of the "Pure" Type, WHO Grade 2). *A.* Axial computed tomography (CT) shows calcifications in the right temporal lobe. *B.* In the same patient, axial T2-weighted image shows the hyperintense tumor in the right temporal lobe to better advantage. *C.* Axial CT shows calcifications in the right parietal region. *D.* Corresponding T2-weighted image shows hyperintense tumor affecting white matter and cortex. As in the previous example, magnetic resonance imaging shows the extent of mass much better than CT, but not the calcifications. *E.* Corresponding postcontrast T1-weighted image shows patchy enhancement in the mass.

continues to be the most common primary brain tumor in adults. In primary brain lymphoma, 8% to 44% of the lesions are multiple. In immunocompetent patients, primary brain lymphoma presents as deep gray or white matter lesions (most common presentation) that are slightly hyperdense on noncontrast CT, have little mass effect or edema, and show mostly prominent contrast enhancement (Fig. 6.21). On T2-weighted images, lymphomas tend to be relatively hypointense, probably reflecting dense cellular packing

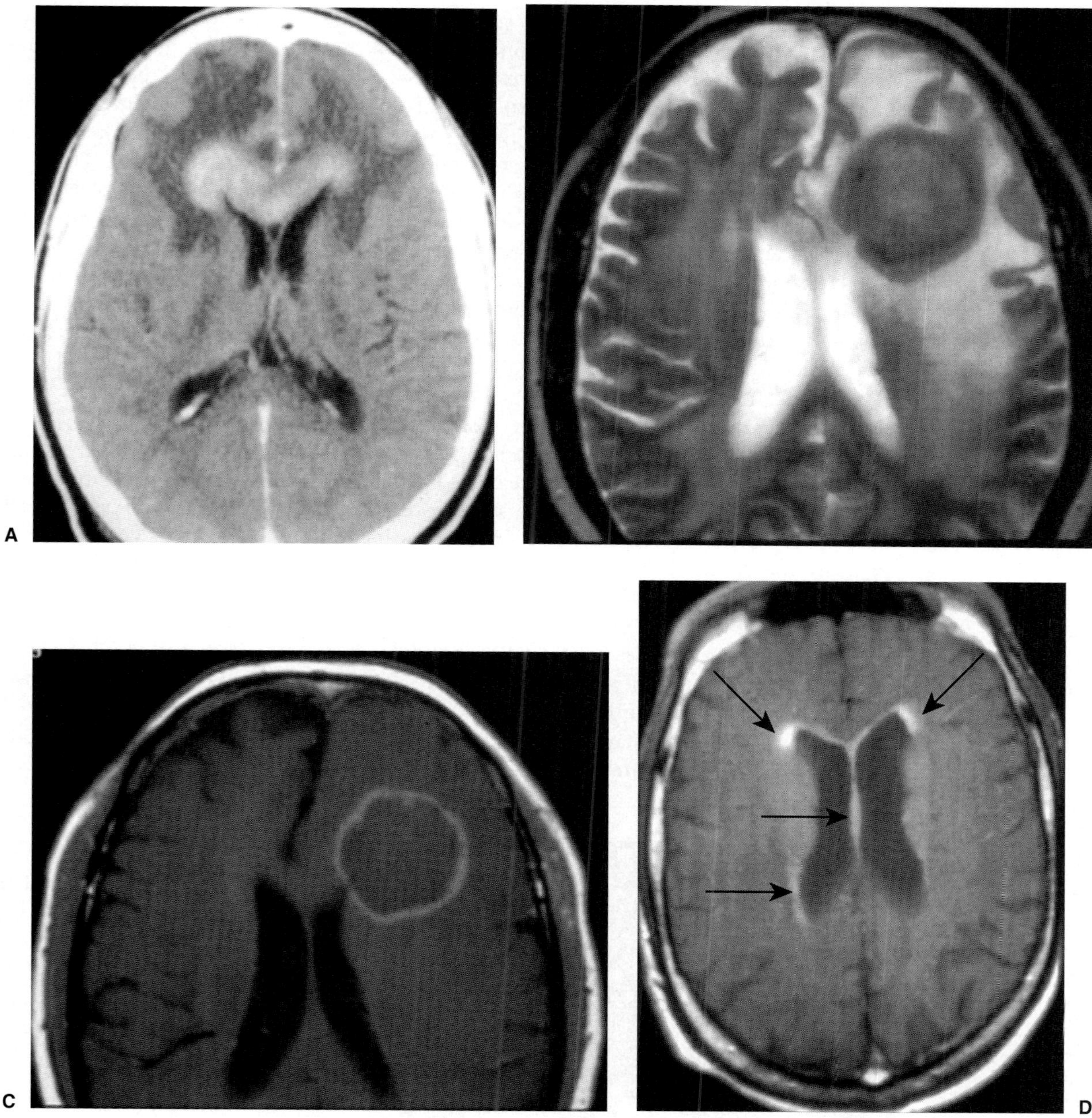

Figure 6.21 *Lymphoma. A.* Contrast-enhanced axial computed tomography shows dense and enhancing lesion with surrounding edema in the genu of the corpus callosum ("butterfly-type" pattern). *B.* Axial T2-weighted image in patient with acquired immunodeficiency syndrome (AIDS) shows dark mass in the left frontal lobe with surrounding edema. The mass is close to the ventricle, a finding typical of lymphoma. There is diffuse hyperintensity in the white matter, probably related to human immunodeficiency virus infection. *C.* Corresponding postcontrast T1-weighted image shows thin peripheral enhancement of the mass. *D.* In an elderly patient without AIDS, axial postcontrast T1-weighted image shows enhancing nodular deposits *(arrows)* of lymphoma along the walls and septum pellucidum of the lateral ventricles.

(56,57) (Fig. 6.21B). In patients with AIDS, primary lymphoma may present as single or multiple ring-enhancing lesions with edema (often indistinguishable from toxoplasmosis, although lymphoma tends to abut the ependymal surfaces). Lymphomas capture thallium-201, whereas infectious processes do not, and this technique is particularly important in patients with AIDS (58). In addition, perfusion studies show higher rCBV in lymphoma compared with infections (59). Proton MR spectroscopy shows significant elevation of choline, reduction of NAA, and presence of lipids/lactate in lymphomas. Unfortunately, toxoplasmosis (as well as other infections) resulting in inflammatory cell infiltrates also may result in elevated choline (45). Placement of the spectroscopy voxel in the presumed central necrosis may provide important information. In lymphoma, only cellular breakdown products are seen, whereas in toxoplasmosis (and other abscesses), the presence of amino acids (e.g., acetate and succinate) may be observed. Diffusion-weighted imaging also plays role in the differentiation of tumor from abscess. Most tumors are dark, whereas most abscesses show central hyperintensity on trace diffusion-weighted studies (60). The central hyperintensity seen in abscess is due to the fact that pus is very complex (containing cellular debris, inflammatory cells, and the like), restricting the motion of extracellular water protons. Secondary brain lymphoma may present as dural, pial, or ependymal thickening (which may be nodular), or as dural-based masses. Lymphoma is one of the few entities that may involve the dura and scalp tissues with a seemingly normal intervening calvarium. Although lymphomas are highly radiosensitive, the median survival for these patients is only 12 months because of the high rate of recurrence.

Central Neurocytoma

The diagnosis of central neurocytoma is receiving increasing attention. Previously, these tumors were thought to be intraventricular oligodendrogliomas, but now they are recognized as a distinct entity. They are very rare, representing less than 0.5% of all intracranial tumors, and most are found in patients 20 to 40 years of age (55). The most common sites are the frontal horns of the lateral ventricles (75%), the lateral and third ventricles (20%), and both lateral ventricles (5%). Because of the intraventricular location, most symptoms are related to increased intracranial pressure due to hydrocephalus (56). When they involve the lateral ventricles, they usually abut the septum pellucidum and the roof of the ventricles (Fig. 6.22). Central neurocytomas are dense on noncontrast CT and of heterogeneous signal intensity on both T1- and T2-weighted images. They are well demarcated and somewhat lobulated masses. Approximately half of central neurocytomas contain calcifications, and approximately half show contrast enhancement.

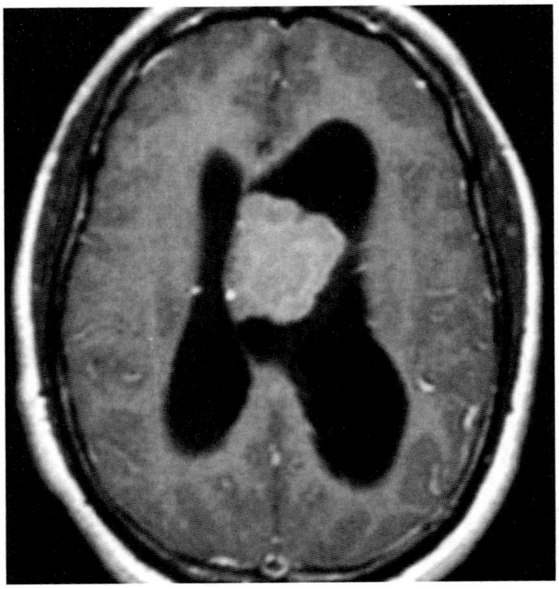

Figure 6.22 *Central Neurocytoma (WHO Grade 2).* Axial postcontrast T1-weighted image shows enhancing mass inside of the left lateral ventricle. The mass is attached to the septum pellucidum and there is hydrocephalus.

Table 6.10: Classifications of Pineal Tumors

Germ Cells	*Pineal Cells*	*From Neighboring Tissues*	*Nontumorous Masses*	*Metastases*
Germinoma (Fig 6.22), teratoma (Fig. 6.24), embryonal carcinoma, choriocarcinoma, endodermal sinus tumor	Pineocytoma (Fig. 6.25), peripheral neuroectodermal tumor (pineoblastoma) (Fig. 6.26), glioma	Glioma, meningioma, lymphoma	Cyst, lipoma, dermoid, epidermoid, vascular lesions	

Pineal Gland Tumors

Tumors arising in the pineal gland account for approximately 1.5% of all intracranial neoplasms (2). The normal pineal gland measures approximately 4 × 8 mm and contains calcifications in approximately 50% of the population. Pineal calcification usually is seen after 10 to 12 years of age, and should never be present before 5 years of age. Once pineal calcification is established, it does not grow or change throughout the life of an individual. Symptoms related to pineal gland masses are as follows (57):

Physiologic pineal gland calcification is not seen before 5 years of age.

- Increased intracranial pressure due to hydrocephalus
- Precocious puberty
- Hypogonadism
- Diabetes insipidus
- Parinaud's syndrome

Pineal gland tumors may be classified according to their origin (57) (Table 6.10).

Table 6.11 addresses the major features of pineal cells tumor originating from germ cells.

Tumors arising from pineal cells account for approximately 15% of all pineal gland tumors. Table 6.12 describes their features.

The specific imaging findings for tumors arising in tissues neighboring the pineal gland are discussed individually throughout this chapter. In addition, the imaging findings for nontumoral masses are addressed elsewhere. One important aspect is the fact that all pineal gland tumors may disseminate through the subarachnoid spaces, and postcontrast imaging of the entire neuraxis may be required in many patients (58). Germinomas and teratomas also may occur in the suprasellar regions. Pineal PNET may be a part of the trilateral retinoblastoma syndrome.

Table 6.11: Salient Features of Germ Cell Pineal Tumors

Tumor Type	*Age of Patients/Sex/ Serum Markers*	*Imaging Features*
Germinoma (most common; Fig. 6.23)	10–20 yr, almost exclusively male	Dense on computed tomography, low T2 signal, marked enhancement, pial metastases
Teratoma (second most common; Fig. 6.24)	Young children, male	Cysts, fat, calcium, areas of enhancement
Choriocarcinoma (<5% of pineal masses)	Young, male	Nonspecific but may contain subacute hemorrhage
Endodermal sinus tumor (yolk sac tumor, very rare)	Newborns and young children, AFP	Nonspecific
Embryonal cell carcinoma (very rare)	Newborns and young children, AFP, human chorionic gonadotropin	Nonspecific

AFP, α-fetoprotein.

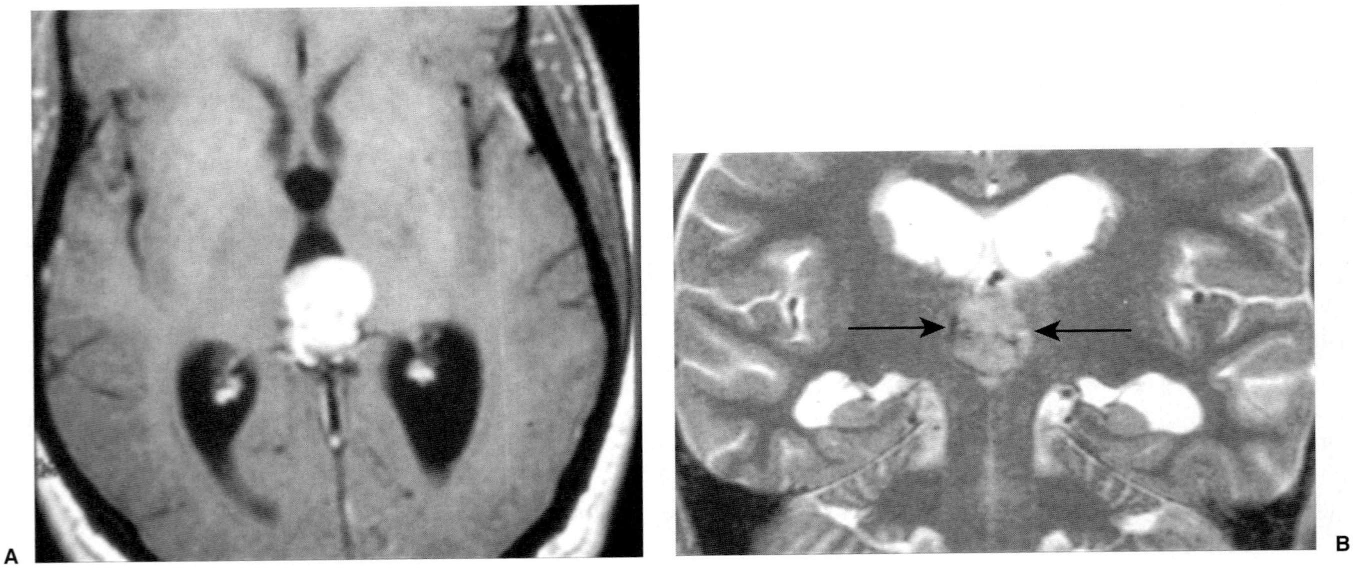

Figure 6.23 *Germinoma. A.* Postcontrast axial T1-weighted image shows nonspecific appearance of enhancing pineal gland germinoma. *B.* In a different patient, a germinoma *(arrows)* is relatively hypointense on this coronal T2-weighted image, a finding typical of germinoma. There is hydrocephalus.

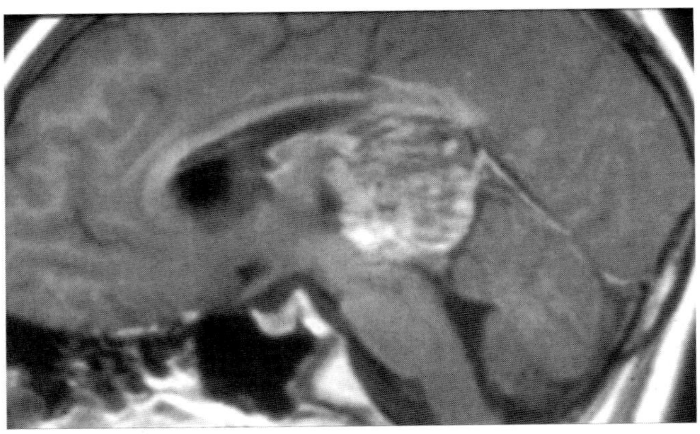

Figure 6.24 *Teratoma.* Sagittal postcontrast T1-weighted image shows large mass in the pineal gland region containing areas of high signal, some of which are fat and others that are true enhancement.

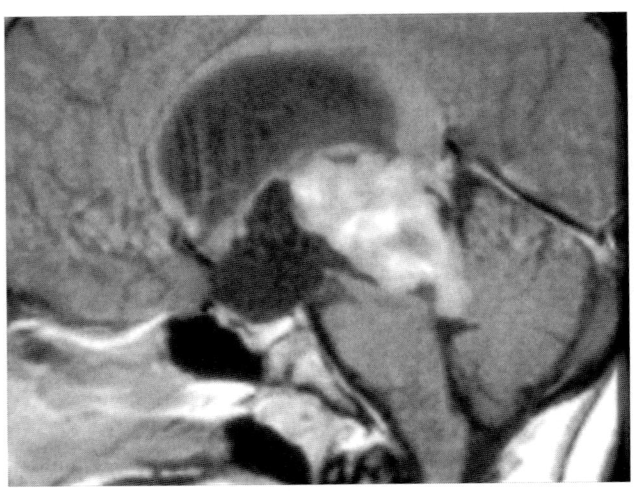

Figure 6.25 *Pineocytoma (WHO Grade 2).* Sagittal postcontrast T1-weighted image shows nonspecific-appearing mass in the pineal gland region. There is hydrocephalus.

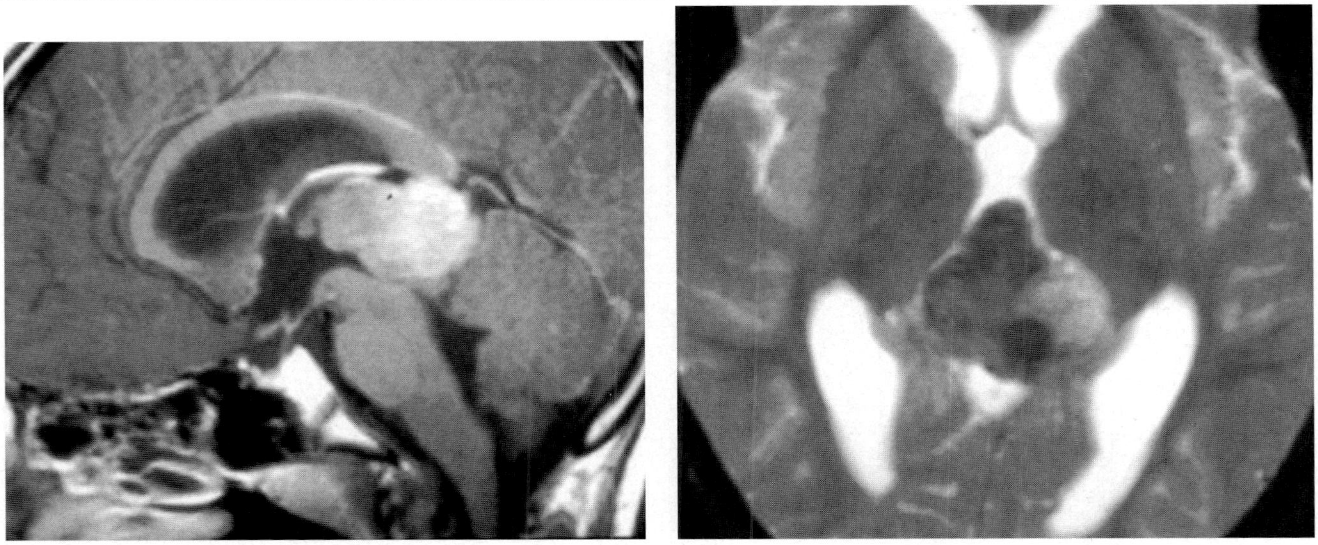

Figure 6.26 *Pineoblastoma (Primitive Neuroectodermal Tumor, WHO Grade 4). A.* Sagittal postcontrast T1-weighted image shows nonspecific-appearing, enhancing mass in the pineal gland region. *B.* On an axial T2-weighted image, the mass is mostly hypointense, a feature typical of these highly malignant hypercellular tumors. There is hydrocephalus.

Meningioma

Meningioma is the most common extraaxial tumor in adults and represents approximately 15% of all intracranial tumors in adults (2). Meningiomas occur mainly in middle-aged women (some authors have suggested a relationship to sex hormones) and in patients with NF-2. In the setting of this phakomatosis, the meningiomas may be multiple, present earlier in life, and have atypical appearances. Common sites for meningiomas include parasagittal/falcine (50%), sphenoid wing (20%), floor of the anterior cranial fossa (10%), parasellar region (10%), tentorium, and cerebellopontine angle cistern region (59) (Fig. 6.27). The main histologic types for meningiomas are typical (90% to 95%), atypical (3% to 5%), and frankly malignant (1%; the WHO now recognizes 15 types of meningiomas according to their histology).

Although multiple meningiomas are seen in NF-2, they are found more commonly in patients without NF-2.

The classic "hyperostosis" of underlying bone is present in only 5% of meningiomas and no longer is commonly encountered because most patients are imaged with MRI. Erosion of bone may occur with atypical and malignant meningiomas, but is still more common with typical meningiomas (Fig. 6.27D). On CT, the tumors are somewhat rounded, well demarcated, and show marked contrast enhancement. Underlying edema may be seen in up to 50% of patients (Fig. 6.27A and B). Meningiomas may be masslike or *en plaque* in configuration. *En plaque* meningiomas are perhaps somewhat more common in the base of the skull. Meningiomas may involve the cavernous sinuses, extend extracranially through skull base foramina, involve the jugular foramen and the foramen magnum, be purely intraosseous, or arise extracranially. On MRI, most meningiomas are isointense to gray matter on both T1- and T2-weighted images (60,61). They show marked enhancement after contrast is given (Fig. 6.27C and D). Their histologic status cannot be predicted based on the imaging features, but bright meningiomas on T2-weighted images tend to have more atypical microscopic features. On MRI, a "dural tail" suggests the diagnosis of meningioma, but is not

Table 6.12: Salient Features of Pineal Cell Tumors

Tumor Type	*Age/Sex*	*Imaging Features*
Pineocytoma (Fig. 6.25)	>20 yr, no sex predilection	Well circumscribed, nonspecific
Peripheral neuroectodermal tumor (pineoblastoma; Fig. 6.26)	<10 yr, no sex predilection	Nonspecific
Mixed tumors and astrocytomas	Nonspecific	Nonspecific

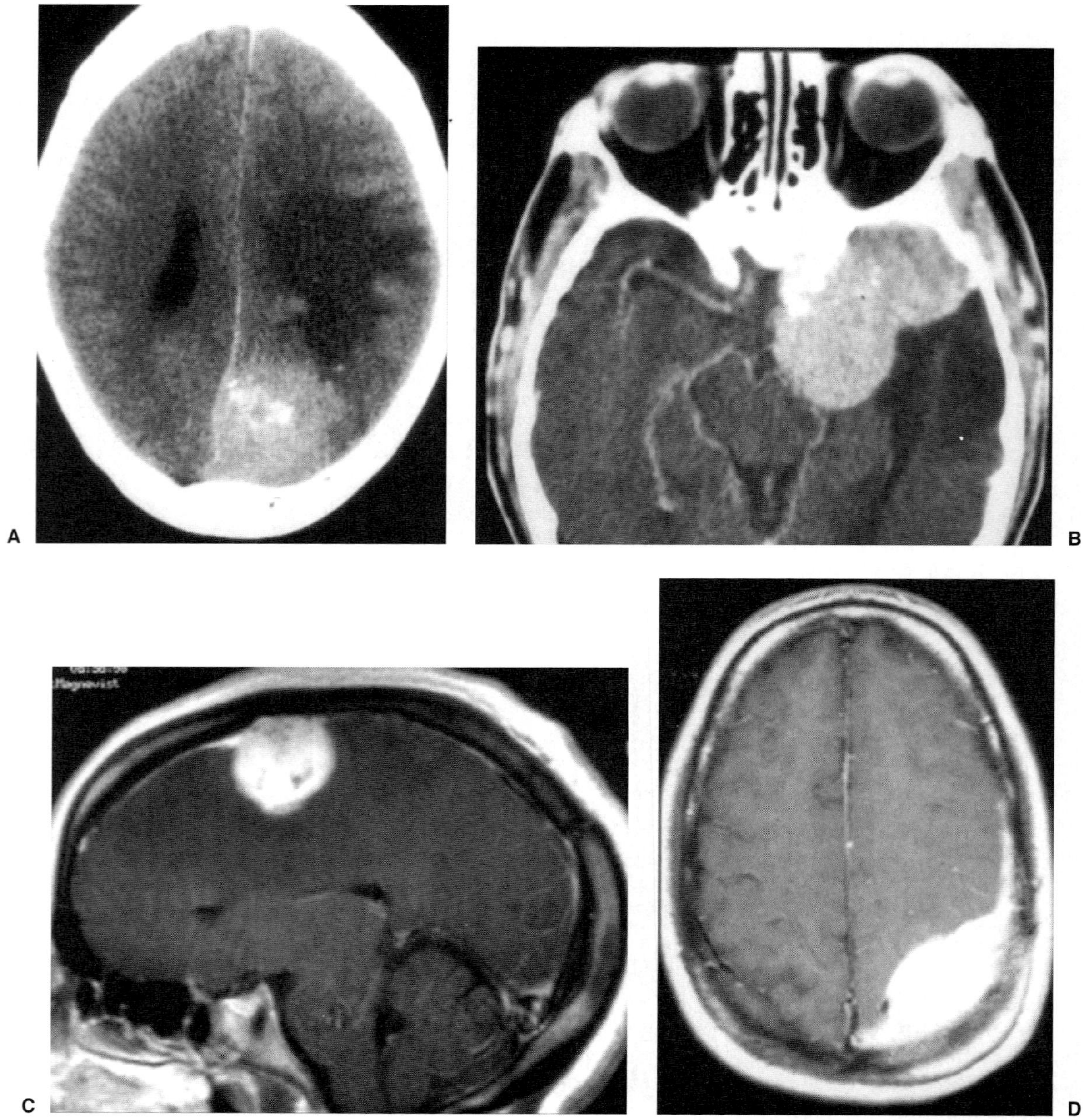

Figure 6.27 *Meningioma. A.* Axial computed tomography (CT) shows left posterior parasagittal, partially calcified meningioma (WHO grade 1) with associated edema. *B.* In a different patient, axial postcontrast CT shows densely enhancing meningioma (WHO grade 1) arising in the left greater sphenoidal wing and extending into the suprasellar region. There is edema in the left temporal lobe. *C.* Parasagittal postcontrast T1-weighted image shows typical enhancing convexity meningioma (WHO grade 1) with short "dural tails" and underlying cerebral edema. *D.* Axial postcontrast T1-weighted image enhancing left parasagittal meningioma with typical dural tails. Note invasion of overlying skull despite this being a WHO grade 1 tumor.

pathognomonic (62). This dural tail may be due to frank meningioma invasion or secondary to reactive changes. In parasagittal meningiomas, MR venography may be needed to assess patency and invasion of the superior sagittal sinus. Some meningiomas are hypervascular and may benefit from preoperative embolization. In adults, cystic meningiomas are rare. Most cystic meningiomas usually have a large dural-based component. The size of the cyst(s) is variable, and their walls may or may not enhance. By proton MR spectroscopy, meningiomas show marked elevation of the choline peak, very low or no NAA, and presence of alanine (at 1.5 ppm) (63,64). Although the presence of alanine is fairly typical for meningioma, it is inconstantly documented. Meningiomas in children deserve special mention. Their features are opposite to those seen in adults; that is, most childhood meningiomas occur in boys, in atypical locations, and have a higher incidence of malignancy.

Metastases

Approximately 25% of all patients with cancer will develop metastases to the brain. Metastases are the second most common brain tumor after GBM (65). They are seen mostly in patients older than 50 years of age. The most common primary tumors in adults to cause bone metastases are breast, prostate, lung, and kidney (always include multiple myeloma in the differential diagnosis). In children, neuroblastoma and Langerhans cell histiocytosis are common causes of bone metastases. The most common primary tumors in adults to cause dural or leptomeningeal metastases are breast, small cell carcinoma, and melanoma (always include lymphoma and leukemia in the differential diagnosis). In children, PNET is a common cause for meningeal metastases. The most common tumors in adults to cause parenchymal metastases (10% to 35% of all brain tumors in adults) are lung, breast, melanoma, kidney, and gastrointestinal tract tumors. Unknown primaries account for 10% to 15% of patients with brain metastases. Most parenchymal metastases occur at gray–white junctions, 80% are supratentorial, and 60% to 80% are multiple (Fig. 6.28A). The average survival for

Metastases are the second most common malignant brain tumor after GBM.

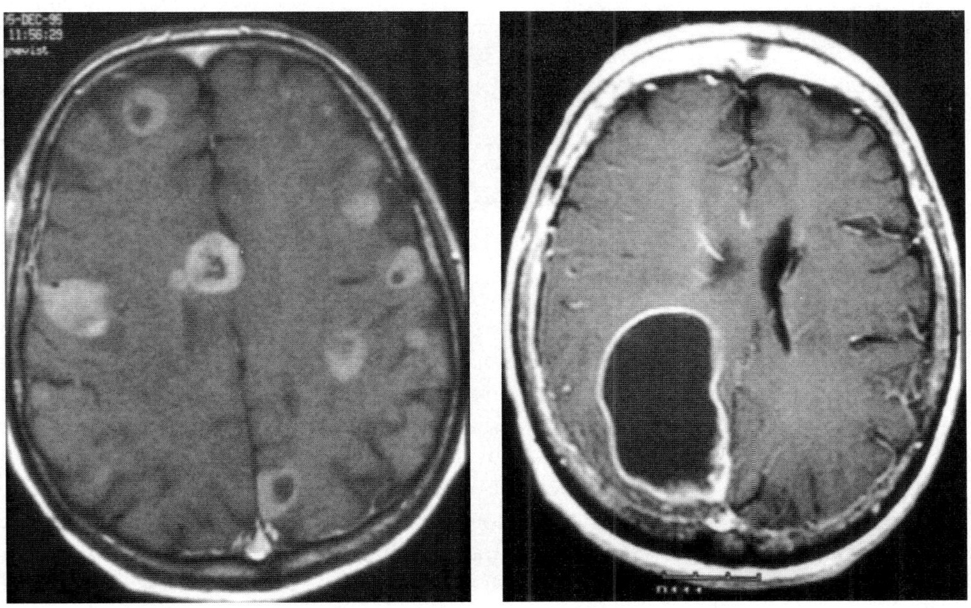
A B

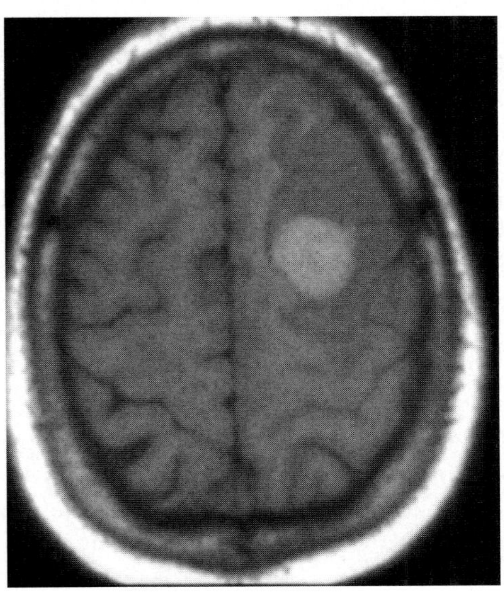
C

Figure 6.28 *Metastases. A.* Axial postcontrast T1-weighted image shows typical multiple, mostly ring-enhancing masses (from primary lung cancer) at the gray–white matter junctions of both cerebral hemispheres. *B.* In a different patient, postcontrast axial T1-weighted image shows large cystic metastasis from breast cancer. *C.* Noncontrast axial T1-weighted image shows bright metastasis from melanotic melanoma.

a patient with brain metastases is 3 to 12 months. Metastases may be large or small, solid or ring enhancing (even cystic), and may show low signal intensity on T2-weighted images (65,66) (Fig. 6.28B). Most metastases have considerable surrounding edema. Metastases with increased T1 signal intensity before contrast administration include melanoma, kidney, lung, choriocarcinoma, and bowel (because of the presence of mucin) (67) (Fig. 6.28C). A single-dose contrast MR study with magnetization transfer is probably as sensitive for detection of brain metastases as a double-dose study (68). Proton MR spectroscopy shows significantly elevated choline and very low NAA (the presence of NAA in many metastases represents contamination from adjacent tissues due to partial averaging) (45). Lactate and lipids usually are high. The tissues surrounding the enhancing mass usually are normal by spectroscopy (unlike high gliomas).

Leukemia

Leukemias represent approximately 3% of cancers in the United States. Nearly one-half of patients with leukemia have complications involving the central nervous system. The imaging features related to this involvement may be classified as shown in Table 6.13 (69). Treatment related complications are addressed in Chapter 11.

Table 6.13: Complications of Leukemia

Direct Involvement	*Cerebrovascular*
Meningeal	Hemorrhages
Brain involvement (chloromas)	Infarction
Extracranial (orbits, nodes, paranasal, sinuses)	Venous thrombosis
Bone marrow	

Nonneoplastic Masses

Arachnoid Cyst. In adults, arachnoid cysts represent approximately 1% of intracranial masses, but they are the most common extraaxial cystic lesions (followed by meningioma and schwannoma). Arachnoid cysts are more common in men. Common locations include the sylvian fissure (50%), suprasellar (10%) and quadrigeminal plate cisterns (10%), cerebellopontine angle (5% to 10%) and supracerebellar cisterns (<5%), and cisterna magna (<5%), prepontine cistern, and convexities (70–73). They may grow slowly and cause adjacent bone remodeling. Specific histologic subtypes include the leptomeningeal and intraarachnoid cysts, which cannot be separated by imaging (probably this is not clinically important). Arachnoid cysts appear as CSF signal/density-equivalent masses by all imaging modalities, with the main differential diagnosis being epidermoid (distinction may require diffusion MRI or FLAIR sequences; Fig. 6.29). The only reliable way to assess communication with the remainder of CSF spaces is through contrast CT cisternography (74). Arachnoid cysts usually are solitary. Multiple arachnoid cysts are seen in glutaric type 1 aciduria, neurocutaneous melanosis, tuberous sclerosis, and mucopolysachari doses (75).

Choroidal fissure cysts deserve special mention because they commonly are found during the evaluation of the hippocampi for seizures (76). They almost always are incidental findings. Although they may compress the hippocampus, they do not commonly produce seizures. On imaging, choroidal fissure cysts are spindle shaped and displace the choroid plexus of the temporal horn laterally. Hippocampal fissure cysts are tiny, multiple, and located between the head of the hippocampus and the subiculum, and often appear as a "string of pearls" on axial T2 images.

Most epidermoids are readily differentiated from arachnoid cysts with the use of proton-density images, CISS images, diffusion-weighted MRI, or proton MR spectroscopy.

Epidermoid. Epidermoids arise from intracranial inclusion of epithelial elements during neural tube closure, and are 10 times more common than intracranial dermoids (77). Epidermoids may contain ectoderm, but have no skin appendages. Most epidermoids are found in early adulthood and grow very slowly. Most are asymptomatic but may result in

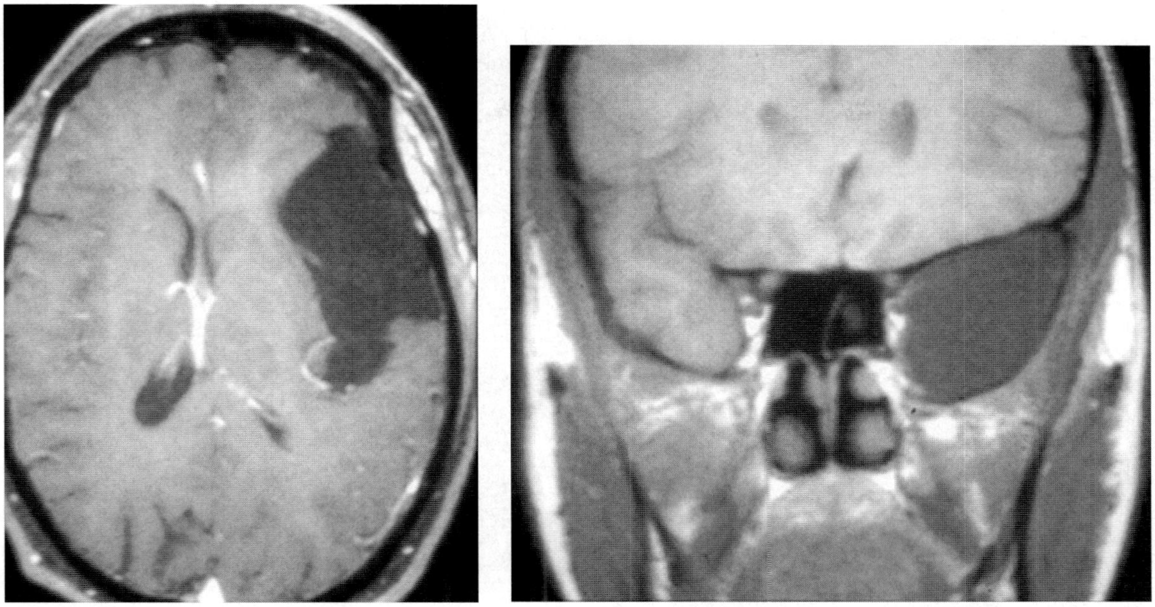

A B

Figure 6.29 *Arachnoid Cyst. A.* Axial postcontrast T1-weighted image shows nonenhancing cyst in the left sylvian cistern. Note lack of mass effect. *B.* Coronal noncontrast T1-weighted image shows that the cyst expands the left middle cranial fossa compared with the right one.

mass effect, cranial neuropathies, and, rarely, seizures. The most common locations for epidermoids include cerebellopontine angle cisterns (50%), sellar and parasellar regions (10% to 15%), fourth ventricle, and prepontine cistern (all epidermoids are located off the midline) (77). Epidermoids also may occur in the diploic space of the skull (10%), giving rise to a lytic lesion with scalloped sclerotic borders (Fig. 6.30A and B). Epidermoids may occur in the middle ear, especially with atresia of the external auditory canal. By MRI and CT, epidermoids may appear similar to arachnoid cysts, and conventional MRI and CT may not be able to distinguish the two lesions. However, epidermoids usually are slightly brighter than arachnoid cysts on T1-weighted, proton-density, and FLAIR images. Epidermoids also contain internal areas of varying signal intensity (flow in arachnoid cysts may result in similar findings, however) (77). High-resolution T2-weighted images using CISS show that epidermoids are of lower signal intensity than arachnoid cysts (78). Diffusion-weighted MRI shows that most epidermoids have increased signal intensity with respect to CSF on trace images (79,80) (Fig. 6.30C and D). Epidermoids do not show contrast enhancement. By proton MR spectroscopy, epidermoids show large peaks of lipids that are not present in arachnoid cysts. Epidermoids may extend into Meckel's cave or arise in it.

Dermoid. Dermoids probably arise from intracranial inclusion of ectodermal elements during neural tube closure. Like epidermoids, dermoids contain ectoderm, but they also contain skin appendages (sweat glands, hair follicles, and sebaceous glands) (2). Dermoids are very rare and represent less than 1% of all intracranial tumors. They present in early to middle adulthood (30 to 50 years of age), with a slight male predominance. The most common sites for dermoids include lumbar spine (associated with spinal dysraphism), parasellar region, floor of the anterior cranial fossa, and posterior fossa (81–83). Almost all dermoids are midline in location (sella, frontobasal region, pineal gland, posterior fossa, anterior fontanelle, and lumbosacral spine) and have the same imaging characteristics as fat because of the liquid cholesterol they contain (epidermoids contain solid cholesterol and thus are T1 hypointense) (83) (Fig. 6.31A). Dermoids may produce chemical meningitis if they rupture and spill their contents into CSF spaces (81,82) (Fig. 6.31B). Differentiating dermoids from midline lipomas may not be possible.

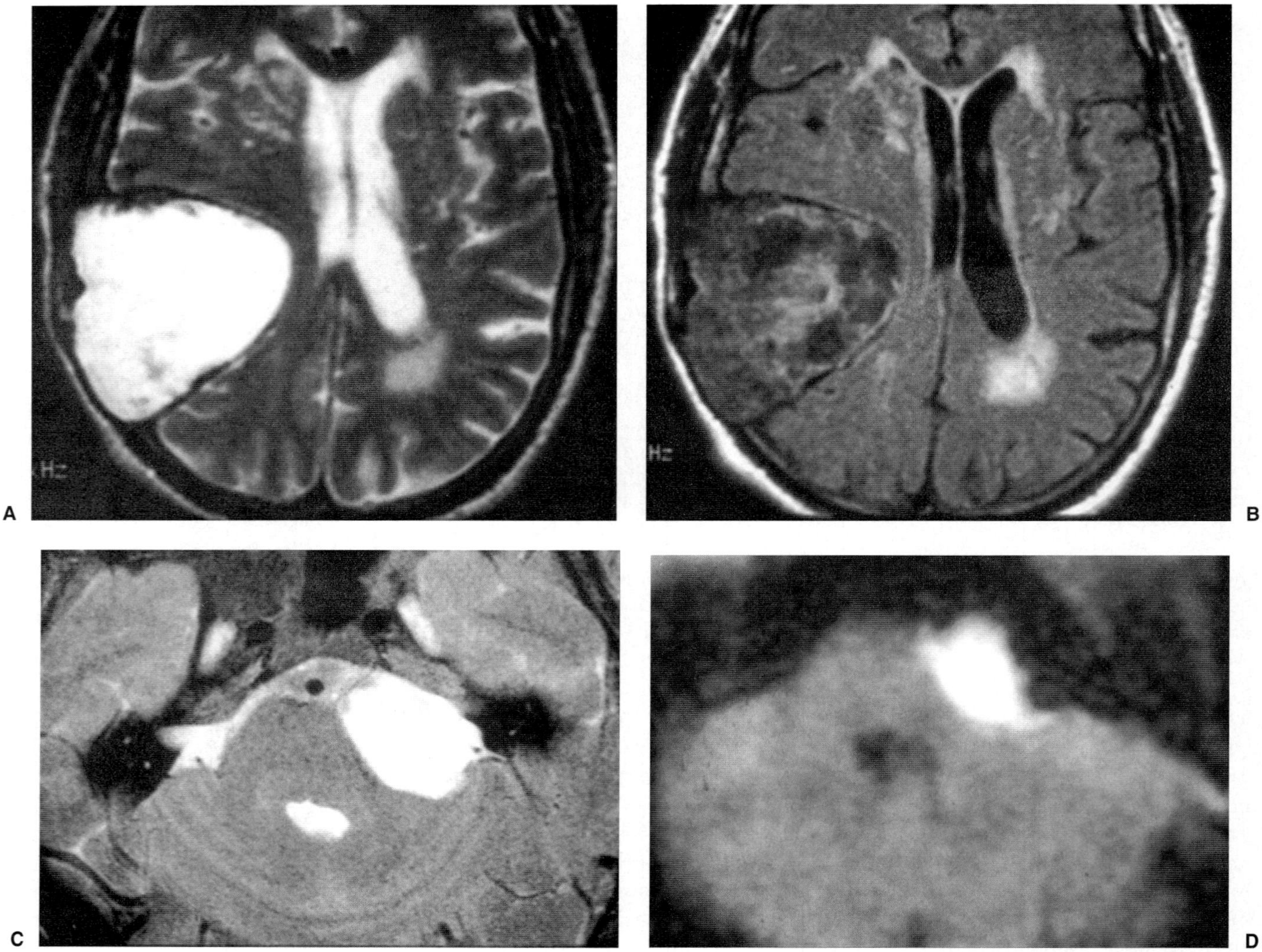

Figure 6.30 *Epidermoid. A.* Axial T2-weighted image shows bright epidermoid presumably arising from the diploë. Note that the tumor is mostly bright on this sequence. *B.* Corresponding fluid attenuation inversion recovery (FLAIR) image shows that the mass is not cystic but has a complex internal architecture. *C.* In a different patient, there is a "cystlike" bright mass in the left cerebellopontine angle cistern on this axial T2-weighted image. *D.* Corresponding diffusion-weighted image shows the mass to be bright, unlike an arachnoid cyst, which would have been darker on this sequence.

Usually, colloid cysts have such a typical appearance that there is no differential diagnosis for them.

Colloid Cyst. Colloid cysts account for less than 1% of all intracranial tumors (84). They usually arise in the anterosuperior portion of the third ventricle, possibly from choroid plexus elements, and obstruct the foramina of Monro, producing hydrocephalus (unilateral or bilateral). Patients present with headache (migraine-like), mental status changes, and nausea and vomiting (which may be particularly severe in the morning) (84). Treatment for colloid cysts includes resection, stereotactic aspiration, and ventricular shunting. By CT, they are hyperdense and usually measure 10 to 20 mm in diameter (Fig. 6.32A). Most colloid cysts are easily identified and are characteristically of high signal intensity on T1- and of very low signal intensity on T2-weighted images (85) (Fig. 6.32B and C). These features probably are due to increased protein content, and some neuroradiologists believe that paramagnetic effects from iron, copper, and magnesium may play a role in determining the imaging features of colloid cysts (84,85). In some cases, colloid cysts are easier to identify on CT than on MRI (86).

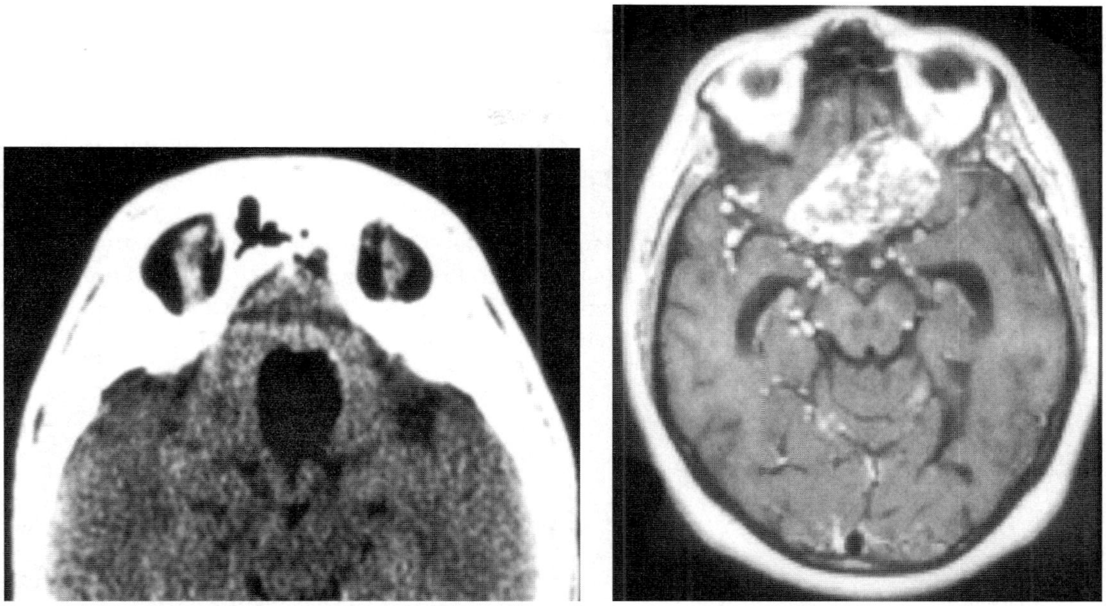

A B

Figure 6.31 *Dermoid. A.* Axial computed tomography shows midline frontobasal fatty-appearing dermoid. *B.* In a different patient, an axial T1-weighted image shows a large midline frontobasal dermoid that has spilled some of its contents into the subarachnoid space (note presence of fat "droplets" in the cisterns and sulci).

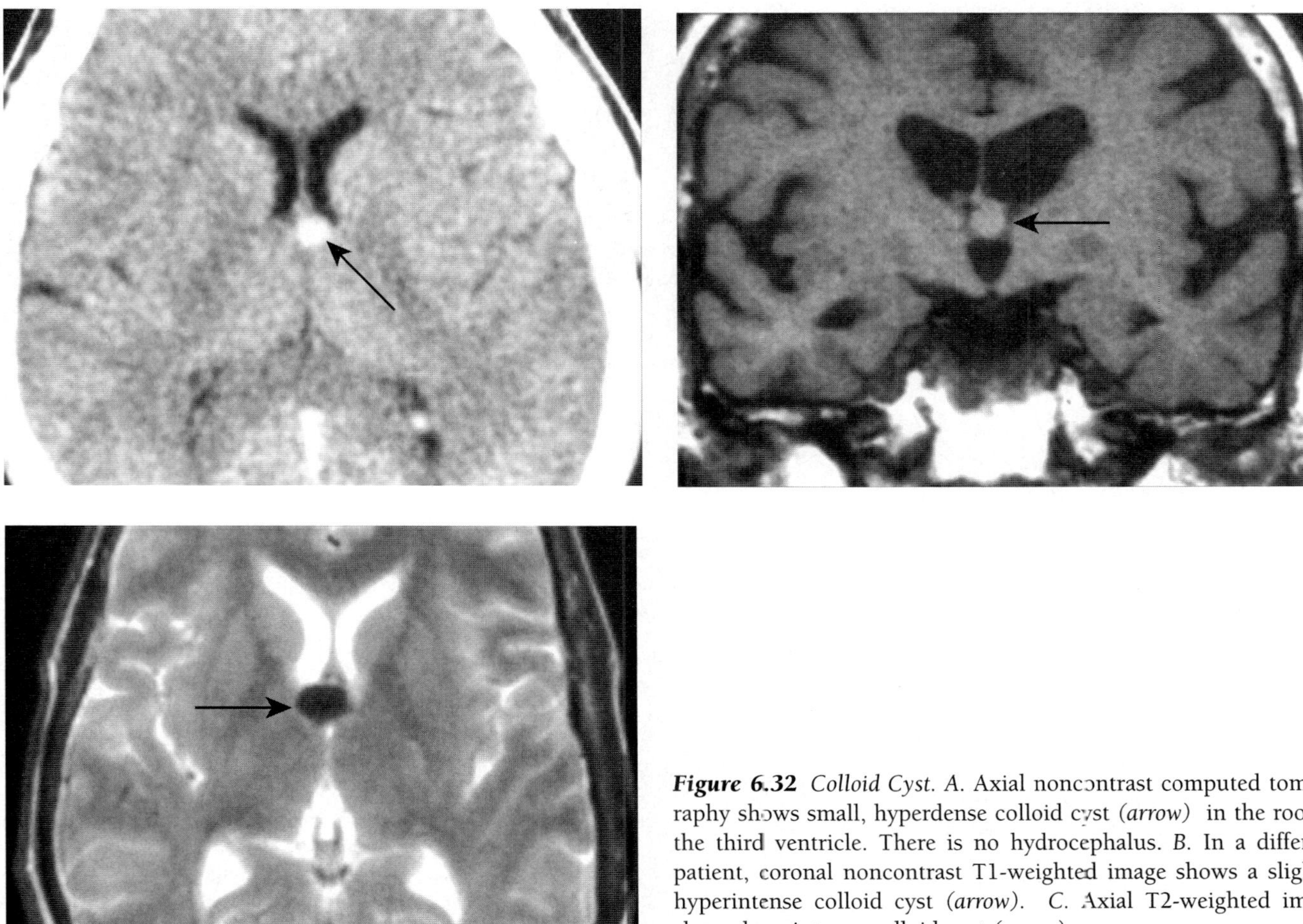

A B C

Figure 6.32 *Colloid Cyst. A.* Axial noncontrast computed tomography shows small, hyperdense colloid cyst *(arrow)* in the roof of the third ventricle. There is no hydrocephalus. *B.* In a different patient, coronal noncontrast T1-weighted image shows a slightly hyperintense colloid cyst *(arrow)*. *C.* Axial T2-weighted image shows hypointense colloid cyst *(arrow)*.

Pineal Cyst. Pineal cysts are found in over 10% of all MRI brain examinations (87). Most of them are small, incidental, asymptomatic, and inconsequential. If larger than 15 mm in diameter, they may result in mass effect and compression of the tectum and aqueduct that may lead to hydrocephalus. Their wall should be thin and smooth, with little enhancement (Fig. 6.33A and B). Occasionally, contrast diffuses into the cyst, making them indistinguishable from solid masses (Fig. 6.33C). This usually is a function of time and seen on delayed images. A pineal cyst may be considered atypical if it is large, enhances immediately, or shows an irregular rim. I like to follow these atypical pineal cysts 6 months after the initial study, and if no change has occurred, then on a yearly basis (87). Patients in whom symptoms develop (see earlier) need to be imaged immediately. Pineal cysts usually remain static in size, but occasionally they grow slightly or even become smaller.

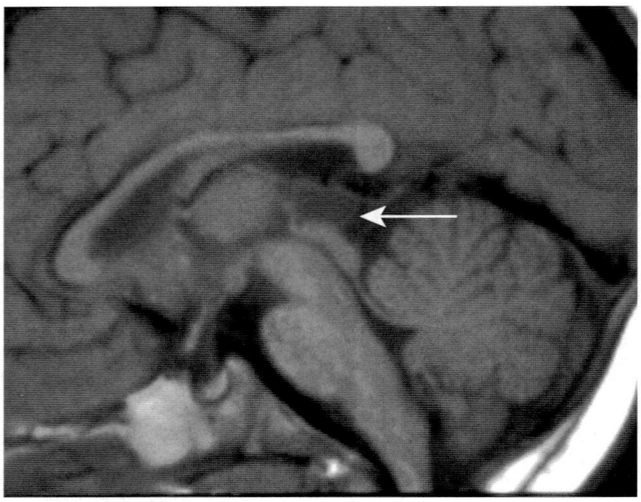

A

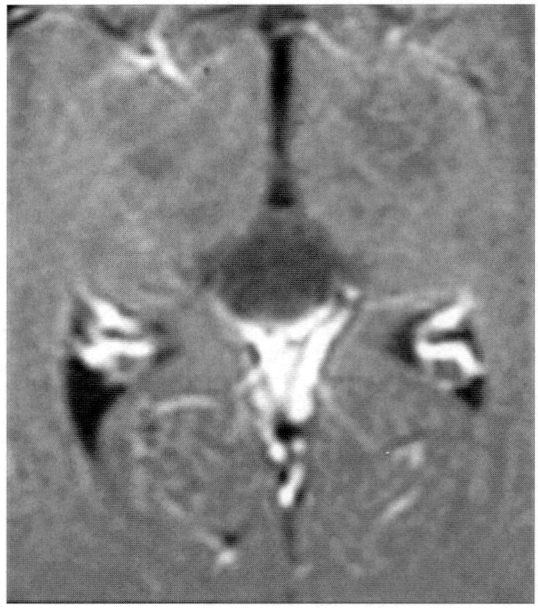

B

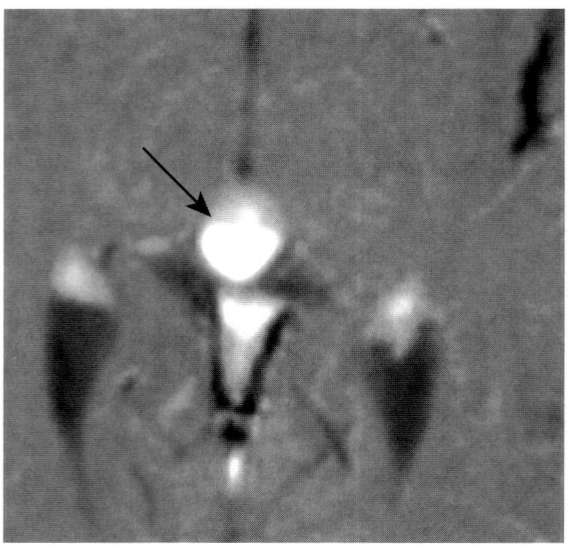

C

Figure 6.33 *Pineal Cyst.* A. Midsagittal noncontrast T1-weighted image shows a 9-mm incidental pineal cyst *(arrow)* in a child. There is no hydrocephalus. *B.* Axial T1-weighted image obtained immediately after contrast administration shows the nonenhancing cyst. *C.* In a different patient, axial T1-weighted image obtained 10 minutes after the administration of contrast shows a pineal cyst *(arrow)* that enhances and thus may be confused with tumor. The contrast probably seeps into the cyst because of the absence of the blood–brain barrier in this region.

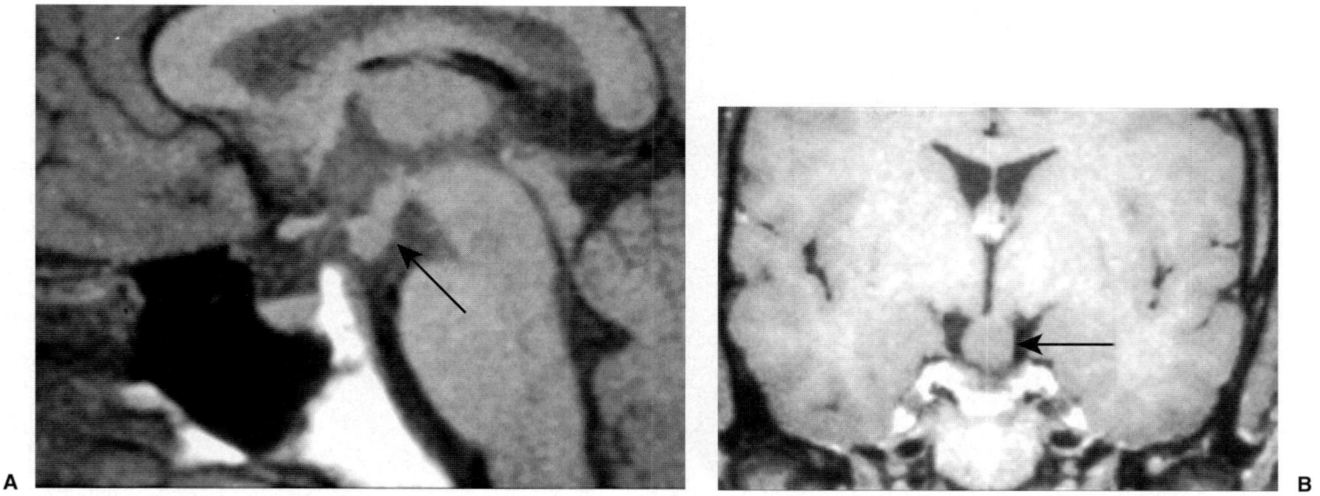

Figure 6.34 *Hamartoma of the Tuber Cinereum. A.* Noncontrast sagittal T1-weighted image shows typical "sessile" appearance of a small presumed hypothalamic hamartoma *(arrow). B.* In a different patient, a coronal noncontrast T1-weighted image shows a more "pedunculated" configuration of a larger hamartoma *(arrow).*

Hamartoma of the Tuber Cinereum. Hamartoma of the tuber cinereum (also called *hypothalamic hamartomas*) are encountered in nearly 20% of autopsies but are rare lesions on imaging studies (2). Most are microscopic, but occasionally they enlarge and become visible on MRI (2). These large hamartomas may result in symptoms. Symptoms from hamartomas of the tuber cinereum include:

- Visual deficits
- Headache
- Precocious puberty
- Gelastic seizures

Most hypothalamic hamartomas are composed of dysplastic neurons. The lesions are attached to the hypothalamus by a narrow or broad stalk (Fig. 6.34). The signal intensity is similar to gray matter on T1-weighted images, but they tend to be slightly brighter than gray matter on T2-weighted images (88,89). They do not enhance after contrast administration. Proton MR spectroscopy shows normal choline and creatine but mildly to moderately decreased NAA.

Lipoma. Lipomas arise from erroneous differentiation of the cells (meninx primitiva; Chapter 1) that eventually form the subarachnoid space (90). Approximately 85% of intracranial lipomas occur in the midline (50% are pericallosal). Other common locations include the quadrigeminal plate, cerebellopontine angle, and suprasellar cisterns. Lipomas usually are asymptomatic, but if midline in location, they may be associated with dysgenesis of the corpus callosum (Chapter 1). Calcification is common in lipomas associated with an anomalous corpus callosum. Lipomas are hypodense on CT and show no contrast enhancement. They are bright on T1-weighted images and fast spin-echo T2-weighted images (Fig. 6.35). Their signal diminishes with fat suppression techniques. Chemical shift artifact is seen on the frequency encoding direction. Lipomas tend to surround the normal structures (blood vessels, cranial nerves) coursing through the subarachnoid space. The diagnosis of lipoma is straightforward, and its differential diagnosis includes a dermoid, the rare "white" epidermoid, hemorrhagic arachnoid cyst, thrombosed aneurysm, neuroenteric cysts (they have a high protein content), and the very rare lipomatous meningioma.

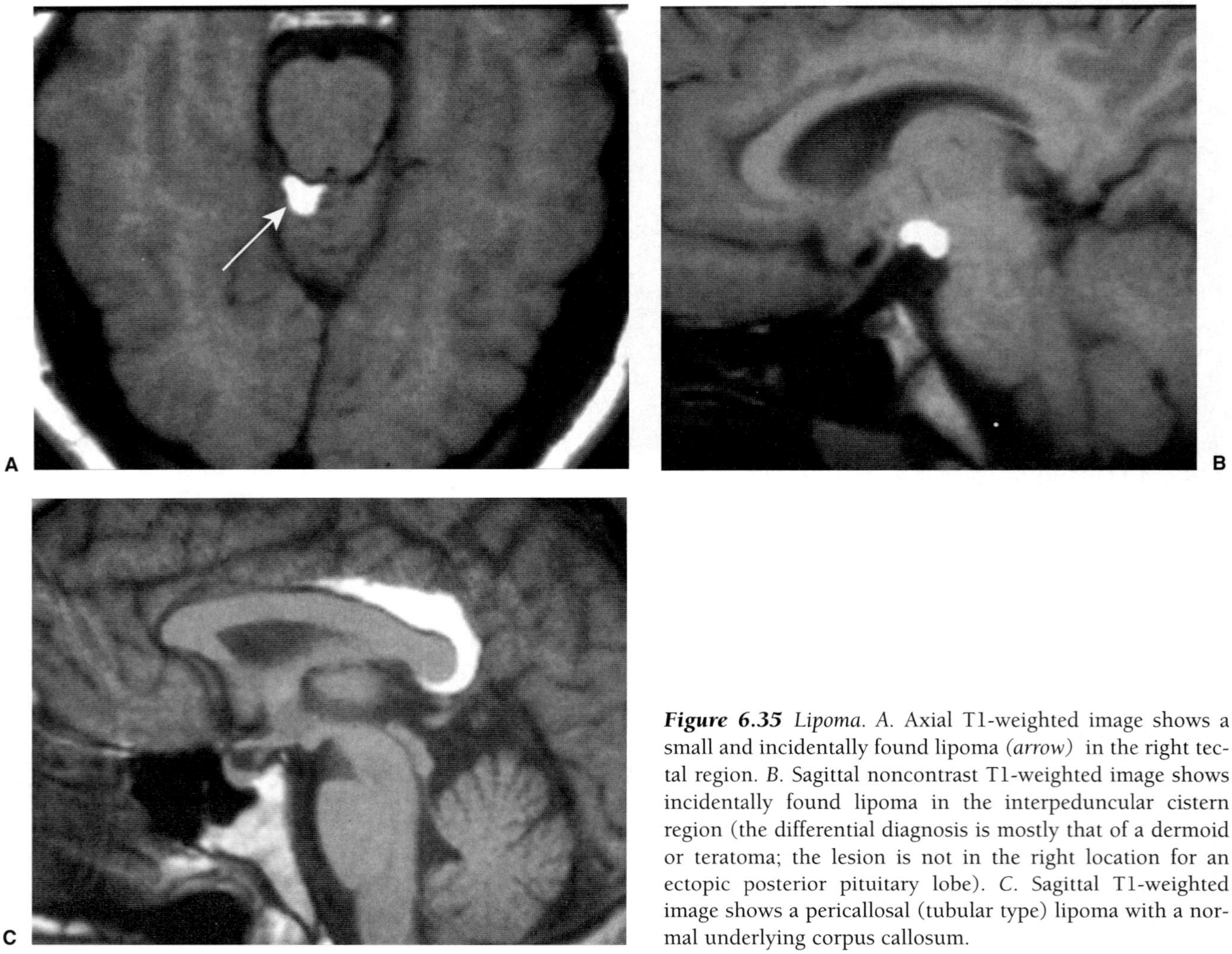

Figure 6.35 *Lipoma. A.* Axial T1-weighted image shows a small and incidentally found lipoma *(arrow)* in the right tectal region. *B.* Sagittal noncontrast T1-weighted image shows incidentally found lipoma in the interpeduncular cistern region (the differential diagnosis is mostly that of a dermoid or teratoma; the lesion is not in the right location for an ectopic posterior pituitary lobe). *C.* Sagittal T1-weighted image shows a pericallosal (tubular type) lipoma with a normal underlying corpus callosum.

References

1. Fulham MJ, Melisi JW, Nishimiya J, et al. Neuroimaging of juvenile pilocytic astrocytomas: an enigma. Radiology 1993;189:221–225.
2. Graham DI, Lantos PL. Greenfield's neuropathology, vol 2, 6th ed. London: Arnold, 1997: 583–795.
3. Strong JA, Hatten HP, Brown MT, et al. Pilocytic astrocytoma: correlation between the initial imaging features and clinical aggressiveness. AJR Am J Radiol 1993;161:369–372.
4. Lee BC, Kneeland JB, Walker RW, et al. MR imaging of brainstem tumors. AJNR Am J Neuroradiol 1985;6:159–163.
5. Bourgouin PM, Tampieri D, Grahovac SZ, et al. CT and MR imaging findings in adults with cerebellar medulloblastoma: comparison with findings in children. AJR Am J Radiol 1992;159: 609–612.
6. Koci TM, Chiang F, Mehringer CM, et al. Adult cerebellar medulloblastoma: imaging features with emphasis on MR findings. AJNR Am J Neuroradiol 1993;14:929–939.
7. Wang Z, Zimmerman RA, Sauter R. Proton MR spectroscopy of the brain: clinically useful information obtained in assessing CNS diseases in children. AJR Am J Radiol 1996;167:191–198.
8. Meyers SP, Wildenhain S, Chess MA, et al. Postoperative evaluation for intracranial recurrence of medulloblastoma: MR findings with gadopentetate dimeglumine. AJNR Am J Neuroradiol 1994;15:1425–1434.
9. Meyers SP, Wildenhain SL, Chang JK, et al. Postoperative evaluation for disseminated medulloblastoma involving the spine: contrast-enhanced MR findings, CSF cytologic analysis, timing of disease occurrence, and patient outcomes. AJNR Am J Neuroradiol 2000;21:1757–1765.

10. Rollins N, Mendelsohn D, Mulne A, et al. Recurrent medulloblastoma: frequency of tumor enhancement on Gd-DTPA MR imaging. AJNR Am J Neuroradiol 1990;11:583–587.
11. Castillo M, Chung C, Mukherji S. Imaging features of atypical teratoid rhabdoid tumors of the central nervous system. Int J Neuroradiol 1997;3:185–191.
12. Spoto GP, Press GA, Hesselink JR, et al. Intracranial ependymoma and subependymoma: MR manifestations. AJNR Am J Neuroradiol 1990;11:89–91.
13. Chiechi MV, Smirniotopoulos JG, Jones RV. Intracranial subependymomas: CT and MR imaging features in 24 cases. AJR Am J Radiol 1995;165:1245–1250.
14. Hoeffel C, Boukobza M, Polivka M, et al. MR manifestations of subependymomas. AJNR Am J Neuroradiol 1995;16:2121–2129.
15. Castillo M, Davis PC, Takei Y, et al. Intracranial ganglioglioma: MR, CT, and clinical findings in 18 patients. AJNR Am J Neuroradiol 1990;11:109–114.
16. Tampieri D, Moumdjian R, Melanson D, et al. Intracerebral gangliogliomas in patients with partial complex seizures: CT and MR imaging findings. AJNR Am J Neuroradiol 1991;12:749–755.
17. Patel U, Pinto RS, Miller DC, et al. MR of spinal cord ganglioglioma. AJNR Am J Neuroradiol 1998;19:879–887.
18. Altman NR. MR and CT characteristics of gangliocytoma: a rare cause of epilepsy in children. AJNR Am J Neuroradiol 1988;9:917–921.
19. Martin DS, Levy B, Awwad EE, et al. Desmoplastic infantile ganglioglioma: CT and MR features. AJNR Am J Neuroradiol 1991;12:1195–1197.
20. Serra A, Strain J, Ruyle S. Desmoplastic cerebral astrocytoma of infancy: report and review of the imaging characteristics. AJR Am J Radiol 1996;166:1459–1461.
21. Meltzer CC, Smirniotopoulos JG, Jones RV. The striated cerebellum: an MR imaging sign in Lhermitte-Duclos disease (dysplastic gangliocytoma). Radiology 1995;194:699–703.
22. Williams DW III, Elster AD, Ginsberg LE, et al. Recurrent Lhermitte-Duclos disease: report of two cases and association with Cowden's disease. AJNR Am J Neuroradiol 1992;13:287–290.
23. Awwad EE, Levy E, Martin DS, et al. Atypical MR appearance of Lhermitte-Duclos disease with contrast enhancement. AJNR Am J Neuroradiol 1995;16:1719–1720.
24. Ahmadi J, Destian S, Apuzzo MLJ, et al. Cystic fluid in craniopharyngiomas: MR imaging and quantitative analysis. Radiology 1992;182:783–785.
25. Davis PC, Hoffman JC Jr, Weidenheim KM. Large hypothalamic and optic chiasm gliomas in infants: difficulties in distinction. AJR Am J Radiol 1984;5:579–585.
26. Castillo M, Scatliff JH, Bouldin TW, et al. Radiologic-pathologic correlation: intracranial astrocytoma. AJNR Am J Neuroradiol 1992;13:1609–1616.
27. Tien RD, Hesselink JR, Duberg A. Rare subependymal giant-cell astrocytoma in a neonate with tuberous sclerosis. AJNR Am J Neuroradiol 1990;11:1251–1252.
28. Buetow PC, Smirniotopoulos JG, Done S. Congenital brain tumors: a review of 45 cases. AJNR Am J Neuroradiol 1990;11:793–799.
29. Anderson DR, Falcone S, Bruce JH, et al. Radiologic-pathologic correlation: congenital choroid plexus papillomas. AJNR Am J Neuroradiol 1995;16:2072–2076.
30. Hopper KD, Foley LC, Nieves NL, et al. The interventricular extension of choroid plexus papillomas [published erratum appears in AJNR 1988;9:556]. AJNR Am J Neuroradiol 1987;8:462–472.
31. Kuroiwa T, Bergey GK, Rothman MI, et al. Radiologic appearance of the dysembryoplastic neuroepithelial tumor. Radiology 1995;197:233–238.
32. Graif M, Pennock JM. MR imaging of histiocytosis X in the central nervous system. AJNR Am J Neuroradiol 1986;7:21–23.
33. Erly W, Carmody RF, Dryden RM. Orbital histiocytosis X. AJNR Am J Neuroradiol 1995;16:1258–1261.
34. Maghnie M, Arico M, Villa A, et al. MR of the hypothalamic-pituitary axis in Langerhans cell histiocytosis. AJNR Am J Neuroradiol 1992;13:1365–1371.
35. Tien RD, Newton TH, McDermott MW, et al. Thickened pituitary stalk on MR images in patients with diabetes insipidus and Langerhans cell histiocytosis. AJNR Am J Neuroradiol 1990;11:703–708.
36. Ho VB, Smirniotopoulos JG, Murphy FM, et al. Radiologic-pathologic correlation: hemangioblastoma. AJNR Am J Neuroradiol 1992;13:986–988.
37. Lee SR, Sanches J, Mark AS, et al. Posterior fossa hemangioblastomas: MR Imaging. Radiology 1989;171:463–468.
38. Eskridge JM, McAuliffe W, Harris B, et al. Preoperative endovascular embolization of craniospinal hemangioblastomas. AJNR Am J Neuroradiol 1996;17:525–531.

39. Swartz, JD. Sensorineural hearing deficit: a systematic approach based on imaging findings. Radiographics 1996;16:561–574.
40. Smirniotopoulos JG, Chang Yue N, et al. Cerebellopontine angle masses: radiologic-pathologic correlation. Radiographics 1993;13:1131–1147.
41. Bonneville F, Sarrazin J, Marsot-Dupuch K, et al. Unusual lesions of the cerebellopontine angle: a segmental approach. Radiographics 2001;21:419–438.
42. Mulkens TH, Parizel PM, Martin J-J, et al. Acoustic schwannoma: MR findings in 84 tumors. AJR Am J Radiol 1993;160:395–398.
43. Meyers SP, Hirsch WL Jr, Curtin HD, et al. Chordomas of the skull base: MR features. AJNR Am J Neuroradiol 1992;13:1627–1636.
44. Earnest F IV, Kelly PJ, Scheithauer BW, et al. Cerebral astrocytomas: histopathologic correlation of MR and CT contrast enhancement with stereotactic biopsy. Radiology 1998;166:823–827.
45. Castillo M, Kwock L. Proton MR spectroscopy of common brain tumors. Neuroimaging Clin North Am 1998;8:733–751.
46. Castillo M, Smith JK, Kwock L. Correlation of myo-inositol levels and grading of cerebral astrocytomas. AJNR Am J Neuroradiol 2000;21:1645–1649.
47. Knopp E, Cha S, Johnson G, et al. Glial neoplasms: dynamic contrast-enhanced T2*-weighted MR imaging. Radiology 1999;211:791–798.
48. Sugahara T, Korogi Y, Kochi M, et al. Correlation of MR imaging–determined cerebral blood volume maps with histologic and angiographic determination of vascularity of gliomas. AJR Am J Radiol 1998;171:1479–1486.
49. Aronen HJ, Gazit IE, Louis DN, et al. Cerebral blood volume maps of gliomas: comparison with tumor grade and histologic findings. Radiology 1994;191:41–51.
50. Yanaka K, Kamezaki T, Kobayashi E, et al. MR imaging of diffuse glioma. AJNR Am J Neuroradiol 1992;13:349–351.
51. Felsberg GJ, Silver SA, Brown MT, et al. Radiologic-pathologic correlation: gliomatosis cerebri. AJNR Am J Neuroradiol 1994;15:1745–1753.
52. Shin YM, Chang KH, Han MH, et al. Gliomatosis cerebri: comparison of MR and CT features. AJR Am J Radiol 1993;161:859–862.
53. del Carpio-O'Donovan R, Korah I, Salazaar A, et al. Gliomatosis cerebri. Radiology 1996;198: 831–835.
54. Bendszus M, Warmuth-Metz M, Klein R. MR spectroscopy in gliomatosis cerebri. AJNR Am J Neuroradiol 2000;21:375–380.
55. Tice H, Barnes PD, Goumnerova L, et al. Pediatric and adolescent oligodendrogliomas. AJNR Am J Neuroradiol 1993;14:1293–1300.
56. Koeller KK, Smirniotopoulos JG, Jones RV. Primary central nervous system lymphoma: radiologic-pathologic correlation. Radiographics 1997;17:1497–1526.
57. Dina TS. Primary central nervous system lymphoma versus toxoplasmosis in AIDS. Radiology 1991;179:823–828.
58. Lee VW, Antonacci V, Tilak S, et al. Intracranial mass lesions: sequential thallium and gallium scintigraphy in patients with AIDS. Radiology 1999;211:507–512.
59. Ernst TM, Chang L, Witt MD, et al. Cerebral toxoplasmosis and lymphoma in AIDS: perfusion MR imaging experience in 13 patients. Radiology 1998;208:663–669.
60. Kim YJ, Chang K, Song IC, et al. Brain abscess and necrotic or cystic brain tumor: discrimination with signal intensity on diffusion-weighted MR imaging. AJR Am J Radiol 1998;171: 1487–1490.
61. Zimmerman RD, Fleming CA, Saint-Louis LA, et al. Magnetic resonance imaging of meningiomas. AJNR Am J Neuroradiol 1985;6:149–157.
62. Tokumaru A, O'uchi T, Eguchi T, et al. Prominent meningeal enhancement adjacent to meningioma on Gd-DTPA-enhanced MR images: histopathologic correlation. Radiology 1990;175: 431–433.
63. Demaerel P, Johannik K, Van Hecke P, et al. Localized H NMR spectroscopy in fifty cases of newly diagnosed intracranial tumors. J Comput Assist Tomogr 1991;15:67–76.
64. Gill SS, Thomas DGT, Van Bruggen N, et al. Proton MR spectroscopy of intracranial tumours: in vivo and in vitro studies. J Comput Assist Tomogr 1990;14:497–504.
65. Sze G, Shin J, Krol G, et al. Intraparenchymal brain metastases: MR imaging versus contrast-enhanced CT. Radiology 1998;168:187–194.
66. Russell EJ, Geremia GK, Johnson CE, et al. Multiple cerebral metastases: detectability with Gd-DTPA-enhanced MR imaging. Radiology 1987;165:609–617.

67. Isiklar I, Leeds NE, Fuller GN, et al. Intracranial metastatic melanoma: correlation between MR imaging characteristics and melanin content. AJR Am J Radiol 1995;165:1503–1512.
68. Boorstein JM, Wong KT, Grossman RI, et al. Metastatic lesions of the brain: imaging with magnetization transfer. Radiology 1994;191:799–803.
69. Ginsberg LE, Leeds NE. Neuroradiology of leukemia. AJR Am J Radiol 1995;165:525–534.
70. Gentry LR, Menezes AH, Turski PA, et al. Suprasellar arachnoid cysts: 2. evaluation of CSF dynamics. AJNR Am J Neuroradiol 1986;7:87–96.
71. Gentry LR, Smoker WR, Turski PA, et al. Suprasellar arachnoid cysts: 1. CT recognition. AJNR Am J Neuroradiol 1986;7:79–86.
72. Bourekas EC, Raji MR, Dastur KJ, et al. Retroclival arachnoid cyst. AJNR Am J Neuroradiol 1992;13:353–354.
73. Robertson SJ, Wolpert SM, Runge VM. MR imaging of middle cranial fossa arachnoid cysts: temporal lobe agenesis syndrome revisited. AJNR Am J Neuroradiol 1989;10:1007–1010.
74. Wolpert SM, Scott RM. The value of metrizamide CT cisternography in the management of cerebral arachnoid cysts. AJNR Am J Neuroradiol 1981;2:29–35.
75. Hald JK, Nakstad PH, Skjeldal OH, et al. Bilateral arachnoid cysts of the temporal fossa in four children with glutaric aciduria type I. AJNR Am J Neuroradiol 1991;12:407–409.
76. Sherman JL, Camponovo E, Citrin CM. MR imaging of CSF-like choroidal fissure and parenchymal cysts of the brain. AJNR Am J Neuroradiol 1990;11:939–945.
77. Tampieri D, Melanson D, Ethier R. MR Imaging of epidermoid cysts. AJNR Am J Neuroradiol 1989;10:351–356.
78. Sakamoto Y, Takahashi M, Ushio Y, et al. Visibility of epidermoid tumors on steady-state free precession images. AJNR Am J Neuroradiol 1994;15:1737–1744.
79. Tsuruda JS, Chew WM, Moseley ME, et al. Diffusion-weighted MR imaging of the brain: value of differentiating between extraaxial cysts and epidermoid tumors. AJR Am J Radiol 1990;155: 1059–1068.
80. Kallmes DF, Provenzale JM, Cloft HJ, et al. Typical and atypical MR imaging features of intracranial epidermoid tumors. AJR Am J Radiol 1997;169:883–887.
81. Roeder MB, Bazan C, Jinkins JR. Ruptured spinal dermoid cyst with chemical arachnoiditis and disseminated intracranial lipid droplets. Neuroradiology 1995;37:146–147.
82. Barsi P, Kenez J, Varallyay G, et al. Unusual origin of free subarachnoid fat drops: a ruptured spinal dermoid tumour. Neuroradiology 1992;34:343–344.
83. Gupta S, Gupta RK, Gujral RD, et al. Signal intensity patterns in intraspinal dermoids and epidermoids on MR imaging. Clin Radiol 1993;48:405–413.
84. Armao D, Castillo M, Chen H, et al. Colloid cyst of the third ventricle: imaging-pathologic correlation. AJNR Am J Neuroradiol 2000;21:1470–1477.
85. Maeder PP, Holtas SL, Basibuyuk LN, et al. Colloid cysts of the third ventricle: correlation of MR and CT findings with histology and chemical analysis. AJNR Am J Neuroradiol 1990;11: 575–581.
86. Mamourian AC, Cromwell LD, Harbaugh RE. Colloid cyst of the third ventricle: sometimes more conspicuous on CT than MR. AJNR Am J Neuroradiol 1998;19:875–878.
87. Barboriak DP, Lee L, Provenzale JM. Serial MR imaging of pineal cysts: implications for natural history and follow-up. AJR Am J Radiol 2001;176:767–743.
88. Burton EM, Ball WS Jr, Crone K, et al. Hamartoma of the tuber cinereum: a comparison of MR and CT findings in four cases. AJNR Am J Neuroradiol 1989;10:497–501.
89. Boyko OB, Curnes JT, Oakes WJ, et al. Hamartomas of the tuber cinereum: CT, MR and pathologic findings. AJNR Am J Neuroradiol 1991;12:309–314.
90. Truwit CL, Barkovich AJ. Pathogenesis of intracranial lipoma: an MR study in 42 patients. AJNR Am J Neuroradiol 1990;11:665–674.

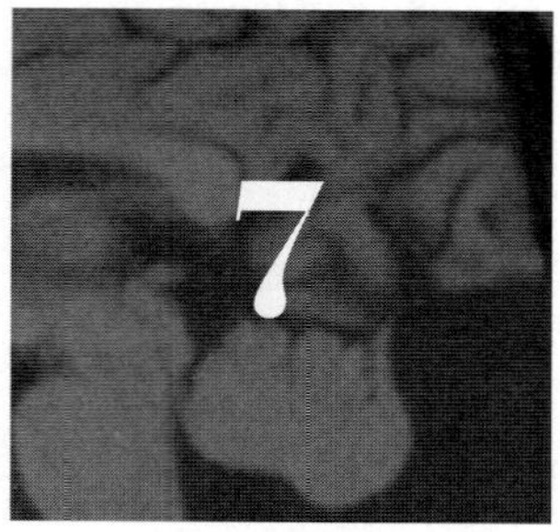

PITUITARY GLAND

- Anatomy and Physiology
- Childhood Lesions
- Adult Lesions

ANATOMY AND PHYSIOLOGY

The pituitary gland is formed by the anterior, intermediate, and posterior lobes (1) (Table 7.1). The anterior lobe (adenohypophysis) constitutes approximately two-thirds of the volume of the gland, the pars intermedia is a sliver of tissue, and the posterior lobe (neurohypophysis) constitutes the posterior one-third of the gland. The gland is encased by the sella, the medial dural walls of the cavernous sinuses, and superiorly by the diaphragma sella. The diaphragma sella contains an opening through which the stalk (infundibulum) of the gland courses. The infundibulum is composed centrally of the stalk proper (which is a part of the neurohypophysis) and an outer core (the pars tuberalis, which is part of the adenohypophysis). The stalk may contain a cerebrospinal fluid (CSF)–filled space centrally (stalk recess) that usually communicates superiorly with the infundibular recess of the third ventricle or may become isolated in cystlike configuration expanding the stalk. The median eminence of the hypothalamus surrounds the stalk at its superior insertion. The hormones produced by the anterior lobe are shown in Table 7.2 (2).

The pars intermedia plays no important role except in pregnancy, where it may be involved in the production of corticotropin, melanocyte-stimulating hormone, and some endorphins. This occurs because pregnancy induces a relative increase in metabolism and the pars intermedia is recruited to "help out" the adenohypophysis. The neurohypophysis contains antidiuretic hormone (vasopressin) and oxytocin. These hormones actually are produced in the hypothalamus and are carried by the stalk into the posterior lobe by a mechanism called *axonal transport*. Vasopressin is carried by neurosecretory granules and is bound to several proteins. The normal high T1 signal commonly seen in the posterior lobe is thought to be due to the presence of these proteins or to lipids contained in the membranes of the neurosecretory granules (2,3). It also is possible that vasopressin itself is responsible for the brightness. Regardless of its etiology, most normal individuals show an intrasellar posterior lobe that is bright on T1-weighted imaging. The size of the posterior lobe correlates with the concentration of vasopressin. During water deprivation, the

The pars intermedia plays an important endocrine role only during pregnancy.

The bright T1 spot of the posterior pituitary lobe diminishes in size with water deprivation and increases in size during overhydration.

Table 7.1: Origin of the Pituitary Gland

Anterior Lobe	*Intermediate Lobe*	*Posterior Lobe*
Rathke's pouch or neuroectoderm	Rathke's pouch (posterior wall) or neuroectoderm	Hypothalamus

Table 7.2: Hormones produced by the Adenohypophysis

Hormone	*Location of Cells Producing the Hormone*
Prolactin	Lactotrophs, lateral wings
Growth hormone	Somatotrophs, lateral wings
Thyroid-stimulating hormone	Thyrotrophs, anterior and central regions
Follicle-stimulating and luteinizing hormones	Gonadotrophs, central region
Corticotropin and melanocyte-stimulating hormones	Corticotrophs, central region

signal intensity and size of the posterior lobe diminish, and during states of adequate hydration or overhydration, the opposite occurs.

The pituitary gland may be slightly and normally enlarged during pregnancy, the postpartum period, neonatal life, adolescence, and the menstrual period.

During the first 2 months of life, the anterior lobe also is bright and the upper border of the gland may bulge slightly superiorly (4). This presumably is due to intense endocrine activity of the gland during the neonatal period (5). At puberty, the gland enlarges again, particularly in girls, but remains of normal signal intensity (6). The gland may show a marked convexity of its superior border during puberty. The gland also increases in height during pregnancy, especially during the third trimester and the immediate postpartum period. After 50 to 60 years of age, the pituitary gland undergoes a progressive loss of volume (7). I use 10 mm as the normal height of the pituitary gland, and allow up to 12 to 13 mm during late pregnancy and the early postpartum period. Just before menses, the gland may bulge superiorly but increases in height very little. The gland may contain the following incidental abnormalities (8):

- Cysts
- Nonfunctioning macroadenomas
- Persistent trigeminal artery
- "Stone"

The gland is surrounded by a vascular plexus called the *pituitary portal system*. This system is very important in collecting the hormones secreted by the gland and carrying them into the systemic circulation. The posterior lobe has a direct blood supply from the internal carotid arteries, and the anterior lobe receives most of its blood supply through the portal system. This arrangement explains the pattern of enhancement seen during dynamic contrast magnetic resonance imaging (MRI). In these studies, the stalk enhances first, followed by the posterior lobe, with the adenohypophysis enhancing last. I use dynamic studies in a coronal projection for microadenoma detection and sagittal dynamic studies when the function of the gland is in question (e.g., hypopituitarism).

Deviation of the pituitary stalk may be normal and physiologic.

Last, a note regarding the appearance of the stalk. Deviation of the stalk often is caused by an underlying tumor displacing it to the opposite side. However, in a large number of patients, infundibular tilt is normal and is related to the development of the gland or sloping of the floor of the sella (9). Infundibular tilting by itself should not be misinterpreted as pathologic.

Childhood Lesions

Absent Pituitary Gland and Hypoplasia

The pituitary gland seldom is truly absent, but may be extremely small. I usually consider the gland small if it measures less than 2 to 3 mm (Fig. 7.1). In these cases, it is important to correlate the imaging findings with the patient's endocrine profile; a small gland in the

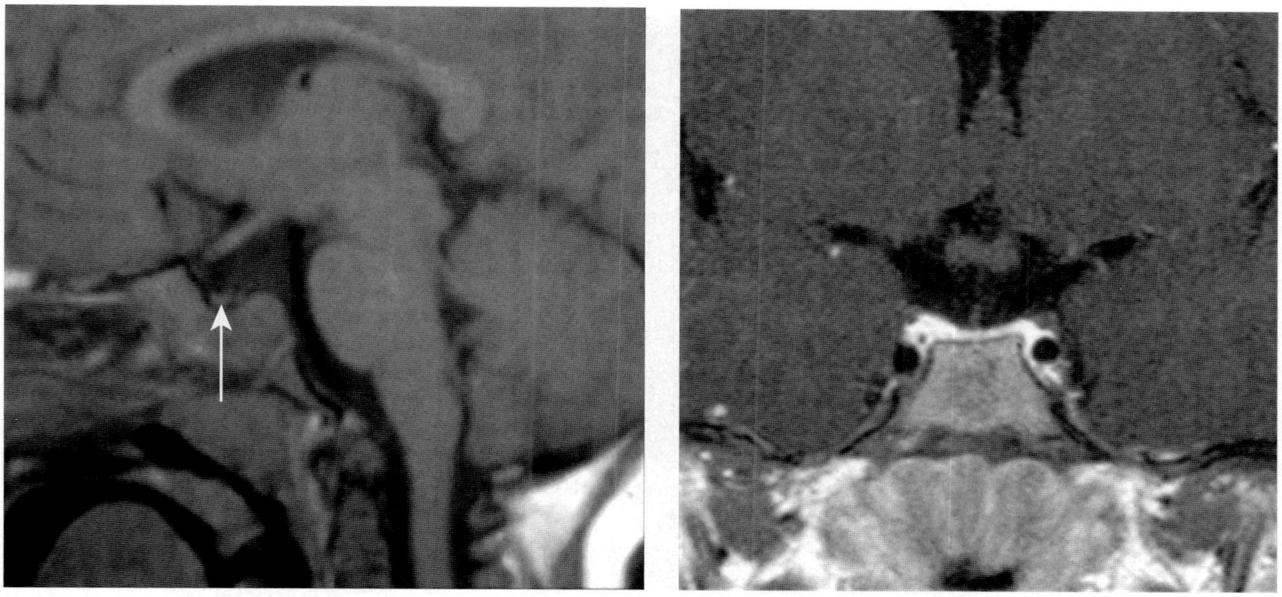

Figure 7.1 *Pituitary Hypoplasia. A.* Sagittal T1-weighted image shows a very small pituitary gland *(arrow)*, sella turcica, and stalk with a normal-appearing optic chiasm. *B.* Coronal postcontrast T1-weighted image shows flat and small but enhancing gland and a thin stalk.

presence of normal hormone levels has little practical significance. During life, the pituitary gland may shrink for the following reasons:

- Pituitary dwarfism
- Postresection
- Postirradiation
- Posttrauma
- Postinfarction or posthemorrhage
- Postinfection
- Midline face and brain anomalies

In most of the aforementioned instances, the gland is hypoactive. However, the gland may not function normally even when its appearance is normal. Primary and secondary hemochromatosis result in a very dark gland on both T1- and T2-weighted images. In hemochromatosis, the gland is only slightly atrophic, but the patients show panhypopituitarism (10). In addition, complete lack of enhancement of the gland has been reported in patients with combined hormone deficiency (11). A small pituitary gland (with ectopic posterior lobe) accompanied by a hypoplastic or absent stalk, hypoplastic optic chiasm, and a normal septum pellucidum probably belongs in the category of the optoinfundibular dysplasia and not septooptic dysplasia (Fig. 7.2).

The differential diagnosis of a dark pituitary gland on T1 and T2 images includes intrasellar aneurysm, intrasellar calcified meningioma, pituitary "stone," and hemochromatosis.

Posterior Ectopic Lobe

In this very interesting entity, the neurohypophysis is "translocated" outside of the sella into the stalk or the median eminence posterior to the insertion of the stalk (12). Ectopia of the posterior lobe may be seen in absence of the gland, with adenomas destroying the gland, and with prior transection of the stalk (usually due to trauma or birth-related injuries). Many patients with an ectopic posterior lobe are asymptomatic or only minimally affected. Absence of the posterior lobe does, however, correlate with diabetes insipidus (13). In the central type of diabetes insipidus, the posterior lobe is absent,

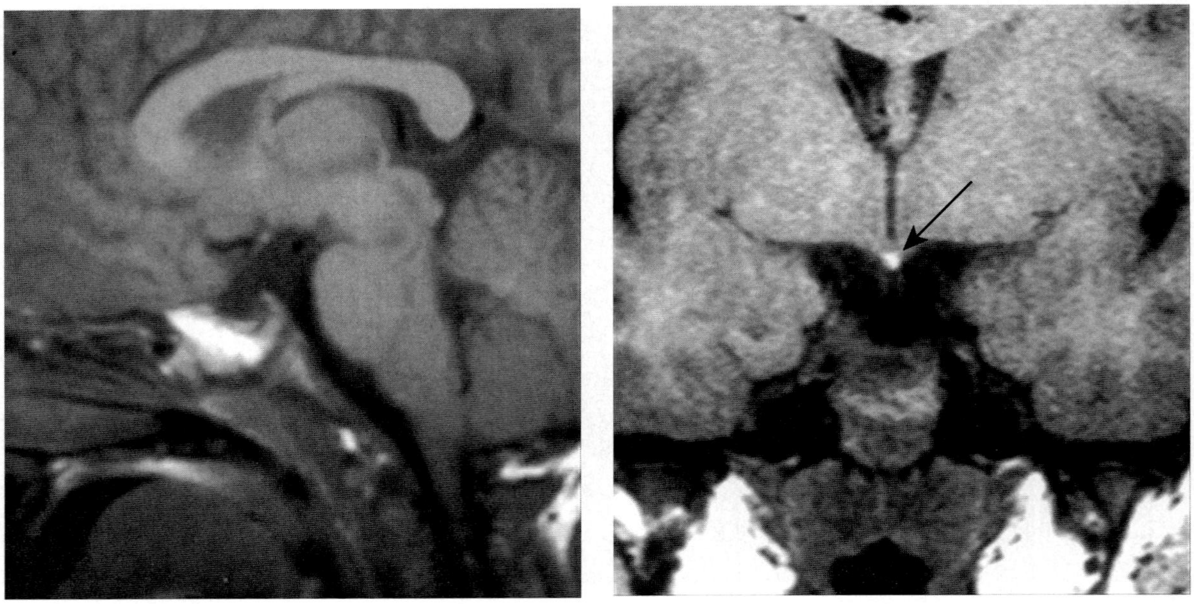

Figure 7.2 *Optoinfundibular Hypoplasia. A.* Sagittal T1-weighted image shows a tiny pituitary gland, absent stalk, and hypoplastic optic chiasm. *B.* Coronal T1-weighted image confirms absent stalk and an ectopic posterior pituitary lobe *(arrow)*. Note that the septum pellucidum is present and hence this is not a case of septooptic dysplasia.

whereas it is present in the nephrogenic type of the disease. In the presence of a normal-appearing stalk/gland, an ectopic posterior lobe is very rare. An ectopic posterior lobe appears as a focal, rounded area of increased signal intensity on precontrast T1 images, usually in the region of the hypothalamus or along the course of the superior aspect of the stalk (Fig. 7.3A and B). If one sees a suprasellar region of increased T1 signal in the presence of a normal-appearing gland and stalk, other entities (e.g., lipoma and dermoid among others) need to be considered (see section on lipomas in Chapter 1). In adults, a tumor may invade the gland and result in translocation of the posterior pituitary lobe because the hormone cannot descend to its normal location (Fig. 7.3C).

Duplication of the Pituitary Gland

Duplication of the pituitary gland is very rare and usually found in children with midline facial clefting syndromes or anomalies such as midline encephaloceles, teratomas, and dermoids (13). Most patients with a duplicated gland have hypertelorism. MRI studies show two enhancing stalks coursing into two discreet glands, or a larger gland that may be only partially separated in the midline (Fig. 7.4). The glands enhance normally. Most of these patients have normal endocrine profiles or profiles that are only minimally abnormal. Thus, the isolated finding of a duplicated pituitary gland has limited clinical importance in most patients. Most patients with a duplicated gland show thickening of the hypothalamus. This thick region is isointense to gray matter on T1- and T2-weighted images and does not enhance. It is presumed to represent a hamartoma of the hypothalamus.

Pituitary Adenomas in Children

Relative to adults, children have an increased incidence of Cushing's syndrome–producing microadenomas and hemorrhagic adenomas.

Pituitary adenomas are very rare in children, and most are found during adolescence. In children there is an increased percentage of Cushing's syndrome–producing adenomas compared with prolactinomas. In addition, there is an increased incidence of hemorrhagic adenomas in children compared with adults (14). The mean age of presentation for pedi-

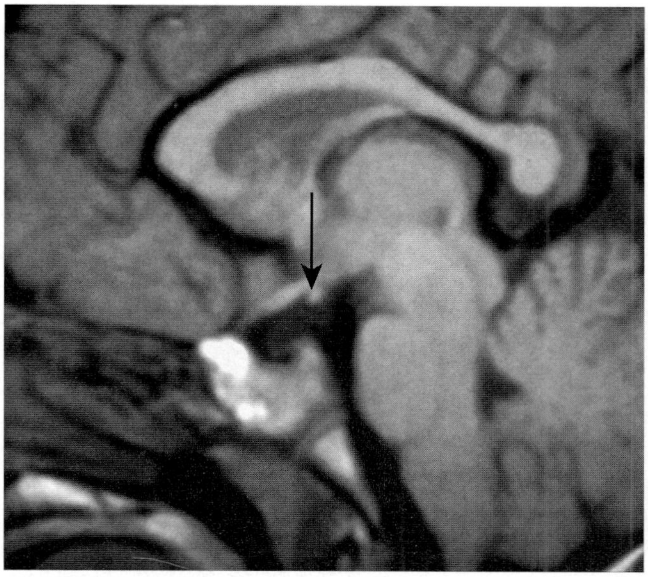

A

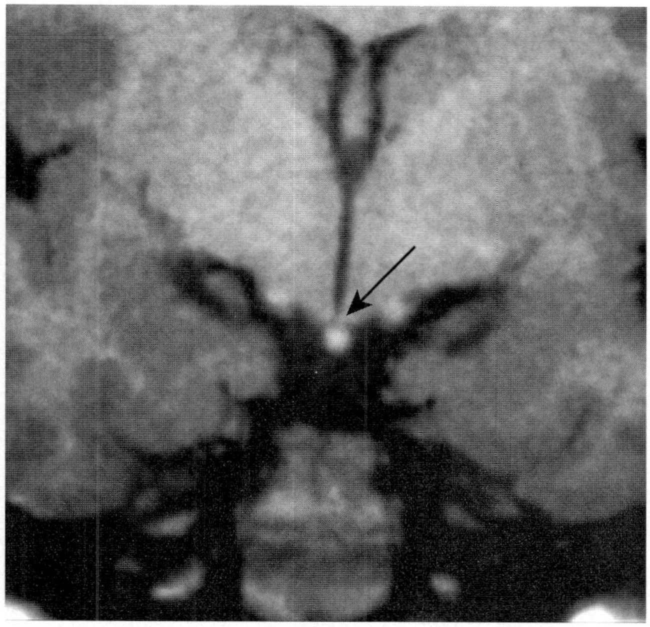

B

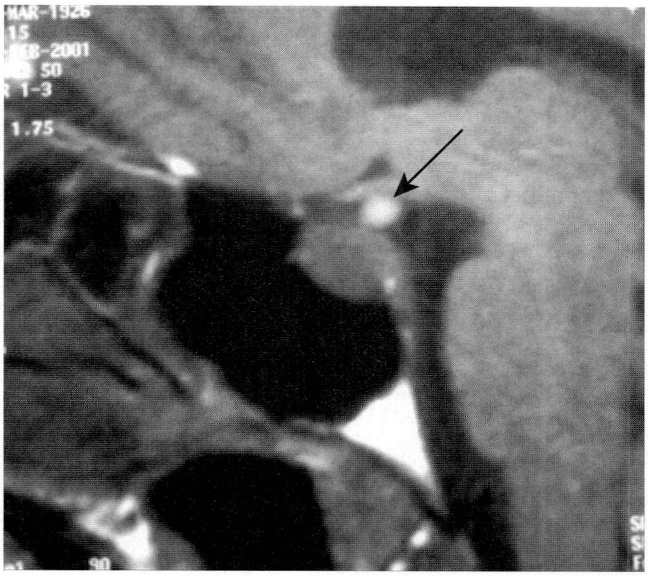

C

Figure 7.3 *Ectopic (Translocated) Posterior Pituitary Lobe. A.* In addition to the hypoplastic pituitary gland and absent stalk, this sagittal T1-weighted image shows a rounded hyperintensity *(arrow)* in the hypothalamus compatible with a neurohypophysis. *B.* The ectopic neurohypophysis *(arrow)* is confirmed on this noncontrast coronal T1-weighted image. *C.* Sagittal noncontrast T1-weighted image in a patient with a pituitary macroadenoma that has replaced the gland shows an ectopic posterior lobe *(arrow)*.

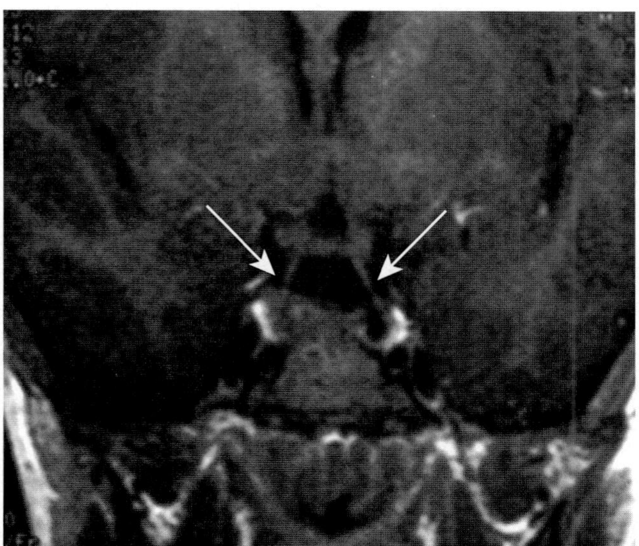

Figure 7.4 *Partially Duplicated Pituitary.* Coronal T1-weighted image shows duplicated stalks *(arrows)* extending into one gland. This patient also had a hypothalamic hamartoma and a midline facial clefting syndrome.

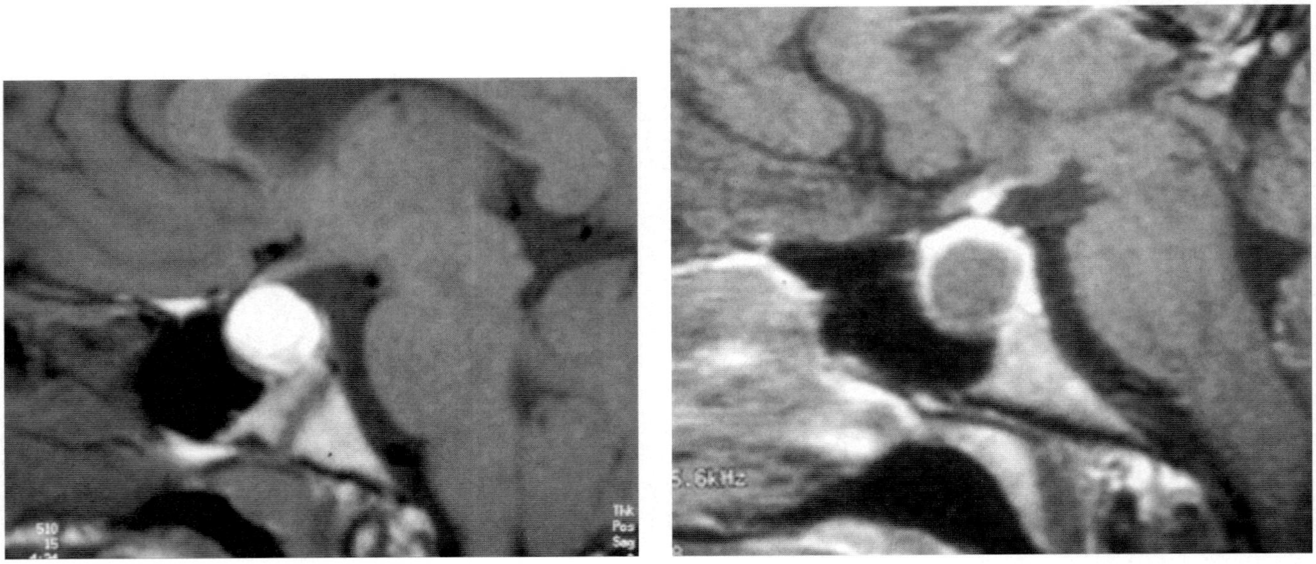

A B

Figure 7.5 *Rathke's Cleft Cyst. A.* Sagittal noncontrast T1-weighted image shows hyperintense mass in the sella turcica of a child. *B.* In a different patient, postcontrast sagittal T1-weighted image shows cystic mass in the pituitary gland. The peripheral enhancement of the mass probably represents the residual gland wrapped around a Rathke's cleft cyst.

atric pituitary adenomas is 14 years. Most children present with visual deficits, headache, and endocrine dysfunction. If the adenomas are hemorrhagic, the lesion may mimic the more common Rathke's cleft cyst or a craniopharyngioma. The treatment of choice is transsphenoidal resection, but some patients require irradiation.

Rathke's Cleft Cyst and Craniopharyngioma

These entities are addressed in this section because they are related to abnormalities in the development of the pituitary gland. Both lesions probably are related and represent the ends of a spectrum. Craniopharyngiomas are addressed in detail in Chapter 6 and are not reviewed here. Rathke's cyst is believed to represent a residue of the stomodeum (15). As such, the pars intermedia of the gland is the most common location (80%) for these cysts. They are common at autopsy, where approximately 30% of pituitary glands show such cysts. They slowly secrete a colloid material that results in growth of the cyst. Most symptomatic cysts measure over 1 cm. Symptoms usually are visual or endocrine. Compression of the stalk may lead to mild prolactinemia ("stalk effect"). When a Rathke's cyst is associated with an adenoma, it is called a *transitional tumor*. Rarely, Rathke's cysts may become infected (and result in the very rare pituitary abscess) or rupture and spill their contents into the subarachnoid space, creating aseptic meningitis. By MRI, Rathke's cysts have varying appearances (Fig. 7.5). They may be isointense or hyperintense on T1-weighted images and hypointense or hyperintense on T2-weighted images. They do not enhance or contain calcifications. Most are intrasellar and midline, but suprasellar extension is not uncommon. Because the pars tuberalis (which is part of the adenohypophysis) surrounds the stalk, Rathke's cysts may be purely suprasellar and arise in the infundibulum.

Adult Lesions

Tumors

Adenomas are the most common tumors of the pituitary gland in adults and represent approximately 10% to 15% of all intracranial tumors. By historical convention, they are

Table 7.3: Types of Pituitary Microadenomas

Tumor Type	*Incidence*
Prolactinoma	30%
Null cell	25%
Growth hormone–producing	15%
Cushing-producing	10%–15%
Gonadotropin-producing	5%–10%
Thyrotropin-producing	1%
Multihormonal	1%

classified as microadenomas (<10 mm in height) and macroadenomas (>10 mm in height) (16). Most tumors are microadenomas. Microadenomas present earlier because they tend to be hormonally active. Macroadenomas usually are not hormonally active and produce symptoms by virtue of mass effect. Adenomas may be seen in a variety of systemic syndromes.

Table 7.3 describes the classification of microadenomas (2) and Table 7.4 describes the symptoms arising from pituitary microadenomas (2).

The amount of prolactin correlates with the imaging findings, as shown in Table 7.5. There are other causes of increased prolactin secretion (2) (Table 7.6). Causes, other than pituitary tumors, for secretion of thyroid-stimulating hormone are hypothyroidism, leading to pituitary gland hypertrophy; for growth hormone, tumors of the pancreas, lung, adrenal gland, ovary, and breast; and for corticotropin, small cell lung cancer, pancreatic islet cell tumors, pheochromocytoma, and ovarian carcinoma.

Nearly all imaging of the pituitary gland for adenomas is done with MRI. However, conventional MRI is not much better than CT in this regard. The overall sensitivity of contrast-enhanced CT in microadenoma detection is approximately 80%, and that of contrast-enhanced MRI is approximately 85% (17,18). Both studies require image sections no greater than 3 mm in thickness. Dynamic MRI studies increase the sensitivity of this technique by approximately 5% to 10% and are particularly helpful in the detection of small adenomas such as those producing Cushing's disease (19) (Fig. 7.6). Dynamic imaging is done after administration of a bolus of contrast. The studies may be done using gradient-echo or fast spin-echo T1-weighted sequences. We obtain three slices (3 mm thick) in coronal projection every 30 seconds for a total of five cycles. We do this in every patient, and then we obtain coronal and sagittal high-resolution spin-echo T1-weighted images. If gradient-echo images are used for the dynamic sequences, magnetic susceptibility artifacts from the floor of the sella and intersphenoid sinus septa may produce areas of decreased signal intensity in the gland that may be mistaken for tumors. Because of this, we use coronal fast spin-echo T1-weighted images for our dynamic studies. An important aspect to remember is that although most microadenomas show less enhancement than the normal gland on conventional imaging, this may not be true of the dynamic sequences (20). Ade-

Although the rate of detection of adenomas for both contrast-enhanced CT and MRI are similar, dynamic contrast-enhanced MRI of the sella increases the sensitivity of MRI considerably.

Table 7.4: Symptoms Produced by Adenomas

Type of Tumor	*Symptoms in Women*	*Symptoms in Men*
Prolactinoma	Amenorrhea, galactorrhea	Decreased libido
Growth hormone–producing	Gigantism in children, acromegaly in adults	Same as in women
Cushing-producing	Cushing's disease	Same as in women
Gonadotropin-producing	Infertility, menstrual abnormalities	None
Thyrotropin-producing	Hyperthyroidism	Same as in women

Table 7.5: Correlations between Prolactin Levels and Magnetic Resonance Imaging (MRI) Findings

Prolactin Level (ngmL)	*MRI Abnormality*
<25	Usually normal
25–100	Adenomas in approximately 50% of patients
100–200	Adenomas in 75%–100%
200–1,000	Adenomas in all
>1,000	Invasion of cavernous sinuses

Table 7.6: Etiologies for Elevated Prolactin Other than Adenoma

Drugs	*Metabolic Disorders*	*Tumors*	*Others*
Phenothiazines, opiates, antihypertensives, estrogens	Kidney failure, liver failure	Suprasellar astrocytoma, craniopharyngioma, chest wall tumors, spinal cord tumors	Sarcoidosis, tuberculosis, histiocytosis

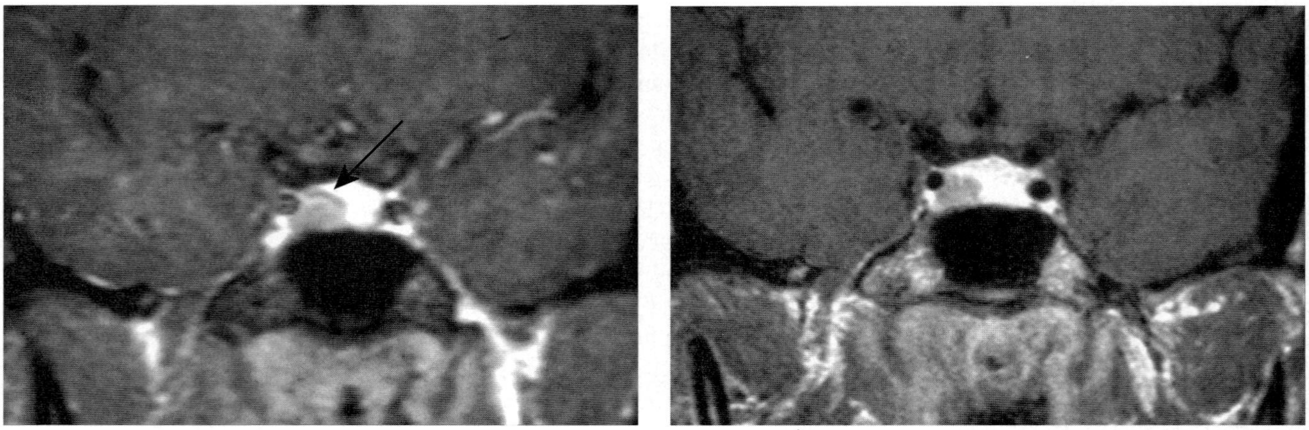
A B

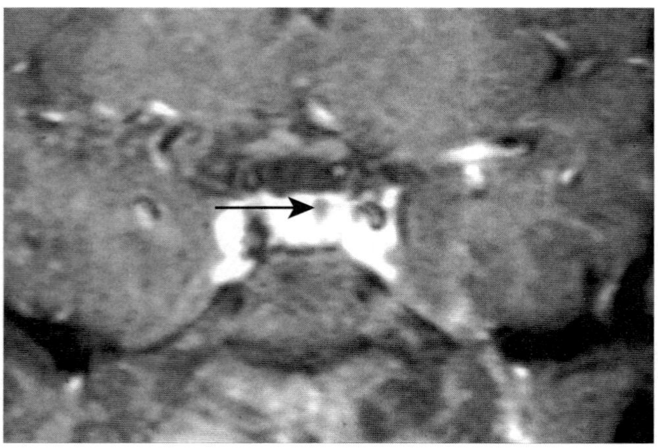
C

Figure 7.6 *Microadenoma. A.* Coronal dynamic T1-weighted image (60 seconds after injection of contrast) clearly shows a nonenhancing, prolactin-producing microadenoma *(arrow)* in the right lateral wing of the gland. *B.* The adenoma also is clearly seen on the coronal, high-resolution delayed T1-weighted image. *C.* In a different patient with Cushing's syndrome, a coronal dynamic T1-weighted image shows a tiny, nearly central microadenoma *(arrow)* that was not visible on the delayed high-resolution images.

nomas have a direct blood supply and thus may enhance earlier and more intensely than the surrounding adenohypophysis, only to become relatively hypointense to the gland as time passes. Unlike microadenomas, most macroadenomas show significant contrast enhancement. Macroadenomas usually have "figure-of-eight" appearance, with intrasellar and suprasellar components separated by a narrow waist where the tumor crosses the sellar diaphragm (Fig. 7.7). These macroadenomas commonly compress the optic chiasm (it sometimes may be difficult to identify the chiasm). Some macroadenomas erode the floor of the sella and extend into the sphenoid sinus. Invasion of the cavernous sinuses is not uncommon (2). By imaging, invasion of the cavernous sinus is certain when tumor is seen located lateral to the internal carotid artery. If tumor is seen superior and inferior, but not lateral, to the internal carotid artery, cavernous sinus invasion is present in only approximately 50% of cases. The only reliable way to exclude cavernous sinus invasion is to visualize a normal but compressed gland between the tumor and the cavernous sinus. Pituitary carcinomas are rare and cannot be distinguished (except in presence of distal metastases)

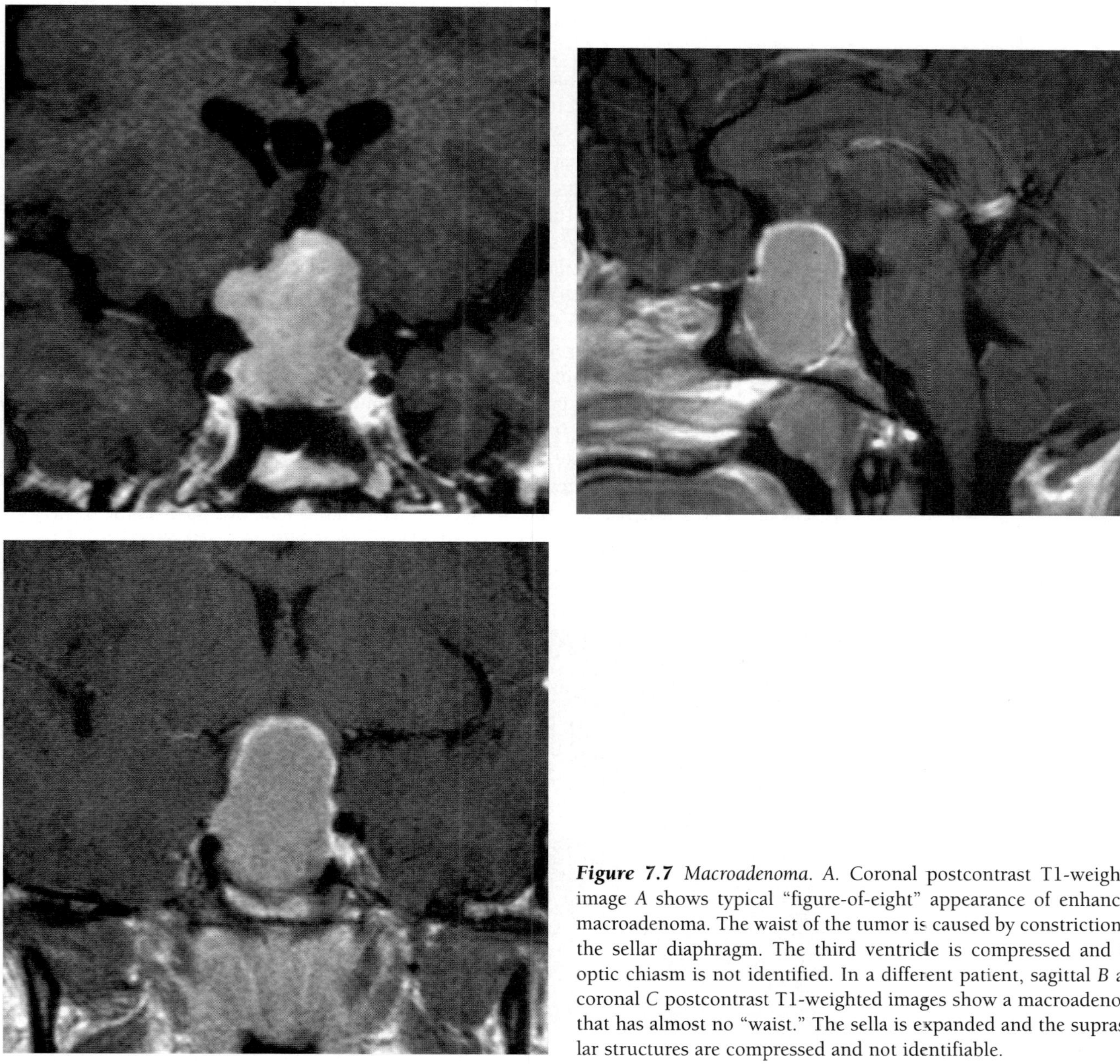

A B C

Figure 7.7 *Macroadenoma. A.* Coronal postcontrast T1-weighted image *A* shows typical "figure-of-eight" appearance of enhancing macroadenoma. The waist of the tumor is caused by constriction by the sellar diaphragm. The third ventricle is compressed and the optic chiasm is not identified. In a different patient, sagittal *B* and coronal *C* postcontrast T1-weighted images show a macroadenoma that has almost no "waist." The sella is expanded and the suprasellar structures are compressed and not identifiable.

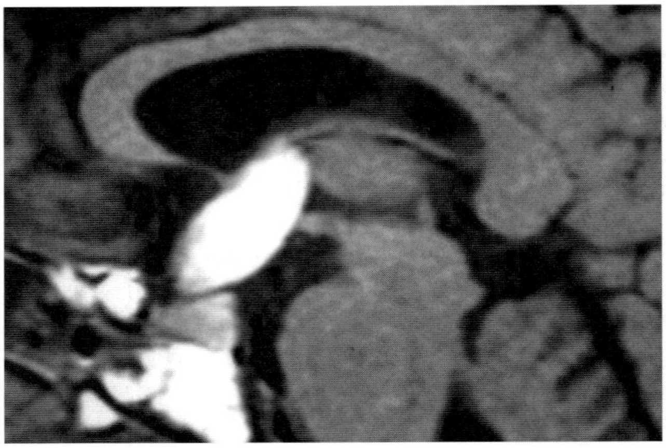

Figure 7.8 *Dermoid.* Sagittal T1-weighted image shows a fatty dermoid with intrasellar and suprasellar extension.

from the more common invasive pituitary adenoma that extends into either the cavernous sinuses or the sphenoid sinus.

Both compression of the optic chiasm by a sellar mass and herniation of the chiasm into an empty sella may result in bitemporal hemianopsia.

At times, a full dose of contrast material results in such a degree of enhancement of the gland that the lesions may not be readily apparent unless they are recorded and analyzed with wide window settings. This has led, in some institutions, to the use of a one-half dose of contrast (21). A smaller dose of contrast also is helpful in the follow-up of treated tumors. In most postoperative studies, it is not possible to determine if the residual sellar enhancing soft tissues represent normal gland, residual tumor, or graft (22). The most important aspect of these studies is to compare them with prior studies to assess increasing soft tissue (suggesting tumor) versus decreasing size of soft tissue (compatible with involuting graft or tumor response to treatment). In some rare cases, a large empty sella (see later) develops after surgery, and the optic chiasm may herniate into it and result in visual deficits.

The utility of contrast-enhanced MRI in patients who will receive medical treatment for suspected microadenomas is questionable. Detailed studies localizing a tumor are needed only when surgery is contemplated. Some authors advocate only coronal noncontrast T1- and T2-weighted images if the patient will be treated with drugs. This excludes invasion of adjacent structures or clinically silent compression of the optic chiasm, all of which may need more aggressive therapies. If the serum hormone level decreases while a patient is taking medication and the symptoms remain stable or improve, the utility of follow-up MRI also is questionable.

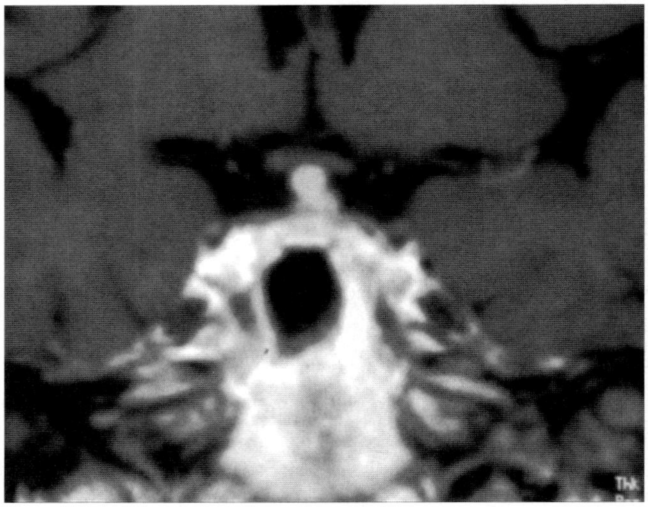

Figure 7.9 *Presumed Breast Metastases.* Coronal postcontrast T1-weighted image shows an enhancing mass in the stalk in a patient with diffuse metastatic disease and sudden onset of hypopituitarism.

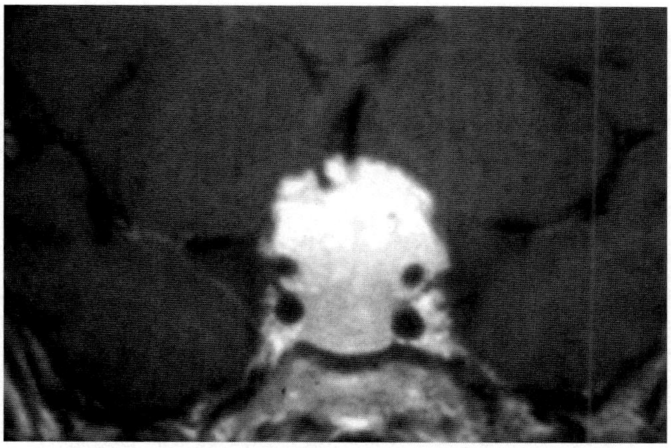

Figure 7.10 *Meningioma.* Coronal postcontrast T1-weighted image shows densely enhancing meningioma with intrasellar and suprasellar extension. There is tumor in the left cavernous sinus.

Other masses affecting the pituitary gland are craniopharyngioma, arachnoid cysts, dermoid/epidermoid, histiocytosis, metastases, ganglion cell tumors, and glandular hyperplasia (Figs. 7.8 and 7.9). Intrasellar meningiomas are very rare, but intrasellar extension of a meningioma arising in the parasellar regions is not unusual (Fig. 7.10). Pituitary metastases are rare, and even fewer result in symptoms (many pituitary metastases are found only at autopsy). The symptoms produced by metastases to the gland are acute and include headaches, visual field defects, and panhypopituitarism. MRI findings are nonspecific, and the studies show metastases as enhancing lesions. Glandular hyperplasia occurs as a response that may be physiologic (see earlier) or pathologic (23). Pathologic pituitary hyperplasia is seen in patients with hypothyroidism, estrogen administration, central precocious puberty, and some hypothalamic lesions. The gland is enlarged and convex superiorly and enhances homogeneously. The gland may return to normal several months after treatment of the underlying abnormality. The pituitary gland may be infiltrated and enlarged in the mucopolysaccharidoses and amyloidosis (2).

Tumors involving the posterior lobe are very rare. These include astrocytoma (pituicytoma), granular cell tumors, ganglion cell tumors, and metastases. The imaging features of these rare tumors are nonspecific, but granular cell tumors show prominent contrast enhancement and may be hypervascular on angiography. Tumors arising in the pituitary stalk are even rarer and include adenoma, Rathke's cysts, astrocytoma (infundibuloma), granular cell tumors, hamartomas, and metastases. Adenomas, cysts, and hamartomas do not enhance, whereas astrocytomas, granular cell tumors, and metastases do enhance.

PITUITARY APOPLEXY

Pituitary apoplexy is not an imaging diagnosis but a clinical syndrome (24). The main imaging finding in this syndrome is pituitary hemorrhage that may or may not result in infarction. Pituitary hemorrhage may be asymptomatic (not apoplectic) or catastrophic (apoplexy). Incidentally found pituitary hemorrhage needs no specific treatment (Fig. 7.11). Pituitary apoplexy is characterized by acute and severe headaches, hydrocephalus (due to compression of the third ventricle), bitemporal hemianopsia, and endocrine dysfunction (Fig. 7.12). Compression of the optic chiasm may result in ischemic necrosis, and decompression of the clot is needed to save vision. Subarachnoid hemorrhage also may be evident after pituitary hemorrhages. Most hemorrhages occur in nonfunctioning macroadenomas, but they may occur in any type of adenoma. Pituitary apoplexy may result from the following causes:

Pituitary apoplexy is a clinical diagnosis and not an imaging one; hemorrhage into the gland may be found in the absence of apoplexy.

- Adenoma
- Treatment with bromocriptine or irradiation
- Pregnancy
- Trauma

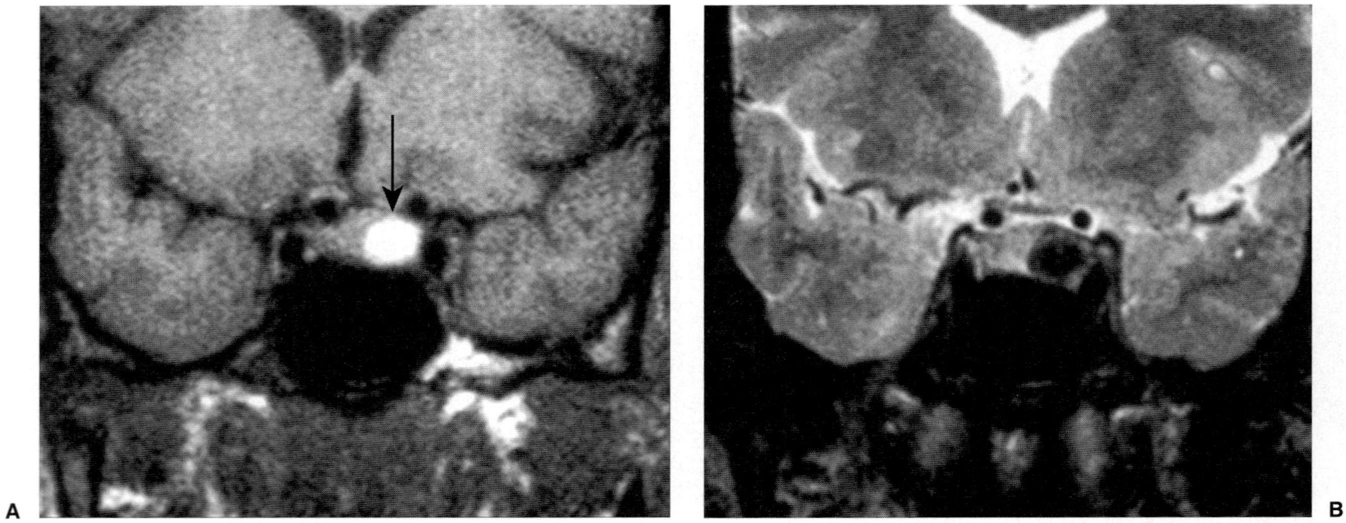

Figure 7.11 *Incidental Hemorrhagic Adenoma. A.* In this patient with no symptoms of pituitary apoplexy, noncontrast coronal T1-weighted image shows a bright adenoma *(arrow)* in the left lateral wing of the gland. The floor of the sella slopes on the side of the tumor. *B.* Corresponding T2-weighted image shows the blood products to be dark (possibly because of the presence of intracellular methemoglobin).

- Hypertension
- Coagulopathy
- Lumbar puncture
- Cerebral angiography

MRI is the modality of choice to evaluate patients suspected of having pituitary hemorrhage. With hemorrhage, the gland is large and upwardly convex. It may be bright on T1 and dark on T2 sequences (Fig. 7.12). A fluid level (as the patient is prone in the MRI unit) may form. Blood in the pituitary gland may not show the same degradation charac-

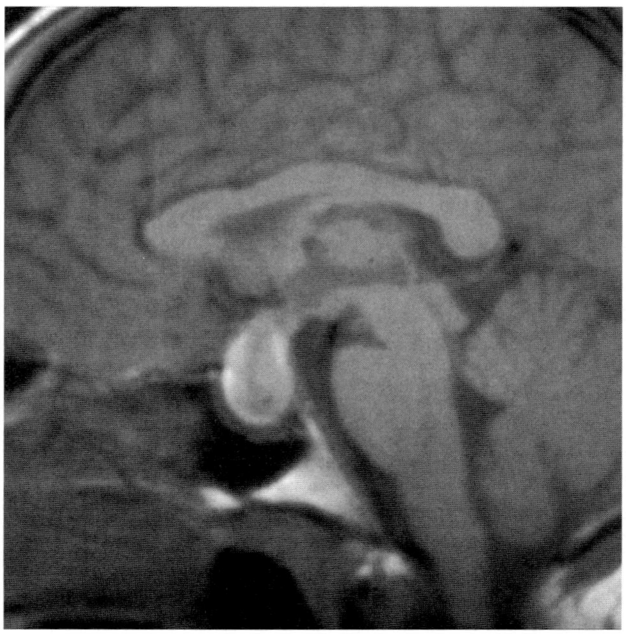

Figure 7.12 *Pituitary Apoplexy.* Sagittal noncontrast image in a patient with sudden onset of blindness and headache shows bright and expanded pituitary gland compressing the optic chiasm.

teristics as an intraaxial hemorrhage because the gland has a high oxygen tension. In patients with large pituitary hemorrhages, imaging of the brain is needed to exclude hydrocephalus. Compression of the optic chiasm may indicate the need for emergent clot evacuation. Patients with pituitary bleeds need to be observed carefully because initially mild symptoms may progress rapidly.

Sheehan's Syndrome

This entity refers to postpartum pituitary gland necrosis that may or may not be hemorrhagic (25). The end result is necrosis of the gland, severe atrophy of the gland, and panhypopituitarism. Most patients experience a hypovolemic shock before or after delivery that is believed to result in circulatory collapse of the pituitary portal system. Occasionally, the optic chiasm and prechiasmatic nerves also may be affected because their blood supply is similar. Symptoms may be acute or take years to present, and occasionally hormone levels may return to normal. The diagnosis of Sheehan's syndrome is a clinical one. The imaging correlates include an acutely enlarged gland that may show only peripheral enhancement (the central portion may be necrotic) and that on follow-up studies becomes progressively atrophied, eventually resulting in an empty or partially empty sella turcica.

Empty Sella

The empty sella syndrome refers to enlargement of the sella turcica caused by pulsations of CSF. The diaphragma sella becomes incompetent, allowing the cerebral pulsations to be transmitted to the fluid in the suprasellar cistern and then to the intrasellar fluid. This results in a "water hammer" effect that may lead to compression of the pituitary gland and remodeling of bone. The sella may be completely empty or, more commonly, only partially empty (residual gland is visualized). The empty sella is a common incidental finding in approximately 20% to 40% of patients older than 40 years of age (26). It nearly always is asymptomatic. The empty sella may be primary (due to intrinsic disease of the pituitary gland) or secondary (due to destruction of gland). Pseudotumor cerebri (idiopathic intracranial hypertension) may be associated with an empty sella. On resolution of the increased intracranial pressure, the gland may return to normal size (26). In cases of a large empty sella, the optic chiasm may herniate into the sella, resulting in visual field deficits (27).

An empty or partially empty sella nearly always is an incidental and asymptomatic finding, but it may be associated with pseudotumor cerebri.

Inflammatory and Histiocytic Lesions of the Pituitary Gland

The inflammatory and histiocytic diseases affecting the gland are shown in Table 7.7. All of these entities are very rare. Abscesses may occur after surgery of the gland or in

Table 7.7 Histiocytic and Inflammatory Disorders of the Pituitary Gland

Histiocytic Infiltration	*Inflammatory Diseases*
Hand-Schuller-Christian disease (Fig.7.13)	Sarcoidosis
Rosai-Dorfman disease	Bacterial infection
Erdheim-Chester disease	Tuberculosis (Fig. 7.14)
	Parasite (mostly cysticercosis) and fungus
	Tolosa Hunt syndrome
	Acute lymphocytic hypophysitis
	Giant cell granuloma
	Wegener granulomatosis

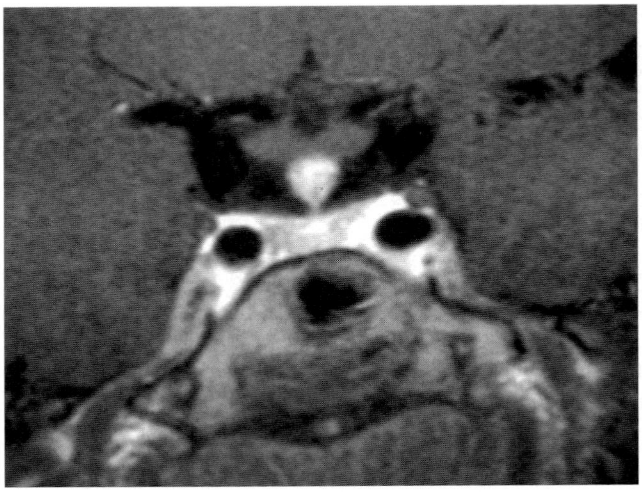

Figure 7.13 *Histiocytosis.* Coronal postcontrast T1-weighted image shows a nonspecific-appearing enhancing mass in the stalk.

patients with septicemia. Their imaging features are not specific and may show a lesion expanding the gland with peripheral enhancement. Tuberculosis is a leading cause of pituitary abscesses in developing countries. With pituitary cysticercosis, there usually are other lesions in the brain and cisterns. All of the histiocytic disorders are very rare and present as solid enhancing lesions affecting the gland, stalk, and hypothalamus (28). Sarcoidosis shows imaging findings similar to those of the histiocytic disorders, but lesions elsewhere in the cisterns and brain usually are present. In cases of Tolosa-Hunt syndrome, solid areas of enhancement that commonly extend into the cavernous sinuses and the superior orbital fissure are present and result in a painful ophthalmoplegia. I have seen giant cell granulomas in the sella turcica only after surgery and as a reaction to foreign tissue in this location. Their appearance is nonspecific.

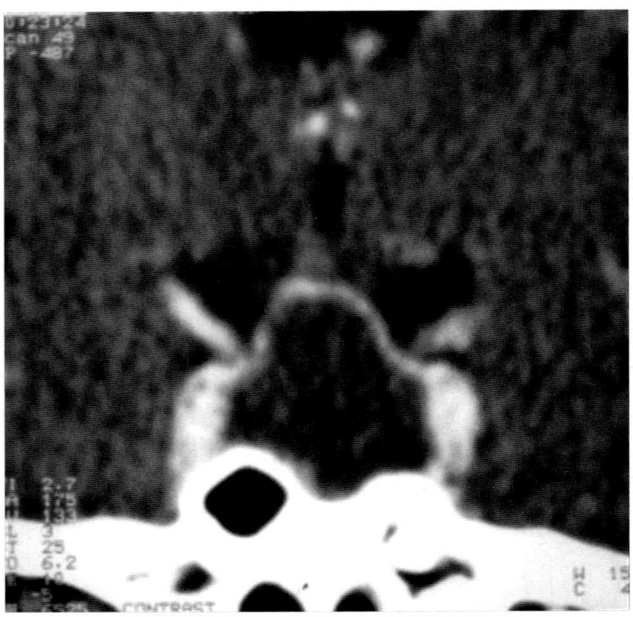

Figure 7.14 *Tubercular Pituitary Abscess.* Coronal postcontrast CT shows cystic mass in the gland with peripheral enhancement.

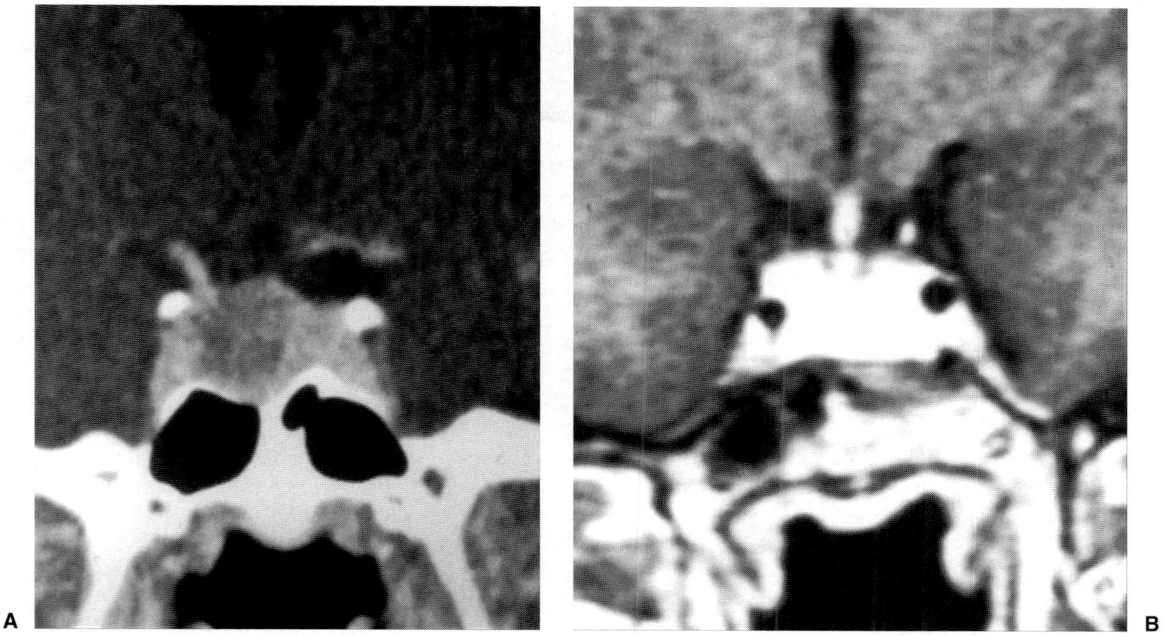

Figure 7.15 *Lymphocytic Hypophysitis. A.* Coronal postcontrast computed tomography shows patchy but significant enhancement of an enlarged gland. This appearance is nonspecific, but the patient was postpartum and acutely developed hypopituitarism. *B.* In a different patient with a similar history, a postcontrast coronal T1-weighted image shows a nonspecific, enlarged, and enhancing mass.

Lymphocytic Hypophysitis

Lymphocytic hypophysitis is a rare and often acute disorder (29). It most commonly involves the adenohypophysis and affects women during pregnancy or the early postpartum period. It may, however, involve the entire gland and also occur in men. Symptoms at presentation include fever, fatigue, headache, decreased libido, diplopia, and diabetes insipidus. When diabetes insipidus is present, involvement of the stalk often is present. On imaging studies, the findings often are nonspecific and include diffuse enlargement and homogeneous enhancement of the gland (Fig. 7.15). On dynamic studies, enhancement of the gland may be delayed. Occasionally, the cavernous sinuses may be involved. A definite diagnosis requires histologic confirmation. Follow-up studies demonstrate improvement after appropriate medical therapy.

References

1. Larsen WJ. Human embryology, 2nd ed. New York: Churchill Livingston, 1997:411–445.
2. Elster AD. Modern imaging of the pituitary. Radiology 1993;187:1–14.
3. Kurokawa H, Fujisawa I, Nakano Y, et al. Posterior lobe of the pituitary gland: correlation between signal-intensity on T1-weighted MR images and vasopressin concentration. Radiology 1998;207:79–83.
4. Teramoto A, Hirakawa K, Sanno N, et al. Incidental pituitary lesions in 1,000 unselected autopsy specimens. Radiology 1994;193:161–164.
5. Ahmadi H, Larsson EM, Jinkins JR. Normal pituitary gland: coronal MR imaging of infundibular tilt. Radiology 1990;177:389–392.
6. Peyster RG, Hoover ED, Viscarello RR, et al. CT appearance of the adolescent and preadolescent pituitary gland. AJNR Am J Neuroradiol 1983;4:411–414.

7. Tsunoda A, Okuda O, Sato K. MR height of the pituitary gland as a function of age and sex: especially physiological hypertrophy in adolescence and in climacterium. AJNR Am J Neuroradiol 1997;18:551–554.
8. Osborn AG. MRI of the sellar/juxtasellar region: juxtasellar and infrasellar masses. Imaging Decis 1994;1:2–11.
9. Ahamdi H, Larsson EM, Jinkins JR. Normal pituitary gland: coronal MR imaging of infundibular tilt. Radiology 1990;177:389–392.
10. Sparacia G, Banco A, Midiri M, et al. MR imaging technique for the diagnosis of pituitary iron overload in patients with transfusion-dependent beta-thalassemia major. AJNR Am J Neuroradiol 1998;19:1905–1907.
11. Falcone S, Sánchez J, Quencer RM. Lack of normal MR enhancement of the pituitary gland: findings in three siblings with combined pituitary hormone deficiency. AJNR Am J Neuroradiol 1998;19:287–289.
12. Kelly WM, Kucharczyk W, Kucharczyk J, et al. Posterior pituitary ectopia: an MR feature of pituitary dwarfism. AJNR Am J Neuroradiol 1988;9:453–460.
13. Sato N, Ishizaka H, Yagi H, et al. Posterior lobe of the pituitary in diabetes insipidus: dynamic MR imaging. Radiology 1993;186:357–360.
14. Poussaint TY, Barnes PD, Anthony DC, et al. Hemorrhagic pituitary adenomas of adolescence. AJNR Am J Neuroradiol 1996;17:1907–1912.
15. Sumida M, Uozumi T, Mukada K, et al. Rathke cleft cysts: correlation of enhanced MR and surgical findings. AJNR Am J Neuroradiol 1994;15:525–532.
16. Kucharczyk W, Davis DO, Kelly WM, et al. Pituitary adenomas: high-resolution MR imaging at 1.5 T. Radiology 1986;161:761–765.
17. Miki Y, Matsuo M, Nishizawa S, et al. Pituitary adenomas and normal pituitary tissue: enhancement patterns on gadopentetate-enhanced MR imaging. Radiology 1990;177:35–38.
18. Bonneville JF, Cattin F, Gorczyca W, et al. Pituitary microadenomas: early enhancement with dynamic CT—implications of arterial blood supply and potential importance. Radiology 1993;187:857–861.
19. Dwyer AJ, Frank JA, Doppman JL, et al. Pituitary adenomas in patients with Cushing disease: initial experience with Gd-DTPA-enhanced MR imaging. Radiology 1987;163:421–426.
20. Yuh WT, Fisher DJ, Nguyen HD, et al. Sequential MR enhancement pattern in normal pituitary gland and in pituitary adenoma. AJNR Am J Neuroradiol 1994;15:101–108.
21. Davis PC, Gokhale KA, Joseph GJ, et al. Pituitary adenoma: correlation of half-dose gadolinium-enhanced MR imaging with surgical findings in 26 patients. Radiology 1991;180:779–784.
22. Knosp E, Herold CJ, Kramer J, et al. Pituitary adenomas: findings in postoperative MR imaging. Radiology 1992;185:521–527.
23. Miki Y, Asato R, Okumura R, et al. Anterior pituitary gland in pregnancy: hyperintensity at MR. Radiology 1993;187:229–231.
24. Post MJ, David NJ, Glaser JS, et al. Pituitary apoplexy: diagnosis by computed tomography. Radiology 1980;134:665–670.
25. Lavallée G, Morcos R, Palardy J, et al. MR of nonhemorrhagic postpartum pituitary apoplexy. AJNR Am J Neuroradiol 1995;16:1939–1941.
26. Zagardo MT, Cail WS, Kelman SE, et al. Reversible empty sella in idiopathic intracranial hypertension: an indicator of successful therapy? AJNR Am J Neuroradiol 1996;17:1953–1956.
27. Bursztyn EM, Lavyne MH, Aisen M. Empty sella syndrome with intrasellar herniation of the optic chiasm. AJNR Am J Neuroradiol 1983;4:167–168.
28. Woodcock RJ Jr, Mandell JW, Lipper MH. Sinus histiocytosis (Rosai-Dorfman disease) of the suprasellar region: MR imaging findings: a case report. Radiology 1999;213:808–810.
29. Sato N, Sze G, Endo K. Hypophysitis: endocrinologic and dynamic MR findings. AJNR Am J Neuroradiol 1998;19:439–444.

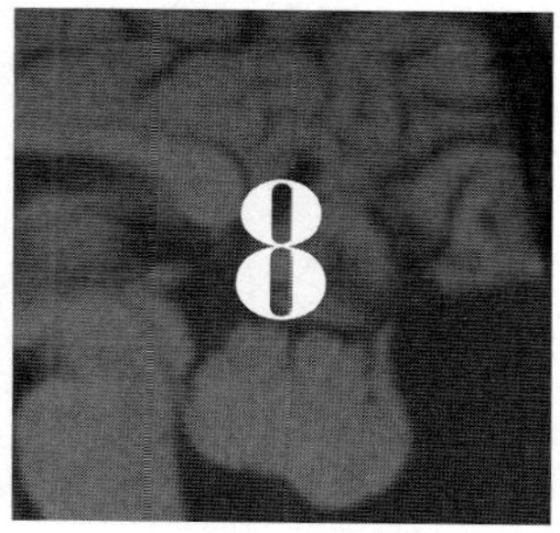

Vascular Occlusive Disorders

- General Facts
- Pathophysiology and Imaging
- Cerebral Infarctions
- Vasculitis
- Moyamoya
- Hypertensive Encephalopathy
- Venous Occlusions
- Vascular Age-Related Changes
- Extracranial Arterial Disease
- Dissection of Extracranial Blood Vessels
- Cerebral Infarction in Children

General Facts

Broadly, the term *stroke* encompasses both transient and permanent neurologic symptoms and signs. Approximately 700,000 patients are diagnosed as having stroke every year in the United States (1). Symptoms that resolve within 24 hours of their onset are referred to as *transient ischemic attacks* (TIA) and those that are fixed or remain for more than 1 day are considered to be secondary to a cerebral infarction (2). This traditional temporal clinical division no longer is completely appropriate because therapy of stroke requires rapid stratification of patients into those with and without cerebral infarctions. The window of opportunity for cerebral thrombolytic therapy varies from 1 to 6 hours (average of 3 hours for the middle cerebral arteries and up to 6 hours for arteries in the posterior circulation) (3). Waiting 24 hours to determine if a patient has had a TIA or a cerebral infarction therefore is no longer appropriate. The aim of imaging in stroke is to:

- Identify patients with cerebral infarction and the extent of these infarctions (delineation of the infracted core and penumbra is now possible)
- Identify hemorrhagic infarctions, which may carry a worse prognosis than nonhemorrhagic infarctions, to prevent unnecessary thrombolytic therapy
- Determine causes other than ischemia for the patient's symptoms (approximately 10% of all strokes are caused by lesions other than vascular occlusion)

Pathophysiology of Stroke and Imaging

Cerebral ischemia is due to diminished blood flow in a focal (regional) or generalized (global) form. Cerebral ischemia may be further subdivided into reversible and irreversible (1). It is traditionally accepted that below a certain threshold of cerebral blood volume, ischemic changes become irreversible infarctions. Ischemia may affect the end-arterial territories or the border (watershed) zones. These zones are formed by the terminal microvascularity between the territories supplied by the major cerebral arteries. The terminal arterial territories often are affected by emboli and atherosclerotic disease, whereas the watershed zones most commonly are affected by hypoxic encephalopathy. In addition

Table 8.1: Outcome of Patients with Cerebral Infarctions

Outcome	*Percentage*
Death	10%–15%
Long-term disabilities	30%–50%
Institutionalization	20%–25%

Cytotoxic edema, secondary to failure of the sodium/potassium pump, begins a few minutes after a significant drop in cerebral blood flow and is responsible for the findings on diffusion-weighted imaging.

to these traditional regions, the brain also responds by selective vulnerability—that is, areas composed of gray matter suffer first in the presence of diminished cerebral blood flow. Vasogenic edema occurs secondary to injury to the endothelial cells in the arterial walls. Leaky capillaries promote the leakage of water and plasma into the extracellular space. Vasogenic edema is first noted 3 to 6 hours after infarction. Cell death occurs after a 40% to 70% reduction in cerebral blood volume and is irreversible a few minutes after vessel occlusion. Alterations at the cellular membrane level [mainly a decrease in adenosine triphosphate (ATP), producing alterations in the sodium/potassium pump] result in influx of water into the cells (cytotoxic edema). There is concomitant loss of the vascular autoregulation that normally protects the brain. Lysis of an intravascular clot results in reestablishment of normal blood flow and the possibility of normal-pressure breakthrough hemorrhages. Based on their imaging features, I classify all infarcts at less than 6 hours as *hyperacute*, infarcts between 6 hours and 3 days as *acute*, between 3 days and 3 months as *subacute*, and older than 3 months as *chronic*. Cerebral infarctions may be stable or unstable (in which the patients either improve or deteriorate). A complete infarction refers to an event in which all the functions assigned to the affected vascular territory are involved. An incomplete infarction is one in which some of the functions controlled by the affected territory remain normal. Treatment of the patient with stroke may include:

- Prophylaxis (with antiplatelet medications or anticoagulation)
- Acute therapy (with thrombolytic drugs, anticoagulation, and calcium channel blockers; and with corticosteroids, which have no proven value)
- Rehabilitation

The prognosis of patients with cerebral infarctions is shown in Table 8.1. Patients who have had one cerebral infarct are at an increased risk for subsequent strokes.

A few seconds after cessation of blood flow, glycogen, glucose, phosphocreatine, and ATP are rapidly depleted. Ischemia occurs when cerebral blood flow is below 60 mL/100 g/minute, oxygen concentration drops below 90 mm Hg, or blood glucose falls below 80 mg/dL (4). With failure of the energy-dependent cell membranes, depolarization occurs, allowing influx of sodium and calcium and efflux of potassium. Intracellular elevation of calcium results in activation of proteases and lipases that release fatty acids that in turn denature proteins. This depolarization also releases large amounts of neurotransmitters at the synapses, and these cause further cellular damage. Neuronal death begins 5 minutes after the cerebral blood flow falls below the critical level. I now address the different imaging methods used in the evaluation of patients with acute cerebral infarctions.

Cerebral Catheter Angiography

Information obtained from cerebral catheter angiography (CCA) is anatomic (including vessel occlusion and narrowing) and physiologic (including cerebral circulation times and development of collateral blood supply). Angiographic signs associated with cerebral infarction include:

- Vasodilatation with increased arteriovenous shunting (earliest sign)
- Slowing of arterial flow

- Collateral circulation
- Mass effect
- Prolonged capillary contrast staining
- Early-draining veins

Persistent vasodilatation, capillary staining, and early venous drainage also are seen in hemorrhagic infarctions. The term *luxury perfusion* is applied to increased blood (and therefore contrast material) flow around the area of infarction and is believed to be secondary to an abnormal vascular autoregulation. Injection of iodinated contrast media into an ischemic cerebral territory is controversial. Experience gathered in the early 1980s reported a detrimental effect of iodinated contrast media in patients with cerebral infarctions. This experience resulted in a restrictive use of iodinated contrast agents in patients with stroke. Because of the recent popularity of techniques such as computed tomographic angiography (CTA), which require injections of relatively large volumes of contrast medium, the effect of these contrast agents on infarcted brain has received further attention. In one article, injection of nonionic iodinated contrast medium into animals that had previously undergone endovascular occlusion of a middle cerebral artery (MCA) resulted in no significant alterations of the infarcted volume or neurologic symptoms (5). Because disruption of the blood–brain barrier (BBB) is one of the last events to occur during cerebral infarction (maximum disruption of the BBB in humans probably occurs 2 to 5 days after the initial ictus), early use of contrast media may not be as toxic as previously thought. This observation, however, is not true of ionic contrast agents. Ionic contrast agents during the acute period may result in increased infarct volumes and worsening of neurologic symptoms. A second factor affecting the performance of CCA in patients with stroke is the inherent risk of the procedure. Approximately 30 years ago, several studies quoted the rate of complications from CCA to be approximately 2.5%, with a mortality rate of 0.5% (6,7). The rate of complications from CCA was found to increase fourfold in patients with stroke. This probably was the result of technical problems, catheter manipulation and navigation, insufficient training and experience, and injection of irritating contrast agents. In view of these observations, the use of CCA in patients with stroke was curtailed. At present, with the use of digital subtraction angiography: smaller, preformed catheters; softer, hydrophilic guidewires; and nonionic contrast media, the overall rate of complications probably is closer to 1.5%, with a mortality rate of less than 0.3% (7). Angiographic evaluation of the patient with a cerebral infarction begins with investigation of the vessels in the neck. Assessment of the degree of stenosis should be done using the criteria set forth by the North American Symptomatic Carotid Endarterectomy Trial (NASCET) (8–10). This requires a minimum of two views of each common carotid artery bifurcation (I obtain three views). The degree of stenosis needs to be calculated on the view showing the most narrowing. Measurements of stenoses are done by measuring residual lumen at the point of maximal narrowing (N) divided by the diameter of the normal internal carotid artery well distal to the bulb (D). The percentage stenosis is calculated as follows (9):

$$[1 - (N/D)] \times 100$$

Stenoses less than 70% usually are considered not to be hemodynamically significant, and most of these patients are not surgical candidates (9,10). However, asymptomatic men with stenoses greater than 60% may benefit from surgery (9,10). Significant lesions in the extracranial carotid arteries are found in only 5% of patients with acute stroke symptoms. Because most cerebral infarctions are thought to be secondary to emboli (presumably arising from a diseased carotid artery bifurcation in the neck), the main finding at CCA is that of an abrupt cutoff of a vessel lumen. Unfortunately, this abnormality is time dependent because many clots lyse rapidly. Therefore, a cerebral infarction may be present even in the face of a normal angiogram. Fibromuscular dysplasia (FMD) is a less common but important cause for strokelike symptoms (see later). FMD is more common in women and may involve any of the three layers (intima, media, and adventitia) that form the wall of an

Internal carotid artery stenoses greater than 70% are hemodynamically significant and benefit from surgery; in men, stenoses greater than 60% also benefit from surgery.

artery. More than 90% of all cases of FMD are due to hyperplasia of the media and result in concentric narrowings of the vessel alternating with focal dilatations, simulating a string of pearls (11). The stenoses tend to involve less than 40% of lumen diameter. The internal carotid artery is affected by FMD predominantly at the C2 level. Bilateral involvement may be seen in up to 75% of patients, and involvement of one or both vertebral arteries occurs in 15% of patients. Both atherosclerotic narrowings and FMD of the internal carotid arteries are now amenable to endovascular treatment.

Indications for carotid endarterectomy include recent symptoms, including TIAs or minor cerebral infarction (lacunar infarction), angiographically proven stenosis between 70% and 99%, and more than a 50% chance of life expectancy greater than 5 years.

Radionuclide Brain Scans

Most nuclear medicine studies of the brain are done using technetium-99m–hexamethylpropylene amine oxime (Tc99m-HMPAO) (12). This radiotracer is lipophilic and its distribution throughout the brain reflects cerebral perfusion at the time of injection. Approximately 70% to 80% of the tracer is removed during its first pass, and it therefore provides a dynamic assessment of cerebral perfusion. Decreased perfusion (which is the first pathophysiologic abnormality in cerebral infarction) is easily assessed by this method. Maximum uptake of drug by the brain occurs 1 to 2 minutes after injection, but an optimal contrast-to-noise ratio is obtained when patients are imaged from 1.5 to 2 hours after the injection (because of clearing of the background). During the first 48 hours after the onset of neurologic symptoms, single-photon emission CT (SPECT) using Tc99m-HMPAO has been shown to have a sensitivity of 79% and a specificity of 95% in the detection of cerebral infarction. In one study, these results were better than those obtained with CT scanning. SPECT is more reliable when the infarctions affect the cortex rather than the deep white matter. This observation reflects the increased blood volume that the cortex normally receives. The defects as seen on SPECT usually are larger than those seen by CT in the same patients (12). In the subacute period, the sensitivity of SPECT decreases considerably, and CT and magnetic resonance imaging (MRI) are better imaging modalities. The size of a defect as seen in early SPECT studies also correlates with the prognosis. Patients with large defects have a poor prognosis. Although SPECT theoretically offers an attractive method with which to evaluate patients with stroke, its relative lack of availability during the night and on the weekend has restricted its more widespread application. Positron emission tomography (PET) also has been used in the patient with stroke. Because of its limited availability and the scope of this review, its applications are not discussed.

Doppler Sonography

A full review of the utility of Doppler sonography of the extracranial carotid arteries is beyond the scope of this review. Clinical applications of transcranial Doppler sonography (TCD) include the diagnosis of intracranial occlusive disease, evaluation of hemodynamic effects of extracranial occlusive disease on intracranial blood flow, documentation of spontaneous or therapeutically induced recanalization of occluded vessels, and evaluation of vessels during anticoagulation or thrombolytic therapies (13). The results of TCD depend on knowing the exact status of the extracranial carotid arteries. TCD provides flow velocity measurements that roughly correlate with cerebral blood flow. The diagnosis of vessel stenosis is based on the presence of increased flow velocity, distal turbulence, low-frequency vibrations, and murmurs. TCD has demonstrated that up to 65% of embolic occlusions of the middle cerebral arteries are completely recanalized within 3 days of the ictus. By 3 weeks, recanalization approaches 80%. In one study, more than 70% of patients with cerebral infarctions showed abnormal blood flow patterns in the proximal middle cerebral arteries, whereas no patients with TIA demonstrated any flow-related anomalies. An interesting combination is that of using TCD and

SPECT together in the evaluation of the patient with acute stroke. In one study, the combination of these two techniques was able to identify the patients with smaller infarctions who responded better to thrombolysis.

Computed Tomography

Conventional Computed Tomography

Using conventional scanning techniques, current CT units are capable of demonstrating abnormalities related to cerebral infarctions as early as 3 to 6 hours after the onset of symptoms (14). Not all cerebral infarctions are seen initially on CT, and its sensitivity increases considerably during the first day after the stroke (13). Therefore, conventional CT is not the ideal method to separate patients with TIAs from those with true cerebral infarctions. CT, however, continues to be a reliable method to identify the presence of clinically significant hemorrhage in patients with acute stroke. CT continues to be the most widely used imaging technique in patients with stroke. In view of the recent emphasis on thrombolytic therapies, CT scanning should be obtained rapidly to exclude the presence of hemorrhage, large infarctions, and mass effect. Contraindications to this type of systemic thrombolysis include hemorrhage, mass effect, and parenchymal hypodensity or cortical sulci effacement of more than 33% in the territory of an MCA (15). Patients who receive systemic thrombolytic drugs during the initial 90 minutes after a stroke have a better prognosis than those who do not undergo this particular therapy. By obtaining only a CT study in these patients, some patients experiencing only TIA will be treated and exposed to the risk of secondary cerebral hemorrhage. This observation accounts for some of the promising initial results in the use of systemic thrombolysis. Heparinization, which is the traditional method of treating cerebral infarctions, has never undergone a formal double-blinded study, and its efficacy is questionable. The initial findings of cerebral infarction on CT depend on the vessel occluded. In the presence of a hemiparetic patient, a negative CT does not rule out infarction. Most infarctions involve the MCA territories, and early CT findings include the following(14):

CT becomes positive in many MCA infarctions at 3 to 6 hours postictus, and always is positive by 24 hours.

- Subtle low density in the putamen and globus pallidus (disappearing lentiform nucleus sign)
- Low density in the insular cortex and underlying white matter (insular low-density sign)
- Hyperdense MCA (due to intraluminal thrombus or embolus)
- Sulcal obliteration
- Effacement of the cortical gray–white matter junction

Unfortunately, up to 40% of patients with cerebral infarction have normal results on conventional CT studies. In all of these patients, CT findings become positive during the first 24 hours (Fig. 8.1). The hypodensity present in infarctions is due to an increase in tissue water. This hypodensity reaches a maximum 3 to 5 days postictus. During the first week, infarctions assume a wedge shape, with their apices pointing to the deep brain structures. Acute and early subacute infarctions have relatively little mass effect for their size. Mass effect is progressive and increases until 2 to 3 weeks postinfarction, and thereafter decreases. Edema and mass effect resolve by 3 weeks. Infarctions involving the anterior cerebral artery (ACA) account for approximately 1% of all occluded cerebral vessels. Most ACA territory infarctions are seen in combination with infarctions involving the MCAs or secondary to midline herniation with clipping of an ACA by the falx. In ACA infarction, CT shows a hypodensity in the medial and superior frontal lobes extending to the parietal lobes. Posterior cerebral artery (PCA) infarctions are the most common ones after those affecting the internal and middle cerebral arteries. They may be embolic, associated with hypertensive encephalopathy, or secondary to downward transtentorial herniation. The most common acute finding in PCA infarction is that of low density involving the medial surface of an occipital lobe.

Isolated ACA infarctions are rare; most infarctions of the ACA territory accompany an MCA infarction.

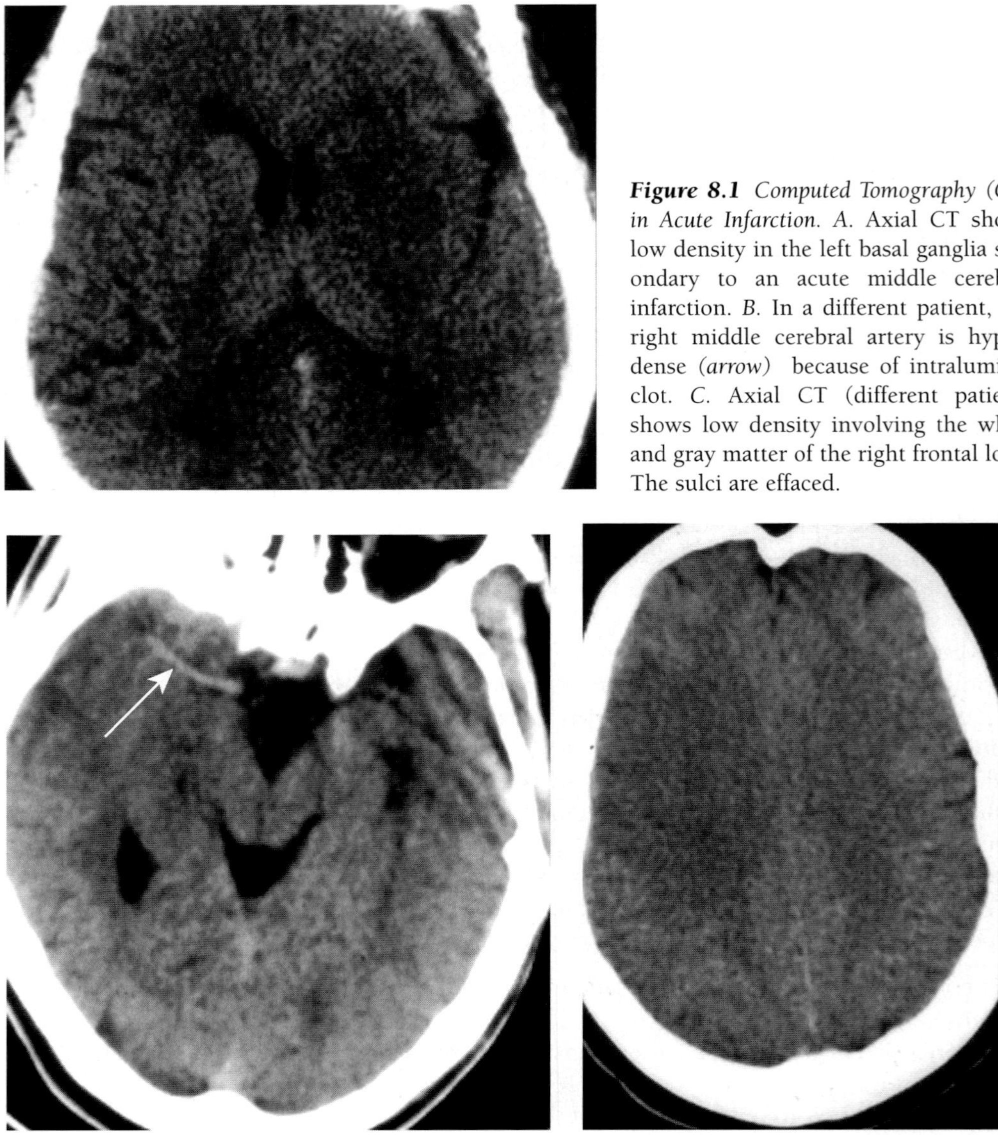

Figure 8.1 *Computed Tomography (CT) in Acute Infarction. A.* Axial CT shows low density in the left basal ganglia secondary to an acute middle cerebral infarction. *B.* In a different patient, the right middle cerebral artery is hyperdense *(arrow)* because of intraluminal clot. *C.* Axial CT (different patient) shows low density involving the white and gray matter of the right frontal lobe. The sulci are effaced.

By CT, only 5% to 10% of all cerebral infarctions contain hemorrhage initially. Most hemorrhagic infarctions represent transformations from ischemic (pale) infarctions. Lysis of the intraarterial clot with sudden reperfusion is responsible for hemorrhagic transformation of infarctions.

Basilar artery thrombosis is an uncommon but catastrophic event (16). Most patients present with nonspecific clinical signs and symptoms and the diagnosis often is delayed. Endovascular thrombolysis may improve their outcome. By CT, a common finding is a hyperdense basilar artery. Hypodensities involving any (or all) of the cerebellar arterial territories or the brainstem are late findings and usually are followed by death (16). Hemorrhagic transformation of posterior circulation infarctions occurs less commonly than in other cerebral infarctions.

Computed Tomographic Angiography

CTA is used to study the carotid bifurcations in the neck, and intracranial aneurysms. Studies are obtained after the injection of high volumes of iodinated 60% contrast material (3 to 5 mL/second for a total of 100 mL) (17). This requires the placement of a wide-bore needle in a large vein. Image acquisition may be begun empirically after waiting approximately 20 to 30 seconds after the initiation of the injection of contrast medium. Drawbacks of this technique include a limited view of the artery in question and the use of intravenous iodinated contrast agents. CTA also has been used in patients with acute stroke. The technique for examination of patients with stroke is similar to the one described previously, but the area imaged is the circle of Willis and above. In patients with acute stroke, cerebral CTA shows acute cutoff of the proximal vessels of the circle of Willis.

Computed Tomographic Perfusion

CT perfusion helps in identifying large infarctions; brainstem and lacunar infarctions may be missed. Subtraction of the precontrast and postcontrast CT studies provides a map of relative cerebral blood volume (rCBV) and readily identifies zones of hypoperfusion (18). These hypoperfused regions correspond with the territory supplied by the occluded vessel. Areas of decreased perfusion (but not absent perfusion) may represent the penumbra at risk (the penumbra usually undergoes a 20% to 40% reduction in cerebral blood flow). Using the time-to-peak parameter of the perfusion curve, over 93% of large infarcts may be identified even before the conventional CT study shows morphologic abnormalities (18,19). Delay in the time-to-peak and slow enhancement indicate hypoperfusion. rCBV can be easily calculated as follows:

rCBV = peak tissue enhancement/peak enhancement in the superior sagittal sinus

Perfusion CT studies usually are of the "first-pass" type and require the administration of a very compact bolus of contrast (no less than 50 mL) through a power injector. Spiral or multislice capabilities are needed; if helical acquisition is used, then only one slice (one location) usually is acquired over a relatively prolonged period (30 seconds). With multidetector units, several slices may be obtained. With the first pass of contrast, a time-to-peak–enhancement curve may be easily generated. The area under this curve is proportional to the rCBV. By selecting a region of interest over a large vessel (in most cases, the MCA), a second time-to-peak curve is generated, and by integrating it into the rCBV curve, one can calculate the relative cerebral blood flow (rCBF). Once rCBF is known, the equation for the mean transit time (MMT) is solved as follows (4):

rCBF = rCBV/MTT

These three parameters are useful in evaluating cerebral perfusion using both CT and MRI. All three parameters are affected in cerebral infarctions. Alterations in rCBF are seen in over 90% of infarcts using CT perfusion.

CT perfusion might be the most reliable and expeditious technique to assess patients suspected of having a cerebral infarction.

Xenon Computed Tomography

A detailed review of the utility of xenon CT is beyond the scope of this chapter. Xenon is a lipophilic molecule that diffuses into the brain, thereby providing a measurement of blood perfusion. Perfusion is calculated by knowing the concentration of the tracer in the blood and its time-dependent accumulation in tissues (20). Data obtained are displayed as quantitative maps of the rCBF and are relatively easy to interpret. Xenon CT demonstrates acute cerebral infarctions within minutes of their onset. Xenon CT also may be used for patients with suspected chronic cerebral ischemia, analysis of cerebral blood flow after temporary test balloon occlusion of an internal carotid artery, ischemia secondary to vasospasm induced by subarachnoid hemorrhage, and alterations of cerebral blood flow after trauma.

Magnetic Resonance Imaging

Conventional Magnetic Resonance Imaging

Studies comparing the utility of CT versus MRI in patients with acute stroke clearly show the superiority of the latter technique (21). Approximately 80% of all cerebral infarctions are seen on MRI by 24 hours after the ictus (22). Administration of contrast (gadolinium chelates) increases the sensitivity of MRI (23). Early MRI abnormalities in acute cerebral infarctions include the lack of normal vascular flow void on noncontrast images, increased intravascular signal on fluid attenuation inversion recovery (FLAIR) images, and the intravascular enhancement sign on contrast enhanced MRI. The former two signs may be present immediately but may be difficult to identify reliably, whereas the latter sign also is present early (<2 hours) after the onset of clinical symptoms and is most obvious when the MCA is affected. The intravascular enhancement sign consists of increased intravascular signal intensity on postcontrast T1-weighted images due to slow intraarterial blood flow (Fig. 8.2A). The second earliest sign is probably a subtle increase in the signal intensity from the affected cerebral cortex on proton-density (balanced) and FLAIR images (Fig. 8.2B). The abnormal cortex also may appear thick. These cortical abnormalities are present as early as 3 hours after the ictus. T2-weighted (including FLAIR) images are more sensitive for the detection of infarctions involving the deep white and gray matter. Brain-

A
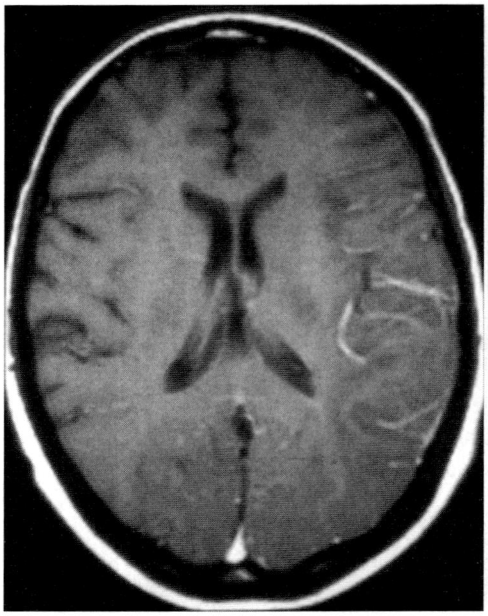

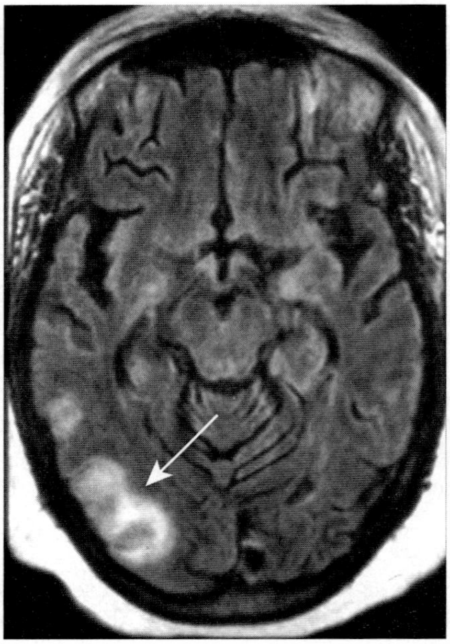
B

C
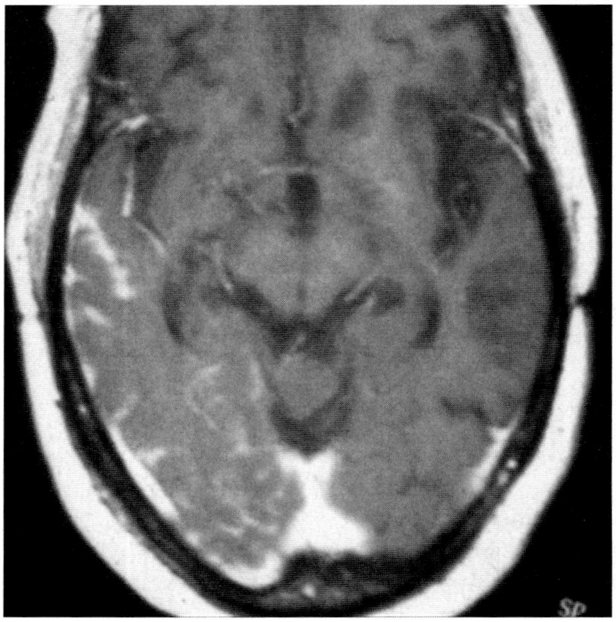

Figure 8.2 *Magnetic Resonance Imaging in Acute Infarction. A.* Axial postcontrast T1-weighted image shows intravascular enhancement in branches of the left middle cerebral artery. Note effacement of sulci in this region secondary to cortical edema. *B.* Axial fluid attenuation inversion recovery (FLAIR) image in a patient with lupus vasculitis shows a right temporooccipital acute infarction *(arrow)*. There is diffuse atrophy. *C.* Postcontrast T1 axial image shows dural and pial enhancement in the right temporooccipital region of a different patient with an acute infarction.

Table 8.2: Findings of Acute Cerebral Infarction on Contrast-Enhanced Magnetic Resonance Imaging

Finding	*Time of Onset*
Intravascular enhancement sign	Very early (<2 hr)
Meningeal enhancement over the infarct	Approximately 24 hr
Mixed phase (meningeal and parenchymal enhancement)	2–3 days
Parenchymal enhancement	After 3–4 days and may persist up to 6 mo

stem infarcts may not be seen well with FLAIR images. Meningeal enhancement overlying the infarct is seen in 30% of patients during the first 24 hours (Fig. 8.2C). Around the second to third day after the infarction, there is a mixed phase in which both intravascular and meningeal enhancement are present. Some lesions that show early and intense enhancement after contrast administration may have a better prognosis than those that do not enhance until later (a fact probably reflecting increased collateral circulation). At approximately the third day after the ictus, meningeal enhancement becomes less prominent and parenchymal enhancement begins. The infarct becomes hyperintense on T2-weighted images. Cerebral contrast enhancement persists for weeks and even up to 6 months. Table 8.2 summarizes the MRI findings in acute infarction (22,23). Conventional magnetic resonance imaging findings in acute cerebral infarction are:

- Lack of normal arterial flow void
- Subtle increased T2 signal intensity in cortex
- Effacement of cortical sulci

Early wallerian degeneration (WD) can be seen as low signal intensity in the corticospinal tract ipsilateral to the infarction (24,25). This is believed to be due to abnormal transport and metabolism of iron. A few days after an infarction, WD is noted as increased T2 signal intensity along the ipsilateral corticospinal tracts and medial thalamus (see below; Fig. 8.3). The importance of these findings is that patients with WD may have a

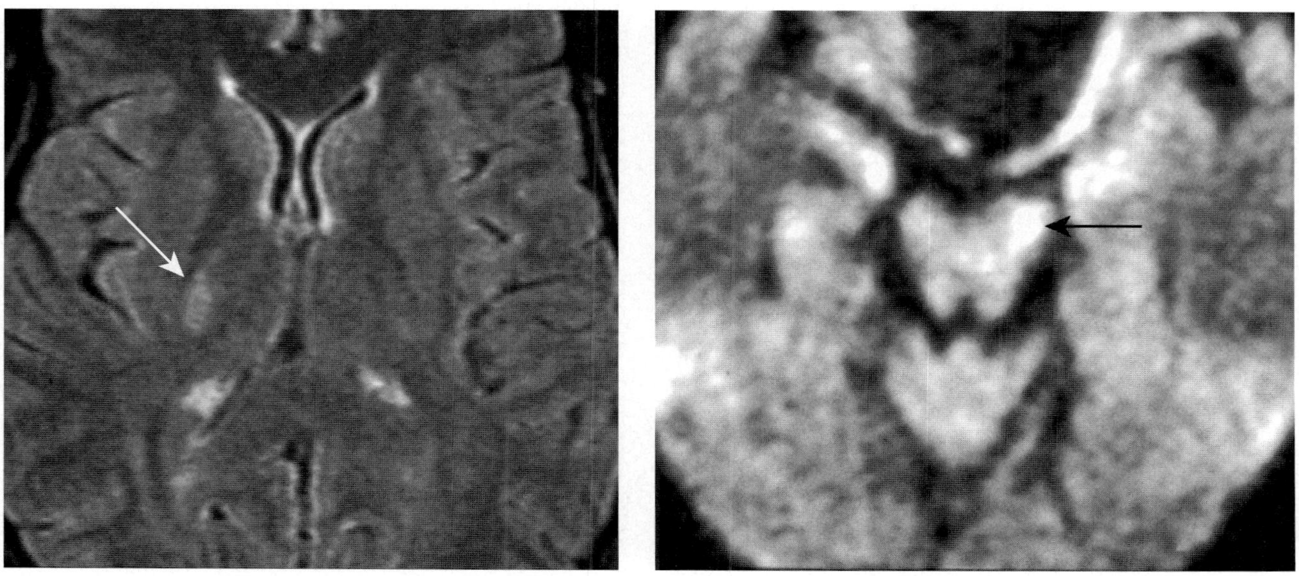

A B

Figure 8.3 *Acute Wallerian Degeneration. A.* Axial fluid attenuation inversion recovery (FLAIR) image shows high signal and swelling of the right corticospinal tract *(arrow)* secondary to an acute infarction located in the convexity (not shown). *B.* Axial diffusion-weighted image shows high signal in the left cerebral peduncle *(arrow)* secondary to an ipsilateral acute middle cerebral artery infarction.

worse prognosis and that this degeneration should not be confused with other, newer infarctions. Acute WD also is detected with diffusion-weighted MRI (DWI) (26). Detection of hemorrhage associated with infarctions is difficult with conventional spin-echo or fast (turbo) spin-echo MRI sequences and usually requires the use of echo planar or gradient (T2*) echo sequences, which are much more sensitive to the presence of magnetic susceptibility artifacts arising from blood products.

Magnetic Resonance Angiography and Venography

Three-dimensional time-of-flight MRA overestimates most stenoses by approximately 20% to 30%.

MR angiography (MRA) may be obtained using time-of-flight (TOF, with or without contrast administration) or phase contrast techniques. We use TOF techniques for evaluation of the vessels in the neck and brain. In the neck, a technique that is sensitive to slow flow (and thereby to the presence of high-grade narrowings) is needed. Two-dimensional (2-D) TOF MRA provides this capability at the expense of slightly lower resolution than other techniques. Because the common carotid artery bifurcation is a relatively large anatomic structure, images with high resolution are not always needed. MRA tends to overestimate all stenoses, and therefore is an ideal screening method (27). The rate of false-positive results is nearly zero. Mild and moderate stenoses are overestimated by approximately 20% to 30%. Distal trickle flow may not be evident on noncontrast TOF MRA. The presence of flow-related enhancement distal to an area of no signal intensity usually signifies a significant stenosis. Normally, there is some loss of flow-related signal intensity in the posterior aspect of the internal carotid artery bulb because of recirculation and turbulence of blood at this level, and this should not be misinterpreted as a stenosis. TOF neck MRA obtained after a bolus of gadolinium decreases this artifact and results in a better depiction of stenoses (we now use it for all neck MRAs). Using a coronal three-dimensional gradient-echo technique, the circulation from the aortic arch to the circle of Willis may be evaluated. The visualization of the aortic origin of the great vessels is very important because after the carotid artery bifurcation in the neck, their aortic ostia are the second most common site of stenosis.

Three-dimensional TOF MRA usually is used to evaluate vessels of the circle of Willis. This technique offers slightly more resolution than its 2-D counterpart, but is less sensitive to slower blood flow. Although visualization of the central intracranial vessels tends to be good, the peripheral circulation is not well displayed. MRA shows vessel narrowing or occlusion in the acute stroke period (Fig. 8.4).

A

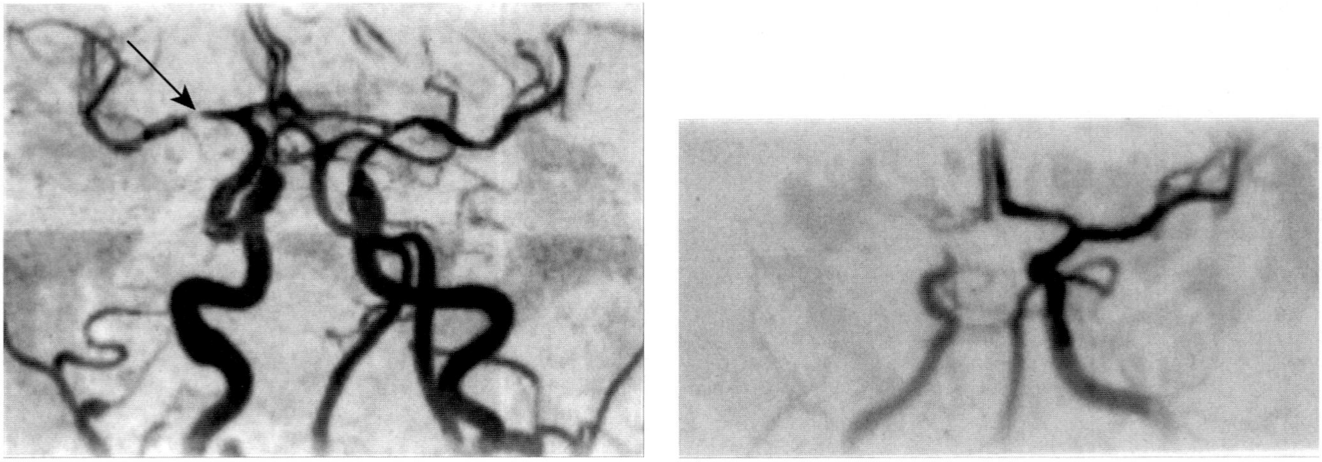

B

Figure 8.4 *Magnetic Resonance Angiography in Stroke. A.* Frontal oblique view shows significant narrowing *(arrow)* of the right middle cerebral artery in this patient with an acute infarction corresponding to this territory. The contralateral middle cerebral artery is irregular. *B.* Frontal view in a patient with a right cerebral hemisphere infarction shows attenuated flow-related signal in the right internal and anterior cerebral arteries and lack of flow in the middle cerebral artery.

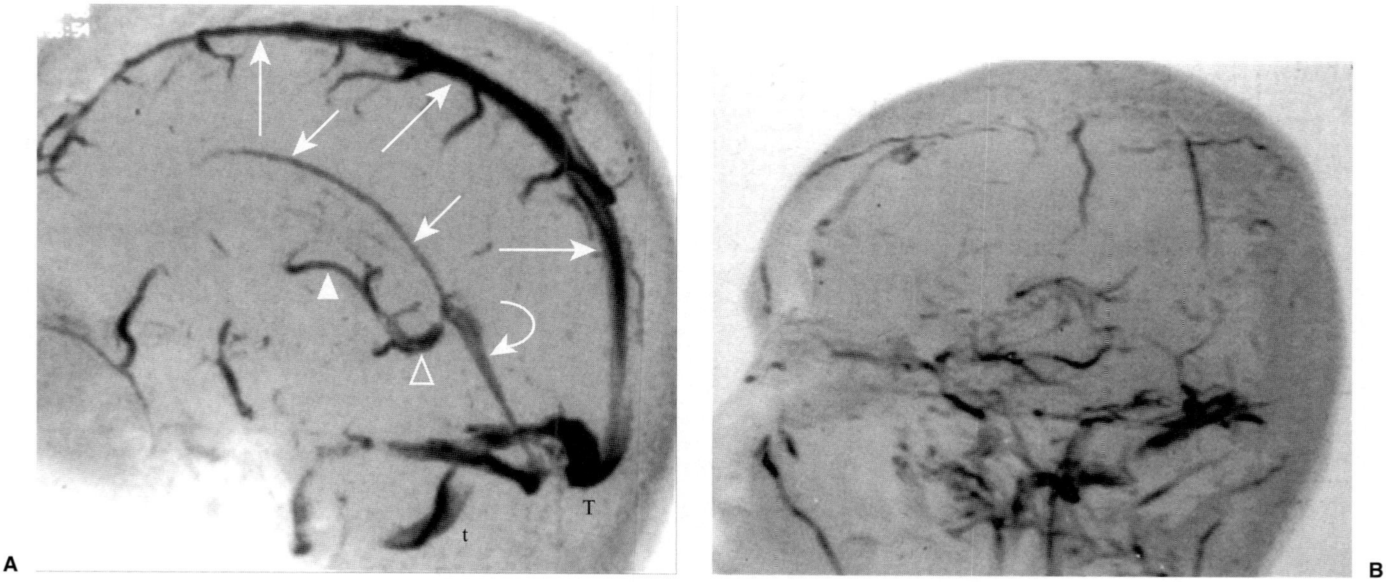

Figure 8.5 *Magnetic Resonance Venography in Venous Thrombosis. A.* Lateral oblique view of a normal venogram shows the major sinuses and the deep venous system (*large arrows*, superior sagittal sinus; *small arrows*, inferior sagittal sinus; *solid arrowhead*, internal cerebral veins; *open arrowhead*, vein of Galen; *curved arrow*, straight sinus; *T*, venous torcular; *t*, transverse sinuses). *B.* Lateral view shows lack of flow in most venous sinuses and deep system (compare with *A*). There is some flow in the transverse and sigmoid sinuses.

Venous thrombosis is more common in patients with infections, but also may be aseptic. Most occlusions affect the superior sagittal and transverse sinuses (Fig. 8.5). The thrombosed sinus is hyperintense on noncontrast T1-weighted images (28). MR venograms may be obtained with 2-D TOF or phase contrast techniques. Bright intraluminal clot may "shine through" in the maximum-intensity projections done for TOF MR venograms and may simulate patency. I obtain TOF MR venograms aligning the source images in two different planes. The first is a coronal plane that allows for visualization of most of the superior sagittal and transverse sinuses. With this projection, the distal aspect of the superior sagittal sinus and proximal transverse sinuses becomes nearly parallel to the axis of the images, and some flow-related enhancement is normally lost. This problem may be compensated by acquiring another TOF venogram with the source images oriented at a slightly oblique sagittal (angled) position. This problem usually is avoided by using phase contrast MR venography.

Proton Magnetic Resonance Spectroscopy

In clinical practice, most MR spectroscopy is obtained using protons (HMRS). Spectroscopy using long echo times (TE) allows for identification of lactate and its confirmation by inverting its peak by switching from a TE of 256 milliseconds to 128 milliseconds. Lactate normally is not present in the brain (except perhaps during the first few hours of life) (29). A conversion of aerobic to anaerobic glycolysis, as seen in cerebral infarctions, induces a buildup of lactate (Fig. 8.6). In addition, the levels of other metabolites such as *N*-acetyl aspartate (NAA), choline, and creatine are decreased in the infarcted zone (29). These metabolic abnormalities may remain present up to 5 weeks postinfarction. The penumbra may be identified and shows low NAA, choline, and creatine but no significant lactate levels, or some lactate but normal concentrations of the other metabolites. HMRS detects cerebral infarctions earlier than does conventional MRI.

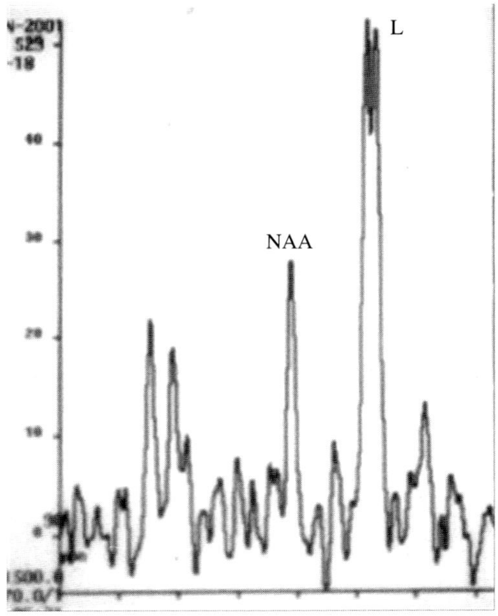

Figure 8.6 *Proton Magnetic Resonance Spectroscopy in Acute Infarction.* Long echo time study shows low N-acetyl aspartate *(NAA)* and a large double peak of lactate *(L)*.

Rarely, some hyperacute infarctions are not appreciated on DWI, but perfusion MRI shows the abnormality in these rare cases.

Diffusion Magnetic Resonance Imaging

DWI provides physiologic information. After cessation of perfusion, alterations in the sodium/potassium pump lead to increased intracellular accumulation of water and restriction of the normal random motion of extracellular fluid (30). It is this restriction in the free movement (Brownian motion) of extracellular water that DWI measures. Echo planar capabilities are desirable to perform DWI. Two diffusion-sensitizing gradients change the phase of water protons (mostly those in the extracellular space) that, when free to move, cancel out their signal intensity (31). The addition of diffusion-sensitizing gradients to echo planar gradient-echo or spin-echo images results in an increased sensitivity to restriction of Brownian motion of water. In the presence of normal water motion, signal intensity is lost because of random dephasing of the spins. Restriction in the motion of these spins results in increased signal intensity. Infarctions are seen as areas of high signal intensity on DWI. DWI identifies cerebral infarctions within 1 hour of onset and possibly within minutes of occurrence, and well before conventional MRI (32) (Fig. 8.7A and B). Therefore, if anticoagulation or thrombolytic therapy is considered, DWI stratifies patients into those with infarctions and those with TIAs. Recently, several articles have described negative DWI in presence of hyperacute infarctions (33,34). All of these patients were scanned 2 to 3 hours after the onset of symptoms. Perfusion MR studies demonstrated these infarctions despite normal DWI results. All patients showed abnormal DWI study results 6 or more hours after the ictus. I have seen this phenomenon in cerebral deep infarcts, but not in major territorial or cortical ones. I also have seen several cases of hyperacute basilar artery thrombosis with initially normal DWI results. From a theoretical standpoint, DWI may both overestimate or underestimate the size of an infarction. In our experience, these differences are minimal and do not affect the clinical management of the patients. DWI abnormalities may reverse after successful thrombolysis. Abnormalities as seen on single-axis and trace DWI reflect both restrictions of water motion as well as shine-through from prolonged T2 relaxation (35). However, with apparent diffusion coefficient (ADC) maps, this T2 shine-through phenomenon is eliminated (Fig. 8.7C). From a practical standpoint, it is easier to visualize the infarctions on trace images than on ADC maps. To assess the amount of shine-through present on the trace diffusion-weighted images, the radiologist needs to evaluate the ADC map (where infarctions appear as dark areas). I always look at the trace images first, and then confirm the presence of an infarction by correlating it with the ADC map.

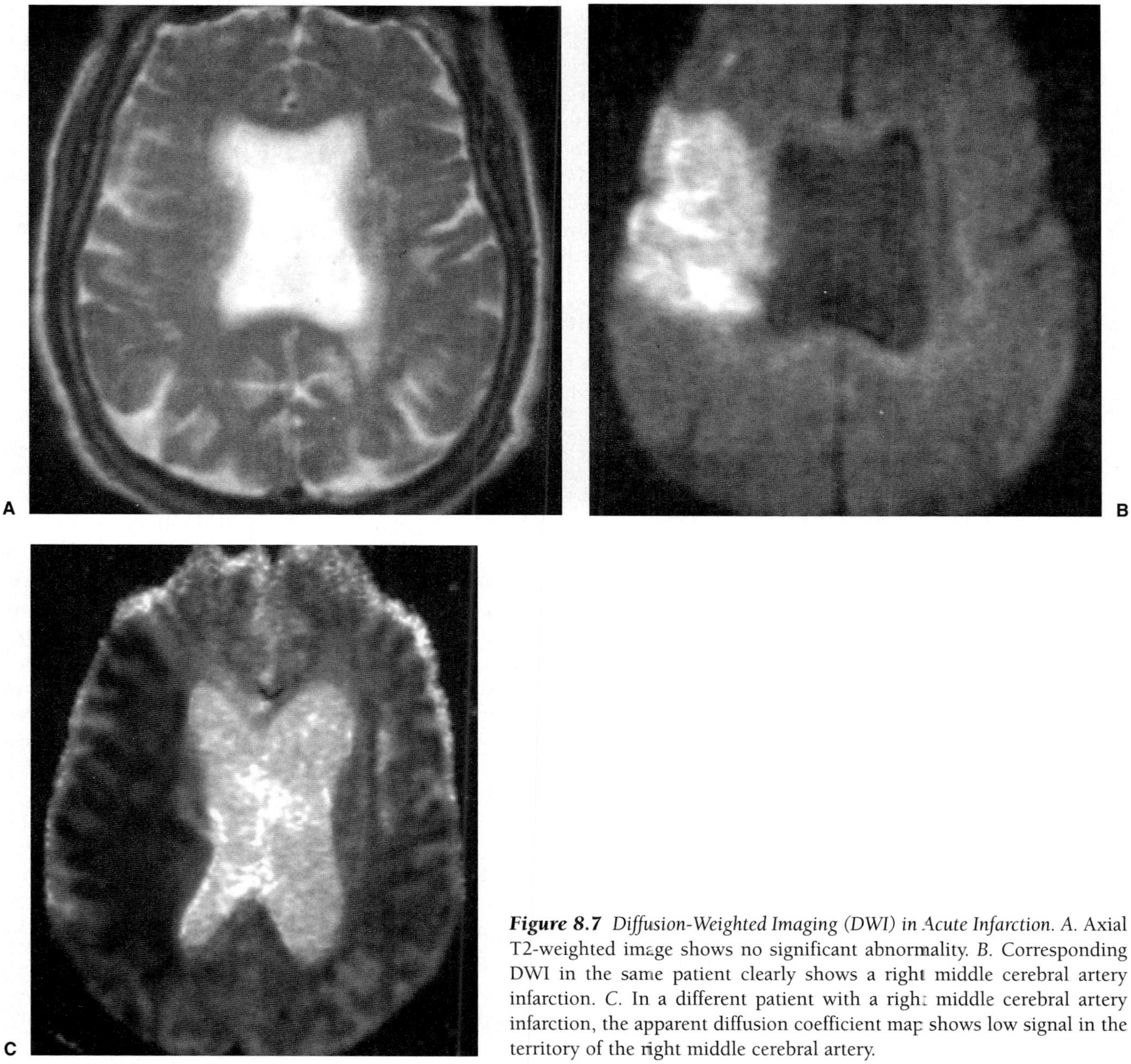

Figure 8.7 *Diffusion-Weighted Imaging (DWI) in Acute Infarction. A.* Axial T2-weighted image shows no significant abnormality. *B.* Corresponding DWI in the same patient clearly shows a right middle cerebral artery infarction. *C.* In a different patient with a right middle cerebral artery infarction, the apparent diffusion coefficient map shows low signal in the territory of the right middle cerebral artery.

Perfusion Magnetic Resonance Imaging

Perfusion MRI may be one of the most reliable studies available with which to demonstrate hyperacute cerebral infarctions. Because the first pathophysiologic alterations in an infarction are decreased or absent blood flow, this technique depicts acute infarctions reliably. Perfusion MRI provides information regarding the status of the cerebral microvasculature. Echo planar spin-echo techniques are better to evaluate smaller vessels (capillary level), and gradient-echo techniques display larger vessels (36). Perfusion MRI provides information regarding rCBV and the vascular mean transit time. A standard dose of MR contrast is given intravenously by power injection. Dynamic spin-echo echo planar susceptibility images or gradient-echo images are then obtained every 2 seconds for 1 minute. Perfusion MRI may be even more sensitive than DWI in the identification of hyperacute cerebral infarction (37). These studies require extensive postprocessing and a pixel-by-pixel analysis to generate perfusion maps that are visually pleasing and easy to interpret. Because gadolinium extravasates to some degree during the first pass, it is not the optimal perfusion agent. Work in progress indicates that labeling the blood spins with a radiofrequency at the level of the neck and imaging them in the brain may be a promising way to depict rCBF. It is important to remember that hypoperfused areas may or may not become infarcted. Thus, the penumbra may be defined as an area of hypoperfusion with normal DWI, whereas the core of an infarction is hypoperfused and shows hyperintensity on DWI (4). The parameters obtained with perfusion MRI (and also CT perfusion) have been discussed previously. The eventual size of the infarct probably is between the size of the DWI abnormality and that of the abnormality as seen on perfusion studies.

Interventional Procedures

These procedures may be used in the arterial or venous circulations. Risks of thrombolysis include rupture or perforation of a vessel, dissection, and aggravation of the disease secondary to hemorrhages. Hemorrhages elsewhere in body (chest and abdomen) also may occur. Recent pregnancy, surgery, or coagulopathies are contraindications to intraarterial thrombolysis. The window of opportunity for occlusions in the anterior circulation probably is approximately 3 hours, whereas it may be as long as 6 hours (or even longer) in the vertebrobasilar arteries (15). Some authors have shown that anterior circulation strokes are amenable to thrombolysis even after 6 hours and that patients with posterior circulation strokes may benefit from thrombolysis beyond the initial 12 hours (15). These observations probably are based on the fact that a "physiologic" window of opportunity exists and that it is only loosely related to the traditional window of opportunity. It is possible that in the future, a combination of functional MRI sequences will identify patients who may benefit from thrombolysis regardless of the traditional window of opportunity. Maximal thrombolysis is achieved if the tip of the microcatheter is embedded in the clot. After lysing the clot, underlying stenoses not uncommonly are found. Some interventional neuroradiologists use angioplasty and stents to enlarge these narrowings. A complete discussion of these procedures is beyond the scope of this book.

Cerebral Infarctions

I now review (at the risk of repeating myself) the imaging features of cerebral infarctions according to the most common sites in which they occur.

Middle Cerebral Artery Infarctions

Acute

Approximately 75% of all cerebral infarctions involve the territory of the MCA (14). Cerebral infarctions are the third most common cause of death in the United States, and the mortality rate with each episode varies between 15% and 35% (1). Emboli originating from atherosclerosis in the common and internal carotid arteries (particularly the bifurcation) are the most common cause of MCA occlusion. Approximately 50% to 60% of patients with an MCA infarction have a negative CT during the initial 12 hours (see earlier) (14). The importance of CT lies in establishing the presence or absence of hemorrhage, therefore determining the prescription of thrombolytic or conservative treatments. Early CT signs (<24 hours) of MCA infarction include hyperdense MCA on noncontrast CT (25% to 50%), "disappearing" lentiform nucleus, and loss of insular cortex (Fig. 8.1).

The most common cerebral infarction involves the territory of an MCA, and most are caused by embolus.

Approximately 80% of MCA infarctions are identified by MRI during the initial 24 hours. The earliest abnormality is the intravascular enhancement sign, which may be seen 2 hours after ictus and probably is caused by slow, bright intraarterial blood flow (see earlier) (23) (Fig. 8.2A). Increased intravascular signal intensity on FLAIR images also is seen very acutely (Fig. 8.2B). Meningeal enhancement overlying infarcted territory is seen in 30% of cases during the first 3 days (Fig. 8.2C). Cortical edema (hyperintensity, increased thickness, and a blurry gray–white matter junction) may be seen as early as 3 hours after a stroke, particularly in proton-density and FLAIR images.

Subacute

Mass effect increases during the first 3 days, and CT shows a wedge-shaped area of low density that involves both gray and white matter (14) (Fig. 8.8). CT has a sensitivity of over 90% in detection of subacute infarcts involving the MCA territory. Gyral enhancement (which may reflect luxury perfusion) begins 3 to 7 days after ictus and may correlate with a better prognosis than infarcts with no gyral enhancement. Hemorrhage (especially in the basal ganglia and cortex) eventually occurs in approximately 15% of all MCA infarctions. Hemorrhagic transformation usually occurs 1 to 4 days after onset of infarction (Fig. 8.9).

The findings on MRI already have been reviewed, and I address them only briefly here. As intravascular and meningeal enhancement become less prominent, they are followed by parenchymal (especially cortex) enhancement that begins 3 to 7 days after ictus and may persist from 1 week to 6 months. The infarctions become markedly hyperintense on proton-density and T2-weighted images (including FLAIR). Approximately 75% of all subacute MCA infarctions show parenchymal contrast enhancement (Fig. 8.10). Chronic changes of malacia (with loss of volume) ensue later, with or without evidence of old blood (hemosiderin) in the region of the infarction. The findings on DWI correlate with the findings on conventional MRI and are shown in Table 8.3 (38).

Chronic infarctions may calcify (39). This calcification is dystrophic and tends to occur in less than 5% of infarctions. Accumulation of intracellular calcium is a part of coagulative necrosis. Once the cell membrane has been damaged, intracellular calcium accumulates.

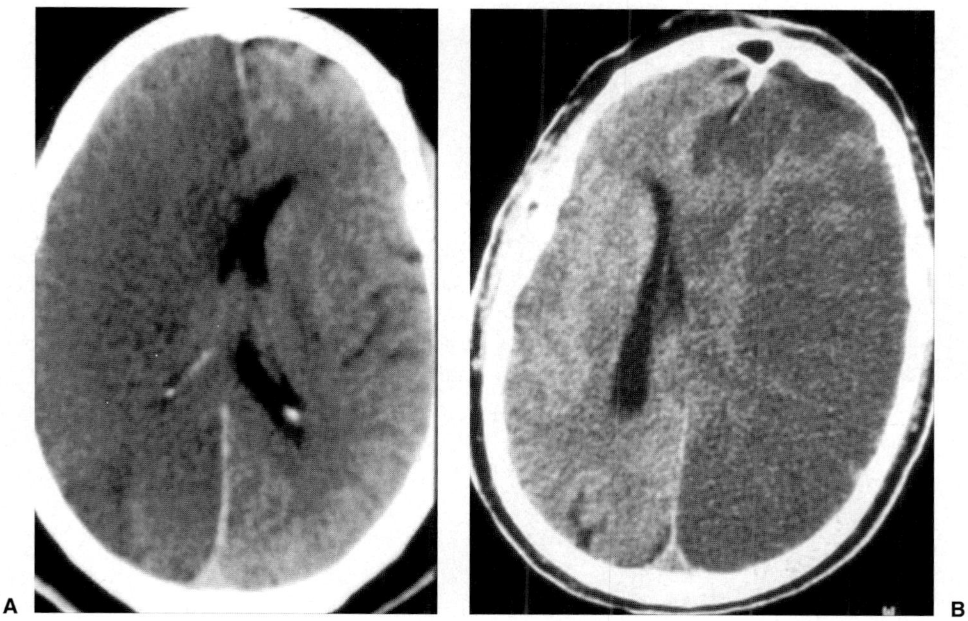

Figure 8.8 *Computed Tomography (CT) in Subacute Infarction. A.* Axial CT shows diffuse low density and sulci effacement in the right cerebral hemisphere. There is mass effect with a mild shift of the midline structures to the left. *B.* Axial CT shows significant swelling of the left cerebral hemisphere with a significant midline shift to the right, resulting in a left anterior cerebral artery infarction.

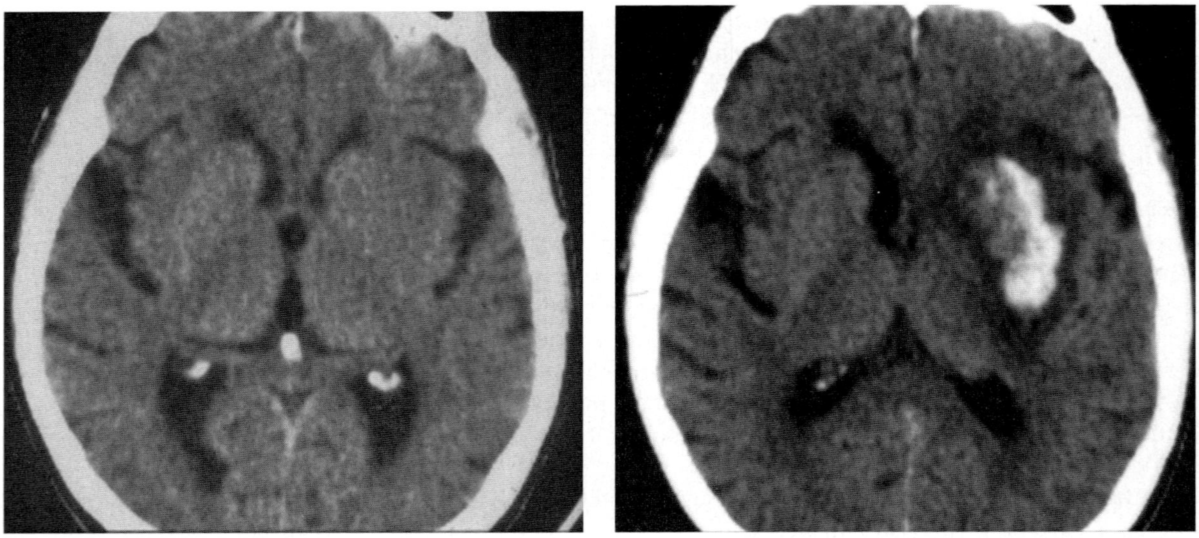

A B

Figure 8.9 *Hemorrhagic Infarction. A.* Computed tomography (CT) during acute period shows only subtle low density in the left basal ganglia in this patient with symptoms of a corresponding middle cerebral artery infarction. *B.* Three days later, CT shows acute clot and surrounding edema in the left basal ganglia due to hemorrhagic transformation.

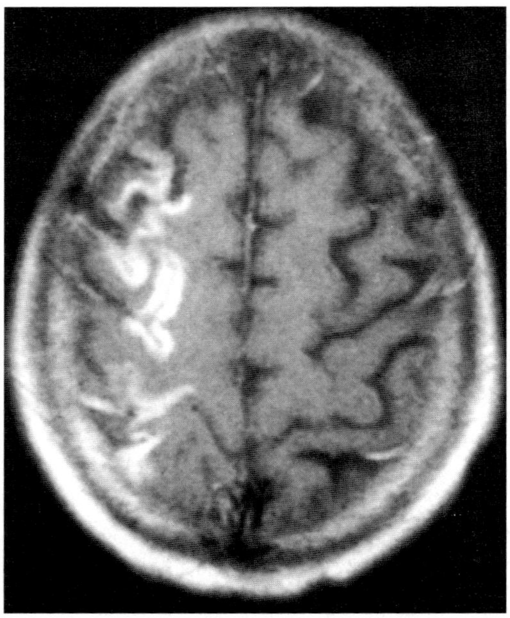

Figure 8.10 *Magnetic Resonance Imaging in Subacute Infarction.* Axial postcontrast T1-weighted image shows cortical enhancement secondary to a right middle cerebral artery infarction.

Table 8.3: Time Course of Signal Intensity Changes of Cerebral Infarctions on Diffusion-Weighted Imaging

Time Period	*Diffusion-Weighted Imaging*	*Magnetic Resonance Imaging*
Hyperacute	Nearly always bright	Normal images, absent flow voids, intravascular enhancement sign
Acute	Bright	Above + increased signal in cortex and sulci effacement
Subacute	Less bright (tends to "pseudonormalize" at approximately 2–3 wk postinfarction)	Above + meningeal and parenchymal enhancement
Late subacute and chronic	Negative (Fig. 8.11)	Parenchymal enhancement + development of loss of volume

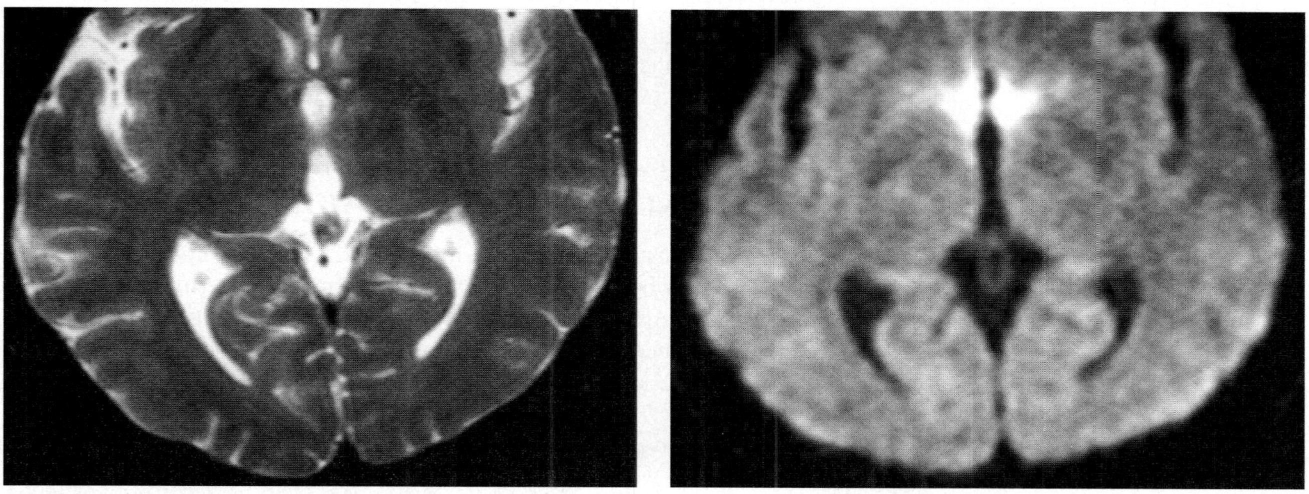

A B

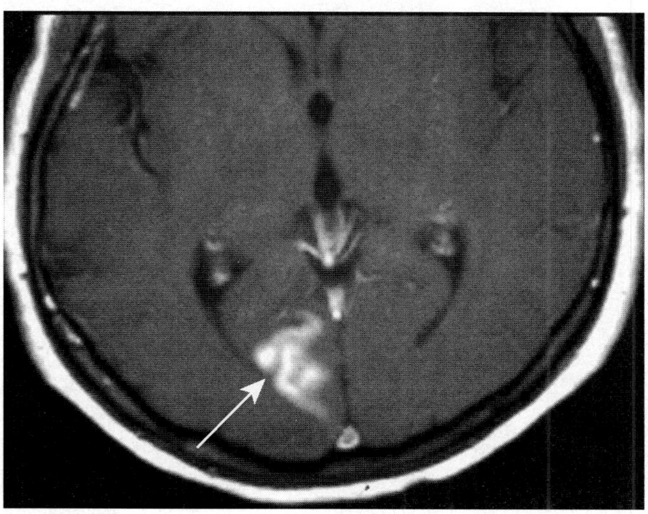

C

Figure 8.11 *Pseudonormalization of Infarction. A.* Axial T2-weighted image shows no significant abnormality approximately 2 weeks after the ictus. *B.* The corresponding diffusion-weighted image also is negative. *C.* Corresponding postcontrast T1-weighted image shows cortical enhancement *(arrow)* in the right occipital lobe.

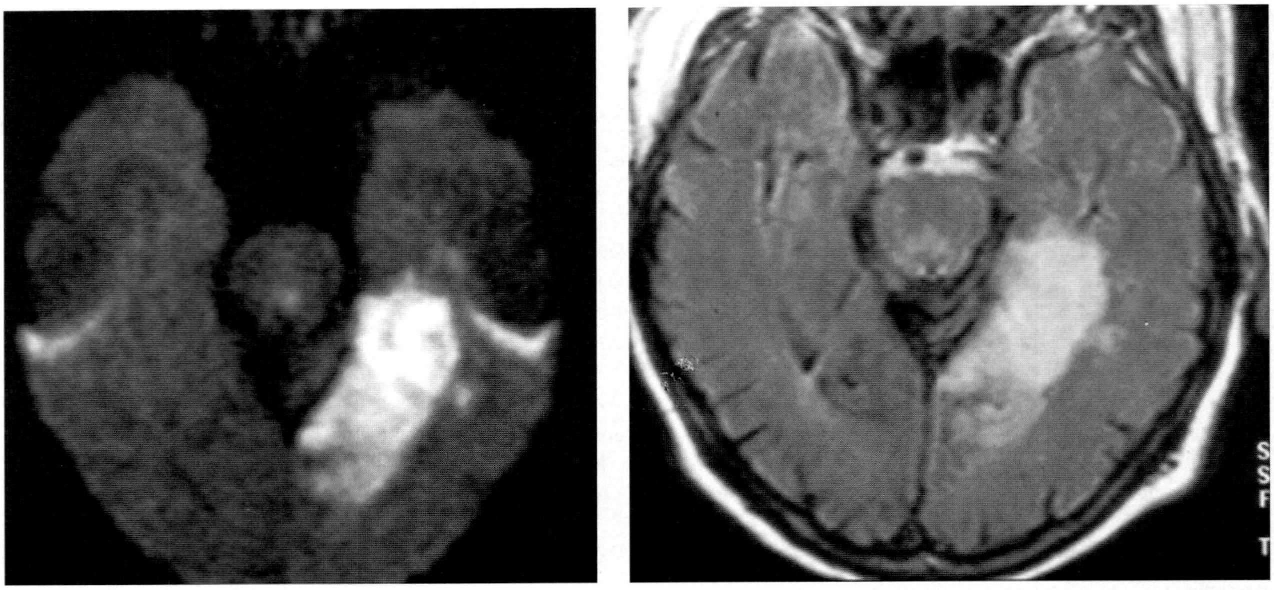

A B

Figure 8.12 *Posterior Cerebral Artery Infarction. A.* Axial diffusion-weighted image shows a bright acute infarction involving the territory of the left posterior cerebral artery. *B.* Corresponding axial fluid attenuation inversion recovery (FLAIR) image shows similar findings.

Posterior and Anterior Cerebral Artery Infarctions

PCA infarctions are the most common after internal carotid artery and MCA infarctions (40). PCA infarcts also may be seen with downward transtentorial herniation secondary to compression of the PCA between the temporal lobe and edge of the tentorium. Transtentorial herniation may produce bilateral PCA infarctions. Involvement of the medial occip-

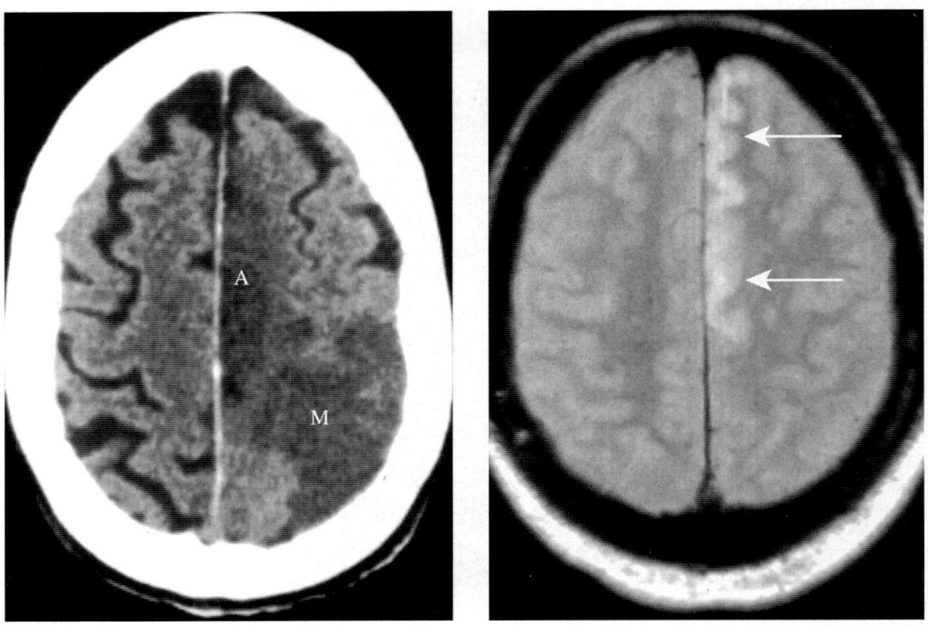

A B

Figure 8.13 *Anterior Cerebral Artery Infarction. A.* Axial computed tomography shows infarctions in the territories of the left middle *(M)* and anterior *(A)* cerebral arteries. *B.* Axial proton-density image shows cortical edema in the territory of the left anterior cerebral artery *(arrows)* due to an acute infarction.

ital lobe causes homonymous hemianopsia. The findings in PCA infarction include hypodensity (CT) or hyperintensity (T2-weighted or FLAIR images) in the medial occipital lobe(s) or involving the entire occipital lobe(s) (Fig. 8.12). An intravascular enhancement sign may be present in both PCA and ACA infarctions.

Most ACA infarctions occur in combination with internal carotid artery occlusion. Isolated ACA infarctions are rare (<1%). Unlike MCA infarctions, most ACA infarctions result from primary vessel disease and not emboli. ACA infarctions also may be secondary to subfalcine herniation and "clipping" of the ACA under the falx cerebri. By imaging, the most the common sign in ACA infarction is hypodensity (CT) or hyperintensity (T2-weighted and FLAIR images) along the medial cerebral convexity (Fig. 8.13). ACA infarcts also may produce edema of the corpus callosum secondary to occlusion of short perforating branches. Although unilateral ACA infarctions carry a relatively good prognosis, bilateral ones are catastrophic. ACA infarcts also may be seen after the clipping of aneurysms arising in the anterior communicating artery. ACA infarctions rarely are hemorrhagic.

Although previously believed to be very rare, infarctions of the corpus callosum are not uncommonly encountered when using DWI.

Hemorrhagic Infarctions

A hemorrhagic infarction is considered as such if it contains blood within 24 hours of the ictus, whereas hemorrhagic transformation of an infarction occurs when blood is identified 2 to 14 days after the ictus (14). Most hemorrhagic infarctions occur as a consequence of underlying ischemic infarctions. Most hemorrhagic infarctions are due to sudden reperfusion (lysis of intraarterial clot) to damaged tissues that include weak blood vessel walls (also called *breakthrough bleeding*). Hemorrhagic infarctions also are common after septic embolism (Fig. 8.14). By CT, only 5% of all cerebral infarctions initially are hemorrhagic (14). CT shows hemorrhage in 15% to 50% of patients with large strokes, especially when the MCA territory is involved initially (Fig. 8.9). Other types of hemorrhagic infarctions include laminar necrosis and venous infarcts. Hemorrhagic infarcts are assumed to have a worse prognosis than nonhemorrhagic infarctions, but this view recently has been challenged and may not be true. CT is an ideal method to evaluate for acute blood. It is conceivable that small amounts of hemorrhage may be missed on conventional MRI. Gradient-echo imaging and echo planar imaging (such as DWI) are extremely sensitive to the presence of acute blood (which nearly always appears as dark areas on both sequences), and, in my experience, clinically significant hemorrhage is not missed if one uses these sequences (41) (Fig. 8.14).

Hemorrhagic infarctions and hemorrhagic transformation of an infarction more commonly involve the territory of an MCA.

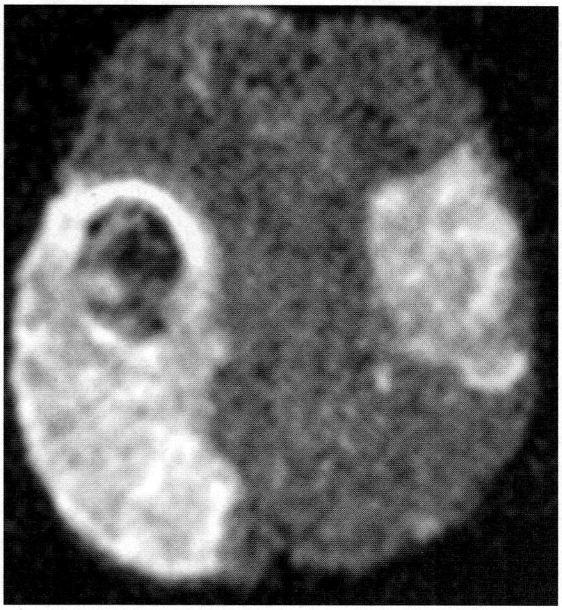

Figure 8.14 *Hemorrhagic Infarction.* Axial diffusion-weighted image shows acute infarctions in territories supplied by both middle cerebral arteries. Note low signal (due to magnetic susceptibility) in a hematoma located amid the right infarction. These infarctions were due to septic emboli.

Cerebellar and Brainstem Infarctions

The posterior inferior cerebellar artery (PICA) is the most commonly occluded cerebellar artery, followed by the superior and anterior inferior cerebellar arteries (40,42) (Fig. 8.15). Occlusion of the PICA may produce Wallenberg's syndrome, in which the lateral medulla and the inferior cerebellar peduncle are involved. In this syndrome,

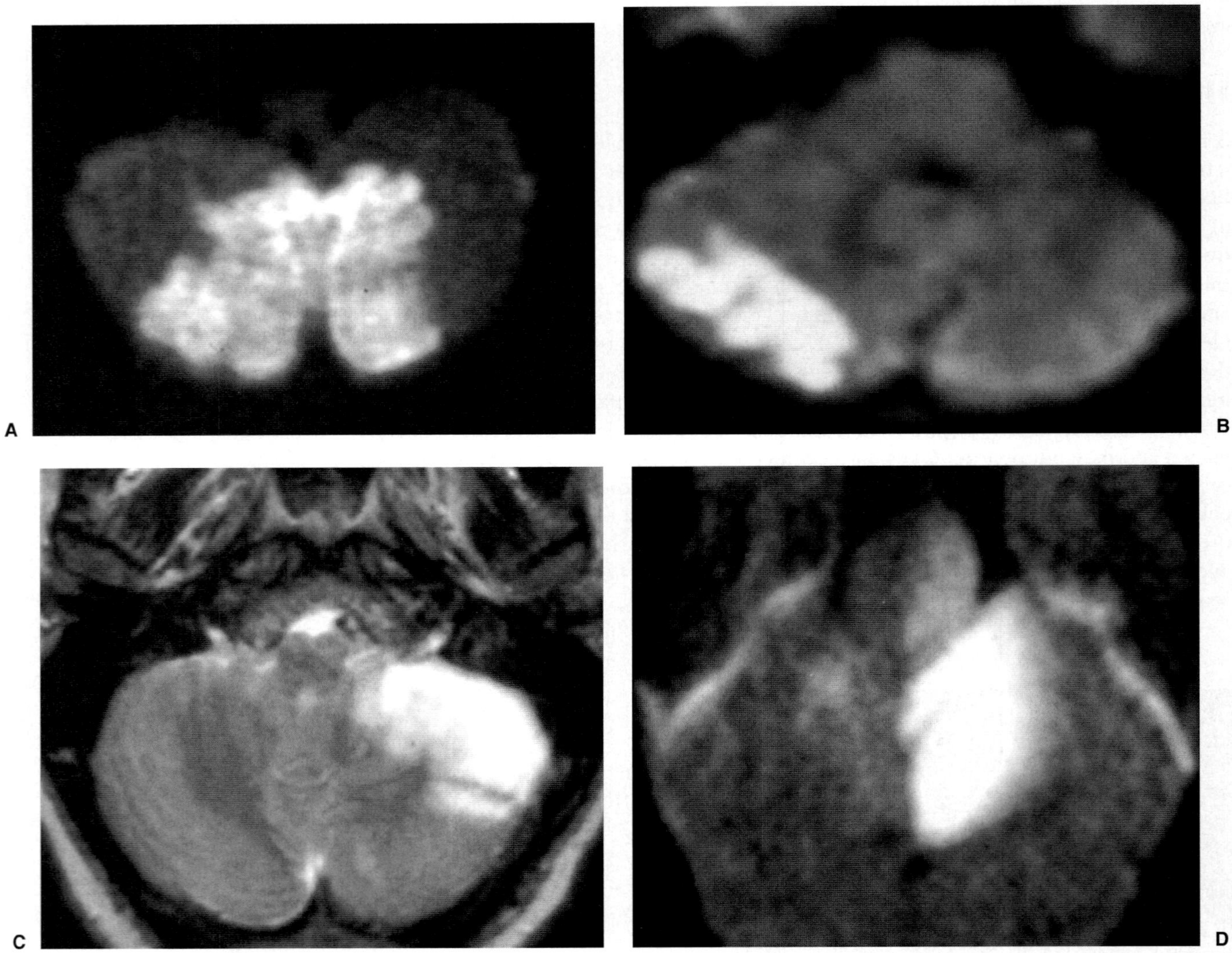

Figure 8.15 *Infarctions in Territories Supplied by the Vertebrobasilar Circulation. A.* Axial diffusion-weighted image (DWI) shows acute infarctions in the territories supplied by both posterior inferior cerebellar arteries. *B.* Axial DWI shows acute infarction in a territory probably supplied by hemispheric branches of the right posterior inferior cerebellar artery. *C.* Axial T2-weighted image shows hyperintensity in the territory of the left anterior inferior cerebral artery. *D.* Axial DWI shows an acute infarction involving the left superior cerebellar artery territory. Note also involvement of the brainstem in this patient, with a clot at the apex of the basilar artery.

there is loss of pain and temperature sensation on the contralateral side of the body, ipsilateral motor findings, ataxia, and nystagmus. Cerebellar infarcts also may occur in association with basilar artery occlusion (see later). Cerebellar infarcts may lead rapidly to death by compression of brainstem and acute obstructive hydrocephalus (secondary to compression of the fourth ventricle). Upward cerebellar herniation (seen as effacement of the quadrigeminal plate cistern) also may occur. Emergency resection of involved cerebellum may be required as a life-saving measure. Cerebellar infarctions may be difficult to image by CT owing to the presence of artifacts, and are better evaluated with DWI and MRI (43). For unknown reasons, cerebellar infarctions almost never are hemorrhagic.

In basilar artery thrombosis, the mortality rate is 2.5 times higher than with occlusion of one internal carotid artery (16). Common etiologies for thrombosis of the basilar artery include embolism, atherosclerosis, vascular malformations of the base of the skull, syphilis, and tuberculous or fungal meningitis. If only the distal portion of the basilar artery is occluded, the "top-of-the-basilar" syndrome is produced, resulting in infarcts of thalami, posterior limbs of internal capsules, and midbrain. Infarcts of the pons may lead to a "locked-in" syndrome that is characterized by retained consciousness and voluntary eye movements with quadriparesis. Because of the high mortality rate associated with basilar artery thrombosis, intraarterial thrombolysis may be attempted despite carrying a mortality/morbidity risk of over 30%. I prefer to classify basilar artery thromboses into two types. The first one is acute and complete thrombosis; these patients usually die immediately and are not imaged. The etiology for these cases may be embolic. The second type may be acute or progressive, and has a slower course. These patients usually have progressive thrombosis due to a variety of reasons, such as heart disease (and low cardiac output), dehydration, and so forth. This group comprises most of the patients imaged for basilar artery thrombosis because they live longer. CT may show a hyperdense basilar artery (16). Unfortunately, basilar artery thrombosis tends to happen in older individuals in whom the basilar artery walls may be calcified, resulting in increased CT density. I always compare the density of the basilar artery with that of the supraclinoid internal carotid arteries. If the basilar artery is denser and the history is appropriate then MRI should be rapidly obtained. The conventional MRI shows lack of flow void in the basilar artery (Fig. 8.16A). DWI shows increased signal intensity in the pons (if this has occurred, the value of thrombolysis is questionable; Fig. 8.16B–D). This high signal intensity may be easier to see on trace DWI than on ADC maps (44). The combined effects of white matter tract anisotropy, T2 shine-through, and water motion restriction makes the lesions quite obvious on single-axis DWI. MRA clearly displays the absence of flow-related enhancement in the basilar artery and its branches.

Brainstem infarctions may be easier to visualize on single-axis DWI than on trace DWI and ADC maps.

Diffuse Hypoxia/Anoxia

Etiologies for diffuse cerebral anoxia in adults include trauma, severe hypotension or hypertension, acute radiation, and venous sinus occlusion (45). In children, the etiologies for diffuse brain anoxia are mainly dehydration, neonatal anoxia, and child abuse (46). Hypoxia/ischemia preferentially and initially involves the gray matter structures because of their higher metabolic rate (this is called *selective vulnerability*). Generalized brain hypoxia also may give rise to watershed (border zone) infarcts or laminar (deep layers of cortex) necrosis. On CT, the brain shows diffuse effacement of the gray–white junctions and the cerebrospinal fluid–containing spaces. Hypodensity in the gray matter (particularly in the basal ganglia) may be seen as early as 24 hours after the insult. I believe that MRI is more sensitive in the evaluation of diffuse brain

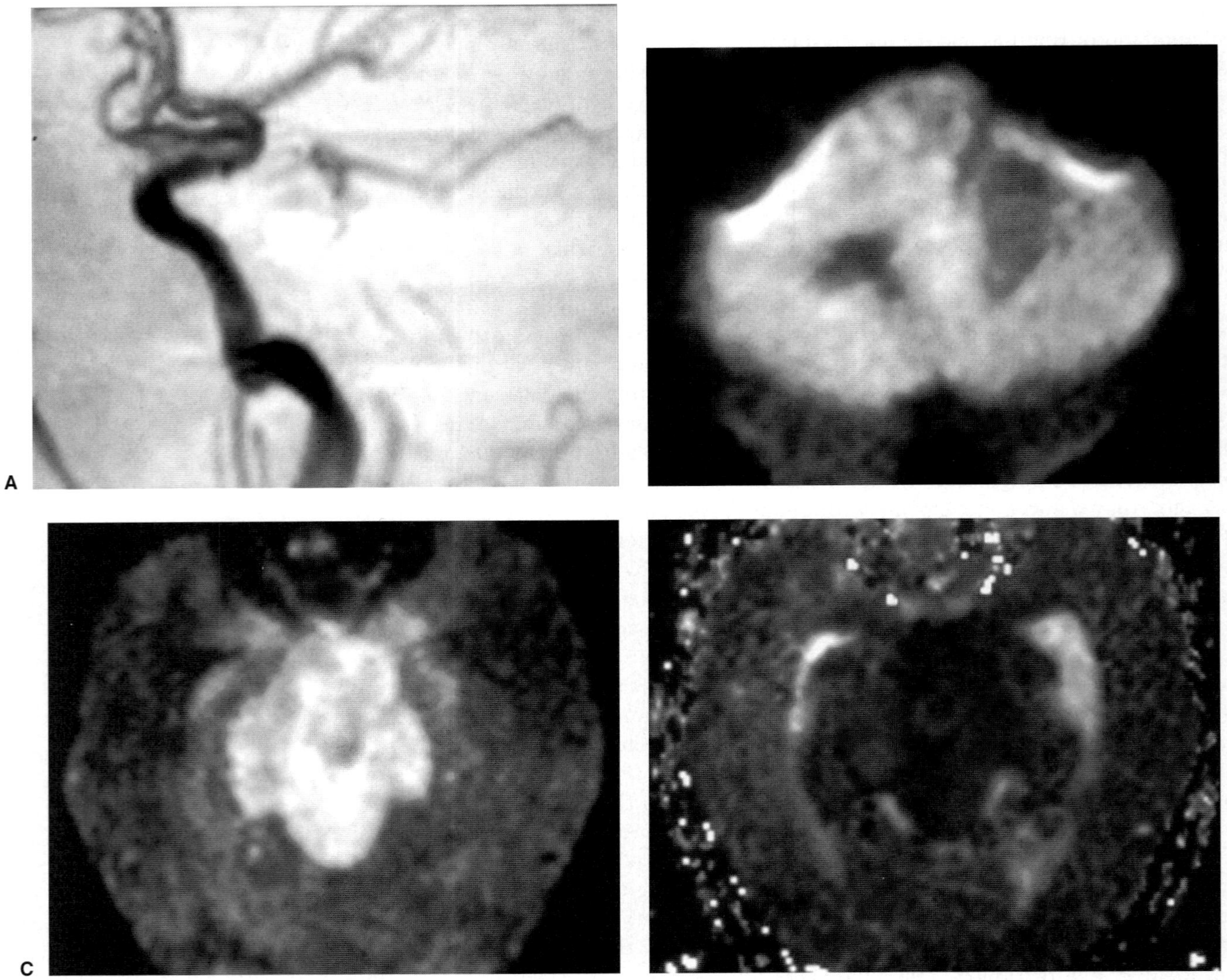

Figure 8.16 *Basilar Artery Thrombosis. A.* Lateral view of a magnetic resonance angiogram shows absence of the body of the basilar artery. There is some flow in the posterior cerebral arteries, presumably established through the posterior communicating arteries. *B.* Axial diffusion-weighted image (DWI) shows acute infarction of the cerebellum and brainstem. *C.* In a different patient, axial DWI shows acute infarction in the cerebellum and brainstem. *D.* Corresponding apparent diffusion coefficient map shows very low signal in that same region, confirming that the signal on the DWI is due to water motion restriction and not T2 shine-through phenomenon.

hypoxia, particularly if DWI is used (Fig. 8.17). The findings on MRI are shown in Table 8.4.

Laminar Necrosis

Laminar necrosis is more commonly a sequela of diffuse anoxia, but also may be seen after focal and territorial infarctions.

Laminar necrosis refers to ischemic changes in the cortex of the cerebrum and cerebellum. Although usually secondary to generalized brain hypoxia, laminar necrosis also may be seen with regional infarctions (47). Layers 3, 5, and 6 of the cortex are very sensitive to ischemia and are affected in laminar necrosis. Usually the watershed zones in the parietal, occipital, and temporal lobes are affected. In the acute and subacute stages, MRI shows cortical enhancement and cortical hyperintensity on noncontrast T1-weighted images

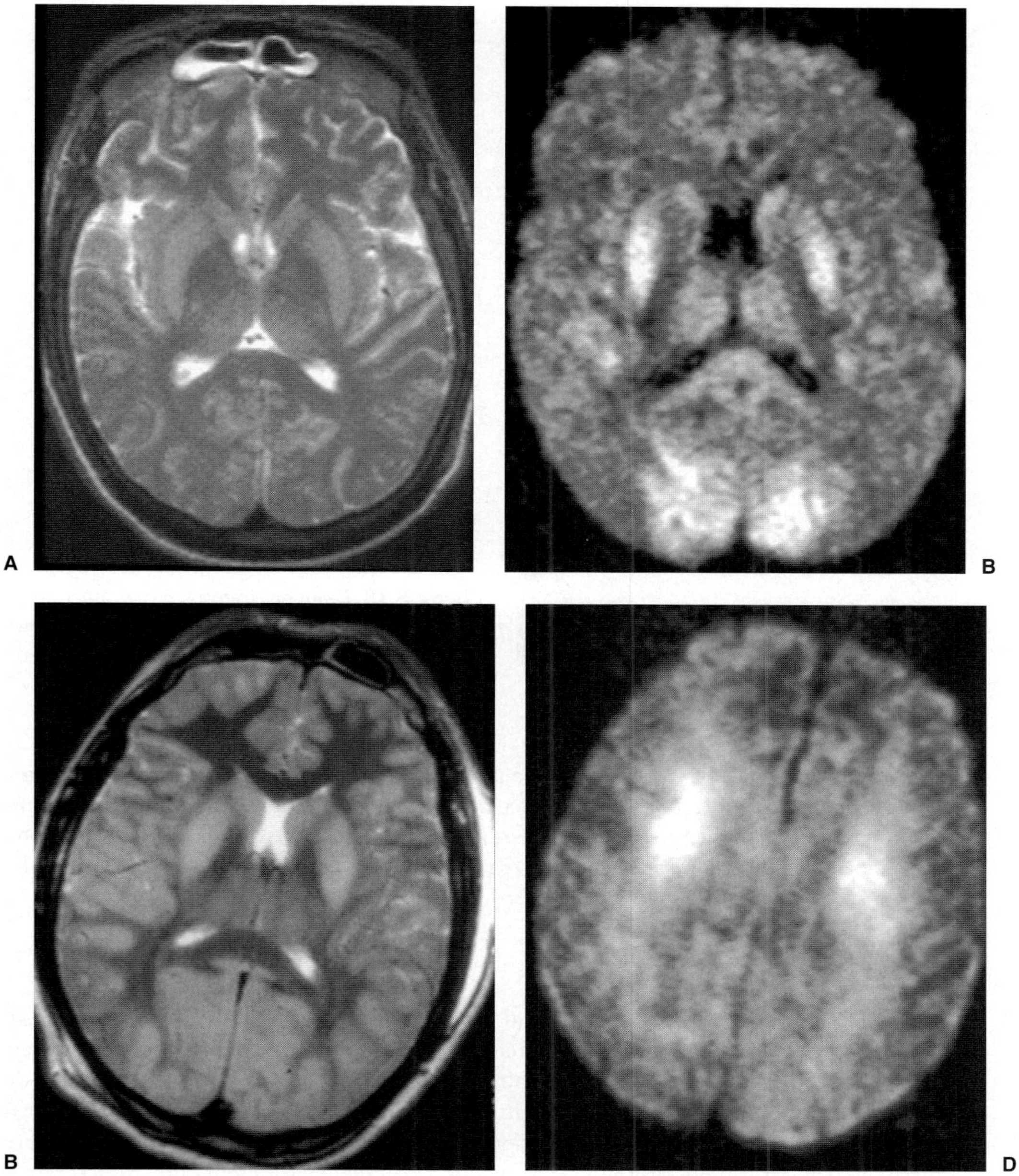

Figure 8.17 *Diffuse Cerebral Anoxia. A.* Axial T2-weighted image 1 hour after cardiac arrest shows subtle increased signal intensity in both basal ganglia. *B.* Corresponding diffusion-weighted image (DWI) shows definite high signal in the basal ganglia and occipital lobes. *C.* Three days later, an axial T2-weighted image shows marked edema of all gray matter structures. *D.* During the subacute period, an axial DWI shows that the signal intensity of the gray matter has "pseudonormalized" and that there is diffuse white matter hyperintensity.

Table 8.4: Magnetic Resonance Imaging (MRI) Findings in Diffuse Brain Anoxia

Time Period	*Noncontrast MRI*	*Contrast MRI*	*Diffusion-Weighted Imaging*
Acute	Subtle high signal in gray matter (T2 and fluid-attenuated inversion recovery) and effacement of cerebrospinal fluid spaces	None	High signal in basal ganglia, thalami, perirolandic gray matter, and cerebellum
Subacute	Increased T2 signal in gray matter, swelling	Enhancement of gray matter	Diffuse high signal in gray matter, increased signal in white matter (early wallerian degeneration?)
Chronic	Atrophy, persistent high signal in gray matter	None	None

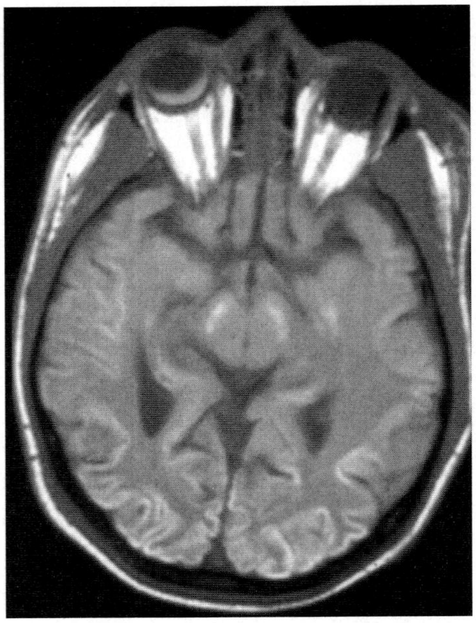

Figure 8.18 *Laminar Necrosis.* Axial noncontrast T1-weighted image shows linear hyperintensities in the cortices and midbrain.

(Fig. 8.18). This finding is believed to be a result of lipid-laden macrophages in the area of necrosis, and is not due to the presence of hemorrhage. Although histologically, laminar necrosis may be a hemorrhagic process, this feature is not visualized by MRI. Atrophy and hypointensity in the same cortical regions on T2-weighted images are seen in the chronic stage.

Wallerian Degeneration

WD has been briefly addressed earlier and is reviewed here for the sake of completeness. WD usually occurs after a cerebral infarction, but also may be seen with hemorrhages, tumors, trauma, and primary white matter disorders (26). WD refers to anterograde degeneration of the axons and their myelin. It usually affects the ipsilateral corticospinal tracts, the medial thalamus, and occasionally the contralateral cerebellar hemisphere (cross-cerebellar atrophy—although this may be a completely different entity). WD rarely is seen during the first month after a stroke. Acute WD is not visible on CT. Chronic WD is seen on CT as atrophy of the cerebral peduncle ipsilateral to the infarction (48). MRI may show WD earlier than CT (Fig. 8.3). In approximately 10% of MCA infarctions, DWI shows increased signal intensity in the ipsilateral cerebral peduncle, which is thought to represent early WD (26). Four weeks after the ictus, a band of T2 hypointensity along the ipsilateral corticospinal tract may be seen, and it is thought to be related to abnormal metabolism of iron (24,25). Approximately 2 to 3 months after a stroke, the ipsilateral corticospinal tract or the medial thalamus become hyperintense on T2 images, and there is associated atrophy that is especially obvious in the ipsilateral cerebral peduncle (49).

Vasculitis

Cerebral vasculitis is characterized by inflammation and fibrinoid necrosis of arterial media and intima, leading to occlusions, infarctions, and hemorrhages (50). Vasculitis may be primary or secondary. Secondary vasculitis may be due to inflammation or may occur postirradiation. Common infectious etiologies for vasculitis include bacterial, mycobacterial, viral (including herpes virus and human immunodeficiency virus), and fungal meningitis (mainly involving vessels at the base of the brain), and syphilis (mainly involving

Table 8.5: Etiologies for Infection-Related Cerebral Vasculitis

Bacterial	*Viral*	*Fungal*	*Granulomatous*	*Rickettsial/Spirochetal*
Hemophilus influenzae, *Streptococcus*, *Staphylococcus*	Herpes virus, human immunodeficiency virus	*Aspergillus*, mucormycosis, *Actinomyces*, coccidioidomycosis	Tuberculosis, sarcoidosis	Rocky Mountain spotted fever, Lyme disease, syphilis

large-caliber vessels) (51). Table 8.5 addresses the infectious causes for cerebral vasculitis, and Table 8.6 describes some common noninfectious etiologies for cerebral vasculitis. Vasculitis also may be associated with the following drugs:

- Cocaine
- Amphetamines
- Heroin
- Ergot derivatives
- Pseudoephedrine
- Phenylpropanolamine

The diagnosis of cerebral vasculitis is a clinical one that may be confirmed in many patients by MRI and angiography (Fig. 8.19). In most patients, T2-weighted and FLAIR images show patchy areas of increased signal intensity in the white matter (both deep and superficial locations) (52). These regions usually do not enhance. Vasculitis may result in cerebral infarctions, which have the findings described previously. The diagnosis of vasculitis may be confirmed by catheter angiography. In my opinion, the diagnosis of vasculitis is difficult to make using MRA unless large-caliber vessels are affected, as is the case in many of the inflammatory vasculitides. Catheter angiograms show irregular narrowing of smaller intracranial vessels distant to branching points, occlusions, or aneurysm formation. Some vasculitides, such as the granulomatous type, affect tiny vessels that are not visible on angiograms, and a biopsy is required to establish the diagnosis. Until a few years ago, we used to think that vasculitis in absence of T2/FLAIR abnormalities was not possible. There now is evidence that in rare instances the MRI studies may be negative and a vasculitis still be present. Vasculitis also may result in intracerebral bleeds that occasionally may be the result of aneurysm formation. The mortality rate after hemorrhage secondary to vasculitis approaches 50%. DWI is particularly helpful in assessing small acute infarctions and in dating infarctions of varying ages.

Vasculitis may be present in the absence of T2 abnormalities; however, in these patients, FLAIR, DWI, and perfusion studies usually show abnormalities. (I recommend Wasserman BA, Sonte JH, Hellman DB, et al. Reliability of normal findings on MR imaging for excluding the diagnosis of vasculitis of the central nervous system. AJR Am J Radiol 2001;177:455–459.)

Table 8.6: Etiologies for Primary Cerebral Vasculitis

Primary angiitis of the central nervous system (PACNS)
Giant cell arteritis
Polyarteritis nodosa
Temporal arteritis
Takayasu's arteritis
Granulomatous angiitis
Rheumatoid arthritis
Lupus erythematosus
Wegener's granulomatosis
Scleroderma
Behçet's disease

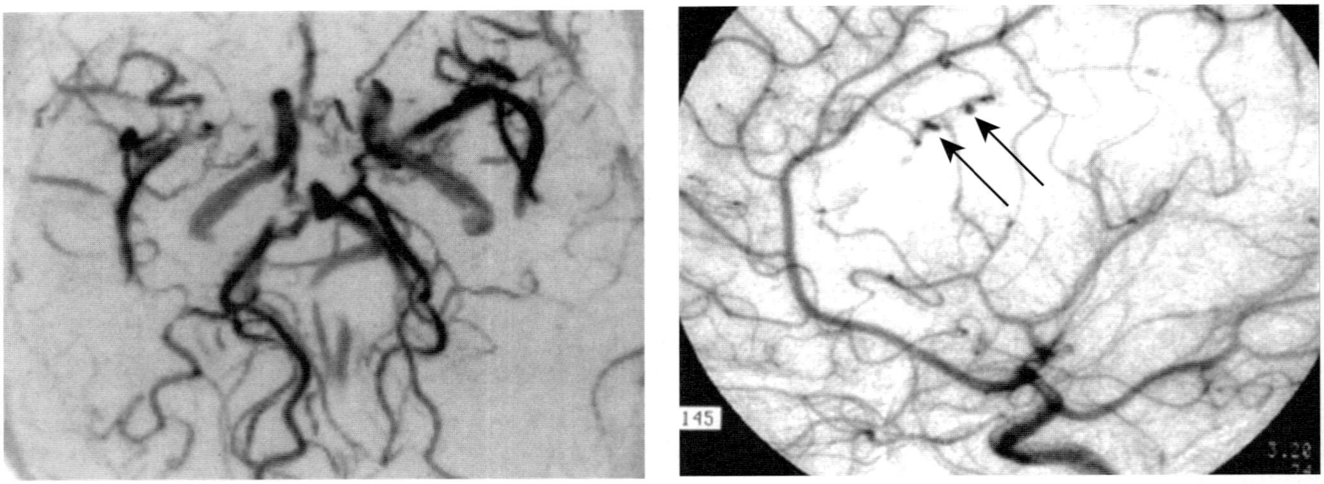

A C

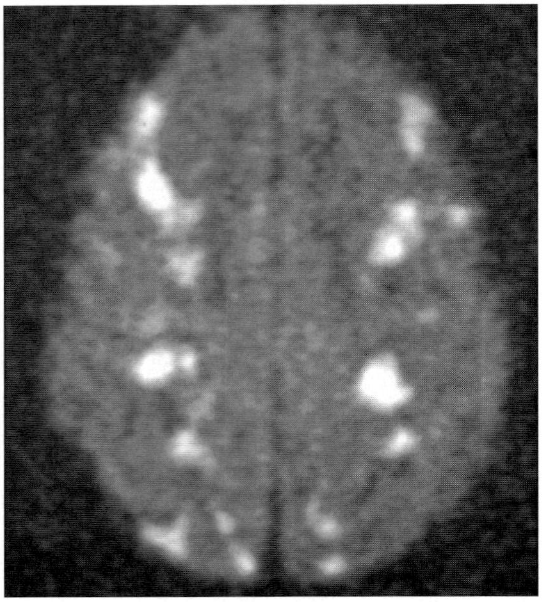

B

Figure 8.19 *Vasculitis. A.* Base view from magnetic resonance angiogram shows multiple narrowings and occlusions predominantly in the middle cerebral arteries. *B.* Axial diffusion-weighted image shows multiple, acute small infarctions in parasagittal distributions. *C.* In a different patient, oblique view from catheter angiogram shows occlusion of the middle cerebral artery and aneurysms *(arrows)* in a branch of the anterior cerebral artery.

MOYAMOYA

The term *moyamoya* refers to different disease processes. Moyamoya *disease* (also known as *idiopathic progressive arteriopathy of childhood*) is a primary arterial disorder leading to occlusion of intracranial internal carotid arteries, and is seen mainly in Japan (53). Moyamoya *syndrome* is a radiographic nonspecific finding that is identical to the disease but seen in association with sickle cell anemia, collagen vascular disorders (e.g., Ehlers-Danlos or Marfan's syndromes, homocystinuria), neurofibromatosis type I, Menkes' kinky hair syndrome, atherosclerosis, and radiation injury. The syndrome is the most common manifestation of this process in the United States. As the internal carotid arteries narrow, collateral circulation develops in the form of hypertrophied perforating arteries (Fig. 8.20). The lenticulostriate arteries are involved initially, but as the disease extends into the posterior communicating and posterior cerebral arteries, the thalamostriate arteries also hypertrophy (note that moyamoya never involves the infratentorial arteries). The blood supply to the brain becomes tenuous, and deep cerebral infarctions are not unusual. By conventional angiography, MRI, or MRA, there is occlusion of the supraclinoid internal carotid artery and proliferation of large and irregular perforating

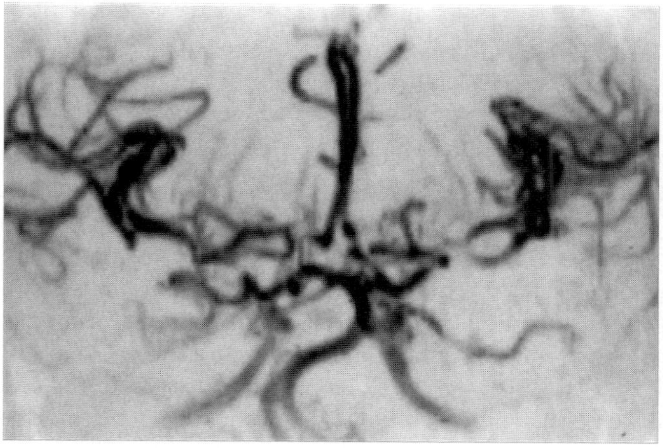

A

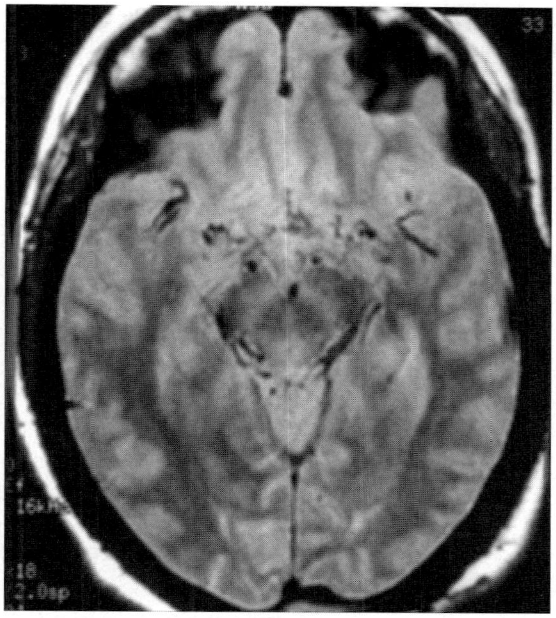

B

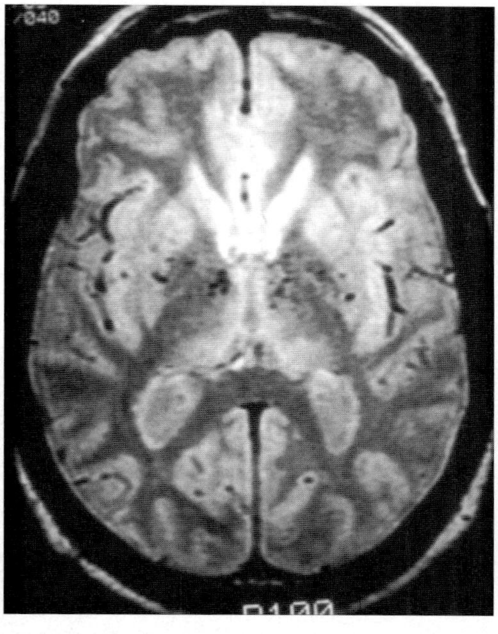

C

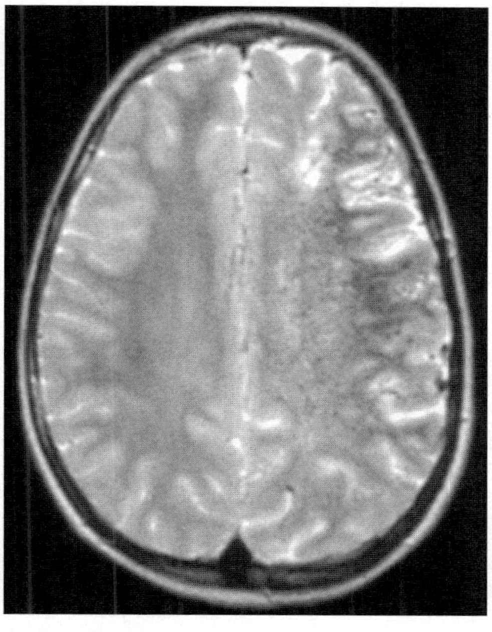

D

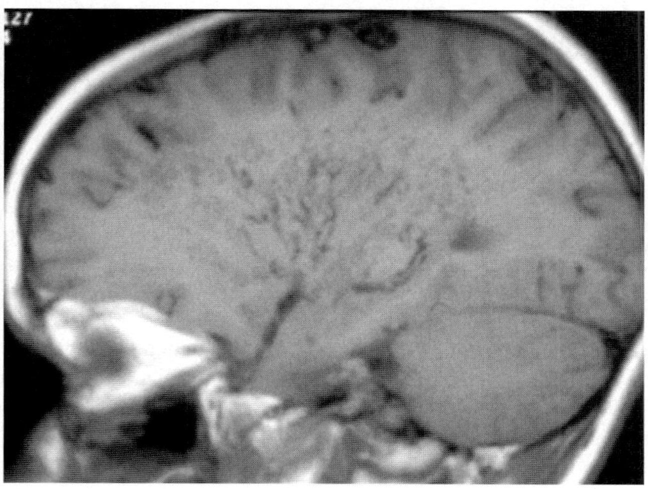

E

Figure 8.20 *Moyamoya Phenomenon. A.* Frontal view from magnetic resonance angiogram shows severely attenuated flow in the internal carotid arteries, including their supraclinoid regions. There is proliferation and increased caliber of the perforating arteries. *B.* In a different patient, axial T2-weighted image shows multiple enlarged perforating arteries in the territories of the middle and posterior cerebral arteries. *C.* In the same patient, hypertrophied lenticulostriate arteries are seen in the basal ganglia. *D.* In a different patient, axial T2-weighted image shows atrophy of the left cerebral hemisphere and multiple enlarged deep perforating arteries throughout the white matter. *E.* In the same patient, parasagittal T1-weighted image confirms the presence of the enlarged deep perforating arteries.

The "ivy sign" refers to proliferation of blood vessels on the pia leading to subarachnoid space enhancement of the convexities.

vessels seen as focal areas of flow void in the basal ganglia (54,55). Transdiploic collaterals from the external carotid artery to the pial circulation develop to supply ischemic brain regions. MRI studies show infarcts in up to 80% of patients (particularly children). The most common initial presentation of moyamoya in adults is intraventricular hemorrhage.

HYPERTENSIVE ENCEPHALOPATHY

For the PRES syndrome, a good review may be found in Port JD, Beauchamp NJ. Reversible intracerebral pathologic entities mediated by vascular autoregulatory dysfunction. Radiographics 1998;18:353–367.

Hypertensive encephalopathy results from a significant acute elevation of the systemic blood pressure and escape of fluids and proteins through vessel walls, leading to diffuse or focal cerebral edema (56). This occurs as a result of abnormal vascular (arterial) autoregulation. Common etiologies for hypertensive encephalopathy include toxemia of pregnancy, renal insufficiency, hemolytic–uremic syndrome, cyclosporine/tacrolimus administration, and thrombotic thrombocytopenic purpura (57,58). Most lesions occur in the distribution of the posterior cerebral circulation and produce seizures and visual disturbances because they affect the cortex (59) (Fig. 8.21). Approximately 90% of the lesions are reversible, but some produce permanent infarctions. The lesions are not hemorrhagic and usually do not enhance after contrast is given. The lesions are bright on T2-weighted and FLAIR images and involve both gray and white matter. They may completely disappear, and some have termed this constellation of findings *posterior reversible leukoencephalopathy syndrome* (PRES; I believe that this is poor term because many patients have lesions in the frontal lobes and basal ganglia and many of them are not reversible). The lesions are bright on DWI, and ADC maps may be used to separate those that are true infarctions from those that are related to transient ischemia. Perfusion MRI may show normal or near-normal rCBV and rCBF in ischemic lesions, but reduction of both parameters in infarctions.

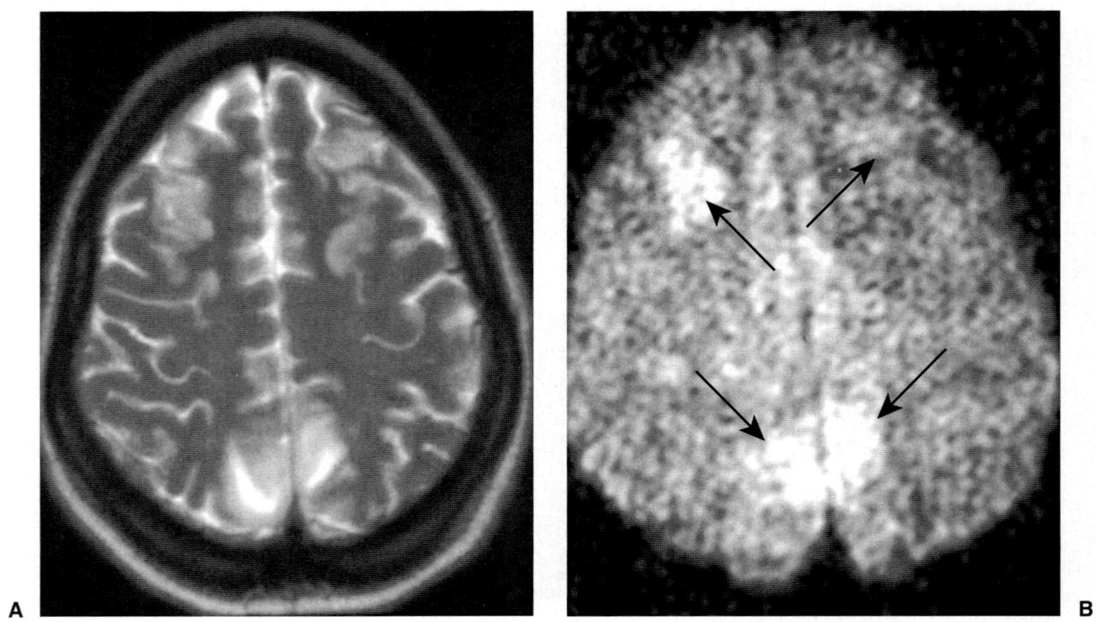

Figure 8.21 *Hypertensive Encephalopathy. A.* Axial T2-weighted image in a patient with preeclampsia shows high signal intensity in the parietal and frontal regions involving both white and gray matter. *B.* Corresponding diffusion-weighted image shows only subtle brightness *(arrows)* in the same regions. The findings resolved completely.

Box 8.1: Venous Sinuses Affected by Thrombosis in Decreasing Order of Frequency

Superior sagittal sinus
Transverse sinus
Sigmoid sinus
Cavernous sinus

Venous Occlusions

Venous thrombosis accounts for approximately 1% of cerebral infarctions (60). In children, venous thrombosis tends to produce less severe symptoms and may resolve spontaneously. In adults, venous thrombosis may have a more aggressive course. Box 8.1 lists the most commonly affected venous sinuses according to their frequency.

The etiologies responsible for thrombosis of the venous sinuses are listed in Table 8.7. Most patients with cerebral venous thrombosis present with headache, altered mental status, seizures, and blurred vision, and these symptoms may progress to coma and death. The presence of diffuse brain edema and hemorrhages carries a poor prognosis. Contrast-enhanced CT may show a "delta" sign, which is due to a filling defect (clot) inside a sinus surrounded by hyperdensity that may be the result of opacified venous blood in the sinus or a proliferation of neovascularity around the sinus (it is known that after venous sinus thrombosis, angiogenic factors are produced that may induce formation of neovascularity about the area of occlusion) (61) (Fig. 8.22A). Noncontrast MRI shows hyperintensity and lack of flow void in the affected sinus (Fig. 8.22B). After contrast is given, there may be enhancement of the involved sinus and striking dural enhancement (Fig. 8.22C). MR venography (2-D TOF or phase contrast) is useful in confirming the diagnosis and shows lack of flow-related enhancement in the affected sinus (Fig. 8.22D). The prognosis of patients with cerebral venous thrombosis can be predicted based on the presence of intracerebral abnormalities. Venous infarctions have a poor prognosis. Infarctions usually are located in a nonarterial distribution, particularly in the parasagittal convexities. These infarctions may be hemorrhagic and typically show little or no contrast enhancement (the reason for this is not known; Fig. 8.22D). The presence of diffuse cerebral edema correlates with a poor outcome. Hydrocephalus also may develop (Chapter 5).

In the absence of cerebral edema and infarctions, the symptoms related to venous sinus thrombosis are not severe, and no aggressive intravascular therapy is indicated.

Table 8.7: Etiologies for Venous Sinus Thrombosis

Aseptic	*Septic*
Idiopathic (25%)	Meningitis
Pregnancy	Paranasal sinusitis
Dehydration (most common cause in children)	Mastoiditis
Oral contraceptives	Orbital cellulitis
Trauma (including child abuse)	Subdural/epidural empyema
Tumors (distant and close or invading the sinuses)	Encephalitis
Polycythemia and hypercoagulable states	
Sickle cell disease	
Leukemia	

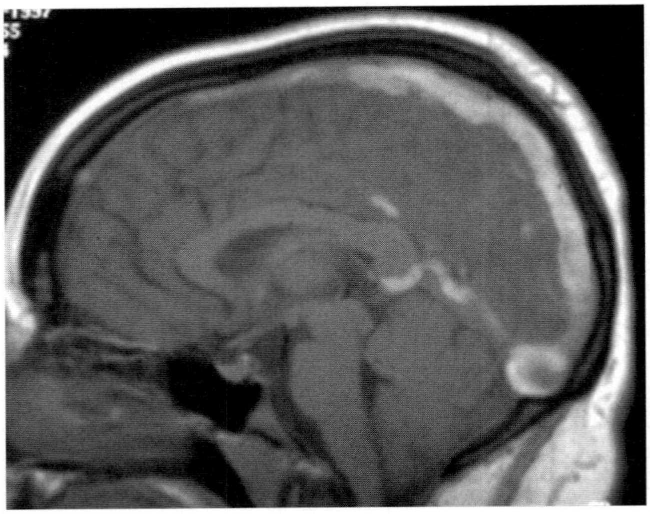
A

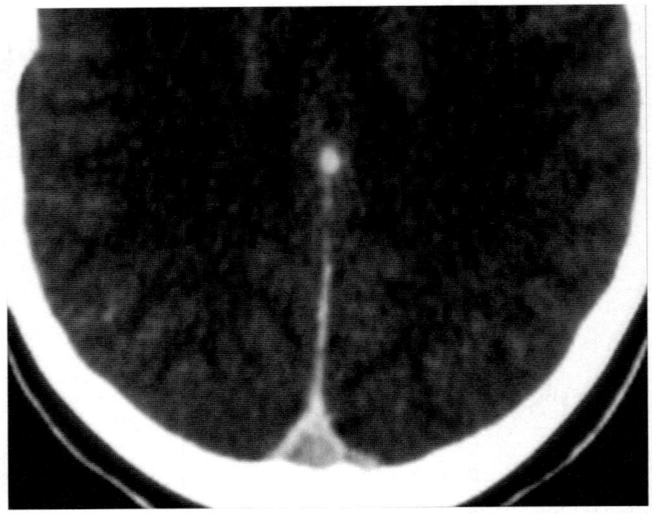
B

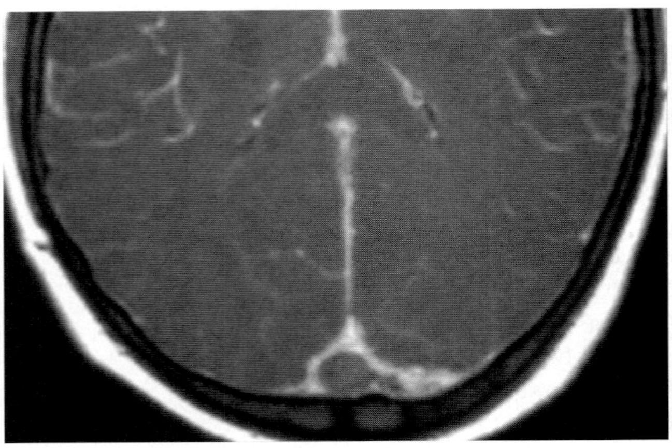
C

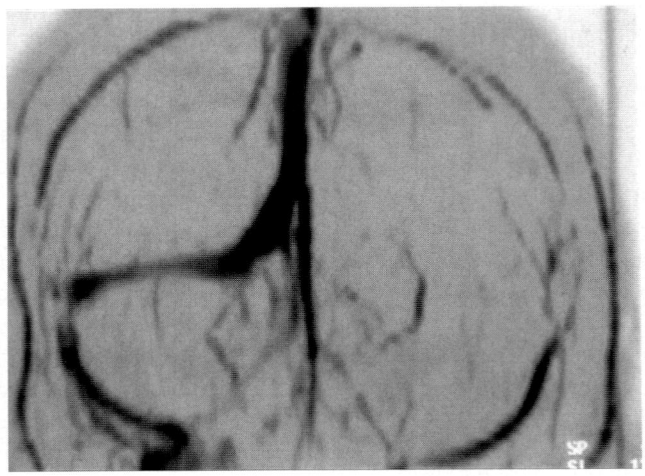
D

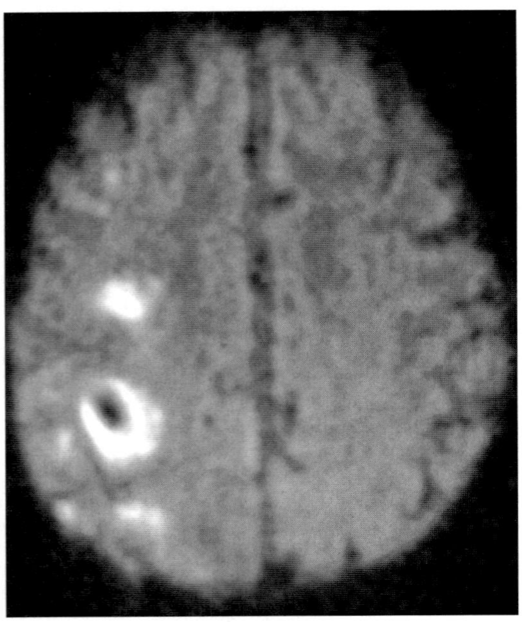
E

Figure 8.22 *Venous Thrombosis. A.* Midsagittal T1-weighted image shows bright clot in the superior and inferior sagittal sinuses, vein of Galen, straight sinus, and torcular. *B.* Axial postcontrast computed tomography (different patient) shows enhancement of the walls of a clot-filled superior sagittal sinus ("delta" sign). *C.* In the same patient, postcontrast T1-weighted image shows similar findings to *B. D.* Frontal view from magnetic resonance venogram shows absence of flow in most of the left transverse sinus due to thrombosis. *E.* In a different patient, axial diffusion-weighted image shows multiple acute subcortical infarctions (note that the largest contains low central signal intensity compatible with hematoma) in a nonarterial distribution in this patient with cortical vein thrombosis.

Deep venous system thrombosis is less common than occlusion of the dural sinuses or the cortical veins. Thrombosis of the deep venous system is more common in children than in adults. The etiologies are similar to those described for venous sinus thrombosis. The deep gray matter nuclei typically are involved, and the findings may simulate generalized anoxia, both clinically and on imaging. The deep infarctions may be hemorrhagic. Deep venous occlusion is an important cause of bilateral thalamic and midbrain infarctions and hemorrhages.

Vascular Age-Related Changes

MRI shows patchy areas of increased T2 and FLAIR signal in the white matter of 20% to 30% of adults, particularly those older than 60 years of age (62). The abnormalities are more prevalent in men. These patients usually are healthy and are not apparently symptomatic from these abnormalities. In the presence of symptoms such as TIAs, the prevalence of these abnormalities is markedly increased (69%) (63). There is little correlation between the presence of lesions and the development of dementia. It is clear, however, that demented patients may have an increased lesion burden compared with "normal" age-matched individuals. The lesions usually are discreet and measure approximately 0.5 cm in diameter (64). The lesions are of high signal on T2-weighted and FLAIR images, do not enhance, and may be confluent. I grade them as mild, moderate, and severe, but this grading is subjective and based on experience. Many of these patients have a history of prolonged hypertension or smoking. The etiology for these abnormalities is not known, and the following possible etiologies have been proposed (65–67):

- Ischemic demyelination
- True infarction
- Venous collagenosis
- Amyloidosis (this may cause focal areas of hypointensity as well)

Extracranial Arterial Disease

Atherosclerotic disease involves, in order of frequency, the common carotid artery bifurcation in the neck, the ostia of the great vessels at the level of the aortic arch, the cavernous and supraclinoid internal carotid arteries, the origin of the vertebral arteries, and the intracranial circulation (both anterior and posterior). It is thought that chronic injury at zones of turbulent blood flow may lead to a reaction characterized by cellular proliferation, development of fibrofatty plaques, and thrombus formation due to platelet aggregation (68). The most common sources of emboli that cause cerebral infarctions include atherosclerotic plaques at the carotid artery bifurcations in the neck and the heart. To produce hemodynamically significant aberrations, the diameter of a vessel needs to be reduced by over 60%. According to NASCET, symptomatic patients with narrowing of the internal carotid artery of between 70% to 99% benefit from surgery (10). According to the Asymptomatic Carotid Atherosclerosis Study (ACAS), men with stenosis of the internal carotid artery of over 60% may benefit from surgery. Ulcers can be diagnosed by angiography in only 50% of stenoses, and they carry an increased risk of cerebral infarction. Methods for measurement of the stenoses were discussed previously. The diagnosis of carotid artery stenosis may be established by conventional angiography, MRA and CT angiography, and Doppler sonography. Here I briefly address some issues regarding CT angiography because this method is becoming popular. There are three methods to generate the images: surface rendering, volume rendering, and maximum-intensity projection. Only the last two are helpful in evaluating stenoses because they allow for visualization of the stenosis even in the presence of significant calcification. The agreement for the measurement of stenoses between catheter and CT angiograms is approximately 90% (69,70).

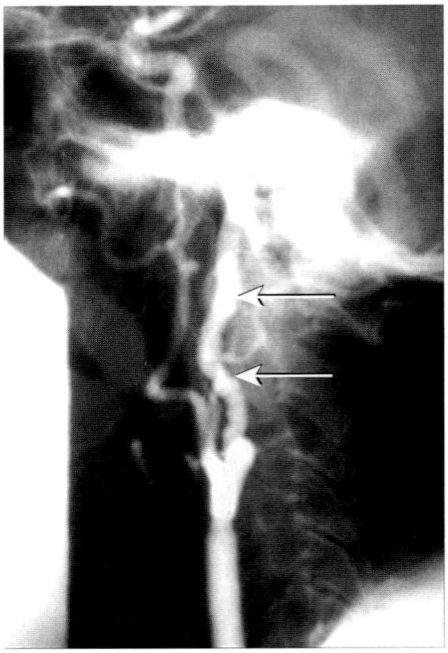

Figure 8.23 *Fibromuscular Dysplasia.* Lateral view from catheter angiogram shows "beaded" appearance *(arrows)* of internal carotid artery due to fibromuscular dysplasia.

FMD may be associated with intracranial aneurysms, spontaneous carotid or vertebral artery dissection, spontaneous arteriovenous fistulas, and renal artery FMD.

FMD is a relatively common disease and is addressed here only briefly because it has been discussed previously. Approximately 90% of patients are women 40 to 60 years of age (71). FMD usually involves the high internal carotid (95%) or vertebral (15% to 25%) arteries (at the C1–C2 level). Bilateral involvement is seen in 60% to 75% of patients. It may be associated with intracranial aneurysms (20% to 50%), spontaneous carotid or vertebral artery dissection, spontaneous arteriovenous fistulas, and renal artery FMD. Although it usually is clinically silent, a bruit and focal neurologic deficits may occur. The medial form (90% to 95%) is much more common than the intimal (5%) or subadventitial (1%) forms. In my opinion, the best method to study patients with suspected FMD remains catheter angiography. FMD may be demonstrated by MRA, but I believe this method makes it difficult to render a definitive diagnosis because motion artifacts may result in similar findings (71) (Fig. 8.23). I am not aware of any publications discussing the use of CT angiography for the diagnosis of FMD. The most common angiographic appearance of FMD is that of areas of narrowing alternating with areas of dilatation. This finding is seen in 80% to 90% of patients with FMD. An area of long and tubular narrowing is seen in approximately 10% to 20% of patients, and less common findings include intraluminal septa and diverticula.

Dissection of the Extracranial Blood Vessels

Dissections involving the carotid and vertebral arteries are not uncommon. There usually is a tear in the intima resulting in extravasation of the blood into the potential space between the media and internal elastica laminae (72). The blood under pressure dissects through this space, resulting in hematoma formation that secondarily narrows the lumen of the artery. The hemorrhage also may be due to rupture of the vasa vasorum into the media. The most common causes for dissections are as follows:

- Idiopathic
- Trauma
- FMD

- Hypertension
- Contraceptive use
- Collagen vascular disorders
- Irradiation

Dissections involving the carotid artery tend to occur at the bifurcation in the neck, in the high cervical portion as it enters the foramen lacerum, and in its supraclinoid portion. The vertebral artery usually is dissected at the level of C6, where it enters the foramen transversarium; at C1, where it wraps around the lateral masses of this vertebra; or as it enters the foramen magnum where it crosses the dura. Most dissections begin extracranially and then extend intradurally. Dissections are well evaluated with catheter angiography (73). The dissected vessel commonly is occluded, and the proximal occlusion may be "flame shaped." This is referred to as the *stenoocclusive* form of a dissection. The artery may be occluded after a short segment of dilatation, and this is called the *aneurysmal* pattern of dissection. MRI clearly shows high T1 signal intensity (clot) in the wall of the artery, with narrowing or disappearance of the central flow void. In the vertebral arteries, which normally are surrounded by the fat of the foramina transversaria, this high–signal-intensity clot may be difficult to see and may require the use of fat suppression techniques (although I also use fat-suppressed images for possible dissections of the internal carotid arteries). MRA usually also shows the narrowing.

Cerebral Infarction in Children

Cerebral infarctions in children are rare and most are found during the neonatal period. Although most of the imaging manifestations are similar to those of adults [with the exception of periventricular leukomalacia (PVL)], the etiologies for cerebral infarctions in children are different. The most common etiologies include the following (74):

- Perinatal hypoxia
- Protein C or S deficiency
- Sickle cell disease
- Vasculitis
- Meningitis
- Idiopathic
- Hypoglycemia
- Mitochondrial disorders
- Carnitine deficiency
- Related to medications (immunosuppressants, antileukemics)
- Trauma
- Congenital or acquired heart disease
- Chronic illnesses (thalassemia, nephrotic syndrome, diabetes)
- Sudden infant death syndrome

The most common symptoms at presentation are seizures, hemiplegia, and nonspecific and nonlocalizing signs. Unfortunately, the most common sequelae are hemiplegia and seizures.

Venous infarctions are perhaps more common in children than in adults. Their imaging findings are similar, however, and have been addressed previously. The most common etiologies for venous infarctions are (74):

- Bacterial meningitis
- Hypercoagulable states
- Hypovolemia and dehydration
- Antineoplastic medications (L-asparaginase)
- Trauma

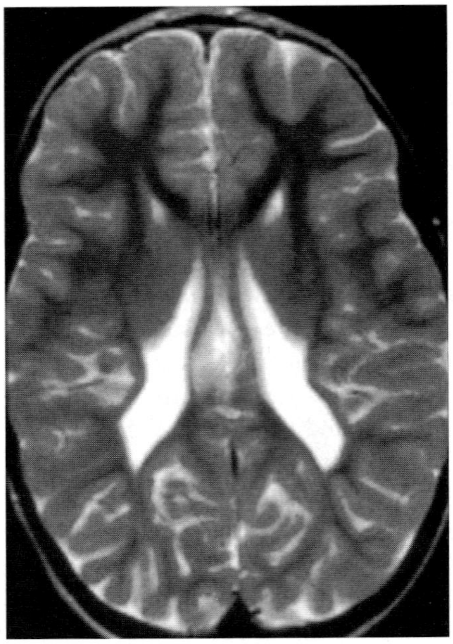

Figure 8.24 *Periventricular Leukomalacia.* Axial T2-weighted image shows prominence of the posterior aspects of the lateral ventricles. The outer walls of the lateral ventricles have a "wavy" appearance. The volume of the posterior white matter is diminished and the gray matter is close to the ventricles. These findings are the chronic sequelae of periventricular leukomalacia.

The most common symptom of a cerebral venous infarction in a child is seizures. The most common sequelae are speech delay, seizures, and mild motor weakness.

Periventricular leukomalacia is the sequela of watershed infarction occurring in premature and low–birth-weight neonates, and is a leading cause of spastic diplegia.

One of the most important sequelae of diffuse neonatal hypoxia is PVL (75,76). The periventricular white matter is a watershed territory found between the ventriculofugal and ventriculopetal arterial circulations of children. Diffuse hypoxia leads to coagulative necrosis and inflammatory changes in the periventricular white matter, particularly posteriorly. PVL occurs in up to 20% of premature infants, especially in those with low birth weight. Aside from the acute symptoms, patients with PVL develop symptoms in the spectrum of cerebral palsy (particularly spastic diplegia). Acute PVL nearly always is detected by cranial sonography. Initially, there is increased echogenicity in the periventricular white matter; 2 to 4 weeks later, cystic changes ensue. Although the posterior white matter is affected more severely, the frontal white matter also commonly is affected. Chronic changes of PVL are seen clearly on CT or MRI studies (Fig. 8.24). These images show that the volume of the white matter (particularly posteriorly) is decreased and may be of high T2 signal intensity. The cortical sulci extend deep and almost touch the outer walls of the lateral ventricles. The posterior aspect of the sylvian fissures may be very prominent. Similar changes, but usually to a lesser degree, may be seen in the frontal white matter. The outer wall of the lateral ventricles may have a "wavy" contour. The trigones of the lateral ventricles are enlarged disproportionately with respect to the rest of the ventricles (so-called colpocephaly). On sagittal images, the posterior body and splenium of the corpus callosum are thin.

References

1. TerPenning B. Pathophysiology of stroke. Neuroimaging Clin North Am 1992;3:389–408.
2. Castillo M. Prethrombolysis brain imaging: trends and controversies. AJNR Am J Neuroradiol 1998;18:1830–1834.
3. Del Zoppo GJ, Poeck K, Pessin MS, et al. Recombinant issue plasminogen activator in acute thrombotic and embolic stroke. Ann Neurol 1992;32:78–86.
4. Sorensen AG, Reimer P. Cerebral MR perfusion imaging: principles and current application. Stuttgart, Germany: Thieme, 2000.
5. Doerfler A, Engelhorn T, von Kummer R, et al. Are iodinated contrast agents detrimental in acute cerebral ischemia? An experimental study in rats. Radiology 1998;206:211–217.

6. Aaron J, Hesselink J, Oot R, et al. Complications of the intravenous SDA performed for carotid artery disease: a prospective study. Radiology 1984;153:675–678.
7. Waugh JR, Sacharias N. Arteriographic complications in the DSA era. Radiology 1992;182: 243–246.
8. Eliasiw M, Fow AJ, Sharpe BL, et al. Carotid artery stenosis: external validity of the North American Symptomatic Carotid Endarterectomy Trial measurement method. Radiology 1997;204: 229–233.
9. Ackerman R, Morelia RC. Identifying clinically relevant carotid disease. Stroke 1994;25:1–10.
10. Fisher M, Martin A, Cosgrove M, et al. The NASCET-ACAS plaque project: North American Symptomatic Carotid Endarterectomy Trial–Asymptomatic Carotid Atherosclerosis Study. Stroke 1993;24:131–132.
11. Furie DM, Tien RD. Fibromuscular dysplasia of arteries of the head and neck: imaging findings. AJR Am J Radiol 1994;162:1205–1209.
12. Baird AE, Austin MC, McKay WJ, et al. Sensitivity and specificity of 99mTc-HMPAO SPECT cerebral perfusion measurements during the first 48 hours of the localization of cerebral infarction. Stroke 1997;28:976–980.
13. Beauchamp N, Barker P, Wang P, et al. Imaging of the acute cerebral ischemia. Radiology 1999; 212:307–324.
14. Weingarten K. Computed tomography of cerebral infarction. Neuroimaging Clin North Am 1992;3:409–420.
15. Ferguson RDG, Ferguson JG. Cerebral intraarterial fibrinolysis at the crossroad: is a phase III trial advisable at this time? AJNR Am J Neuroradiol 1994;15:1201–1206.
16. Castillo M, Falcone S, Naidich TP, et al. Imaging in acute basilar artery thrombosis. Neuroradiology 1994;36:426–426.
17. Castillo M, Wilson JD. CT angiography of the common carotid artery bifurcation: comparison between two techniques and conventional angiography. Neuroradiology 1994;36:602–604.
18. Reichenbach JR, Rother J, Jonetz-Mentzel L, et al. Acute stroke evaluated by time-to-peak mapping during initial and early follow-up perfusion CT studies. AJNR Am J Neuroradiol 1999;20:1842–1850.
19. Koenig M, Klotz W, Luka B, et al. Perfusion CT of the brain: diagnostic approach for early detection of ischemic stroke. Radiology 1998;209:85–93.
20. Fukui MB, Johnson DW, Yonas H, et al. Xe/CT cerebral blood flow evaluation of delayed symptomatic cerebral ischemia after subarachnoid hemorrhage. AJNR Am J Neuroradiol 1992;13: 265–270.
21. Bryan RN, Levy LM, Whitlow WD, et al. Diagnosis of acute cerebral infarction: comparison of CT and MR imaging. AJNR Am J Neuroradiol 1991;12:611–629.
22. Yuh WTC, Crain MR, Loes DJ, et al. MR imaging of cerebral ischemia: findings in the first 24 hours. AJNR Am J Neuroradiol 1991;21:621–629.
23. Elster AD, Moddy DM. Early cerebral infarction: gadopentetate dimeglumine enhancement. Radiology 1990;177:627–632.
24. Kuhn M, Mikulis D, Ayoub D, et al. Wallerian degeneration after cerebral infarction: evaluation with sequential MR imaging. Radiology 1989;172:79–182.
25. Kuhn M, Johnson K, Davis K. Wallerian degeneration: evaluation with MR imaging. Radiology 1988;168:199–202.
26. Castillo M, Mukherji S. Early abnormalities related to postinfarction wallerian degeneration: evaluation with MR diffusion-weighted imaging. J Comput Assist Tomogr 1999;23:1004–1007.
27. Heiserman J, Drayer B, Keller P, et al. Intracranial vascular stenosis and occlusion: evaluation with three-dimensional time-of-flight MR angiography. Radiology 1992;85:667–673.
28. Mattle HP, Wentz KU, Edelman RR, et al. Cerebral venography with MR. Radiology 1991;178: 453–458.
29. Barker PB, Gillard JH, van Zijl PCM, et al. Acute stroke: evaluation with serial proton MR spectroscopic imaging. Radiology 1994;192:723–732.
30. Sevick RJ, Kanda F, Mintorovich J, et al. Cytotoxic brain edema: assessment with diffusion-weighted MR imaging. Radiology 1992;185:687–690.
31. Provenzale J, Sorensen G. Diffusion-weighted MR imaging in acute stroke: theoretic considerations and clinical applications. AJR Am J Radiol 1999;173:1459–1467.
32. Gonzalez R, Schaefer P, Buonanno F, et al. Diffusion-weighted MR imaging: diagnostic accuracy in patients imaged within 6 hours of stroke symptom onset. Radiology 1999;210:155–162.
33. Lefkowitz D, LaBenz M, Nudo SR, et al. Hyperacute ischemic stroke missed by diffusion-weighted imaging. AJNR Am J Neuroradiol 1999;20:1871–1875.

34. Wang PYK, Barker PB, Wityk RJ, et al. Diffusion-negative stroke: a report of two cases. AJNR Am J Neuroradiol 1999;20:1876–1880.
35. Burdette J, Elster A, Ricci P. Acute cerebral infarction: quantification of spin-density and T2 shine-through phenomena on diffusion-weighted MR images. Radiology 1999;212:333–339.
36. Patel M, Siewert B, Warach S, et al. Diffusion and perfusion imaging techniques. Magn Reson Imaging Clin N Am 1995;3:425–438.
37. Tzika AA, Massoth RJ, Ball WS, et al. Cerebral perfusion in children: detection with dynamic contrast-enhanced T2*-weighted MR images. Radiology 1993;187:449–458.
38. Burdette J, Ricci P, Petitti N, et al. Cerebral infarction: time course of signal intensity changes on diffusion-weighted MR images. AJR Am J Radiol 1998;171:791–795.
39. Kapila A. Calcification in cerebral infarction. Radiology 1984;153:685–687.
40. Cormier P, Long E, Russell E. MR imaging of posterior fossa infarctions: vascular territories and clinical correlates. Radiographics 1992;12:1079–1096.
41. Ebisu T, Tanaka C, Umeda M, et al. Hemorrhagic and nonhemorrhagic stroke: diagnosis with diffusion-weighted and T2-weighted echo-planar MR imaging. Radiology 1997;203:823–828.
42. Schwaighofer B, Klein M, Lyden P, et al. MR imaging of vertebrobasilar vascular disease. J Comput Assist Tomogr 1990;14:895–904.
43. Beauchamp N, Ulug A, Passe T, et al. MR diffusion imaging in stroke: review and controversies. Radiographics 1998;18:1269–1283.
44. Chong J, Lu D, Aragao F, et al. Diffusion-weighted MR of acute cerebral infarction: comparison of data processing methods. AJNR Am J Neuroradiol 1998;19:1733–1739.
45. Arbelaez A, Castillo M, Mukherji S. Diffusion-weighted MR imaging of global cerebral anoxia. AJNR Am J Neuroradiol 1999;20:999–1007.
46. Provenzale J, Barboriak D. Brain infarction in young adults: etiology and imaging findings. AJR Am J Radiol 1997;169:1161–1168.
47. Takahashi S, Higano S, Ishii K, et al. Hypoxic brain damage: cortical laminar necrosis and delayed changes in white matter at sequential MR imaging. Radiology 1993;189:449–556.
48. Stovring J, Fernando L. Wallerian degeneration of the corticospinal tract region of the brains stem: demonstration by computer tomography. Radiology 1983;149:717–720.
49. Ogawa T, Yoshida Y, Okudera T, et al. Secondary thalamic degeneration after cerebral infarction in the middle cerebral artery distribution: evaluation with MR imaging. Radiology 1997;204: 255–262.
50. Harris KG, Tran DD, Sickels WJ, et al. Diagnosing intracranial vasculitis: the roles of MR and angiography. AJNR Am J Neuroradiol 1994;15:317–330.
51. Gillams AR, Allen E, Hrieb K, et al. Cerebral infarction in patients with AIDS. AJNR Am J Neuroradiol 1997;18:1581–1585.
52. Greenan T, Grossman R, Goldberg H. Cerebral vasculitis: MR imaging and angiographic correlation. Radiology 1992;182:65–75.
53. Fujisawa I, Asato R, Nishimura K, et al. Moyamoya disease: MR imaging. Radiology 1987;164: 103–107.
54. Yamada I, Suzuki S, Matsushima Y. Moyamoya disease: comparison of assessment with MR angiography and MR imaging versus conventional angiography. Radiology 1995;196:211–218.
55. Yamada I, Matsushima Y, Suzuki S. Moyamoya disease: diagnosis with three-dimensional time-of-flight MR angiography. Radiology 1992;184:773–778.
56. Weingarten K, Barbut D, Filippi C, et al. Acute hypertensive encephalopathy: findings on spin-echo and gradient-echo MR imaging. AJR Am J Radiol 1994;162:665–670.
57. Mantello M, Schwartz R, Jones K, et al. Imaging of neurologic complication associated with pregnancy. AJR Am J Radiol 1993;160:843–847.
58. Sanders T, Clayman D, Sanchez-Ramos L, et al. Brain in eclampsia: MR imaging with clinical correlation. Radiology 1991;180:475–478.
59. Port JD, Beauchamp NJ. Reversible intracerebral pathologic entities medicated by vascular autoregulatory dysfunction. Radiographics 1998;18:353–367.
60. Vogl T, Bergman C, Villringer A, et al. Dural sinus thrombosis: value of venous MR angiography for diagnosis and follow-up. AJR Am J Radiol 1994;162:1191–1198.
61. Virapongse C, Cazenave C, Quisling R, et al. The empty delta sign: frequency and significance in 76 cases of dural sinus thrombosis. Radiology 1987;162:779–785.
62. Kirkpatrick J, Hayman L. White-matter lesions in MR imaging of clinically healthy brains of elderly subjects: possible pathologic basis. Radiology 1987;162:509–511.
63. Yetkin F, Fischer M, Papke R, et al. Focal hyperintensities in cerebral white matter on MR images

of asymptomatic volunteers: correlation with social and medical histories. AJR Am J Radiol 1993;161:855–858.

64. Drayer B. Imaging of the aging brain. Part II: pathologic conditions. Radiology 1988;166: 797–806.
65. Krischeff I. Arteriosclerosis ischemic cerebrovascular disease. Radiology 1987;162:101–109.
66. Bryan R, Wells S, Miller T, et al. Infarctlike lesions in the brain: prevalence and anatomic characteristics at MR imaging of the elderly—data from the Cardiovascular Health Study. Radiology 1997;202:47–54.
67. Moody D, Brown W, Challa V, et al. Periventricular venous collagenosis: association with leukoaraiosis. Radiology 1995;194:469–476.
68. Consigny P. Pathogenesis of atherosclerosis. AJR Am J Radiol 1995;164:553–558.
69. Dillon E, van Leeuwen M, Fernandez M, et al. CT angiography: application to the evaluation of carotid artery stenosis.
70. Marcus C, Ladam-Marcus V, Bigot J, et al. Carotid arterial stenosis: evaluation at the CT angiography with the volume-rendering technique. Radiology 1999;211:775–780.
71. Furie DM, Tien RD. Fibromuscular dysplasia of arteries of the head and neck: imaging findings. AJR Am J Radiol 1994;162:1205–1209.
72. Shin J, Suh D, Choi C, et al. Vertebral artery dissection: spectrum of imaging findings with emphasis on angiography and correlation with clinical presentation. Radiographics 2000;20: 1687–1696.
73. Houser OW, Mokri B, Sundt TM, et al. Spontaneous cervical cephalic arterial dissection and its residuum: angiographic spectrum. AJNR Am J Neuroradiol 1984;5:27–34.
74. Thompson J, Castillo M, Barrow M, et al. Imaging features and clinical correlation in 60 consecutive children with cerebral infarctions (other than periventricular leukomalacia). Int J Neuroradiol 1996;2:414–421.
75. Siegle M, Shackelford G, Perlman J, et al. Hypoxic-ischemic encephalopathy in term infants: diagnosis and prognosis evaluated by ultrasound. Radiology 1984;152:395–399.
76. Bowerman R, Donn S, DiPietro M, et al. Periventricular leukomalacia in the pre-term newborn infant: sonographic and clinical features. Radiology 1984;151:383–388.

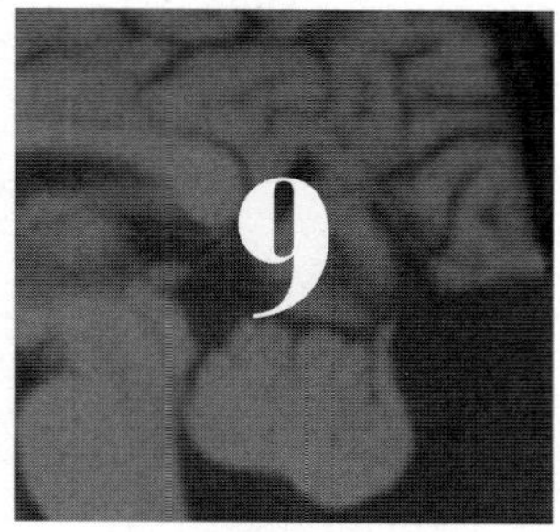

Non-occlusive Cerebral Vascular Disease

- Intraaxial Hemorrhage
- Extraaxial Hemorrhage
- Hemorrhage on Diffusion-Weighted Images
- Hypertensive Hemorrhages
- Germinal Matrix Hemorrhage
- Aneurysms
- Vascular Malformations

One of the most common intracranial lesions is hemorrhage. Its appearance varies according the imaging modality used. I first review the appearance of intracranial bleeds according to their location and imaging modality used; then I review the different types of hemorrhages, aneurysms, and vascular malformations.

Intraaxial Hemorrhage

Computed Tomography

The density of hemorrhage on computed tomography (CT) scans depends on the globin moiety of hemoglobin (1). Acute retracted clot is formed by 90% hematocrit and thus is very dense on CT. Iron and metals contribute less than 0.5% of the CT density of blood (and therefore play no important role in determining the CT density of blood). Clot on CT usually measures 60/80 to 120/150 density units. Acute clot is considered to range from the time of bleeding to 1 week and is dense by CT (2). Subacute clot is considered to range from 1 to 6 weeks old and becomes progressively isodense with the brain. Ring enhancement around a clot begins at 3 days and may last up to 3 to 6 months. The chronic sequelae of hemorrhage are:

- Foci of low attenuation (37%)
- Slitlike low-density lesions (25%)
- Calcifications (10%)

Magnetic Resonance Imaging

The signal characteristics of hyperacute intracerebral hematomas are determined by their water content, not by the state of their hemoglobin molecules.

During the first few hours (hyperacute period), the appearance of intracerebral blood is due to the presence of intracellular oxyhemoglobin that contains no unpaired electrons (it is diamagnetic); thus, its appearance at this time depends on the water content of blood

(3) (Fig. 9.1). Diamagnetism refers to a reduction of an applied magnetic field resulting in low T1 signal intensity. The long relaxation time of water overshadows this diamagnetism on T2-weighted images, and hyperacute blood appears bright. In summary, by magnetic resonance imaging (MRI) a hyperacute clot is slightly hypointense on T1- and hyperintense on T2-weighted images.

By MRI, acute clot is considered as such if it is 4 to 48 hours old. Intracellular deoxyhemoglobin forms during this period because of dissociation of oxygen in nonperfused tissues (4). Although paramagnetic, deoxyhemoglobin is shielded, and neighboring water cannot get close enough to it to alter its relaxation time. Because of the differences between the environments inside and outside of the erythrocytes, there is magnetic susceptibility resulting in some signal loss (particularly in susceptibility-sensitive sequences such as gradient-echo or echo planar imaging). In summary, by MRI acute clot is low on T1 and very low on T2 (especially T2*) images (5).

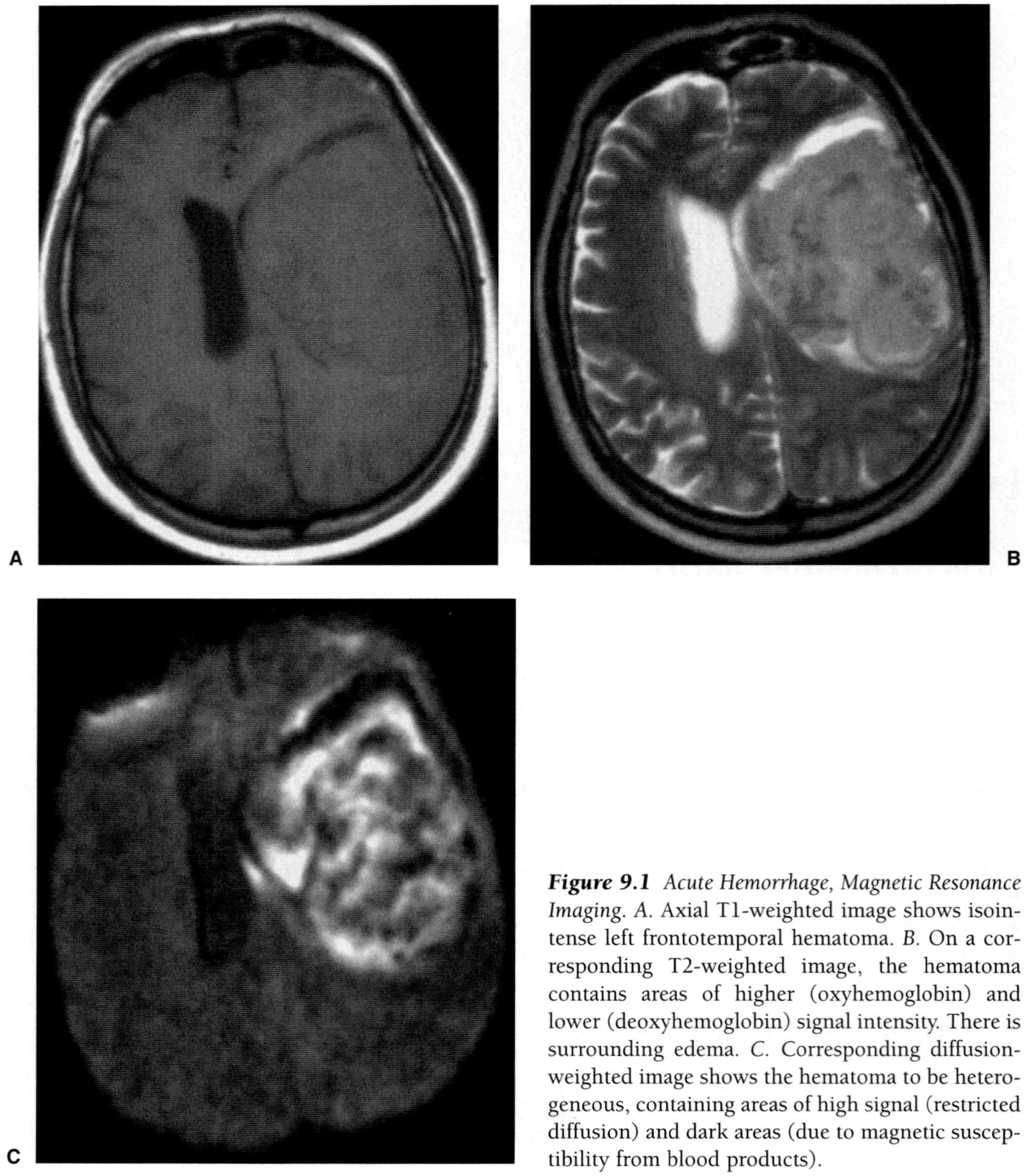

Figure 9.1 *Acute Hemorrhage, Magnetic Resonance Imaging. A.* Axial T1-weighted image shows isointense left frontotemporal hematoma. *B.* On a corresponding T2-weighted image, the hematoma contains areas of higher (oxyhemoglobin) and lower (deoxyhemoglobin) signal intensity. There is surrounding edema. *C.* Corresponding diffusion-weighted image shows the hematoma to be heterogeneous, containing areas of high signal (restricted diffusion) and dark areas (due to magnetic susceptibility from blood products).

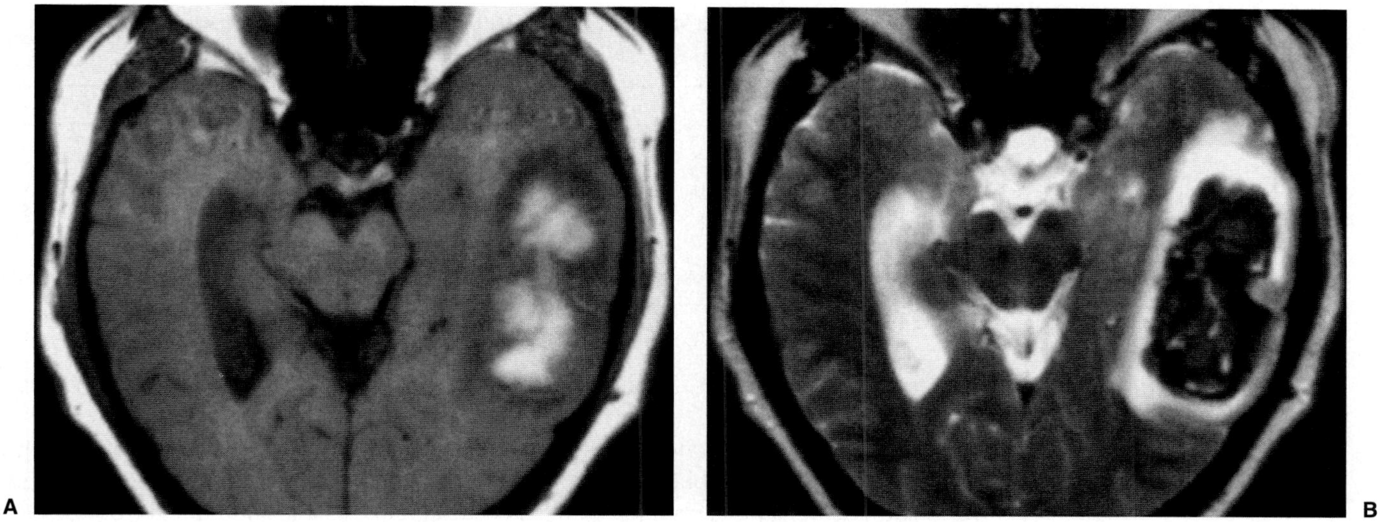

Figure 9.2 *Subacute Hemorrhage, Magnetic Resonance Imaging. A.* Axial T1-weighted image shows a left temporal hematoma to be mostly hyperintense. *B.* Corresponding T2-weighted image shows the hematoma to be dark. The findings are due to presence of intracellular methemoglobin.

Early subacute intracerebral hemorrhage is that which is imaged during the first few days after the bleed. During this period, there is oxidation of deoxyhemoglobin because of loss of intracellular energy, resulting in the formation of intracellular methemoglobin. In this paramagnetic state, water gets close to the iron, but magnetic susceptibility still exists leading to high signal on T1- and low signal on T2-weighted images (6) (Fig. 9.2).

The late subacute period is considered to be days to weeks after the bleed. Methemoglobin becomes extracellular owing to cell lysis. In this paramagnetic state, iron is exposed to water and reduces its relaxation time, leading to high signal on T1 and T2 imaging (6) (Fig. 9.3).

The chronic stage includes the period from weeks to years after the bleed. Heme proteins are phagocytized and stored mostly as ferritin by macrophages. If their capacity to store ferritin is exceeded, the heme proteins are then stored as hemosiderin. Water cannot get close to these compounds and they induce magnetic susceptibility, leading to low sig-

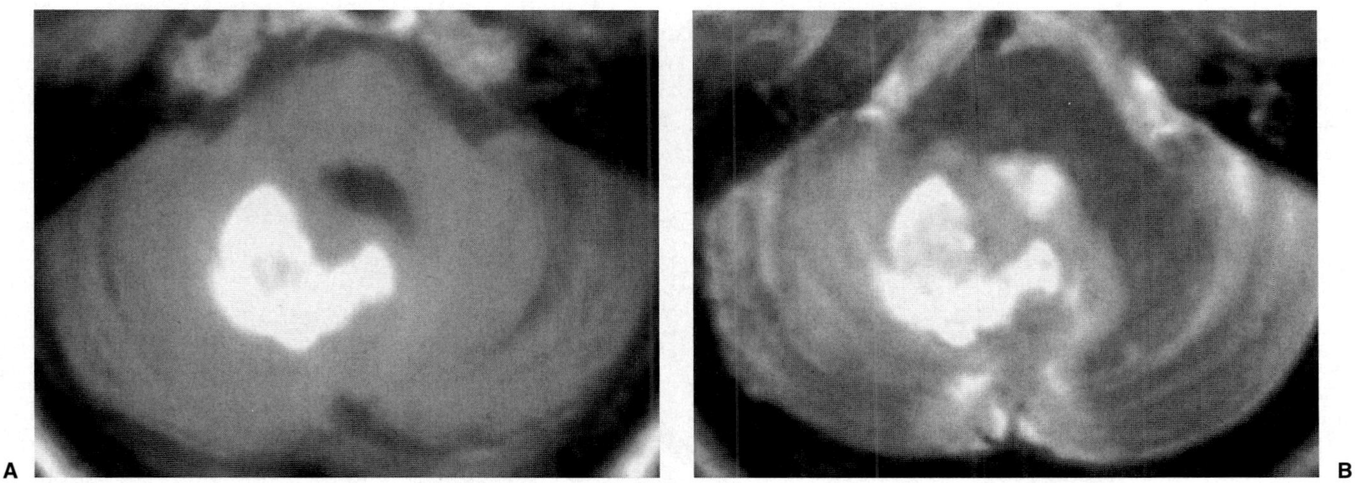

Figure 9.3 *Subacute Hemorrhage, Magnetic Resonance Imaging.* Axial T1- *A* and T2-weighted *B* images show a right cerebellar hematoma that is bright on both sequences. This finding is due to presence of extracellular methemoglobin.

Table 9.1: Appearance of Intraaxial Hemorrhage at 1.5-T Magnetic Resonance Imaging (MRI)

Stage	*T1*	*T2 (and T2*)*
Hyperacute	Isointense	Hyperintense
Acute	Isointense to low	Hypointense
Early subacute	Hyperintense	Hypointense
Late subacute	Hyperintense	Hyperintense
Chronic	Very hypointense	Very hypointense

nal on T1 and T2 images (particularly on gradient-echo T2-weighted and echo planar images).

All of the aforementioned steps are seen when imaging at 1.5 T. The different stages usually begin in the periphery of the hematoma, progress centrally, and follow an organized pattern. Deviations from this pattern occur in rebleeds and should make one suspect an underlying lesion, such as a vascular malformation or a tumor. To review, the appearance of intracerebral hemorrhage by MRI is shown in Table 9.1.

Extraaxial Hemorrhage

Subarachnoid Hemorrhage: Computed Tomography

CT is still the imaging method of choice for the evaluation of the patient suspected to have an acute subarachnoid hemorrhage.

CT permits visualization of subarachnoid hemorrhage (SAH) in more than 90% of patients during the initial 24 hours (7). The volume of blood is grossly related to the underlying etiology, with larger amounts of blood when SAH is due to a ruptured aneurysm and a lesser amount in posttrauma cases. The sensitivity of CT decreases sharply after the initial day and after 3 days, less than 50% of SAHs are identified. Acute subarachnoid blood appears hyperdense by CT and follows the configuration of the subarachnoid spaces (Fig. 9.4).

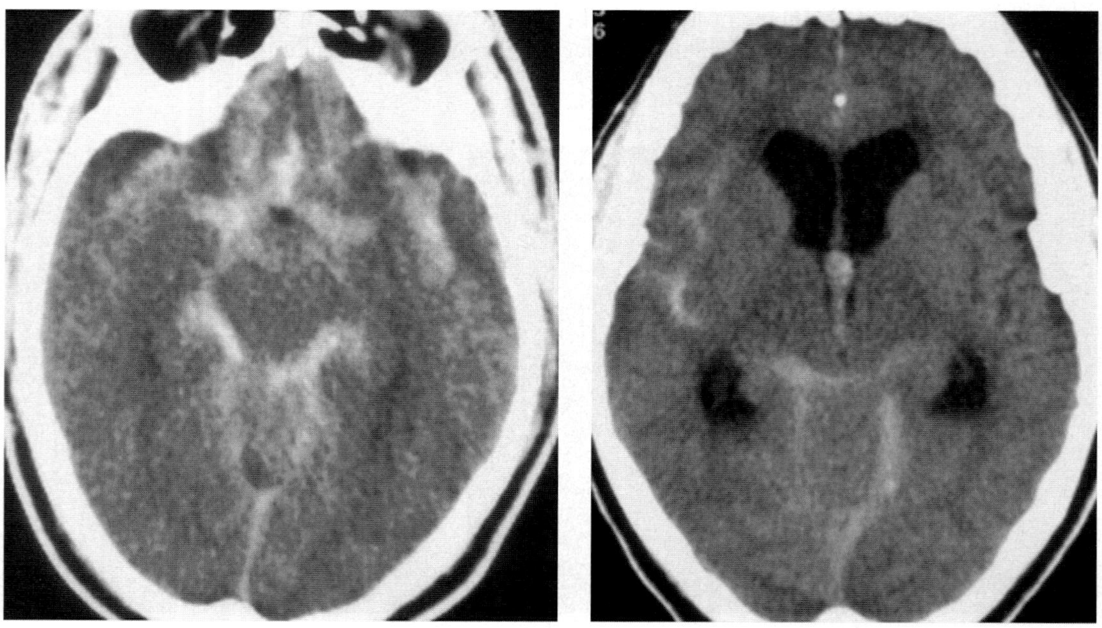

Figure 9.4 *Subarachnoid Hemorrhage, Computed Tomography (CT). A.* Axial CT shows high density due to presence of acute blood filling the basilar and sylvian cisterns. *B.* In a different patient, CT shows acute high-density blood in the quadrigeminal plate and sylvian cisterns. There has been reflux of blood into the third ventricle and development of hydrocephalus.

Table 9.2: Appearance of Extraaxial Bleeds by Computed Topography(CT)

Time Period	*Relative CT Density*	*Enhancement*
Acute	Hyperdense (>80)	No
Subacute	Isodense to brain	Yes, peripheral
Chronic	Hypodense to brain	+/–
Rebleeds	Mixed	+/–

Subdural and Epidural Hematomas: Computed Tomography

The appearance of extraaxial hematomas by CT is listed in Table 9.2 (8) and shown in Figs. 9.5 and 9.6. Visualization of smaller extraaxial bleeds is easier using intermediate window CT settings.

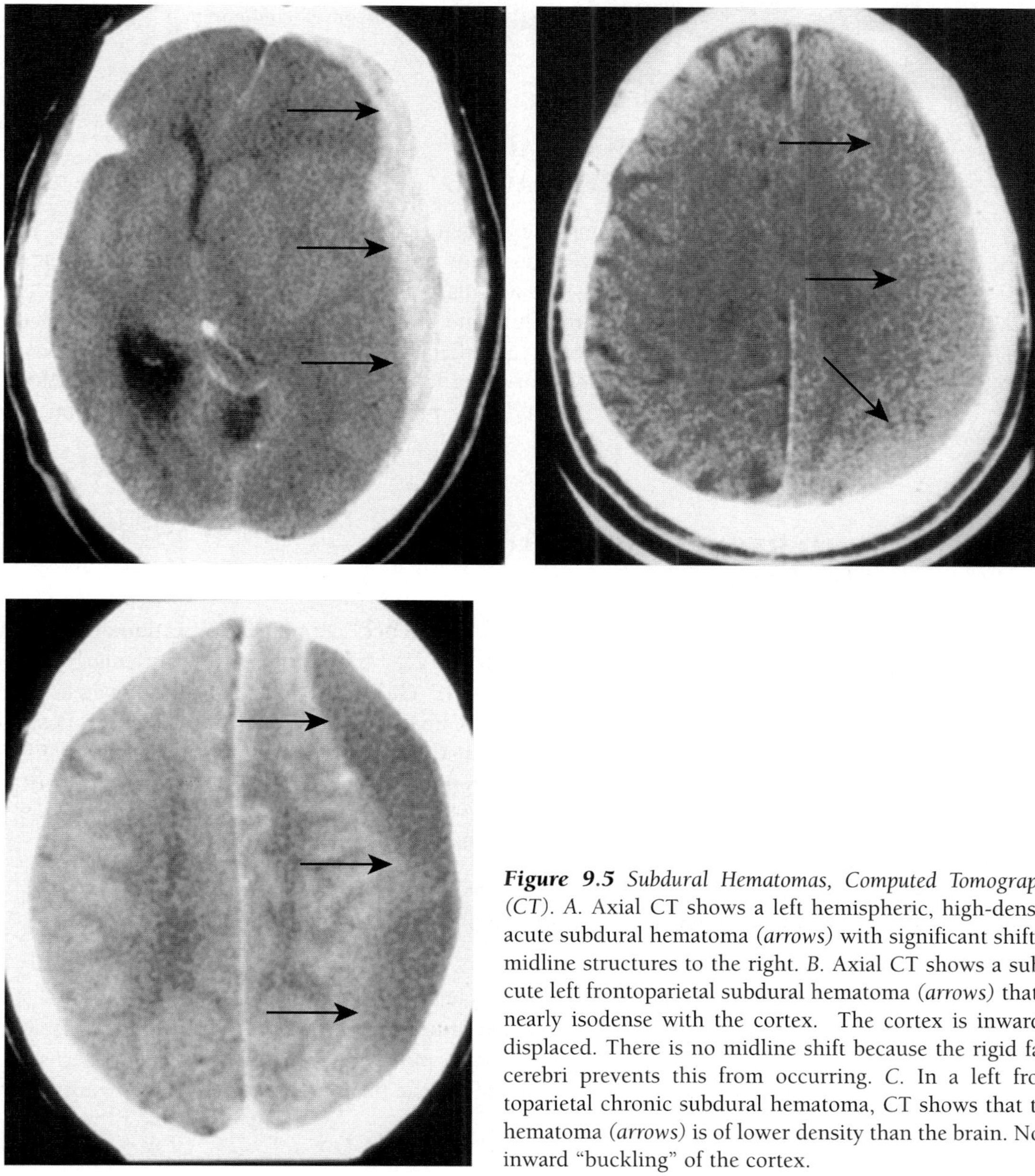

A B C

Figure 9.5 *Subdural Hematomas, Computed Tomography (CT). A.* Axial CT shows a left hemispheric, high-density acute subdural hematoma *(arrows)* with significant shift of midline structures to the right. *B.* Axial CT shows a subacute left frontoparietal subdural hematoma *(arrows)* that is nearly isodense with the cortex. The cortex is inwardly displaced. There is no midline shift because the rigid falx cerebri prevents this from occurring. *C.* In a left frontoparietal chronic subdural hematoma, CT shows that the hematoma *(arrows)* is of lower density than the brain. Note inward "buckling" of the cortex.

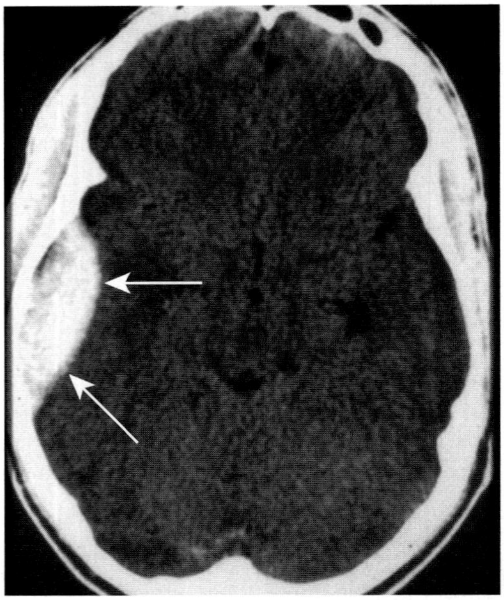

Figure 9.6 *Epidural Hematoma, Computed Tomography (CT).* Axial CT shows right temporal epidural hematoma *(arrows)* with typical biconvex configuration.

Subarachnoid Hemorrhage: Magnetic Resonance Imaging

On conventional MRI techniques, the oxygen tension of cerebrospinal fluid (CSF) is too high to permit degradation of blood, and thus acute SAH is not well seen (9). Chronic SAH may be seen as superficial siderosis (black margins on T2- and T2*-weighted images), particularly on the surface of the cerebellum and brainstem (10). Repeated bleeds are needed for superficial siderosis to occur (11). Superficial siderosis is toxic and results in ataxia and cranial neuropathies. If the etiology for superficial siderosis is not found on brain MRI, the spine needs to be examined to exclude the presence of a vascular malformation or an ependymoma.

Subarachnoid Hemorrhage: FLAIR Images

FLAIR (fluid attenuation inversion recovery sequence) permits identification of acute SAH during the acute and the subacute periods (12). FLAIR images are particularly helpful when SAH is suspected but the CT is negative. On FLAIR images, SAH appears as bright CSF (Fig. 9.7). Detection of SAH by FLAIR images is somewhat limited in the posterior fossa and around the circle of Willis because of motion artifacts in the cisterns. FLAIR imaging is ideal for SAH surrounding the cerebral hemispheres. Bright CSF on FLAIR is a nonspecific finding and may be due to (13):

- SAH
- Increased proteins in CSF, including infections
- Increased oxygen tension in patients on ventilators
- Anesthesia with propofol

On FLAIR images, the CSF may be bright in patients on ventilation devices (14). This is presumed to be due to increased oxygen saturation of the fluid. This finding is seen better in the cortical sulci and ventricles and is not well seen in the basilar cisterns. It is believed that increased oxygenation of CSF by the pia mater and ependyma results in this finding.

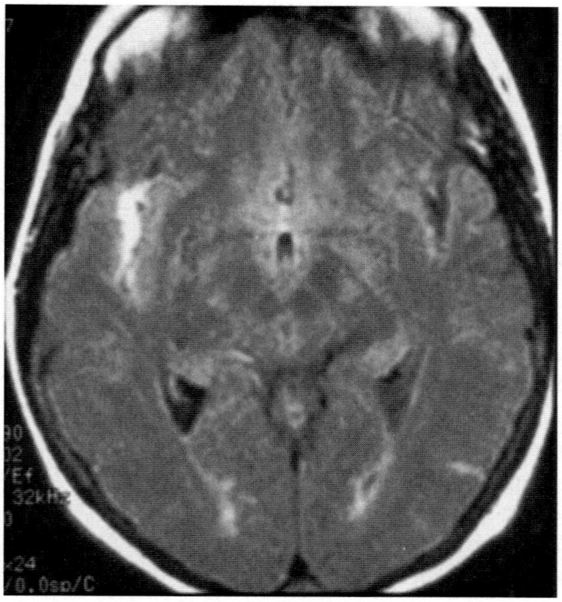

Figure 9.7 *Subarachnoid Hemorrhage, Magnetic Resonance Imaging.* Axial fluid attenuation inversion recovery (FLAIR) image show high signal in cortical sulci, right sylvian fissure, and suprasellar cistern in the presence of blood (and thus, increased proteins) in the cerebrospinal fluid.

Subdural and Epidural Hematomas: Magnetic Resonance Imaging

The blood contained in acute and subacute extraaxial hematomas appears similar to intraaxial blood on MRI studies (Fig. 9.8). Chronic extraaxial hematomas are bright because of the presence of methemoglobin, but become progressively less bright (they are, however, always bright on T2-weighted images). Peripheral deposition of hemosiderin does not commonly occur in extraaxial hematomas. Peripheral enhancement may be present in subacute or chronic extraaxial hematomas. The inner membrane of a subdural

Rarely, subdural hematomas enhance after gadolinium administration, and this may be due to seepage of contrast from the vascularized membranes or to the presence of vascularized clot.

A

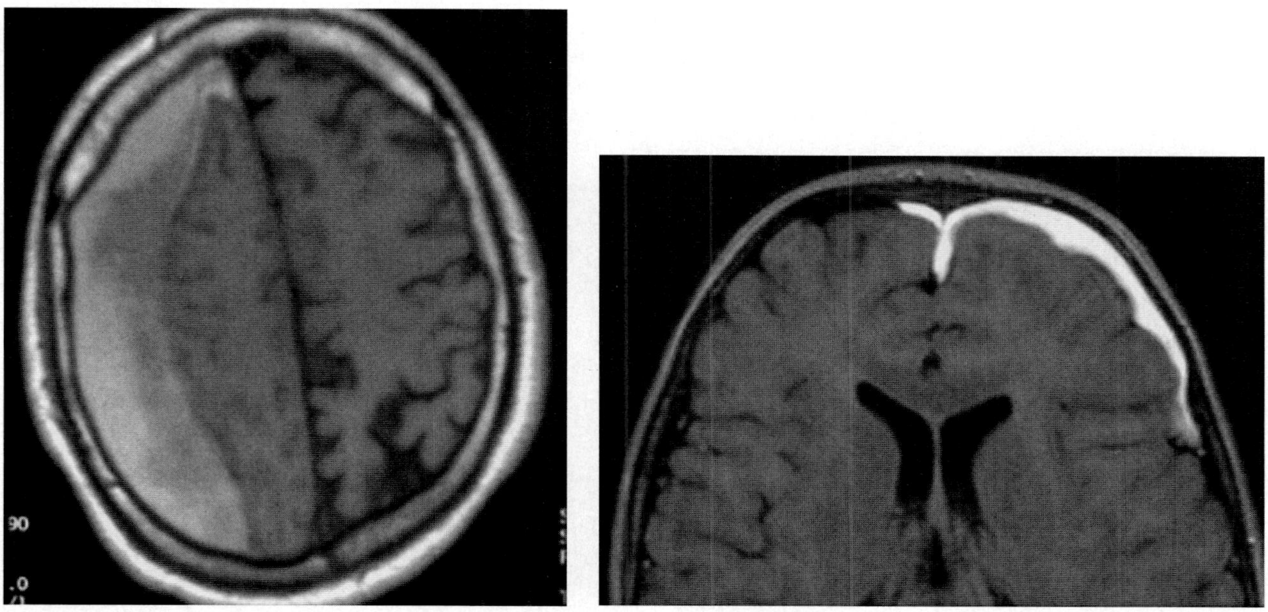

B

Figure 9.8 *Subdural Hematoma, Magnetic Resonance Imaging. A.* Axial T1-weighted image shows high-signal right frontoparietal subdural hematoma. *B.* In a different patient, an axial T1-weighted image shows a thin, high-signal subdural hematoma in the left frontal region and a smaller and similar one in the right frontal region.

hematoma usually is thicker than its outer membrane. Subdural and epidural hematomas are addressed in Chapter 10.

Hemorrhage on Diffusion-Weighted Imaging

Hematomas that are very dark on T2 also may appear dark on ADC maps, and this is an artifact due to the so-called T2 blackout effect. I suggest reading the following: Maldjian JA, Listerud J, Moonis G, et al. Computing diffusion rates in T2-dark hematomas and areas of low T2 signal. AJNR Am J Neuroradiol *2001;22:112–118* (Fig. 9.9).

The appearance of intraaxial hemorrhage on diffusion-weighted imaging depends mostly on the state of the erythrocytes (intact versus lysed). Water contained in the complex intracellular environment has less random motion than water outside of the lysed red blood cells. As such, diffusion is restricted while the erythrocytes remain intact (hyperacute, acute, and early subacute stages) (15). Thus, during these periods, intraaxial hematomas are bright on trace images and dark on apparent diffusion coefficient (ADC) maps. They may be difficult to differentiate from infarctions without studying the conventional MRI sequences. Once the erythrocytes lyse (late subacute and chronic stages) and water is free to move, the diffusion increases, leading to lower signal intensity on trace images and increased signal on the ADC maps (15). Although this behavior is true of most acute and chronic hematomas, I have noticed that many hematomas often display a complex pattern of signal intensity, particularly during the acute period (Fig. 9.1C). This is likely due to the combined magnetic susceptibility effects from blood products superimposed on abnormal diffusion of water.

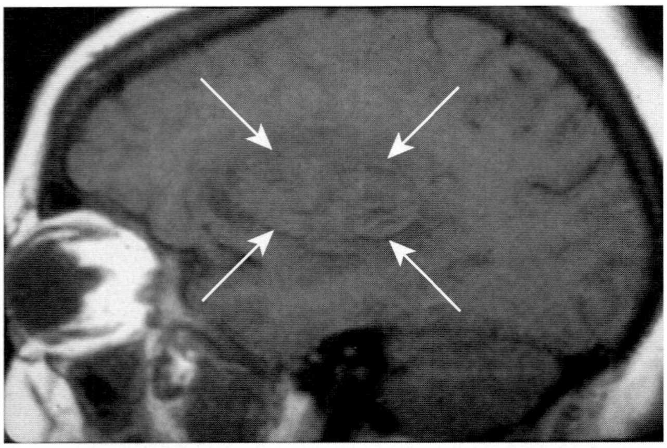

A

Figure 9.9 *Acute Hematoma, DWI. A.* Parasagittal T1-weighted image shows a left temporal acute hematoma *(arrows)* to be nearly isointense with the brain. *B.* Axial T2-weighted image shows that the hematoma is very dark because of the presence of deoxyhemoglobin. Some hyperintense surrounding edema is present. *C.* Corresponding apparent diffusion coefficient map shows that the hematoma is mostly very dark. This is due to magnetic susceptibility and "blackout" effect, and is not due to restriction of water motion.

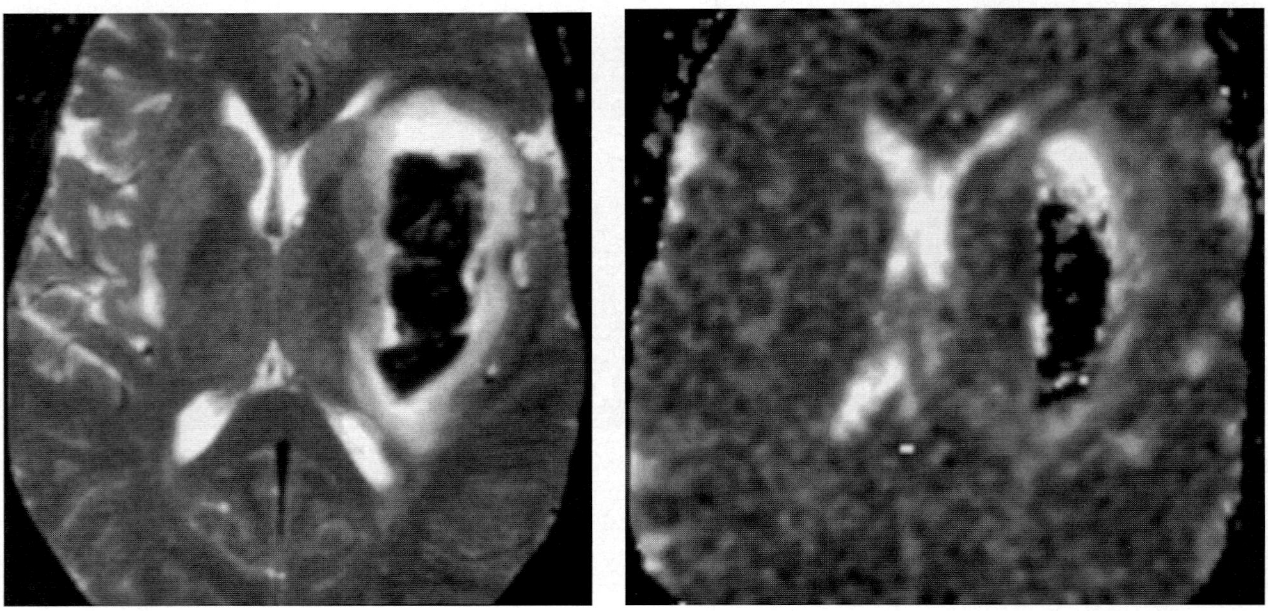

B C

Table 9.3: Location and Frequency of Hypertensive Hemorrhages

Location	Incidence
Basal ganglia (Fig. 9.10A)	60%–70%
Thalami (Fig. 9.10B)	10%–20%
Brainstem (Fig. 9.10C)	5%–10%
Medial cerebellum (Fig. 9.10D)	<5%
Cerebral hemispheres	1%

Hypertensive Hemorrhages

The most common types of brain hemorrhages are posttraumatic and hypertensive. Hypertensive bleeds are more common in men, especially those 60 to 80 years of age. The most common locations are listed in Table 9.3 (16).

Hypertensive bleeds are the underlying cause for 10% of all clinical "strokes," and their mortality rate is as high as 50%. These types of hemorrhages are more common in African-American individuals. In younger patients, a transient elevation of the blood pressure due to drugs (e.g., cocaine, amphetamine, phenylpropanolamine, and phencyclidine) may result in intracerebral bleeds. In older patients it traditionally has been thought that the hypertension causes rupture of small (miliary) aneurysms (called *Charcot-Bouchard aneurysms*). These microaneurysms arise from weakening of the walls of the small perforating arterioles, particularly in the region of the basal ganglia. The relationship between these aneurysms and intracerebral hematomas is questionable (17).

Germinal Matrix Hemorrhage

The germinal matrix (Chapter 1) is located in the outer aspect of the ventricles and is a vascular structure. The germinal matrix involutes throughout late pregnancy, and at 32 weeks' gestation the only remnant is at the level of the caudothalamic notch (18). Hemorrhage arising from the germinal matrix commonly is seen in premature infants (28 to 32 weeks) and in those of low birth weight. The precipitating event tends to be an ischemic event. It traditionally has been believed that germinal matrix hemorrhage is arterial in origin; however, that point of view has been challenged. It appears that most germinal matrix hemorrhages are venous (19). The veins of the germinal matrix are immature and rupture easily. Venous thrombosis that is secondary to hemorrhage and compression of the brain parenchyma results in increased venous pressure that results in even more hemorrhage. Germinal matrix hemorrhages are classified into four grades (Table 9.4).

Most germinal matrix hemorrhages are now thought to be of venous rather than arterial origin.

Grade 1 and 2 hemorrhages have a relatively good prognosis. Grade 3 bleed has a poor prognosis, and many patients develop hydrocephalus. Grade 4 bleeds have a 90% mortality rate. A complicating event is that many patients with germinal matrix hemorrhages also have periventricular leukomalacia (Chapter 8).

Aneurysms

General Information

The overall incidence of intracranial aneurysms is approximately 2% to 8% (20). Approximately 0.5% of aneurysms rupture and bleed per year. This observation applies to patients with aneurysms less than 10 mm in size and no prior history of SAH. The risk of bleeding in patients with a history of prior SAH also is 0.5% per year. However, if the size of the

The most common causes for subarachnoid hemorrhage are trauma and rupture of an intracranial aneurysm.

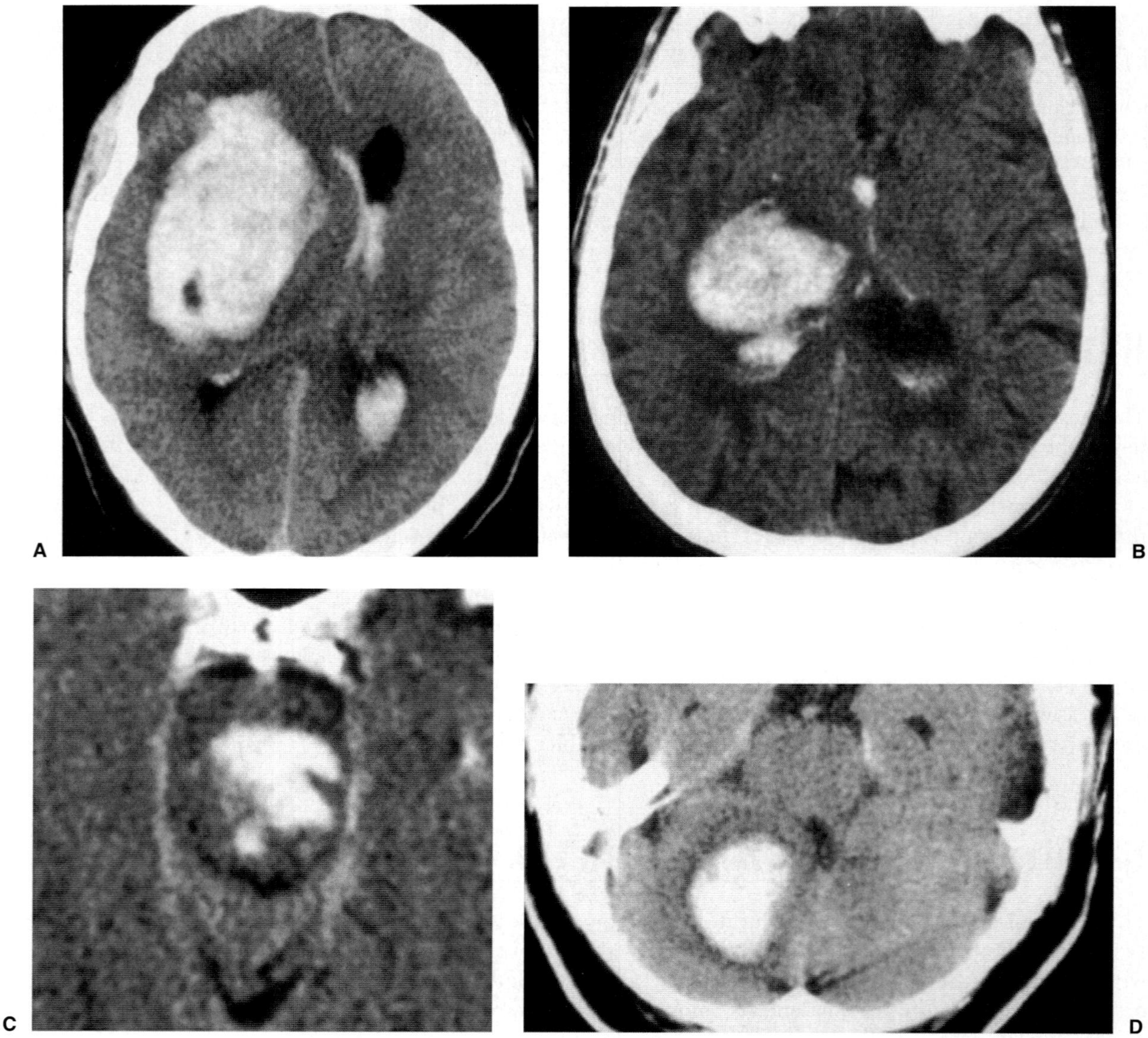

Figure 9.10 *Acute Hypertensive Hematomas. A.* Axial computed tomography (CT) shows acute dense clot in the region of the right lentiform nucleus. There is midline shift to the left and the clot has dissected into the ventricles. *B.* In a different patient, there is an acute and dense hematoma originating from the right thalamus. The hematoma dissected into the ventricles and there is acute blood in the third ventricle and the occipital horns of the lateral ventricles. *C.* Axial CT shows an acute and dense hypertensive hematoma in the brainstem. *D.* In a different patient, axial CT shows a hematoma in the medial (region of the dentate nucleus) right cerebellar hemisphere. There is compression of the fourth ventricle.

Table 9.4: Classification of Germinal Matrix Bleeds

Grade 1	*Grade 2*	*Grade 3*	*Grade 4*
Confined to the germinal matrix at the caudothalamic notch region (Fig. 9.11A)	Grade 1 + extension into the ventricles without hydrocephalus (Fig. 9.11B)	Grade 2 + hydrocephalus (Figs. 9.11C and D)	Grade 3 + intracerebral hematoma (Fig. 9.11E)

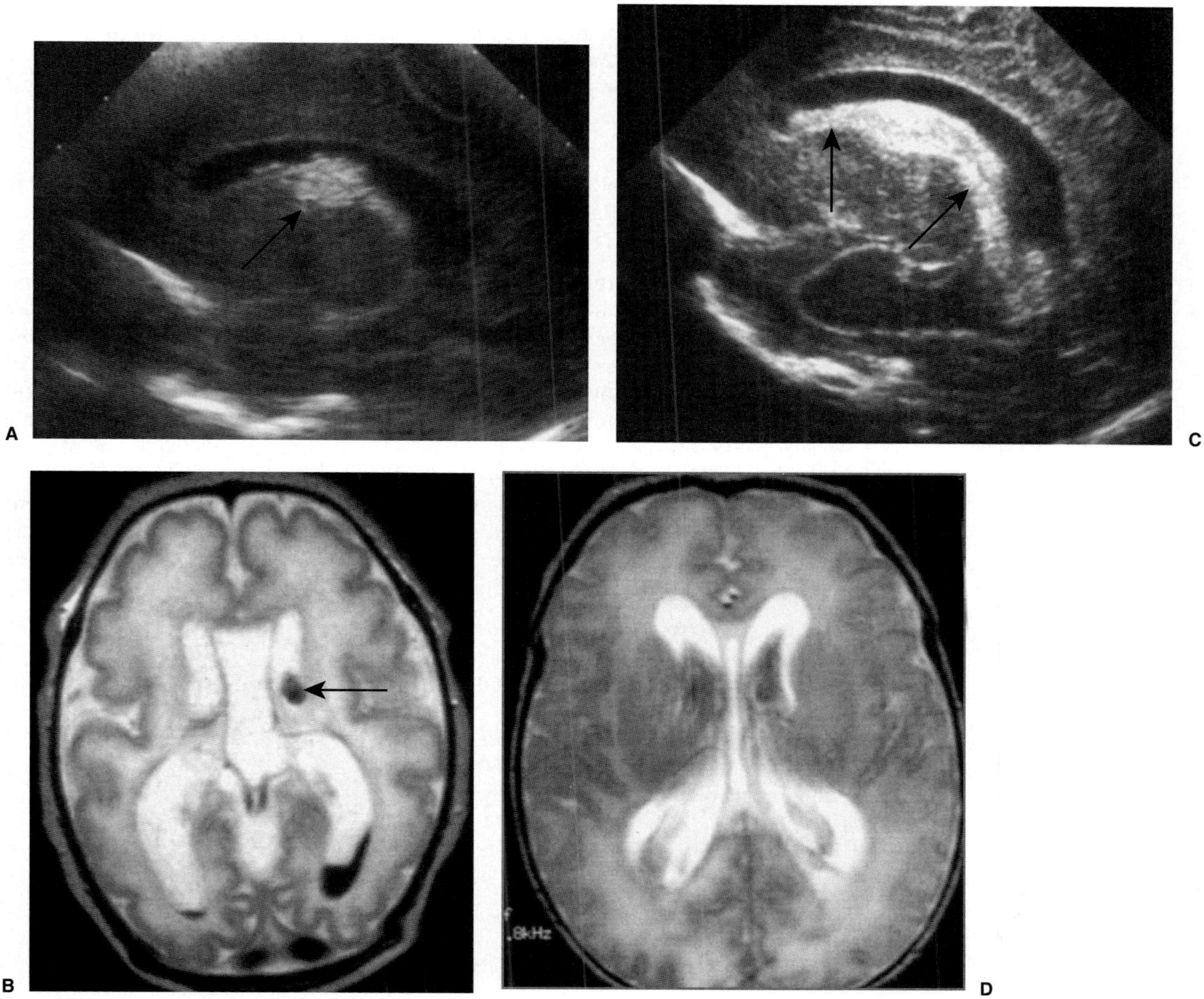

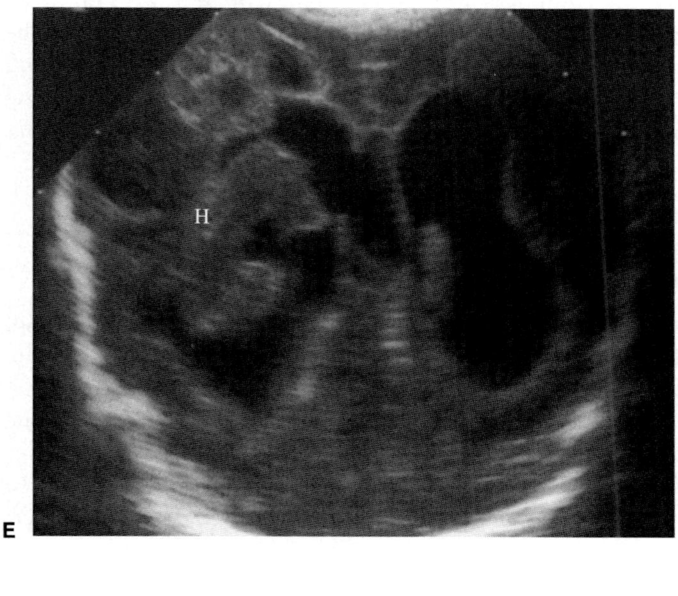

Figure 9.11 *Germinal Matrix Hemorrhages. A.* Parasagittal sonogram shows an echogenic clot *(arrow)* confined to the region of the germinal matrix at the level of the caudothalamic groove (grade 1 hemorrhage). *B.* Axial T2-weighted image shows a dark (due to presence of deoxyhemoglobin) hematoma *(arrow)* in the left caudothalamic groove and also dark blood in the occipital horns of the lateral ventricles (grade 2 hemorrhage). The relative lack of sulcation and prominent ventricles are due to the low gestation age of the child. *C.* Parasagittal sonogram shows echogenic clot *(arrows)* in a dilated lateral ventricle (grade 3 hemorrhage). *D.* In a different patient with a grade 3 hemorrhage, an axial T2-weighted image shows dilated lateral ventricles containing casts of dark blood. *E.* Coronal oblique sonogram shows a complex hematoma *(H)* in and outside of the right lateral ventricle, and hydrocephalus (grade 4 hemorrhage).

aneurysm is over 25 mm, the risk of bleeding increases to 6% per year (cumulative risk of bleeding in 20 years is over 20%). Approximately 90% of intracranial aneurysms arise in the circle of Willis, and 10% in the vertebrobasilar system (21). Approximately 90% of aneurysm ruptures occur in patients 30 to 70 years of age, and all sites rupture with equal frequency (22). The risk of bleeding is closely related to the size of the aneurysm, as follows:

- Less than 5 mm: unlikely to rupture (this observation is debatable and many believe that all aneurysms less than 6 mm should be aggressively treated)
- More than 8 mm: rupture is more common

Despite these general rules, many neurosurgeons believe that there is no safe size and that all aneurysms should be treated. Factors predisposing to aneurysm rupture are increasing age, female gender, hypertension, alcohol, smoking, history of spontaneous dissections (due to deficiency of neural crest cells?), and genetic factors. Intracranial aneurysms probably are not congenital because only 2% of them are found in children. There is a 9.5% incidence of aneurysms in patients with a family history. Some patients with aneurysms may have elevated serum lipoprotein and elastase, and detection of these substances may become a screening test in the future. Most intracranial aneurysms have significant inflammatory changes and are biochemically active lesions, and their parent vessels show increased blood flow and pulsatility index. Thus, aneurysms are not static entities but are dynamic and constantly changing lesions. Intracranial aneurysms may be associated with other disorders, including:

- Fibromuscular dysplasia
- Polycystic kidney disease (autosomal dominant)
- Connective tissue disorders (Ehlers-Danlos syndrome, neurofibromatosis type 1, not Marfan's syndrome)
- Congenitally anomalous vessels (absent, solitary, fenestrated, aortic coarctation)
- Arteriovenous malformations (AVMs)
- Tumors (glioblastoma multiforme, meningioma)
- Vasculitis
- Infections
- Metastases

Anterior Communicating Artery Aneurysm

Aneurysms arising in the anterior communicating artery represent 30% to 35% of all intracranial aneurysms (23). When they bleed, the most commonly affected sites are the gyrus rectus, third ventricle, septum pellucidum, anterior interhemispheric fissure, and basilar cisterns (Fig. 9.12). Aneurysms also may arise in the anterior cerebral artery distal to the anterior communicating artery. Pericallosal artery aneurysms most commonly are posttraumatic, infectious, or associated with an azygos anterior cerebral artery (24).

Posterior Communicating Artery Aneurysm

Aneurysms arising from the posterior communicating artery represent 30% to 35% of all intracranial aneurysms (25) (Fig. 9.13). The most common symptoms at presentation are third cranial nerve palsy and SAH that is diffuse or localized to the basilar cisterns. Perimesencephalic bleeds are a particular type of SAH that are considered benign in the absence of a demonstrable aneurysm on initial angiography (26). It is presumed to represent bleeding from small veins or arteries on the surface of the brainstem. There is no need to repeat the angiogram if the initial one was negative and the SAH conforms to the perimesencephalic cisterns on CT.

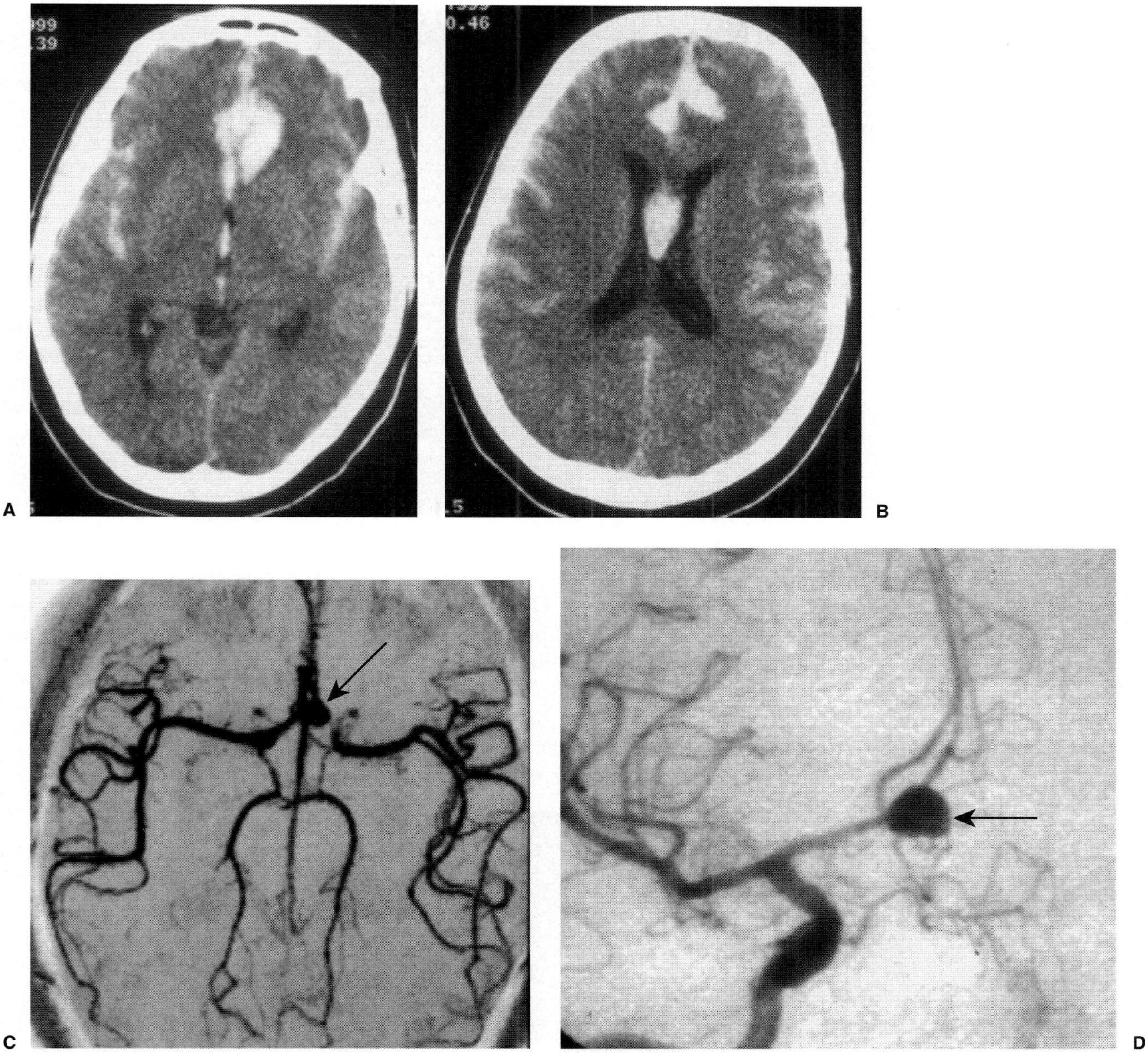

Figure 9.12 *Anterior Communicating Artery Aneurysm. A.* Axial computed tomography (CT) shows typical hematoma resulting from a ruptured anterior communicating artery aneurysm. There is acute dense blood mostly in the anterior interhemispheric fissure and also in the third ventricle and in the sylvian cistern. *B.* In a different patient, axial CT also shows typical hemorrhage caused by ruptured anterior communicating artery aneurysm with acute blood mostly in the anterior interhemispheric fissure and septum pellucidum. There also is subarachnoid blood in cortical sulci and mild hydrocephalus. *C.* Base view from magnetic resonance angiogram (MRA) in an incidentally found anterior communicating artery aneurysm *(arrow)*. *D.* In the same patient, oblique view from a catheter angiogram shows the aneurysm *(arrow)* to be slightly larger than seen on MRA.

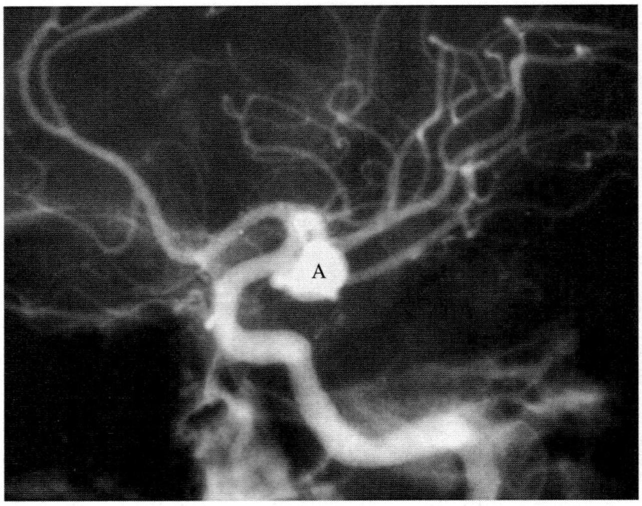

Figure 9.13 *Posterior Communicating Artery Aneurysm.* Lateral oblique projection from a conventional catheter angiogram shows a large aneurysm *(A)* arising in the region of the posterior communicating artery.

Middle Cerebral Artery Aneurysm

Aneurysms from the middle cerebral, anterior communicating, and posterior communicating arteries occur with nearly the same frequency.

Aneurysms arising from the middle cerebral artery (MCA) represent 20% to 30% of all intracranial aneurysms. These aneurysms involve the MCA where it divides (bifurcation or trifurcation) (27) (Fig. 9.14). The bleeds are located in the sylvian fissure, frontal operculum, and basilar cisterns. Approximately 10% of aneurysm ruptures (regardless of their site of origin) present with hydrocephalus.

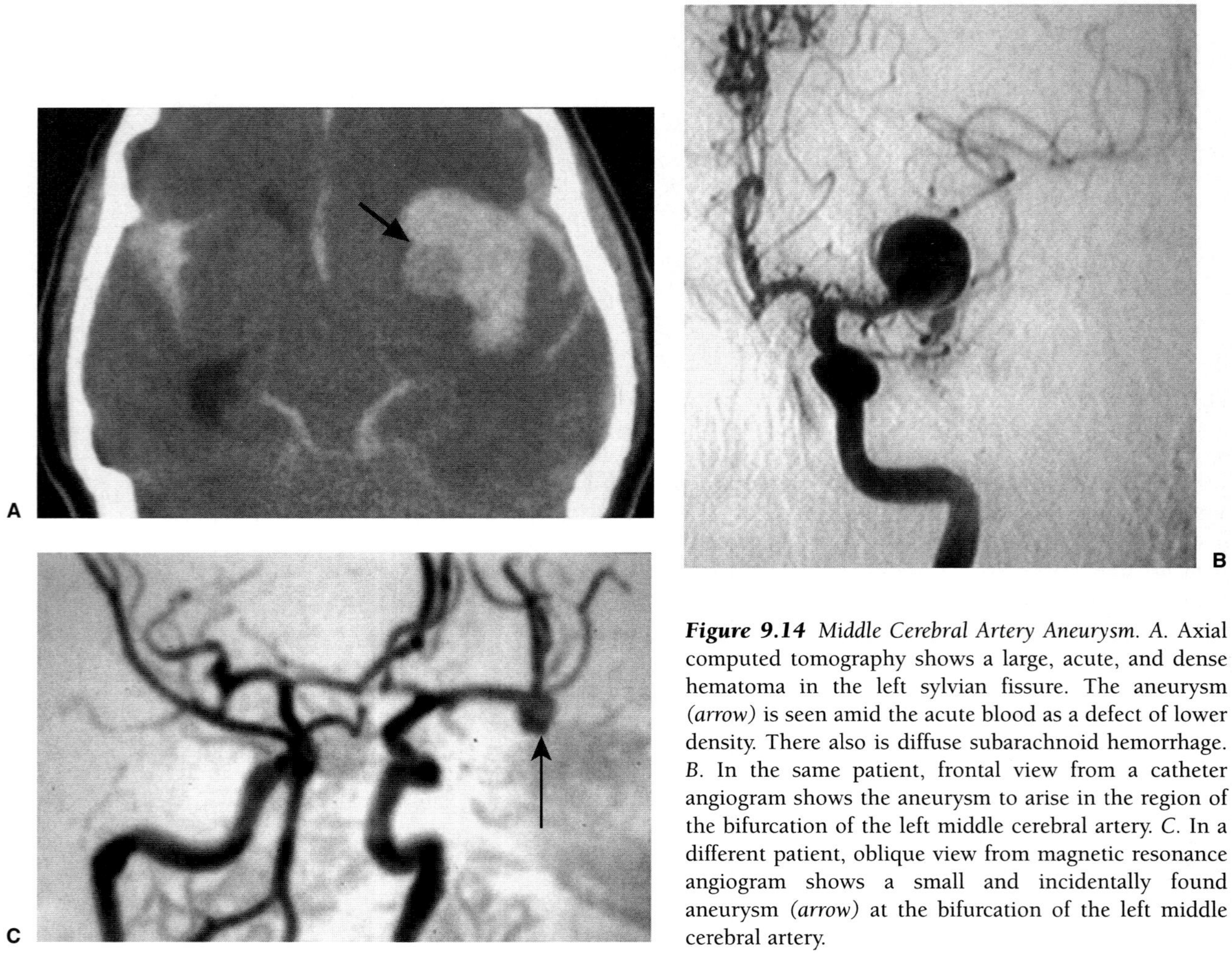

Figure 9.14 *Middle Cerebral Artery Aneurysm. A.* Axial computed tomography shows a large, acute, and dense hematoma in the left sylvian fissure. The aneurysm *(arrow)* is seen amid the acute blood as a defect of lower density. There also is diffuse subarachnoid hemorrhage. *B.* In the same patient, frontal view from a catheter angiogram shows the aneurysm to arise in the region of the bifurcation of the left middle cerebral artery. *C.* In a different patient, oblique view from magnetic resonance angiogram shows a small and incidentally found aneurysm *(arrow)* at the bifurcation of the left middle cerebral artery.

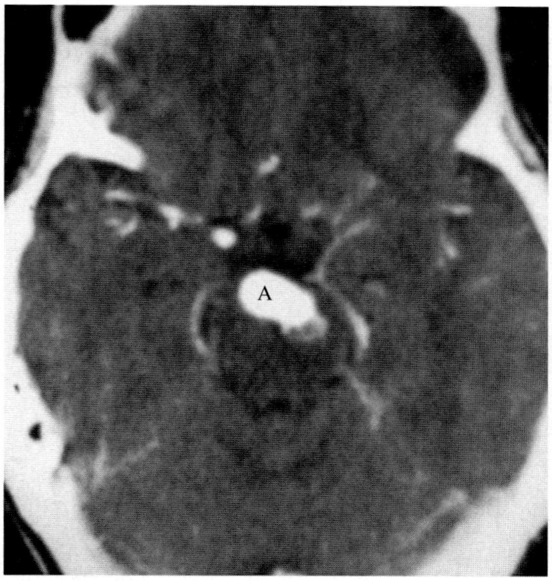

A

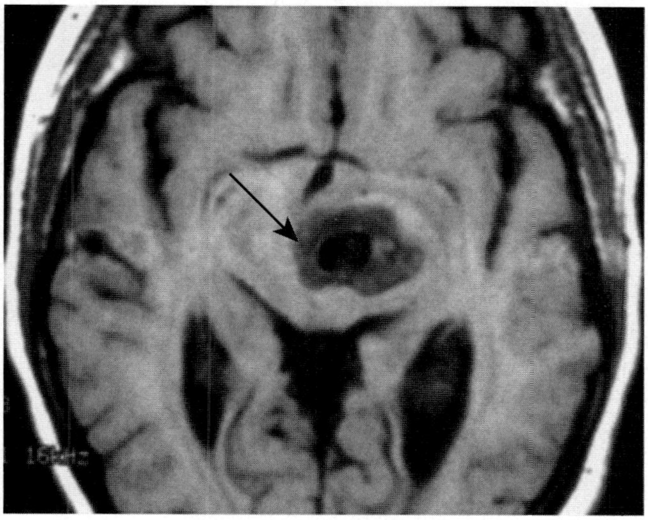

B

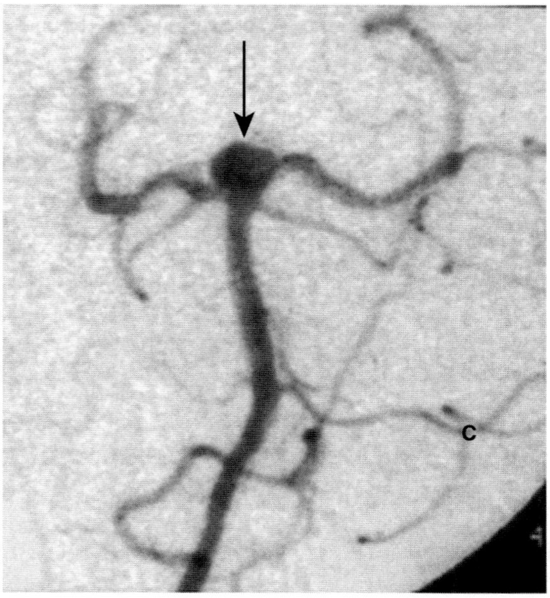

C

Figure 9.15 *Basilar Artery Apex Aneurysm. A.* Axial postcontrast computed tomography shows enhancing mass *(A)* in the interpeduncular cistern caused by an aneurysm of the tip of the basilar artery. *B.* In a different patient, an axial T1-weighted image shows dark mass (*arrow*; due to flow void) in the region of the midbrain. Note somewhat laminated wall of this basilar artery tip aneurysm. *C.* In a different patient, frontal view of conventional angiogram after injection of the right vertebral artery shows an aneurysm *(arrow)* arising in the apex of the basilar artery.

Basilar Artery Apex Aneurysm

Aneurysms arising at the termination of the basilar artery represent 5% to 10% of all intracranial aneurysms. The basilar artery tip is the most common location for aneurysms from the vertebrobasilar circulation, and the fourth most common supratentorial location for aneurysms (28). When they rupture, the bleeds tend to be located in the basilar cisterns and the posterior aspect of the third ventricle. Aneurysms of the basilar artery apex may simulate third ventricular masses (Fig. 9.15).

Infratentorial Aneurysms

Infratentorial aneurysms represent 1% to 3% of all intracranial aneurysms. The most common sites are the posterior inferior cerebellar artery, the body of the basilar artery, and the anterior inferior cerebellar artery (29) (Fig. 9.16). When aneurysms in these sites rupture, the bleeds are located in posterior fossa or fourth ventricle.

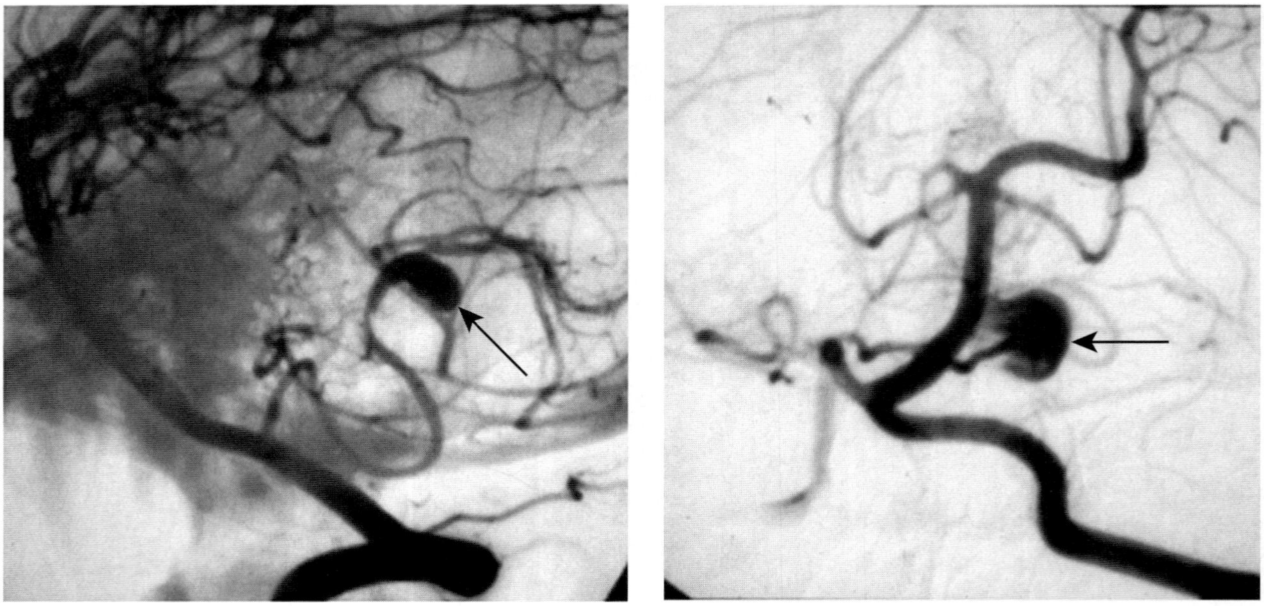

A B

Figure 9.16 *Intratentorial Aneurysms. A.* Lateral view from a conventional angiogram shows an aneurysm *(arrow)* arising at the choroidal point of a posterior inferior cerebellar artery. *B.* In a different patient, frontal view after injection of the left vertebral artery shows an aneurysm *(arrow)* arising at the takeoff of the left anterior inferior cerebellar artery.

Multiple Aneurysms

Approximately 10% to 25% of patients with SAH have multiple aneurysms (30) (Fig. 9.17). There is an increased incidence of multiple aneurysms in women. Of patients with multiple aneurysms, 75% have two aneurysms, 15% have three aneurysms, and 10% have four or more aneurysms. The following criteria may be used to attempt to determine which aneurysm bled when multiple ones are present:

- Largest
- Most irregular
- Lobulated
- Aneurysm adjacent to clot or vasospasm
- Demonstration of active extravasation (very rare)

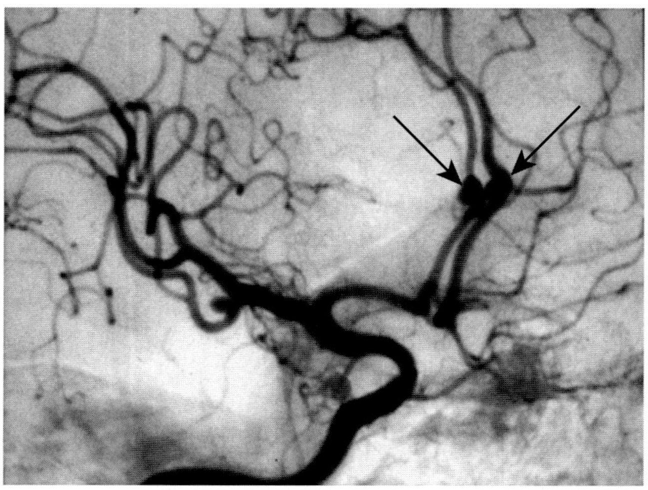

Figure 9.17 *Multiple Aneurysms.* Oblique view from a conventional angiogram shows aneurysms *(arrows)* in the A2 segments of the anterior cerebral arteries, at the bifurcation of the right middle cerebral artery, and in a sylvian artery.

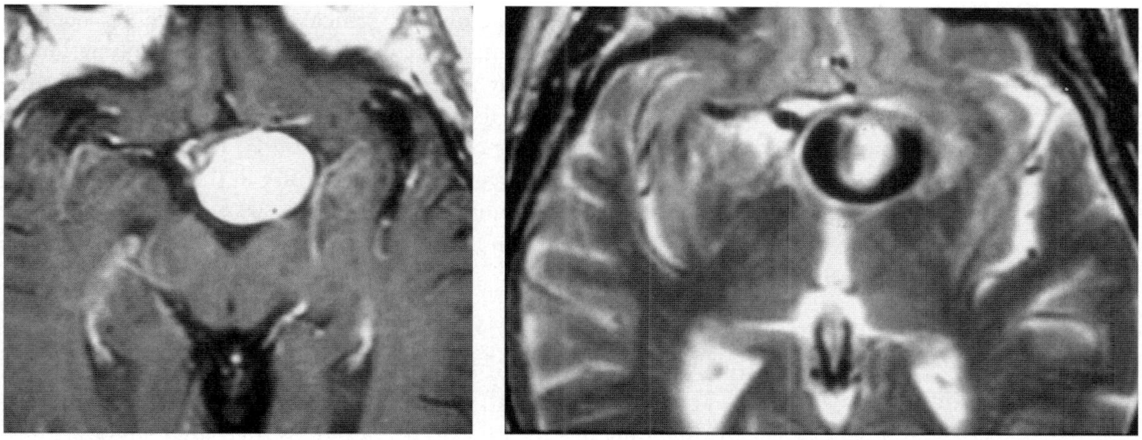

Figure 9.18 *Giant Aneurysm. A.* Axial postcontrast T1-weighted image shows an intense mass in the suprasellar region. *B.* Corresponding T2-weighted image shows complex signal intensity in the mass corresponding to a giant aneurysm arising from the supraclinoid segment of the left internal carotid artery.

Giant Aneurysms

Giant aneurysms are defined as those that measuring greater than 2.5 cm in diameter (31). Their incidence is increased in middle-age women. They tend to rupture less often than smaller aneurysms, and their symptoms commonly are due to mass effect. The most common sites for giant aneurysms are the bifurcation of internal carotid artery (ICA), the intracavernous portion of the ICA, and basilar artery apex (Fig. 9.18). Spontaneous thrombosis of these aneurysms is seen in 13% to 20% of cases. These aneurysms probably grow by intramural hemorrhage, and this is reflected by their imaging appearance. Their MRI characteristics are typical and show concentric layers of blood in different stages of varying signal intensities (32).

Posttraumatic Aneurysms

Posttraumatic aneurysms are rare, accounting for less than 1% of all intracranial aneurysms (24). They commonly are the result of closed head injury or gunshot wounds. Closed head injuries result in aneurysm formation at the base of the skull or in the anterior cerebral artery as it travels under the falx cerebri. The falx then shears the vessels, and many of these aneurysms are indeed "pseudoaneurysms" and not true aneurysms. Posttraumatic aneurysms present in a delayed fashion, with recurrent neurologic symptoms (presumably due to recurrent emboli), SAH, or mass effect. Intraaxial hematomas also may occur after rupture of a posttraumatic aneurysm.

"Blood Blister–Like" Aneurysms

These recently described aneurysms are small focal deficiencies of the entire arterial wall thickness and are covered by only a thin layer of fibrous tissues (33,34). They are broad based, hemispheric in shape, and located on the superior surface of the immediate supraclinoid internal carotid arteries. The underlying vessel may show atherosclerotic changes. Because they are true pseudoaneurysms, their prognosis is poor. Inflammatory changes in their vicinity and their broad base make them very difficult to treat successfully.

Detection of Intracranial Aneurysms

Catheter angiography (using digital subtraction technique) is still the gold standard for the diagnosis of aneurysms. Three-dimensional angiography is playing an increasingly important role, particularly before endovascular therapy, because it displays the neck of an aneurysm well. Angiography may be used to define the optimal ratio between the neck

Both CT and MR angiography may obviate up to 50% of conventional catheter angiograms in patients with acute subarachnoid hemorrhage.

and dome of the aneurysm, and these factors are critical for endovascular occlusion. Today, even some aneurysms with a wide neck are being embolized in combination with remodeling of their neck. MR angiography may show aneurysms down to 3 to 5 mm in size, and three-dimensional time-of-flight techniques are good for screening for "central" aneurysms (those arising from the vessels of the circle of Willis) (35). MR angiography detects more than 85% of aneurysms larger than 5 mm (36). CT angiography detects aneurysms down to 2 mm in size (sensitivity, 88%; specificity, 89%). CT angiography also is good to assess the neck of the aneurysm and detects approximately 96% of aneurysms over 5 mm in size (37).

Vascular Malformations

Cerebral vascular malformations may be divided according to their angiographic appearance as overt (AVMs, venous angiomas) or cryptic (cavernous angiomas, capillary telangiectasia), but in reality such a classification has little clinical utility and significance. This classification stems from the era when catheter angiography was the only diagnostic test used in the evaluation of cerebrovascular lesions, and today has little meaning because MRI shows all of the vascular malformations (hence, cryptic ones no longer are common). Cerebral vascular malformations also may be divided according to their histologic features. From a practical and therapeutic standpoint, it is better to divide them according to their blood flow (Table 9.5).

The importance of this classification is that vascular malformations with arteriovenous shunting need to be treated, those without shunting need no treatment, and those that are partially thrombosed may need to be treated, whereas some may be handled conservatively. I now address each type of malformation.

Arteriovenous Malformations

AVMs are the third most common type of cerebral vascular malformation, but they are discussed first because of their clinical importance. AVMs account for approximately 25% of all cerebral vascular malformations (38). They are primitive communications between arteries and veins devoid of capillary network. The brain surrounding them shows atrophy and gliosis, and these tissues may be considered as nonfunctioning. Over 65% of patients with AVMs present after 40 years of age. When they arise early in life, the function of the brain may be displaced owing to cerebral plasticity. Hemorrhage is common and occurs in 1% to 4% of patients per year. Smaller AVMs bleed more commonly than larger ones. Large AVMs usually present with symptoms related to mass effect. Other symptoms include seizures and headaches. Most AVMs are supratentorial, particularly in the frontal and parietal lobes. Most AVMs are solitary. Multiple AVMs are seen in the Osler-Weber-Rendu and Wyburn-Mason syndromes (39–41).

By CT, AVMs are of high density before contrast administration and show a high degree of enhancement after contrast is infused (42) (Fig. 9.19A). Many AVMs contain

Table 9.5: Division of Cerebral Vascular Malformations According to Their Blood Flow

With Arteriovenous Shunt	*No Arteriovenous Shunt*	*Partially Thrombosed Vascular Malformations*
Arteriovenous malformation	Venous angioma	Postembolization
Arteriovenous fistula	Cavernous angioma	Postirradiation
High-flow hemangioma	Capillary telangiectasia	Postsurgery
	Low-flow hemangioma	Spontaneously thrombosed

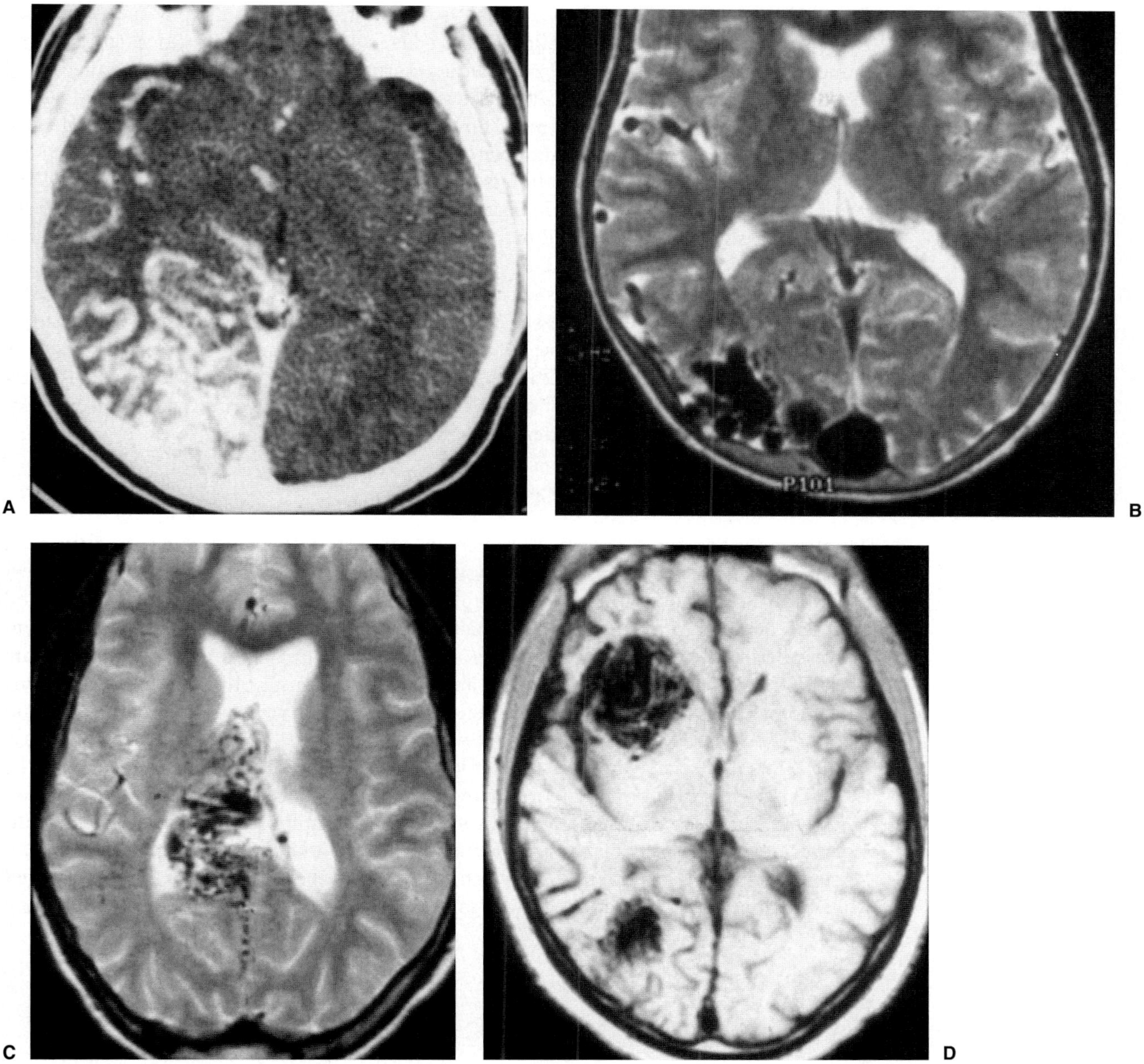

Figure 9.19 *Arteriovenous Malformations (AVM). A.* Axial postcontrast computed tomography shows multiple, serpiginous, high-density vessels in the right occipitotemporal region. Note large diameter of the right middle cerebral artery that partly supplied this AVM. *B.* In a different patient, axial T2-weighted image shows multiple, somewhat rounded flow void defects in the right occipital region. These are mostly the veins draining an AVM. Note the enlarged superior sagittal sinus. *C.* Axial T2-weighted image (different patient) shows a complex AVM inside of the right lateral ventricle. The drainage of this AVM was into the deep venous system. *D.* Axial T1-weighted image shows dual AVMs, one in the right frontal region and another in the right occipital region.

calcifications. The neighboring tissues show atrophy (nearly always present). AVMs tend to be wedge shaped, with their apex pointing toward a ventricle. Small AVMs have fewer feeding arteries than larger ones. Catheter angiography is needed for better definition, establishing feeding vessels, draining veins, and establishing the presence of associated aneurysms. The diagnosis of shunting (and thus of AVM) is made when the arterial, capillary, and venous phases are seen simultaneously on an angiogram. The central aspect of the AVM is called the *nidus*. AVMs have a greater risk of bleeding when their venous drainage is central, when intranidal aneurysms are present, or in the presence of venous hypertension. Most AVMs are called *pial* because they receive their blood supply from branches of the ICA. Contributions from the external carotid artery (ECA, so-called dural blood supply) or contralateral ICA are seen in 30% of large AVMs. On MRI, AVMs show as areas of signal void due to rapidly flowing blood (Fig. 9.19B–D). Time-of-flight MR angiography underestimates the number of feeding vessels, shows the nidus only partially, and in the absence of contrast administration, does not allow clear visualization of the draining veins (43). MRI shows the location and extent of the AVM better than CT. Phase contrast MR angiography is useful in identifying the different components of an AVM, but catheter angiography continues to be the gold standard for diagnostic evaluation.

At present, most deep cerebral AVMs are better treated with a combination of embolization with liquid adhesives and surgery, with or without subsequent stereotactic irradiation.

The association of aneurysms and AVMs deserves special mention because it increases the risk of bleeding. Aneurysms associated with AVMs may be intranidal, in a pedicle feeding the nidus, or remote (44). The first two types probably are flow related, whereas the etiology of the third type is unknown. The flow-related aneurysms are perhaps better treated before resection of the AVM. Most of these aneurysms shrink (and may even disappear) after the AVM has been treated successfully.

Arteriovenous Fistula

Arteriovenous fistulas (AVF) are arteriovenous connections between branches of the ECA or ICA (high-pressure systems) and venous structures (low-pressure system) (45). Most AVF are of the dural type. Dural AVF probably are due to venous sinus thrombosis and represent an attempt by arteries to recanalize that sinus. Many of these arteries represent neovascularity induced by local production of angiogenic factors. Dural AVF are more common in the regions of the transverse and cavernous sinuses (46). Trauma is an important etiology for AVF and is responsible for formation of cavernous sinus fistulas and meningeal fistulas. Rupture of an intracavernous aneurysm gives rise to a fistula. Cavernous sinus fistulas may be direct (a tear in the ICA) or indirect (through branches of the ECA). This classification is important from a practical standpoint because direct cavernous sinus fistulas are treated by occlusion of the rent in the arterial wall, whereas indirect ones require packing and at least partial thrombosis of affected cavernous sinus (47). Most direct fistulas occur in young men. Most indirect fistulas occur in middle-aged women. Patients with direct or indirect cavernous sinus fistulas may show the following signs:

- Exophthalmos
- Conjunctival injection
- Periorbital swelling
- Bruit
- Cranial nerve palsies
- Enlargement of the superior ophthalmic vein

The imaging findings of a cavernous sinus fistula include proptosis, thick sclera, enlarged extraocular muscles, stranding of the retroocular fat, enlarged superior ophthalmic vein (I consider a vein definitely enlarged when it is twice the diameter of the contralateral one), a large cavernous sinus that may contain multiple flow voids, and enlargement of the transcavernous channels and the basilar plexus. The contralateral cavernous sinus also may be enlarged. Visualization of cortical veins implies venous hypertension and carries a worse prognosis.

Most dural fistulas outside of the cavernous sinus remain asymptomatic for many years or throughout the life of the individual. Occasionally, venous hypertension develops and patients have headaches (45,48). Many patients have tinnitus, but a fistula is found mostly in those in whom the tinnitus is objectively heard by the examiner. Hemorrhage may occur, and when it does, it may involve several cranial compartments (epidural, subdural, subarachnoid, intraaxial). These fistulas are very difficult to identify by MRI, and most MRI studies are negative (48,49).

Vein of Galen malformations also are a type of AVF, and are discussed in Chapter 1.

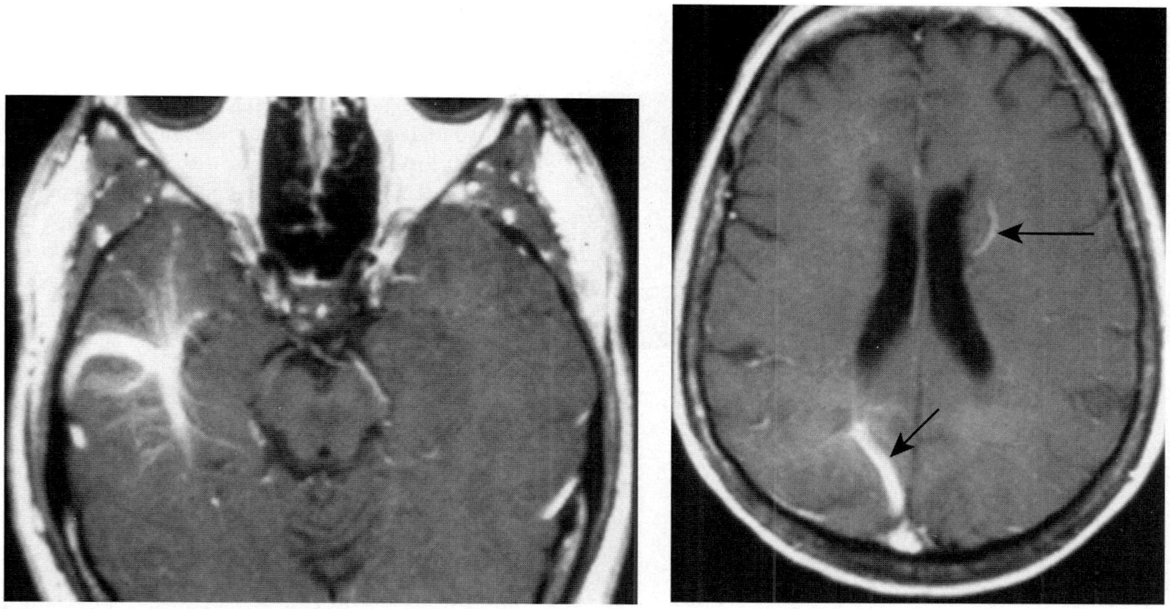

Figure 9.20 *Venous Angioma (Developmental Venous Anomaly). A.* Postcontrast axial T1-weighted image shows typical appearance of right temporal venous angioma draining presumably into the superior middle cerebral vein. *B.* In a different patient, postcontrast axial T1-weighted image shows a right parietal venous angioma *(large arrow)* draining into the superior sagittal sinus. There is smaller venous angioma *(smaller arrow)* in the region of the left caudate nucleus.

Venous Angioma (Developmental Venous Anomaly, Venous Malformation).

Multiple venous angiomas may be seen in the blue rubber bleb syndrome.

Venous angiomas are the most common vascular cerebral malformation and are nearly always incidentally encountered (most often on MRI of brain) (50). They consist of an anomalous group of deep medullary veins draining into a transcerebral vein, which then empties into a cortical vein, venous sinus, ependymal veins, or large deep cerebral vein (51) (Fig. 9.20). The brain surrounding them is normal. Today, they often are called *development venous anomalies*. Most venous angiomas are asymptomatic, but rarely they result in headaches. Most venous angiomas are solitary and located in the frontal lobes, but they can occur anywhere in the brain, including the brainstem (51). Seizures, focal neurologic deficits, and hemorrhages may occur when venous angiomas are associated with a cavernous angioma or located in the posterior fossa (although the latter observation is questionable).

Cavernous Angioma

Cavernous angiomas are the second most common type of cerebral vascular malformation, and most are found incidentally at MRI (52). They are composed of dilated vascular channels containing low-pressure and slow-flowing blood without intervening brain tissue. Cavernous angiomas tend to be associated with subclinical bleeds that account for their appearance on MRI. They may produce seizures, headaches, and focal neurologic deficits, and occasionally they may overtly bleed. Most cavernous angiomas are supratentorial (80%), but they may be seen anywhere, including the brainstem and the spinal cord (53). They usually are found in younger and middle-aged adults, and they have no sex predilection. On CT, they are slightly hyperdense before contrast administration and enhance slightly after contrast administration. Tiny calcifications may be present. On MRI, they typically have a "salt-and-pepper" appearance with a rim of very low signal intensity (Fig. 9.21). Their internal features are due to slow-flowing blood and partially thrombosed vascular channels. The rim is due to deposition of hemosiderin and ferritin (54). The mag-

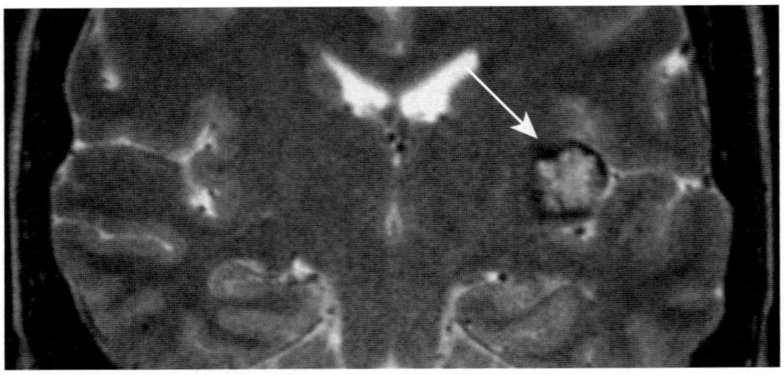

A

Figure 9.21 *Cavernous Angioma. A.* Coronal T2-weighted image shows typical cavernous angioma *(arrow)* in the left insula in this patient with seizures. Note mottled internal architecture surrounded by a hypointense rim. *B.* In a different patient, axial T2-weighted image shows a cavernous angioma in the inferior aspect of the right cerebellar hemisphere. *C.* Corresponding postcontrast T1-weighted image shows that the lesion contains some areas of enhancement.

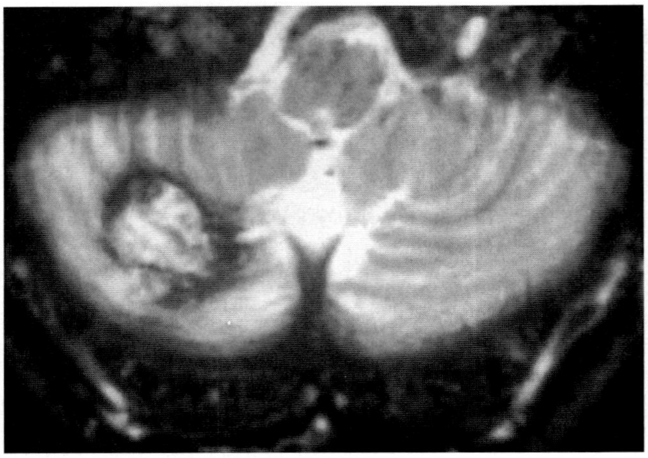

B

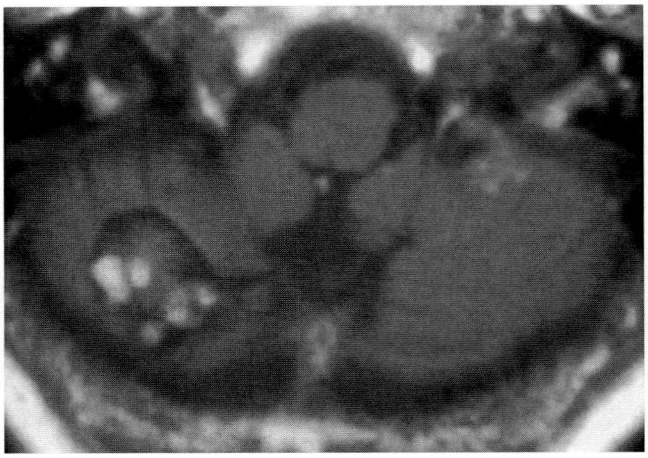

C

netic susceptibility effect caused by the ferritin and hemosiderin is best appreciated on gradient-echo T2-weighted images, where the lesion appears to "bloom." The differential diagnosis for these lesions is shown in Box 9.1.

Cavernous angiomas usually are solitary lesions, but they may be multiple and associated with a familial syndrome (deletion in chromosome 7q) (55). Up to 30% of cavernous angiomas are accompanied by other vascular malformations, particularly venous angiomas (this combination may be seen as a larger vein draining the cavernous malformation). Cavernous angiomas may develop after whole-brain irradiation (particularly low-dose radiation for children with leukemia) (56–58).

Last, a word about nomenclature. The terms *cavernous angioma* and *cavernous hemangioma* have fallen out of favor with some authors. Many prefer to call these lesions *cavernous malformations*. The reason for this is that many believe that *angioma* and *hemangioma* imply growth, and in reality most of these lesions are static. I still use the terms *cavernous angioma* and *cavernous hemangioma* because everyone is familiar with them and because I do believe that these lesions change over time. They are very uncommon in chil-

Box 9.1: Differential Diagnosis of T2 Hypointense Lesions May "Bloom" on Gradient-Echo Images

Cavernous angioma	Cysticercosis
Capillary telangiectasia	Amyloidosis
Shearing injuries	Small hypertensive hemorrhages
Metastases	

dren, but we see them arise *de novo* after brain irradiation (so they do grow). In addition, they are very rare in the elderly (think of all the MRI studies of the brain in older adults you see in your practice, and how many of them had cavernous angiomas). Thus, it is conceivable that some cavernous angiomas involute with age.

Capillary Telangiectasia

Capillary telangiectases are found incidentally in nearly 1% of autopsies but are not commonly encountered in clinical practice (59). They are more common in the pons and upper medulla, but may occur anywhere in the brain. They are a conglomeration of small vessels similar to capillaries containing low-pressure, slow-flowing blood. These vessels are separated by normal brain. Capillary telangiectases contain no gross hemorrhage, gliosis, or calcifications. They almost always are found in the base of the pons, produce no mass effect, and usually do not grow (60). They show no abnormalities (or only a minimal drop) of signal intensity on T2 images, and some show mild enhancement in a brush-like or stipple pattern after gadolinium is given (Fig. 9.22A). The low T2 signal intensity is better appreciated on gradient-echo images and is thought to be related to the presence of deoxygenated blood in the lesion. Blood oxygenation level–dependent (BOLD) imaging and diffusion-weighted imaging which accentuate the presence of deoxyhemoglobin, may be helpful in detection of these lesions and in mapping their extension (61) (Fig. 9.22B). Capillary telangiectases also may develop after low-dose whole-brain radiation, or may be congenital.

Transitional Vascular Malformations

It is becoming obvious that many cerebral vascular malformations are mixed, and some have termed them *transitional malformations*. Capillary telangiectases not uncommonly are associated with cavernous angiomas, venous angiomas, and even AVMs (62,63). It is possible that capillary telangiectasias are not congenital lesions but are acquired secondary to venous drainage obstruction of a venous angioma. Similarly, cavernous angiomas may be found in the vicinity of a venous angioma and may form secondary to venous drainage restriction. Transitional malformations also develop after brain irradiation. The importance of these transitional malformations is that they have an increased risk of bleeding compared with those of only one type.

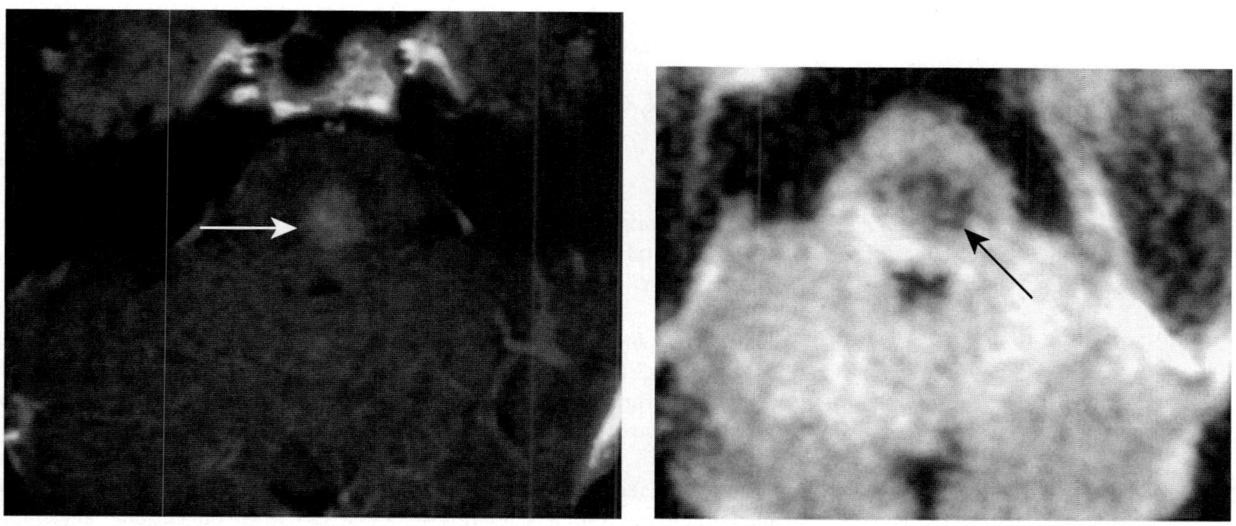

A B

Figure 9.22 *Capillary Telangiectasia (Presumed). A.* Axial post contrast T1-weighted image shows a faintly enhancing lesion *(arrow)* in the pons. *B.* On a diffusion-weighted image, the lesion is hypointense *(arrow)* because of the presence of deoxygenated blood.

References

1. New PFJ, Aronow S. Attenuation measurements of whole blood and blood fractions in computed tomography. Radiology 1976;121:635–640.
2. Scott WR, New PFJ, Davis KR, et al. Computerized axial tomography of intracerebral and intraventricular hemorrhage. Radiology 1974;112:73–80.
3. Brooks R, Di Chiro G, Patronas N. MR imaging of cerebral hematomas at different field strengths: theory and applications. J Comput Assist Tomogr 1989;13:194–206.
4. Clark R, Watanabe A, Bradley W, et al. Acute hematomas: effects of deoxygenation, hematocrit, and fibrin-clot formation and retraction on T2 shortening. Radiology 1990;175:201–206.
5. Atlas S, Mark A, Grossman R, et al. Intracranial hemorrhage: gradient-echo MR imaging at 1.5 T. Radiology 1988;168:803–807.
6. Bradley W. MR appearance of hemorrhage in the brain. Radiology 1993;189:15–26.
7. Norman D, Price D, Boyd D, et al. Quantitative aspects of computed tomography of the blood and cerebrospinal fluid. Radiology 1977;123:335–338.
8. Forbes GS, Sheedy PF, Piepgras DG, et al. Computed tomography in the evaluation of subdural hematomas. Radiology 1978;126:143–148.
9. Atlas S. MR imaging is highly sensitive for acute subarachnoid hemorrhage . . . not! Radiology 1993;186:319–322.
10. Bracchi M, Savoiardo M, Triulzi F, et al. Superficial siderosis of the CNS: MR diagnosis and clinical findings. AJNR Am J Neuroradiol 1993;14:227–236.
11. Mamourian AC. MR of superficial siderosis. AJNR Am J Neuroradiol 1993;14:1445.
12. Noguchi K, Ogawa T, Seto H, et al. Subacute and chronic subarachnoid hemorrhage: diagnosis with fluid-attenuated inversion-recovery MR imaging. Radiology 1997;203:252–262.
13. Melhem E, Jara H, Eustace S. Fluid-attenuated inversion recovery MR imaging: identification of protein concentration thresholds for CSF hyperintensity. AJR Am J Radiol 1997;169:859–862.
14. Deliganis A, Fisher D, Lam A, et al. Cerebrospinal fluid signal intensity increase on FLAIR MR images in patients under general anesthesia: the role of supplemental O_2. Radiology 2001;218: 152–156.
15. Atlas S, DuBois P, Singer M, et al. Diffusion measurements in intracranial hematomas: implications for MR imaging of acute stroke. AJNR Am J Neuroradiol 2000;21:1190–1194.
16. Gokaslan ZL, Narayan RK. Intracranial hemorrhage in the hypertensive patient. Neuroimaging Clin North Am 1992;2:171–195.
17. Challa VR, Moody DM, Bell MA. The Charcot-Bouchard aneurysm controversy: impact of a new histologic technique [see comments]. J Neuropathol Exp Neurol 1992;51:264–271.
18. Blankenberg F, Norbash A, Lane B, Stevenson D, et al. Neonatal intracranial ischemia and hemorrhage: diagnosis with US, CT, and MR imaging. Radiology 1996;199:253–259.
19. Ghazi-Birry HS, Brown WR, Moody DM, et al. Human germinal matrix: venous origin of hemorrhage and vascular characteristics. AJNR Am J Neuroradiol 1997;18:219–229.
20. Ronkainen A, Puranen M, Hernesniemi J, et al. Intracranial aneurysms: MR angiographic screening in 400 asymptomatic individuals with increased familial risk. Radiology 1995;195: 35–40.
21. Klein G, Szolar D, Leber K, et al. Basilar tip aneurysm: endovascular treatment with Guglielmi detachable coils: midterm results. Radiology 1997;205:191–196.
22. McCormick P, McCormick J, Zimmerman R, et al. The pathophysiology of acute subarachnoid hemorrhage. BNI Q 1991;7:18–26.
23. Cognard C, Weill A, Castaings L, et al. Intracranial berry aneurysms: angiographic and clinical results after endovascular treatment. Radiology 1998;206:499–510.
24. Nakstad P, Nornes H, Hauge HN. Traumatic aneurysms of the pericallosal arteries. Neuroradiology 1986;28:225–331.
25. Korogi Y, Takahashi M, Mabuchi N, et al. Intracranial aneurysms: diagnostic accuracy of three-dimensional, Fourier transform, time-of-flight MR angiography. Radiology 1994;193:181–186.
26. Rinkel G, Wijdicks E, Vermeulen M, et al. Nonaneurysmal perimesencephalic subarachnoid hemorrhage: CT and MR patterns that differ from aneurysmal rupture. AJR Am J Radiol 1991;157:829–834.
27. Korogi Y, Takahashi M, Katada K, et al. Intracranial aneurysms: detection with three-dimensional CT angiography with volume rendering—comparison with conventional angiographic and surgical findings. Radiology 1999;211:497–506.
28. Kallmes D, Clark H, Dix J, et al. Ruptured vertebrobasilar aneurysms: frequency of the nona-

neurysmal perimesencephalic pattern of hemorrhage on CT scans. Radiology 1996;201: 657–660.
29. Friedman D. Abnormalities of the posterior inferior cerebellar artery: MR imaging findings. AJR Am J Radiol 1996;160:1257–1263.
30. Wilson FMA, Jaspan T, Holland IM. Multiple cerebral aneurysms: a reappraisal. Neuroradiology 1989;31:232–237.
31. Olsen W, Brant-Zawadzki M, Hodes J, et al. Giant intracranial aneurysms: MR imaging. Radiology 1987;163:431–435.
32. Atlas S, Grossman R, Goldbert H, et al. Partially thrombosed giant intracranial aneurysms: correlation of MR and pathologic findings. Radiology 1987;162:111–114.
33. Ogawa A, Suzuki M, Ogasawara K. Aneurysms at nonbranching sites in the supraclinoid portion of the internal carotid artery: internal carotid artery trunk aneurysms. Neurosurgery 2000;47:578–583.
34. Wrobel CJ, Taubman K. Blood-blister-like aneurysms [letter; comment]. J Neurosurg 2000;92: 1076–1077.
35. White P, Wardlaw J, Easton V. Can noninvasive imaging accurately depict intracranial aneurysms? A systematic review. Radiology 2000;217:361–370.
36. Huston J, Rufenach D, Ehman R, et al. Intracranial aneurysms and vascular malformations: comparison of time-of-flight and phase-contrast MR angiography. Radiology 1991;181:721–730.
37. Schwartz R, Tice H, Hooten S, et al. Evaluation of cerebral aneurysms with helical CT: correlation with conventional angiography and MR angiography. Radiology 1994;192:717–722.
38. Edelman R, Wentz K, Mattle H, et al. Intracerebral arteriovenous malformations: evaluation with selective MR angiography and venography. Radiology 1989;173:831–837.
39. Willinsky RA, Lasjaunias P, Terbrugge K, et al. Multiple cerebral arteriovenous malformations (AVMs). Neuroradiology 1990;32:207–210.
40. Kikuchi K, Kowada M, Sakamoto T, et al. Wyburn-Mason syndrome: report of a rare case with computed tomography and angiographic evaluations. J Comput Tomogr 1988;12:111–115.
41. Patel U, Gupta SC. Wyburn-Mason syndrome. Neuroradiology 1990;31:544–546.
42. Brunelle F, Harwood-Nash D, Fitz C, et al. Intracranial vascular malformation in children: computed tomographic and angiographic evaluation. Radiology 1983;149:455–461.
43. Atlas S, Mark A, Fram E, et al. Vascular intracranial lesions: applications of gradient-echo MR imaging. Radiology 1988;169:455–461.
44. Marks M, Lane B, Steinberg G, et al. Intranidal aneurysms in cerebral arteriovenous malformations: evaluation and endovascular treatment. Radiology 1992;183:355–360.
45. Cognard C, Gobin Y, Pierot L, et al. Cerebral dural arteriovenous fistulas: clinical and angiographic correlation with a revised classification of venous drainage. Radiology 1995;194: 671–680.
46. Peeters F, Kroger R. Dural and direct cavernous sinus fistulas. AJR Am J Radiol 1979;132: 599–606.
47. Francis P, Flom R, Zabramski J, et al. Treatment of carotid-cavernous fistulas: Part I. Interventional neuroradiology. BNI Q 1991;7:2–8.
48. DeMarco J, Dillon W, Halbach V, et al. Dural arteriovenous fistulas: evaluation with MR imaging. Radiology 1990;175:193–199.
49. Chen J, Tsuruda J, Halbach V. Suspected dural arteriovenous fistula: results with screening MR angiography in seven patients. Radiology 1992;183:265–271.
50. Truwit C. Venous angioma of the brain: history, significance and imaging findings. AJR Am J Radiol 1992;159:1299–1307.
51. Cammarata C, Han J, Haaga J, et al. Cerebral venous angiomas imaged by MR. Radiology 1985; 155:639–643.
52. Sigal R, Krief O, Houtteville J, et al. Occult cerebrovascular malformations: follow-up with MR imaging. Radiology 1990;176:815–819.
53. Gomori J, Grossman R, Goldberg H, et al. Occult cerebral vascular malformations: high-field MR imaging. Radiology 1986;158:707–713.
54. Kim J, Kucharczyk W, Henkelman R. Cavernous hemangiomas: dipolar susceptibility artifacts at MR imaging. Radiology 1993;187:735–741.
55. Brunereau L, Labauge P, Tournier-Lasserve E, et al. Familial form of intracranial cavernous angioma: MR imaging findings in 51 families. Radiology 2000;214:209–216.
56. Alexander M, DeSalles A, Tomiyasu U. Multiple radiation-induced intracranial lesions after treatment for pituitary adenoma. J Neurosurg 1998;88:111–115.

57. Larson J, Ball W, Bove K, et al. Formation of intracerebral cavernous malformations after radiation treatment for central nervous system neoplasia in children. J Neurosurg 1998;88:51–56.
58. Novelli P, Reigel D, Gleason P, et al. Multiple cavernous angiomas after high-dose whole-brain radiation therapy. Pediatr Neurosurg 1997;26:322–325.
59. Lee R, Becher M, Benson M, et al. Brain capillary telangiectasia: MR imaging appearance and clinicohistopathologic findings. Radiology 1997;205:797–805.
60. Barr R, Dillon W, Wilson C. Slow-flow vascular malformations on the pons: capillary telangiectasis? AJNR Am J Neuroradiol 1996;17:71–78.
61. Lee B, Vo K, Kido D, et al. MR high-resolution blood oxygenation level-dependent venography of occult (low-flow) vascular lesions. AJNR Am J Neuroradiol 1999;20:1239–1242.
62. Rigamonti D, Johnson PC, Spetzler RF, et al. Cavernous malformations and capillary telangiectasia: a spectrum within a single pathological entity. Neurosurgery 1991;28:60–64.
63. Huddle D, Chaloupka J, Sehgal V. Clinically aggressive diffuse capillary telangiectasia of the brain stem: a clinical radiologic-pathologic case study. AJNR Am J Neuroradiol 1999;20:1674–1677.

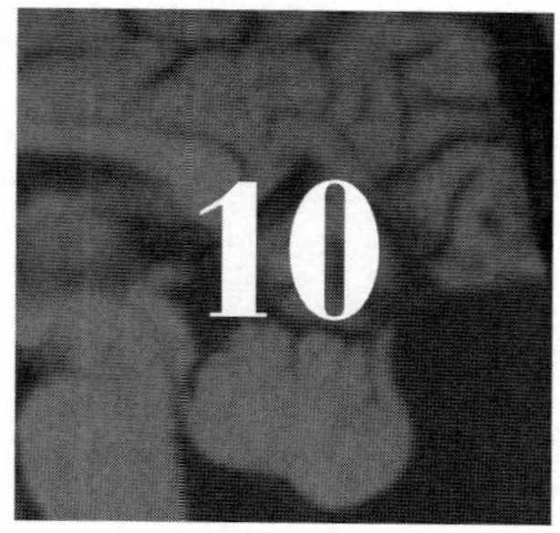

CRANIAL TRAUMA

- General Facts and Classification
- Intracranial Lesions
- Extracerebral Lesions
- Child Abuse
- Skull Fractures
- Injury to the Pituitary Stalk
- Penetrating Injuries
- Chronic Lesions

GENERAL FACTS AND CLASSIFICATION

Computed tomography (CT) continues to be the imaging method of choice in most traumatic brain injuries, particularly during the acute period (1). Magnetic resonance imaging (MRI) is indicated when CT does not provide the information needed for the management of the patient or when the clinical signs and symptoms do not correlate with the CT findings (this is especially true of patients with shearing injuries, in whom CT underestimates the extent of the injury). Understanding the meaning of the imaging findings is critical in the management of the traumatized patient because brain injuries are the most common cause of death in children and young adults. Clinically, the most important factor determining the prognosis of the patient is elevated intracranial pressure. I divide traumatic injuries into intracerebral (primary and secondary), extracerebral but intracranial, and those affecting the bones. Isolated extracranial injuries, such as fractures, have little clinical significance by themselves, and hence plain radiographs no longer are used in the routine evaluation of these patients. Extracranial injuries are however, important in the diagnosis of child abuse. Traumatic brain injuries may be classified as primary or secondary (Table 10.1).

Many of the entities addressed in this chapter have been discussed previously and illustrated in Chapter 9, so I have tried to keep the illustrations at a minimum here. I urge the reader to peruse Chapter 9 as a complement to this one.

INTRACRANIAL LESIONS

PRIMARY INJURIES

Diffuse Axonal (Shearing) Injuries

Diffuse axonal injuries or shear injuries are the most common cause of significant morbidity and mortality after head trauma (1). Unfortunately, CT underestimates their extent because most individual lesions are small and initially nonhemorrhagic (2). The underlying responsible mechanism for shearing injuries is a combination of acceleration, deceleration, and rotation. As such, portions of the brain where tissue density differs (such as the gray–white junctions) and rigid structures (brainstem and corpus callosum) are affected most commonly (Figs. 10.1 to 10.3). The most common locations for these injuries are as follows:

- Cerebral hemispheres (gray–white matter junction)
- Basal ganglia
- Splenium of the corpus callosum
- Dorsal midbrain

Table 10.1: Classification of Traumatic Injuries to the Brain

Primary	*Secondary*
Diffuse axonal or "shearing" injuries	Cerebral edema
Cerebral contusions	Infarctions
Shearing of ventricular ependyma and subependymal veins	Aneurysm and pseudoaneurysm formation
Shearing of choroid plexus	Herniations
	Arterial dissection
	Arteriovenous fistula

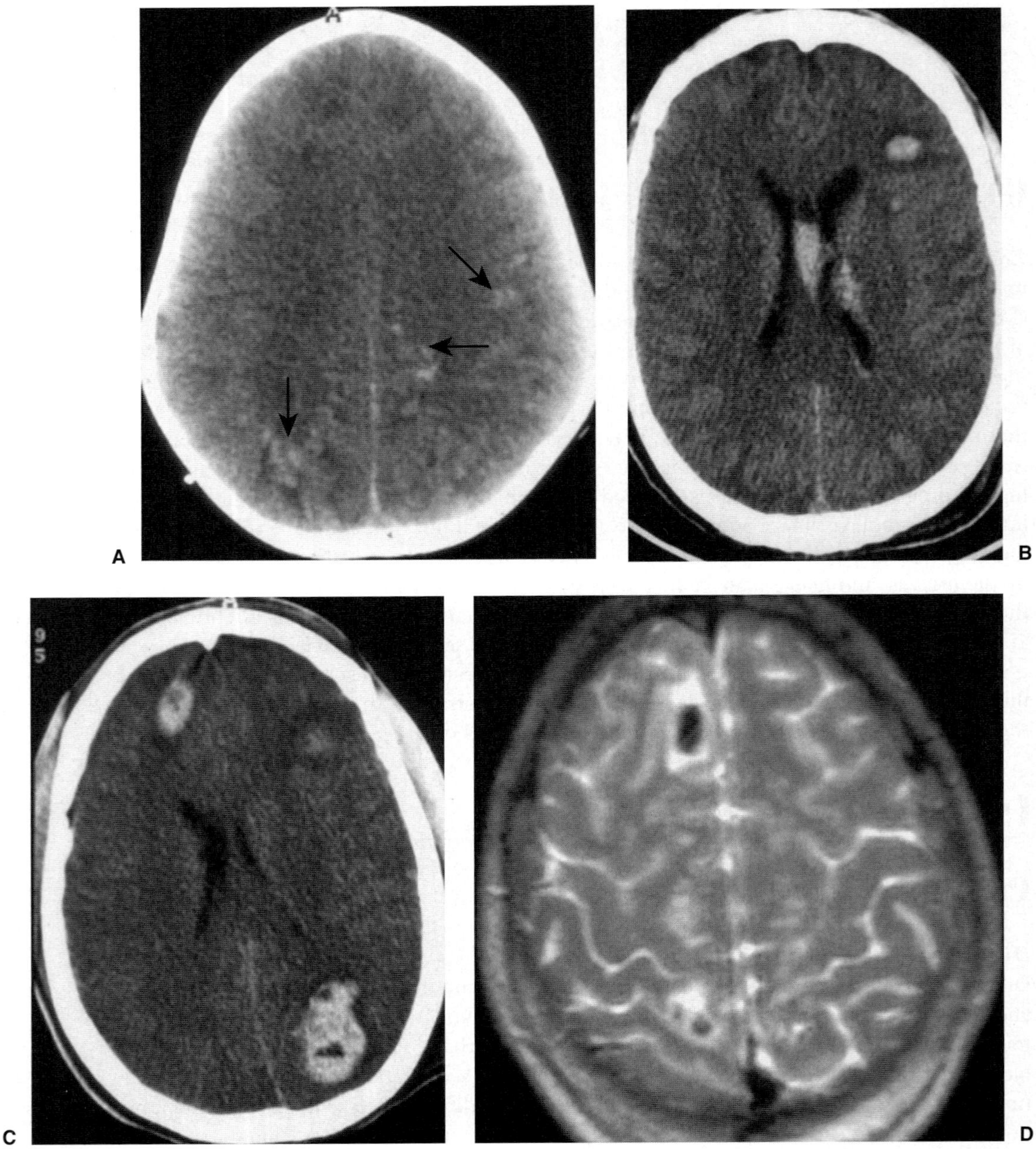

Figure 10.1 *Shearing Injuries. A.* Axial computed tomography (CT) shows multiple punctuate hemorrhagic injuries *(arrows)* at the gray–white matter junctions, predominantly in the parietal regions. *B.* CT shows hemorrhagic shears in the left frontal region, septum pellucidum, and ependyma of the left lateral ventricle. *C.* CT shows large hemorrhagic shears. Note blood–fluid level in the posterior-most one. *D.* Axial T2-weighted image shows dark (owing to presence of deoxyhemoglobin) shears in the right frontal and parietal lobes.

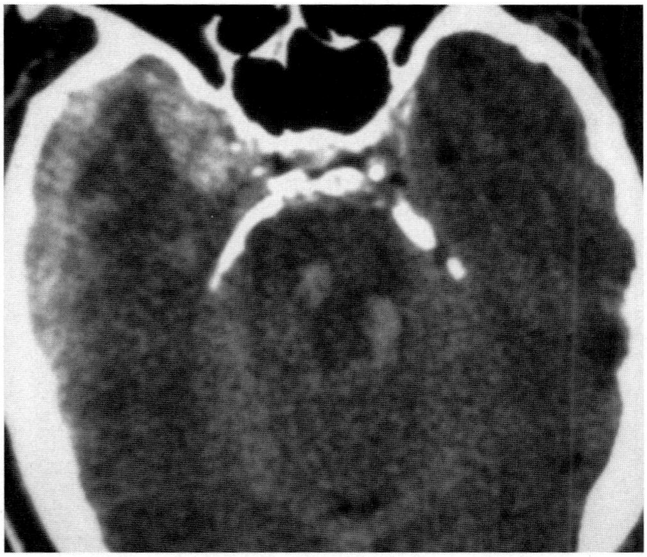

Figure 10.2 *Brainstem Shearing Injury.* Axial computed tomography shows hypodense and swollen brainstem with focal hemorrhagic lesions.

Intermediary injuries are a specific type of shearing injuries affecting the basal ganglia and carrying a poor prognosis.

The frontal and temporal lobes are affected in over 59% of patients with shearing injuries. Only approximately 20% to 30% of patients show shearing injuries on initial CT (thus, CT is negative in up to 80% of cases). As time progresses, CT demonstrates more injuries as they become edematous. Only 10% of shearing injuries are initially hemorrhagic (Fig. 10.1A–C). MRI is helpful in the detection of subtle hemorrhagic lesions, especially when using susceptibility-sensitive imaging such as gradient-echo (T2*) or echo planar techniques that demonstrate the full extent of the injuries (3) (Fig. 10.1D). Conventional T2-weighted images also are useful for detection of edematous lesions but less sensitive in the detection of minute hemorrhages [particularly fast spin-echo and HASTE

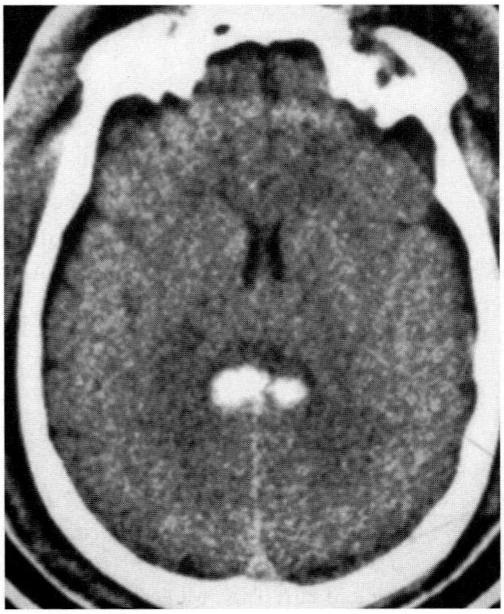

A

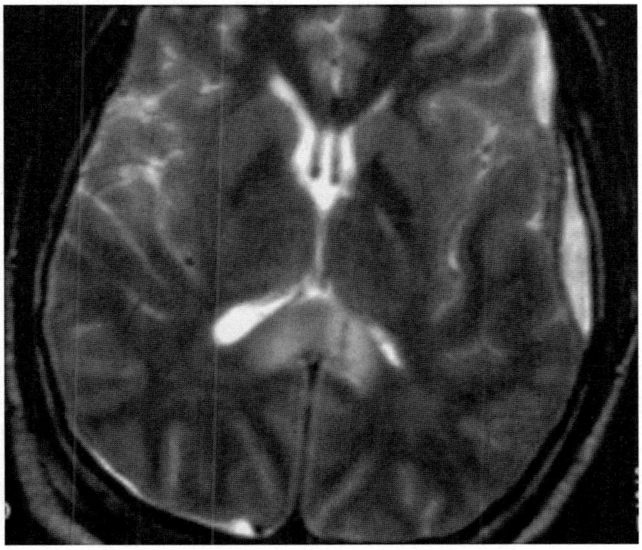

B

Figure 10.3 *Shearing Injuries of the Corpus Callosum. A.* Axial computed tomography shows hemorrhagic injury in the splenium of the corpus callosum. *B.* In a different patient, axial T2-weighted image shows nonhemorrhagic injury in the posterior callosum as well as a small epidural hematoma in the left temporal region. Nonhemorrhagic injuries of the corpus callosum are easier to visualize with magnetic resonance imaging.

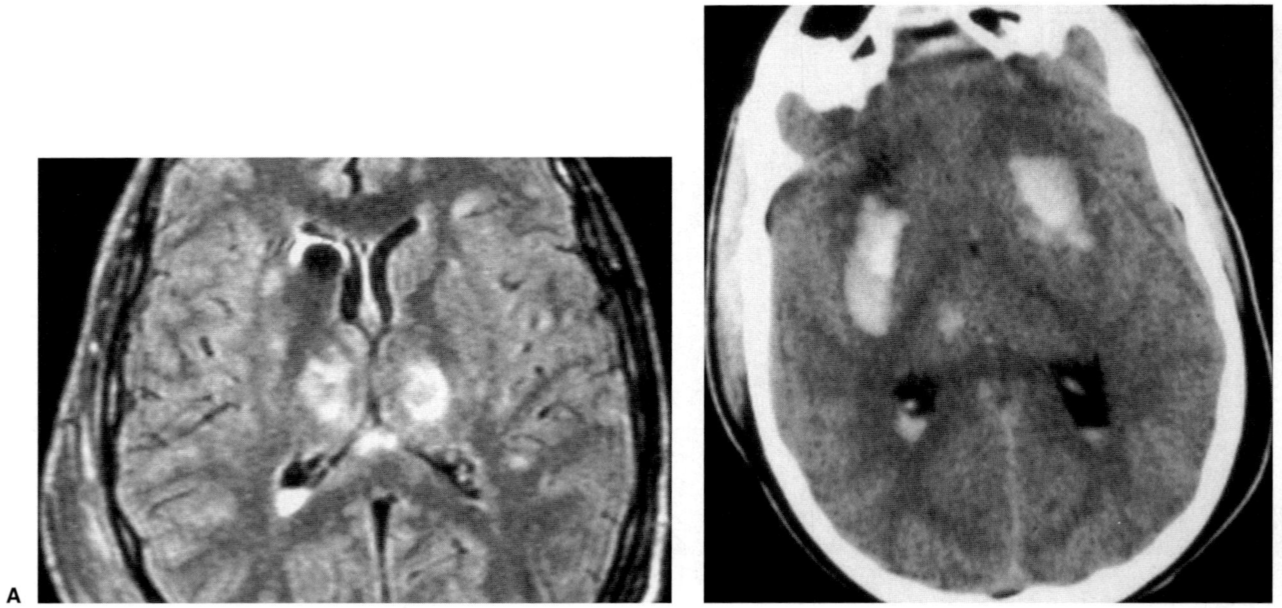

Figure 10.4 *Intermediary Shearing Injuries. A.* Axial fluid attenuation inversion recovery (FLAIR) image shows significant nonhemorrhagic shears in the thalami and to a lesser extent in the basal ganglia. Note shear of the callosal splenium blood level in the occipital horns. The artifact in the right caudate nucleus head is due to the presence of a ventriculostomy. *B.* Axial computed tomography shows large hemorrhagic shears in both basal ganglia and a smaller one in the right thalamus. Note blood levels in the lateral ventricles.

(half-Fourier acquisition single-shot turbo spin-echo) images; Fig. 10.3B]. From a biochemical standpoint, the following are the mechanisms responsible for the damage associated with diffuse axonal injuries:

- Excess release of excitatory amino acids
- Generation of free radicals
- Release of inflammatory cytokines
- Cellular apoptosis
- Calpain proteolysis (destruction of the cytoskeleton)
- Axonal stretch

A less common type of shear is the so-called *intermediary injury* (4). This injury occurs as consequence of shearing of the deep perforating lenticulostriate and thalamostriate arteries at the level of the basal ganglia. CT shows unilateral or, more commonly, bilateral hematomas in the lentiform nuclei (Fig. 10.4A). Occasionally, these lesions contain a fluid level (Fig. 10.4B). These patients have a poor prognosis.

Contusions

Most cortical contusions involve the frontobasal, anterior temporal, and temporobasal regions.

Cortical contusions are the second most common type of primary intraaxial traumatic lesion. They result from contact of the brain surfaces on ridges and crests of bone and as such commonly involve the frontobasal and anterior temporal regions (1) (Fig. 10.5). As the brain "glides" over these excrescences of bone, it becomes bruised. Cerebral contusions also can be the result of a contrecoup injury, and therefore the side of the brain opposite to skull and scalp injuries always should be checked carefully. Most cerebral contusions are subtle on initial CT scanning but tend to become larger and more obvious during the first 3 days posttrauma because of progressive edema and hemorrhage. Many superficial contusions initially are hemorrhagic, reflecting the rich vascular supply of the cortex. Multiple contusions are found in over 30% of patients (5). MRI is more sensitive in the

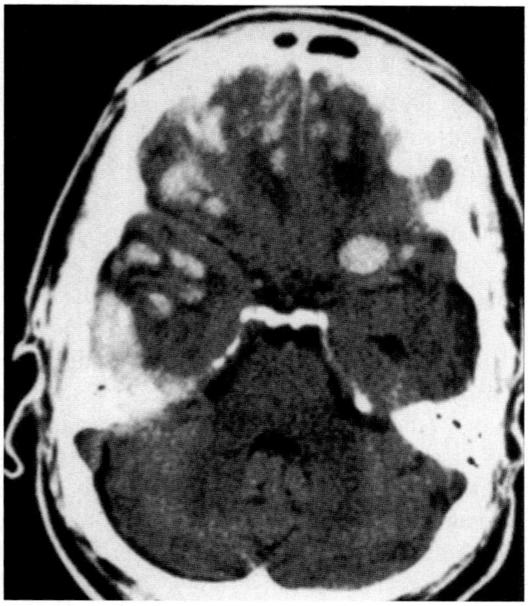
A

Figure 10.5 *Cerebral Contusions. A.* Axial computed tomography (CT) shows typical acute and hyperdense hemorrhagic contusions in the basal aspects of the frontal and temporal lobes. *B.* In a different patient, axial CT shows hemorrhagic contusions in both frontal lobes, and subarachnoid hemorrhage. *C.* Axial CT shows hemorrhagic contusions predominantly in the portion of the temporal lobes overlying the petrous bones.

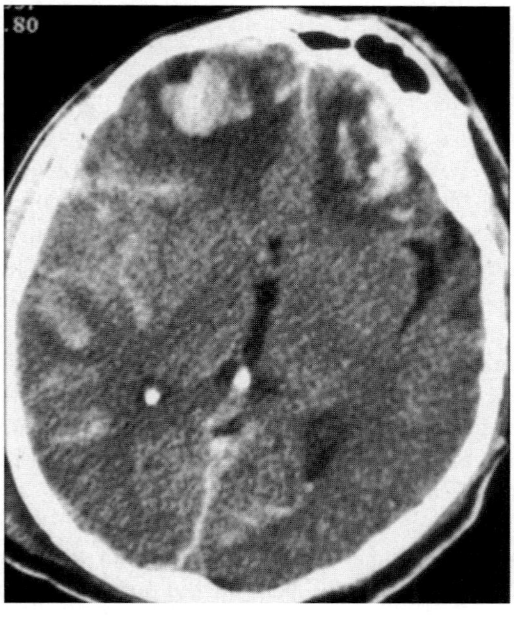
B

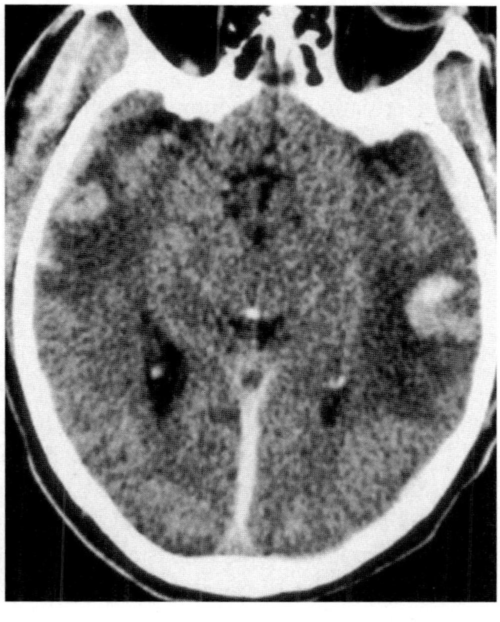
C

detection of cortical contusions because of the absence of artifacts (beam hardening) arising from adjacent bones that commonly are present on CT.

Choroid Plexus and Ventricular Ependyma Injuries

A relatively uncommon type of injury is that affecting the ventricles and the choroid plexuses. Posttrauma intraventricular hemorrhage is not rare and most often is the sequela of subarachnoid hemorrhage (SAH) reflux (see later). At times, primary intraventricular hemorrhage results from tearing of the subependymal veins (1) (Fig. 10.1B). The choroid plexus also may be torn, resulting in intraventricular hemorrhage or localized periventricular hematomas. Without hydrocephalus, these two types of injuries have little clinical significance when they are isolated. Unfortunately, most patients with ventricular/choroid plexus hemorrhages have other significant brain injuries, and their prognosis is poor.

Secondary Injuries

As their name implies, these injuries are secondary to primary intracerebral or extracerebral lesions. Diffuse cerebral edema may be secondary to shearing injuries or to generalized anoxia. Overhydration used in resuscitation efforts also occasionally may result in cerebral edema, although this more commonly results in significant scalp swelling. Cerebral edema also may be primary without accompanying lesions.

Focal cerebral edema and infarctions result from transection, dissection, and occlusion of vessels, mostly arteries but occasionally also veins. Both penetrating and nonpenetrating injuries may produce focal ischemia. Focal ischemia also may be secondary to herniations. Uncal herniation may occlude one or both posterior cerebral arteries and subfalcine herniation may occlude one anterior cerebral artery. Generalized ischemia usually is the result of cardiac arrest, and posttrauma vasospasm usually is not significant enough to result in ischemia. Aneurysm or pseudoaneurysm formation is a rare event (Chapter 9). Most posttrauma aneurysms (and pseudoaneurysms) occur in the distal branches of the anterior cerebral arteries and in the supraclinoid portions of the internal carotid arteries. Other vascular injuries arising from traumatic brain injuries are arteriovenous fistulas and thrombosis. The most common type of posttrauma arteriovenous fistula is the cavernous sinus–internal carotid artery fistula. Fistulas between meningeal arteries and veins usually are seen in combination with skull fractures, and by themselves are not clinically significant.

Herniations

Herniations resulting in cerebral infarctions include subfalcine (resulting in occlusion of the anterior cerebral artery) and uncal transtentorial (resulting in occlusion of the posterior cerebral artery) herniations.

Herniations are common in the trauma patient. The most common type of herniation is subfalcine herniation (6), in which a cingulate gyrus is forced under the falx cerebri, resulting in midline shift. The opposite lateral ventricle may be dilated because of entrapment and occlusion of its foramen of Monro. The anterior cerebral artery may be "clipped" by the falx cerebri and result in an infarction. The second most common type of brain herniation is the descending transtentorial herniation, in which the uncus of a temporal bone descends medially to the tentorial incisura. This leads to obliteration of the basilar cisterns (particularly the suprasellar and perimesencephalic cisterns) and to compression of the brainstem. Duret hemorrhages are secondary to compression and shearing of the deep brainstem-perforating arterioles (1). Note that Duret hemorrhages are very difficult to identify by CT. A *Kernohan notch* is an indentation caused by the tentorium on the lateral aspect of the brainstem opposite the side of uncal herniation. This term is borrowed from the pathology literature and has little significance from an imaging standpoint. When bilateral uncal transtentorial herniation occurs, the thalami also may descend through the tentorial incisura. This is called *downward* or *central herniation*. In this type of severe herniation, the third ventricle is inferiorly displaced and the belly of the pons is flattened against the clivus. The brainstem is then pushed posteriorly, and this results in stretching of the perforating arterioles and may give rise to Duret hemorrhages. The aqueduct also is compressed and hydrocephalus may ensue. If the herniation continues, the entire cerebellum may be caudally displaced and the cerebellar tonsils may herniate inferiorly through the foramen magnum. This is a rare occurrence, and most cerebellar tonsillar herniations are associated with space-occupying lesions in the posterior fossa.

Upward or *ascending transtentorial herniation* are terms usually reserved for the superior displacement of the cerebellar vermis and the medial aspect of the cerebellar hemispheres through the tentorial incisura. These portions of herniated cerebellum compress the quadrigeminal plate and its cistern. The aqueduct is compressed, giving rise to hydrocephalus. This type of herniation usually is secondary to space-occupying lesions in the cerebellum.

External or *transcalvarial herniation* refers to herniation of brain through a skull defect. It is unlikely to happen after trauma and skull fractures, and is seen most commonly when edematous brain herniates through a surgical defect. The herniated brain assumes a mushroom shape and may contain hemorrhage.

Extracerebral Lesions

Subdural Fluid Collections

Subdural hematomas are the most common type of acute extracerebral injury and also the most lethal one (7). They are the result of tearing of the bridging veins (located between the cortical veins and the dural sinuses, mostly in the region of the superior sagittal sinus). Hence, subdural hematomas are seen more commonly in the elderly, in whom cerebral atrophy widens the subarachnoid spaces, exposing these veins to trauma. These hematomas also commonly are seen in victims of child abuse. Subdural hematomas are located between the dura and the arachnoid, a space that is easily dissected. These hematomas commonly are extensive and may involve one (common) or both (less common) hemispheres (Fig. 10.6A and B). They also may be parafalcine or located in the posterior fossa (Fig. 10.6C). Midline interhemispheric subdural hematomas are typical of child abuse. If a hematoma crosses a dural sinus, it is epidural in location and not subdural. Although most subdural hematomas are seen easily by plain CT, identification of some subacute and isodense subdural hematomas may necessitate injection of contrast material or use of MRI (8). Subdural hematomas are crescent shaped and tend to extend widely over one hemisphere. Subdural hematomas result in significant mass effect. When bilateral, the midline brain structures may remain in a normal position. For the first week (acute period), subdural hematomas are homogeneously hyperdense by CT. From 1 to 3 weeks (subacute period), the clot begins to liquefy and the CT density of subdural hematomas becomes patchy. At this time, a subdural hematom may develop a fluid level, with its inferior aspect being hyperdense and the supernatant hypodense. Between the acute and subacute periods, there is a stage in which a subdural hematomas may be isodense with the underlying gray matter and difficult to identify (Fig. 10.6D). In this situation, the gray–white matter junction is displaced inwardly ("buckled"). After contrast administration, there is enhancement of the inner wall of the hematoma, which is hypervascular. Septations inside the hematoma also may form and enhance. Weeks to months later, a subdural hematoma becomes hypodense and easy to visualize. Approximately 25% of chronic subdural hematomas are bilateral. Subdural hematomas resorb slowly and become smaller with time. Rarely, their inner and outer membranes may calcify. When the CT findings are compatible with a chronic (low-density) subdural hematoma, the following entities need to be considered in the differential diagnosis:

Subdural hematomas have a worse prognosis than epidural hematomas.

- Chronic subdural hematoma
- Subdural hygroma
- Subdural effusion secondary to meningitis (particularly *Hemophilus influenzae*).

MRI is not the method of choice for diagnosis of acute subdural hematomas, although it does help to differentiate a chronic one from the other entities mentioned in the preceding list (8). Acute subdural hematomas may be isointense to brain on T1-weighted and hypointense on T2-weighted images (reflecting the presence of deoxyhemoglobin). Subacute and chronic subdural hematomas are bright on T2-weighted images and may be dark on echo planar images (because of magnetic susceptibility effects). Most patients with subdural hematomas have intracerebral injuries and as such have a poor prognosis, with mortality rates ranging from 30% to 80%. Subdural hematomas also occur after decompression of the ventricles by shunting.

A subdural hygroma is a collection of nonbloody cerebrospinal fluid (CSF) (1). It is located in the subdural space, similar to hematomas. A rent in the arachnoid membranes allows CSF to escape and accumulate in the subdural space. In the absence of arachnoid lacerations, injury to the blood vessels may result in leakage of fluid and its accumulation (9). Subdural hygromas are found in <5% of patients with head trauma and are more common in children and the elderly. By CT, chronic subdural hematomas may be indistinguishable from subdural hygromas. However, the walls of hygromas do not

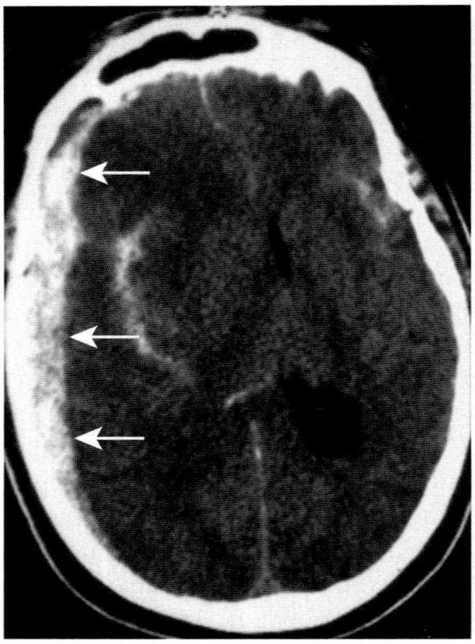
A

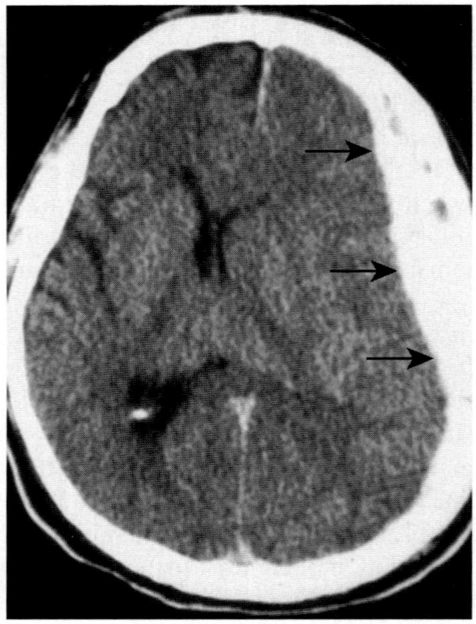
B

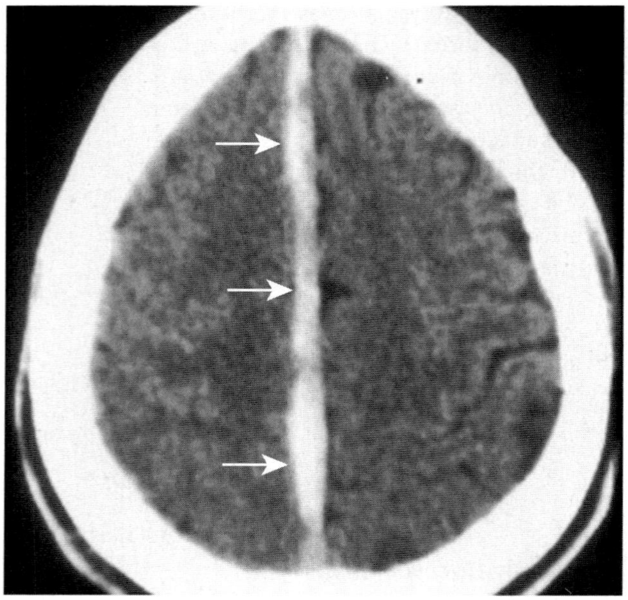
C

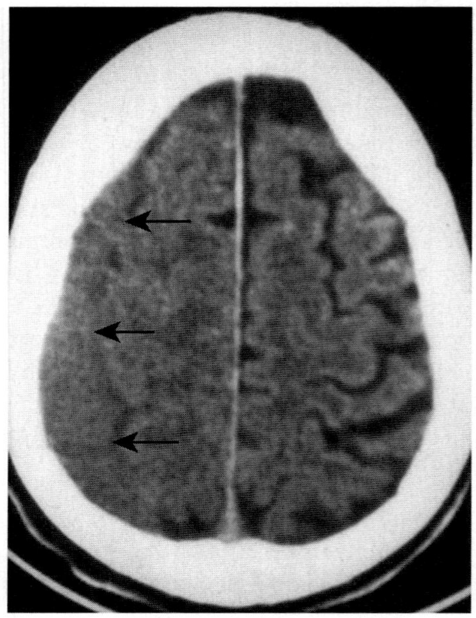
D

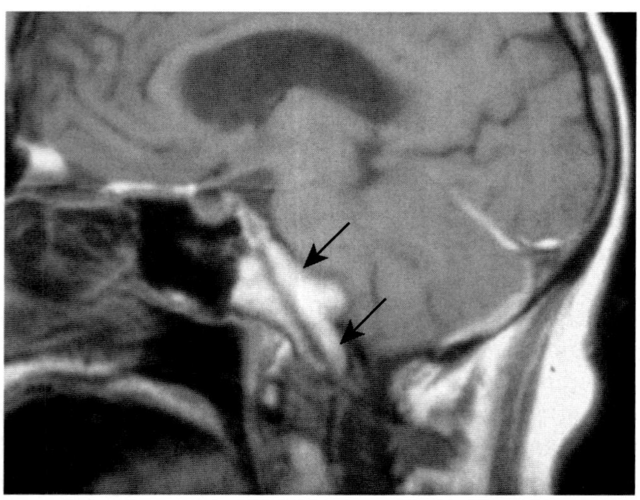
E

Figure 10.6 *Subdural Hematoma. A.* Axial computed tomography (CT) shows right hemispheric acute subdural hematoma *(arrows)* with midline shift to the left and subarachnoid hemorrhage in both sylvian fissures. *B.*Axial CT shows left frontotemporal acute subdural hematoma *(arrows)* with midline shift to the right. *C.* Axial CT shows interhemispheric acute subdural hematoma *(arrows)* along the right side of the falx cerebri. *D.* Axial CT shows right-sided subacute isodense subdural hematoma *(arrows).* Note inward "buckling" of the gray matter. *E.* Sagittal T1-weighted image shows bright subdural hematoma (arrows) along the clivus. Note also bright subdural hematoma above and below the vermis.

enhance. MRI shows that hygromas have a signal intensity very similar to that of CSF in all sequences, including fluid attenuation inversion recovery (FLAIR) images. Approximately one-fifth of all patients with subdural hygromas show traumatic lesions in the brain.

Epidural Hematoma

Most epidural hematomas occur in the temporal squama region and are due to laceration of the middle meningeal artery.

Epidural hematomas are the second most common type of acute extracerebral injury, and have a better prognosis than subdural hematomas (1). Delayed extraaxial hematomas also occur, but are rare (10). Most epidural hematomas are seen in patients with fractures involving the squamosal portion of the temporal bones. These fractures lacerate the middle meningeal artery and result in accumulation of blood between the outer dural layer (periosteum) and the bone. Unlike subdural hematomas, nearly all epidural hematomas are unilateral and encountered in younger individuals. Brain herniations are more common with epidural than with subdural hematomas. Most epidural hematomas are easy to diagnose by CT, and MRI does not play a primary role in the management of these patients. Also, epidural hematomas are more common in the posterior fossa than are subdural hematomas. Epidural hematomas are localized (because the dura anchors their edges) and biconvex in shape (Fig. 10.7A). Only lesions located in the epidural space can cross a venous sinus. Convexity epidural hematomas are rare and difficult to identify. If an epidural hematoma crosses a venous sinus, a tear in the sinus must be considered as the source of bleeding (Fig. 10.7B). Most epidural hematomas in the posterior fossa are venous. Most epidural hematomas are hyperdense on CT, and the stages previously described for subdural hematomas are not seen because epidural hematomas usually are evacuated emergently. Smaller epidural hematomas may be managed conservatively (11). These show decreasing density and size with time. The walls of a chronic epidural hematoma also may calcify.

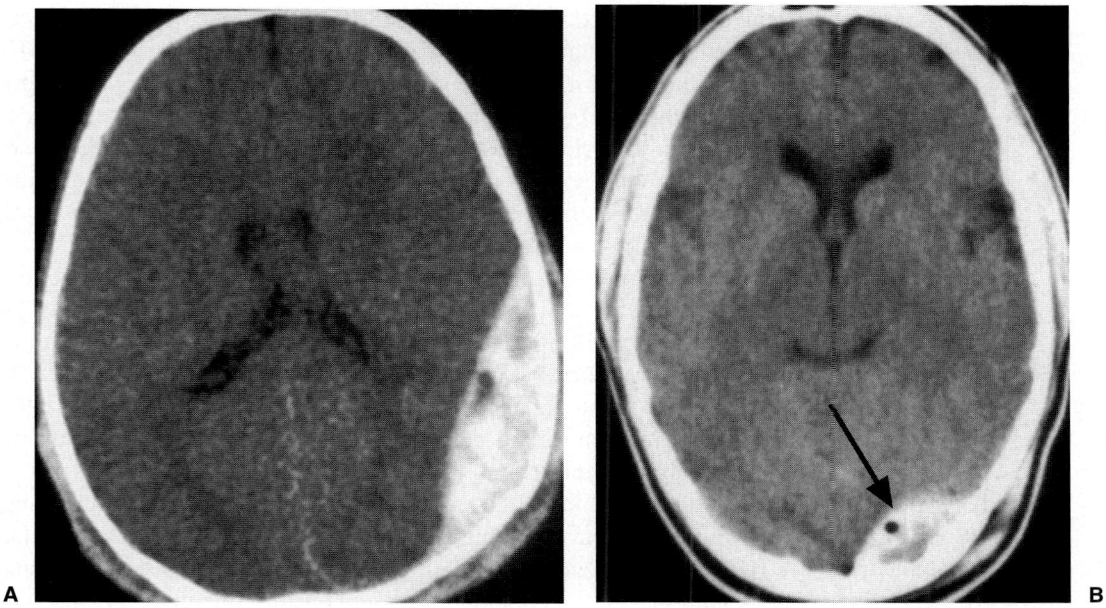

Figure 10.7 *Epidural Hematoma. A.* Axial computed tomography (CT) shows acute, dense, right parietotemporal epidural hematoma. *B.* In a different patient, axial CT shows biconvex, dense, acute epidural hematoma *(arrow)* over the region of the left transverse sinus. This venous epidural hematoma also contains gas because of an open skull fracture.

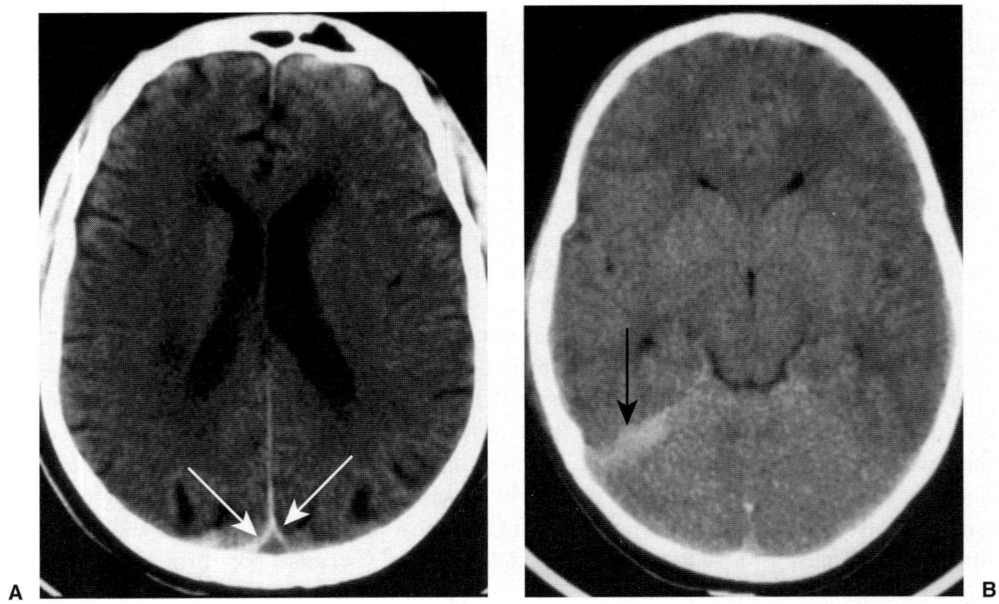

Figure 10.8 Subarachnoid Hemorrhage. *A.* Axial computed tomography (CT) shows acute subarachnoid hemorrhage (*arrows*) layering in the occipital regions and outlining the posterior aspect of the superior sagittal sinus ("pseudo delta sign"). *B.* In a child, axial CT shows dense acute subarachnoid blood (*arrow*) layering on the right tentorium.

Subarachnoid Hemorrhage

Acute posttrauma SAH is very common, but often it is subtle and difficult to visualize by CT. It probably originates from tearing of small blood vessels on the surface of the brain (1). The dense-appearing cortical sulci seen in cases of diffuse brain edema may appear identical to SAH. Excessive amounts of intravenous or intraarterial iodinated contrast material may be excreted into the subarachnoid space and also simulate SAH. Outlining of the dependent portion of the superior sagittal sinus by SAH is referred to as *pseudo delta sign* (conversely, a true delta sign is the outlining of an intrasinus clot by contrast material; Fig. 10.8A). The pseudo delta sign is a common manifestation of posttrauma SAH. Other locations for posttrauma SAH include the surface of the tentorium, the prepontine cistern, the sylvian fissures, the interhemispheric fissure, and cortical sulci in the convexities (12) (Fig. 10.8B). SAH in the sylvian fissures may be due to laceration of the superficial cortical veins. The hemorrhage may reflux into the ventricles and lead to acute hydrocephalus. Occasionally, a mild and chronic hydrocephalus leading to headaches may develop in patients with posttrauma SAH.

Pneumocephalus

Although most cases of pneumocephalus do not require a specific treatment, tension pneumocephalus and expanding pneumatoceles in the brain or ventricles may need to be promptly evacuated.

Pneumocephalus is the result of an abnormal communication between an air-containing structure (most commonly the paranasal sinuses and temporal bones) and the subarachnoid space through a tear in the meninges and a fracture of the skull base (13) (Fig. 10.9). Most pneumocephalus poses no immediate danger to the patient, but occasionally its rapid expansion may lead to brain compression (so-called tension pneumocephalus). Tension pneumocephalus is more common after base-of-skull fractures, fractures involving the paranasal sinuses, and craniotomy. Accumulation of gas in the temporomandibular joints may due to a fracture of the temporal bone. Accumulations of air inside the brain are rare and termed *pneumatoceles* (14). Pneumatoceles and tension pneumocephalus may necessitate emergent treatment. An unrecognized fracture presenting with pneumocephalus may be the cause of later meningitis. Intraarterial air may be difficult to differentiate from air in the subarachnoid spaces, but intraarterial gas never rises to the uppermost aspect of the cranium, as subarachnoid air commonly does. Uncomplicated

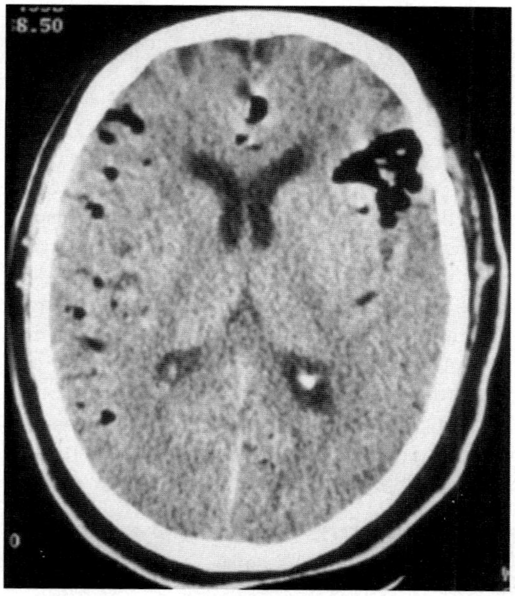

Figure 10.9 *Pneumocephalus.* Axial computed tomography after a gunshot wound to the base of skull shows gas in many cortical sulci.

pneumocephalus (regardless of its etiology) decreases considerably by 10 to 15 days and almost never is present by 3 weeks. Intracranial infections almost never produce pneumocephalus.

Child Abuse

I address child abuse separately because of its importance, although many of its imaging manifestations have been addressed previously. Brain injury is the leading cause of death secondary to child abuse (15). Brain injuries are found in over 40% of abused children and are more common in the youngest ones. Child abuse is more common before 2 years of age, in mentally retarded children, and in those with chronic illnesses. The incidence of child abuse also is increased among families of low socioeconomic status. Box 10.1 lists the causes of injury to the brain in abused children.

By CT, the most commonly identified abnormalities are SAH (75%) and diffuse brain edema (65%) (16). The third most common injury is subdural hematoma. When these hematomas contain blood of different ages or are located along the interhemispheric fissure, they are highly suggestive of child abuse (Fig. 10.10A and B). Not uncommonly, parafalcine subdural hematomas may extend to the surface of the tentorium. Epidural hematomas are rare in child abuse, probably reflecting the compliance of the young skull (Fig. 10.10C). Fractures are not rare, may be simple or complex, and may be seen in 50% to 80% of abused children. Overlying scalp swelling may indicate that a fracture is acute. Strangulation may lead to diffuse cerebral anoxia or dissection of a carotid artery, resulting in cerebral infarction. Diffuse cerebral edema is more common in younger children

Box 10.1 Causes of Brain Injury in Child Abuse

Direct injury
Shaking
Asphyxia
Nutritional deprivation

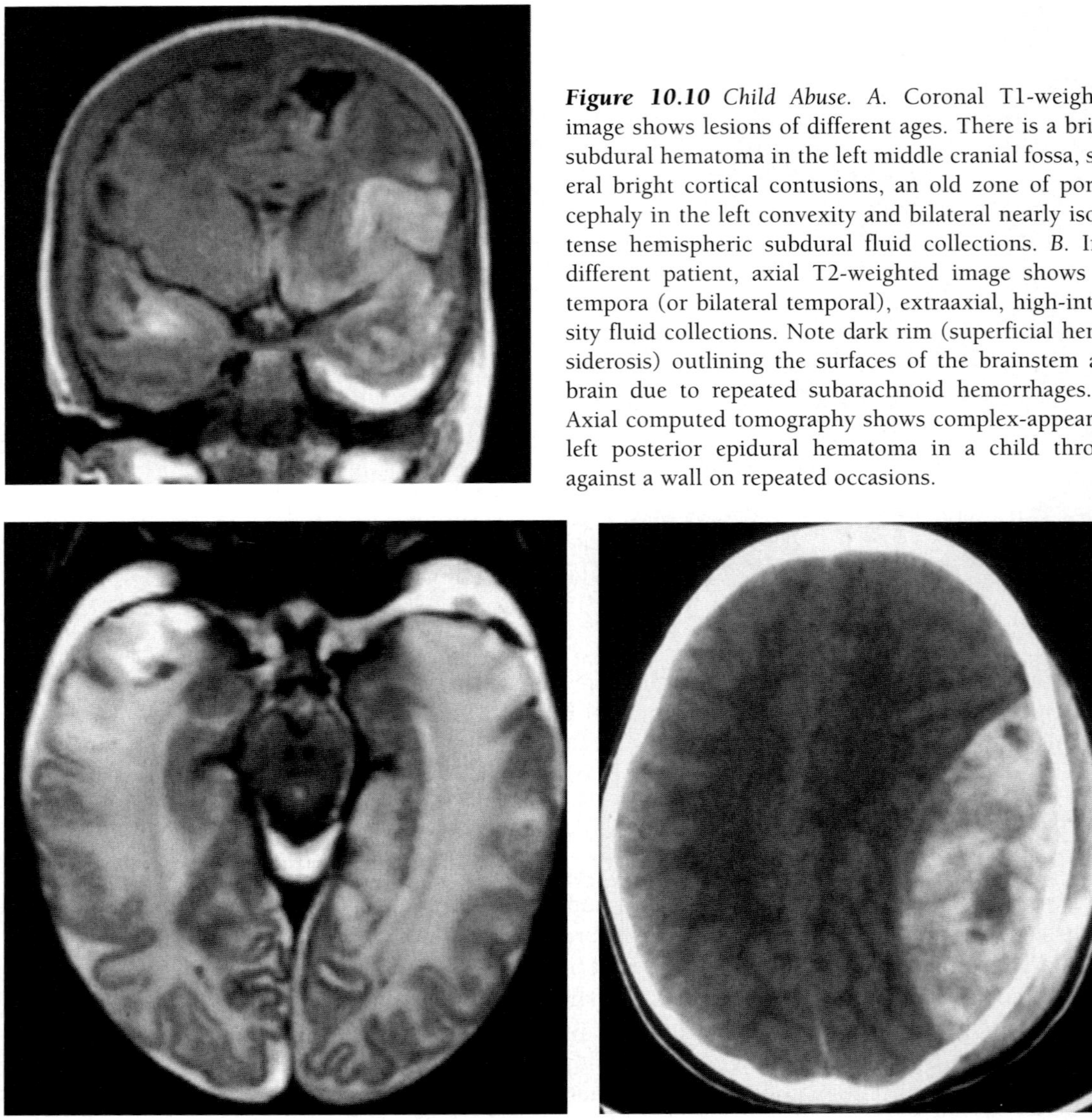

A B C

Figure 10.10 *Child Abuse. A.* Coronal T1-weighted image shows lesions of different ages. There is a bright subdural hematoma in the left middle cranial fossa, several bright cortical contusions, an old zone of porencephaly in the left convexity and bilateral nearly isointense hemispheric subdural fluid collections. *B.* In a different patient, axial T2-weighted image shows bitempora (or bilateral temporal), extraaxial, high-intensity fluid collections. Note dark rim (superficial hemosiderosis) outlining the surfaces of the brainstem and brain due to repeated subarachnoid hemorrhages. *C.* Axial computed tomography shows complex-appearing left posterior epidural hematoma in a child thrown against a wall on repeated occasions.

(17). In child abuse, most cerebral infarctions involve the territory of a middle cerebral artery. Cortical contusions and shearing injuries also are common and may be of varying ages. Although retinal hemorrhages commonly are found on funduscopy, they are not seen readily on imaging studies. MRI is better at dating the injuries than is CT, and has the advantage of being able to examine the cervical spine, where the spinal cord also may be injured. The prognosis of the abused child is grave, with many patients developing mental retardation, cerebral palsy, developmental delay, and behavioral abnormalities.

Skull Fractures

- Skull fractures may be classified as follows:
- Simple or linear
- Complex (diastatic, depressed, comminuted, open)
- Combined

Linear fractures are the most common ones and may involve the calvarium or the base of the skull (1). Calvarial linear fractures in the absence of brain injuries have little clinical significance. Linear fractures of the base of the skull are associated with significant trauma and fractures elsewhere in the cranium and face (18). Skull base fractures commonly extend into the region of the foramen magnum. Temporal bone fractures may be oriented in the long axis of the petrous pyramid (longitudinal fractures) or perpendicular to it (transverse fractures) (19). In reality, most temporal bone fractures are mixed or oblique. Longitudinal temporal bone fractures cause ossicular disruptions (most commonly malleoincudal and incudostapedial dislocations) and result in conductive hearing loss. Facial nerve palsy is common with longitudinal fractures but often resolves spontaneously. Facial nerve palsy in association with a longitudinal fracture commonly is due to edema and compression of the nerve as it travels downward in its bony canal. Conversely, transverse temporal bone fractures often disrupt the osseous and membranous labyrinth and result in permanent neurosensory hearing loss. They also cause a facial nerve palsy that tends to be permanent because of transection of the nerve. All base-of-skull fractures may be associated with pneumocephalus (see earlier) and result in CSF leaks and meningitis. Sphenoidal fractures may involve the greater wings, the walls of the sphenoid sinus, and the pterygoid plates (20,21). They may cross the carotid canals and the apices of the orbits. A fluid level in the sphenoid sinus may be the only indication of the underlying fracture affecting this bone. These patients may sustain dissection of the internal carotid arteries.

Although most petrous temporal bone fractures traditionally are classified as longitudinal and transverse, in reality most are oblique or mixed.

Complex skull fractures may be diastatic, depressed, comminuted, or open (22). Most of these fractures are significant and require treatment. Diastatic fractures imply a separation of a cranial suture(s). Children are more commonly affected. The suture commonly is splayed by at least 2 mm. Sutural diastasis may occur when a fracture located elsewhere extends into a suture. Depressed fractures are due to a high-force impact in a small area. They are considered significant when the bone fragment is depressed by more than the normal width of the calvarium. They may result in meningeal tears and cortical contusions. They also may need to be lifted to avoid future cosmetic defects. Comminuted skull fractures are similar to depressed fractures but contain multiple bone fragments. Indeed, the combination of depression and comminution is quite common. Both depressed and comminuted fractures are more common in adults, in whom the calvarium is rigid compared with that of children. The third variation is that of "compound" or "open" fractures that are characterized by skin lacerations allowing for communication with the environment or with one of the sinonasal cavities. Contamination is common in this type of fracture, and because of the risk of infection they need to be treated acutely. Most compound fractures also are comminuted and depressed.

Injury to the Pituitary Stalk

An uncommon sequela of trauma is that of diabetes insipidus as a consequence of transection of the pituitary stalk (Chapter 7). This type of injury is seen most commonly in severe head-on automobile collisions or in newborns after difficult breech deliveries (23). Absence of the bright posterior pituitary lobe and parainfundibular hematomas may aid in making the correct diagnosis in the right clinical setting.

Penetrating Injuries

Penetrating injuries are addressed separately because they usually involve both the extracranial and intracranial compartments (24). Most are due to gunshot wounds and are more common in young men. Bullet tracts crossing both cerebral hemispheres or an injury to the brainstem nearly always are fatal (25,26) (Fig. 10.11). Superficial injuries, including those that affect only the cortex, have a better prognosis. Unfortunately, most bullets used today are high-velocity ones and produce significant damage and perforation of the skull at their exit site.

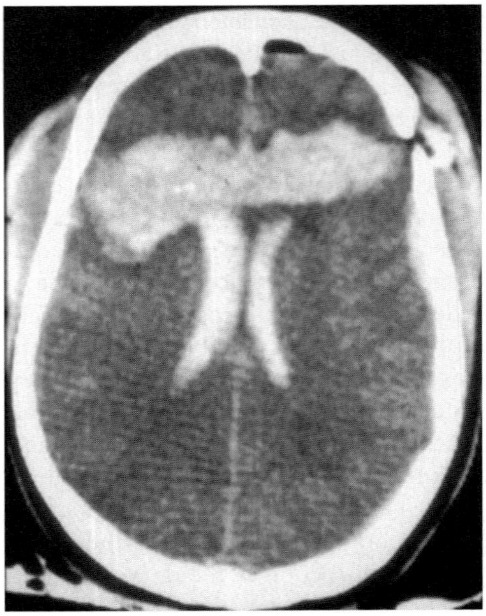

Figure 10.11 *Gunshot Wound.* Axial computed tomography shows thick blood track in the frontal lobes, skull fractures, and scalp hematomas. There is blood in the lateral ventricles and diffuse brain edema.

Chronic Lesions

Because this review deals mostly with the sequelae of acute brain trauma, chronic lesions are mentioned only briefly. With the conservative treatment of many patients with subdural and epidural hematomas, the chronic phase and sequelae of these lesions are becoming more common (see earlier). As is well known, both types of hematomas lose density with time. As the borders of a subdural hematoma collapse, its shape may change and it may become indistinguishable from an epidural hematoma. The rim of chronic extraaxial hematomas may calcify. Encephalomalacia is the most common sequela of intraaxial trauma. Malacia commonly is accompanied by neighboring atrophy. CSF leaks are not uncommon after severe craniofacial trauma. Most of these CSF leaks occur during the first week posttrauma, but usually are not evaluated until later. Meningitis is their most common complication. Diabetes insipidus and cranial nerve palsies also may occur in the chronic period. Posttrauma encephaloceles may occur acutely and usually are encountered in association with CSF leaks and significant fractures. Most posttrauma encephaloceles are found in the chronic period. Leptomeningeal cysts (growing fractures) are rare. They result from herniation of the pia and arachnoid into a fracture and subsequent accumulation of CSF at this level, leading to the formation of a cyst that erodes the margins of the original fracture. Vascular injuries, including dissection, occlusion, and formation of pseudoaneurysms, are addressed in Chapter 8.

References

1. Gentry LR. Imaging of closed head injury. Radiology 1994;191:1–17.
2. Mittl RL, Grossman RI, Hiehle JF, et al. Prevalence of MR evidence of diffuse axonal injury in patients with mild head injury and normal head CT findings. AJNR Am J Neuroradiol 1994;15: 1583–1589.
3. Gentry LR, Thompson B, Godersky JC. Trauma to the corpus callosum: MR features. AJNR Am J Neuroradiol 1988;9:1129–1138.
4. Gean AD. Imaging of head trauma. New York: Raven Press, 1994:165–166.
5. Klufas RA, Hsu L, Patel MR, et al. Unusual manifestations of head trauma. AJR Am J Roentgenol 1996;166:675–681.
6. Laine FJ, Shedden AI, Dunn MM, et al. Acquired intracranial herniations: MR imaging findings. AJR Am J Roentgenol 1995;165:967–973.

7. Gean AD. Imaging of head trauma. New York: Raven Press, 1994:75–146.
8. Sipponen JT, Sepponen RE, Sivula A. Chronic subdural hematoma: demonstration by magnetic resonance. Radiology 1984;150:79–85.
9. McCluney KW, Yeakley JW, Fenstermacher MJ, et al. Subdural hygroma versus atrophy on MR brain scans: "the cortical vein sign." AJNR Am J Neuroradiol 1992;13:1335–1339.
10. Domenicucci M, Signorini P, Strzelecki J, et al. Delayed post-traumatic epidural hematoma: a review. Neurosurg Rev 1995;18:109–122.
11. Hamilton M, Wallace C. Nonoperative management of acute epidural hematoma diagnosed by the CT: the neuroradiologist's role. AJRN Am J Neuroradiol 1992;13:853–859.
12. Yeakley JW, Patchall LL, Lee KF. Interpeduncular fossa sign: CT criterion of subarachnoid hemorrhage. Radiology 1986;158:699–700.
13. Mendelsohn DB, Hertzanu Y. Intracerebral pneumatoceles following facial trauma: CT findings. Radiology 1985;154:115–118.
14. Bhimani S, Virapongse C, Sabshin JK, et al. Intracerebral pneumatocele: CT findings. Radiology 1985;154:111–114.
15. Kleinman PK. Diagnostic imaging in infant abuse. AJR Am J Roentgenol 1990;155:703–712.
16. Petitti N, Williams DW. CT and MR imaging of nonaccidental pediatric head trauma. Acta Radiol 1998;5:215–223.
17. Han BK, Towbin RB, de Courten-Myers G, et al. Reversal sign on CT: effect of anoxic/ischemic cerebral injury in children. AJNR Am J Neuroradiol 1989;10:1191–1198.
18. Hackney D. Skull radiography in the evaluation of acute head trauma: a survey of current practice. Radiology 1991;181:711–714.
19. Momose KJ, Davis KR, Rhea JT. Hearing loss in skull fractures. AJNR Am J Neuroradiol 1983; 3:781–785.
20. West OC, Mirvis SE, Shanmuganathan K. Transsphenoid basilar skull fracture: CT patterns. Radiology 1993;188:329–338.
21. Unger JM, Gentry LR, Grossman JE. Sphenoid fractures: prevalence, sites, and significance. Radiology 1990;175:175–180.
22. Gean AD. Imaging of head trauma. New York: Raven Press, 1994:27–74.
23. Mark AS, Phister SH, Jackson DE, et al. Traumatic lesions of the surprasellar region: MR imaging. Radiology 1992;182:49–52.
24. Stone JA, Slone HW, Yu JS, et al. Gunshot wounds of the brain: influence of ballistics and predictors of outcome by computed tomography. Emerg Radiol 1997;4:140–149.
25. Hollerman JJ, Fackler ML, Coldwell DM, et al. Gunshot wounds: 1. bullets, ballistics, and mechanisms of injury. AJR Am J Roentgenol 1990;155:685–690.
26. Hollerman JJ, Fackler ML, Coldwell DM, et al. Gunshot wounds: 2. radiology. AJR Am J Roentgenol 1990;155:691–702.

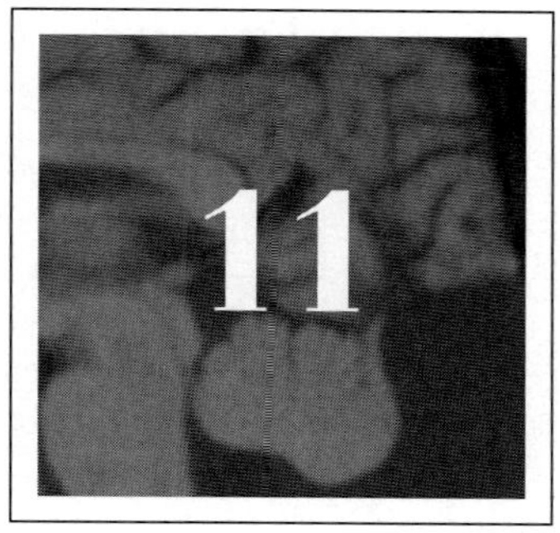

Infectious and Inflammatory Processes

- Meningitis and Its Complications
- Human Immunodeficiency Virus Infection
- Progressive Multifocal Leukoencephalopathy
- Herpes Simplex Virus Infection
- Rasmussen's Encephalitis
- Fungal Infections
- Cysticercosis
- Toxoplasmosis
- Syphilis
- Lyme Disease
- Creutzfeldt-Jakob Disease
- Sarcoidosis
- Tuberculosis

Meningitis and Its Complications

Meningitis is an infectious or inflammatory process affecting the subarachnoid space (1). The most common symptoms of meningitis are fever, headaches, photophobia, nausea, vomiting, lethargy, altered mental status, and cranial nerve dysfunction. The diagnosis is established by these clinical signs in combination with appropriate cerebrospinal fluid (CSF) findings (Table 11.1).

I will limit this discussion to bacterial meningitis. The most common implicated pathogens in bacterial meningitis are listed in Table 11.2.

There is no indication to image patients with uncomplicated bacterial meningitis (2). The only imaging finding in these patients is that of nonspecific leptomeningeal enhancement (3) (Fig. 11.1A). Fluid attenuation inversion recovery (FLAIR) images may show the CSF to have increased signal intensity. Imaging studies should be reserved for those patients suspected of harboring complications. The most common clinical sign of complicated bacterial meningitis is an enlarging head. The complications associated with bacterial meningitis are (2):

There is no indication for imaging studies in simple and complicated bacterial meningitis; imaging studies should be reserved for patients with complicated meningitis.

- Hydrocephalus
- Subdural effusions
- Subdural empyemas
- Ventriculitis
- Venous thrombosis
- Arteritis and cerebral infarctions
- Cerebritis and abscesses

Hydrocephalus is the most common complication of bacterial meningitis, and imaging studies usually show dilatation of all the ventricles (2). Sterile subdural effusions may occur with most pathogens, but most are found in children infected with *Hemophilus influenzae*, and they occur at any age (although most are seen before 18 months of age). The incidence of subdural effusions varies from 10% to 60% in patients with meningitis.

Table 11.1: Cerebrospinal Fluid Findings in Different Types of Meningitis

Parameter	*Bacterial*	*Viral*	*Tuberculosis*	*Fungal*
Cell number	High	Normal to high	High	Normal to high
Cell type	Polymorphonuclear lymphocytes	Lymphocytes	Lymphocytes	Mixed
Proteins	High	Normal to mildly high	Normal to high	Normal to high
Glucose	Low	Normal to mildly low	Normal to mildly low	Normal to mildly low

These collections tend to be large and hemispheric, resulting in significant mass effect (Fig. 11.2). Sterile subdural collections are likely to result from meningeal inflammation and increased permeability of blood vessels. Smaller subdural effusions may resolve spontaneously, but the larger ones may require drainage.

Approximately 2% of all subdural collections become infected and form subdural empyemas (Fig. 11.3). Epidural empyemas (collections of pus) also may occur secondary to sinusitis, surgery, or infection of an epidural hematoma. However, empyemas also may be subdural in location. In adults, most extraaxial empyemas are due to sinusitis; in children, most are seen in the setting of meningitis. Extraaxial empyemas carry a mortality rate (despite antibiotic treatment) of 10% to 100%. Differentiating a sterile from an infected subdural collection by imaging may be very difficult. The rim of both types of collections enhances after contrast administration (4) (Figs. 11.2 and 11.3). Both types of collections are bright on T2-weighted images and hypointense on T1 images. At times, collections may show mildly increased signal intensity on T1-weighted images, a finding that correlates with increased proteins and usually is seen with infections. Infected collections also may be bright on trace diffusion-weighted imaging (DWI) and on FLAIR images (Fig. 11.3B). Apparent diffusion coefficient maps show that these infected collections are of low signal intensity, indicating a restriction in the motion of the free water in the empyema. In very young patients, transcranial sonography shows that infected collections are hyperechoic, contain septa, and have multiple floating regions of increased echogenicity (none of these is seen in sterile subdural collections). Complications of empyemas are venous thrombosis, cerebritis, abscesses, and infarctions.

Cerebral abscesses are rare today because of early antibiotic treatment (5). Approximately 25% of cerebral abscesses occur in patients younger than 15 years of age, and most are seen in men before the age of 30 years. Despite aggressive use of antibiotics, approximately 20% of patients with cerebral abscesses die. Most cerebral abscesses are bacterial and are found in the territory of the middle cerebral arteries (reflecting hematogenous dissemination). Abscesses may be a complication of meningitis, may be bloodborne, or may be secondary to sinonasal, middle ear, and mastoid infections or due to trauma or surgery. Ventriculitis may be the result of a ruptured abscess or secondary to meningitis (Fig. 11.4). The imaging features of abscesses are listed in Table 11.3 (5).

Nearly all pyogenic cerebral abscesses are bright on single-axis and trace diffusion-weighted imaging.

Abscesses usually have considerable surrounding edema and mass effect (Fig. 11.5A and B). Their rim of enhancement tends to be thicker where it abuts the cortex, reflecting the increased vascularity of the gray matter. It is not uncommon to find a part of the abscess capsule adjacent to a ventricle. Rupture into a ventricle, resulting in a ventriculi-

Table 11.2: Common Bacteria Producing Meningitis

Immunocompetent Patients	*Immunodeficient Patients*	*Children*
Streptococcus pneumoniae	*Escherichia coli*	*Staphylococcus agalactiae*
Haemophilus influenza type B	*Klebsiella pneumoniae*	*E. coli*
Neisseria meningitis	*Pseudomonas aeruginosa*	*K. pneumoniae*

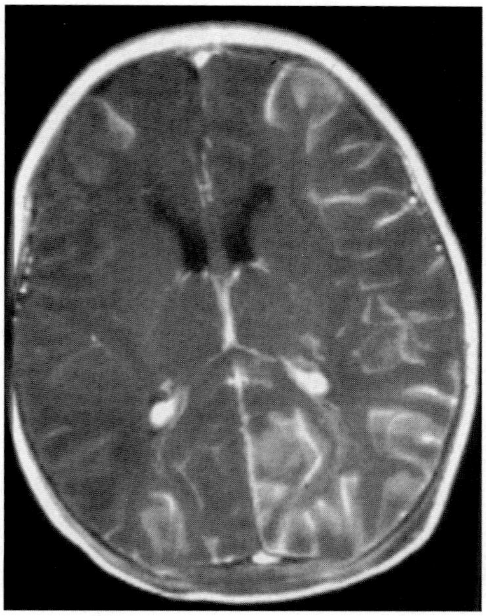

Figure 11.1 *Meningitis, Uncomplicated.* Axial postcontrast T1-weighted image shows leptomeningeal enhancement predominantly in the left hemisphere, and no hydrocephalus.

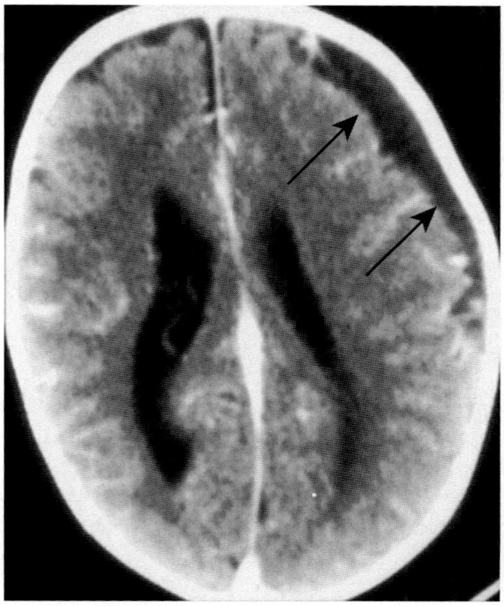

A

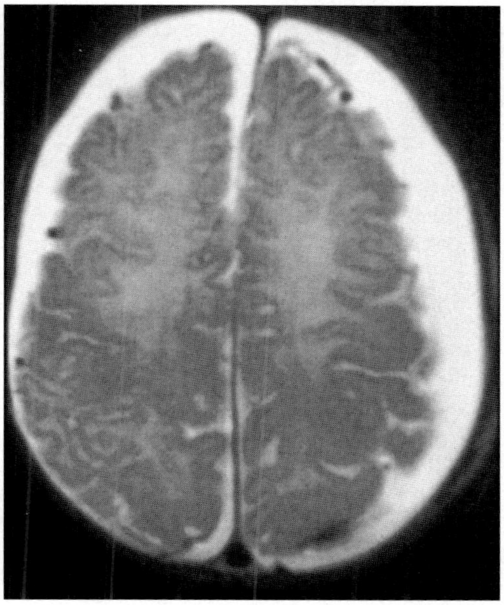

B

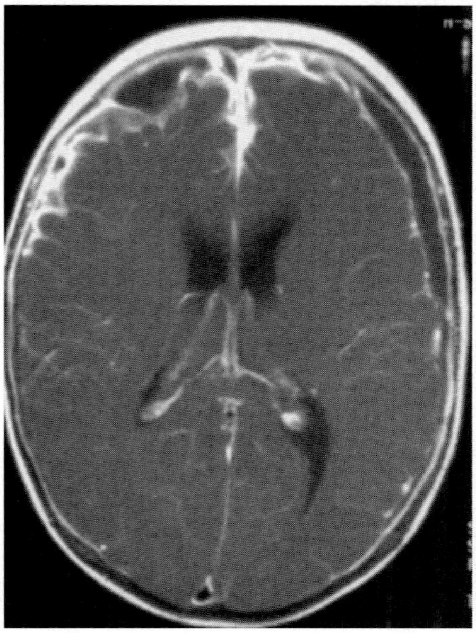

C

Figure 11.2 *Subdural Sterile Collections Secondary to Meningitis. A.* Postcontrast computed tomography shows a left frontal subdural effusion *(arrows)*. *B.* In a different patient, an axial T2-weighted image shows bilateral bright hemispheric subdural fluid collections. Because of their mass effect, they were tapped and were found to be sterile. Note inward displacement of cortical veins typical of subdural collections. *C.* In a different patient, postcontrast axial T1-weighted image shows bifrontal fluid collections of low intensity. Note enhancing margins that lead to aspiration. The diagnosis was that of sterile subdural effusions.

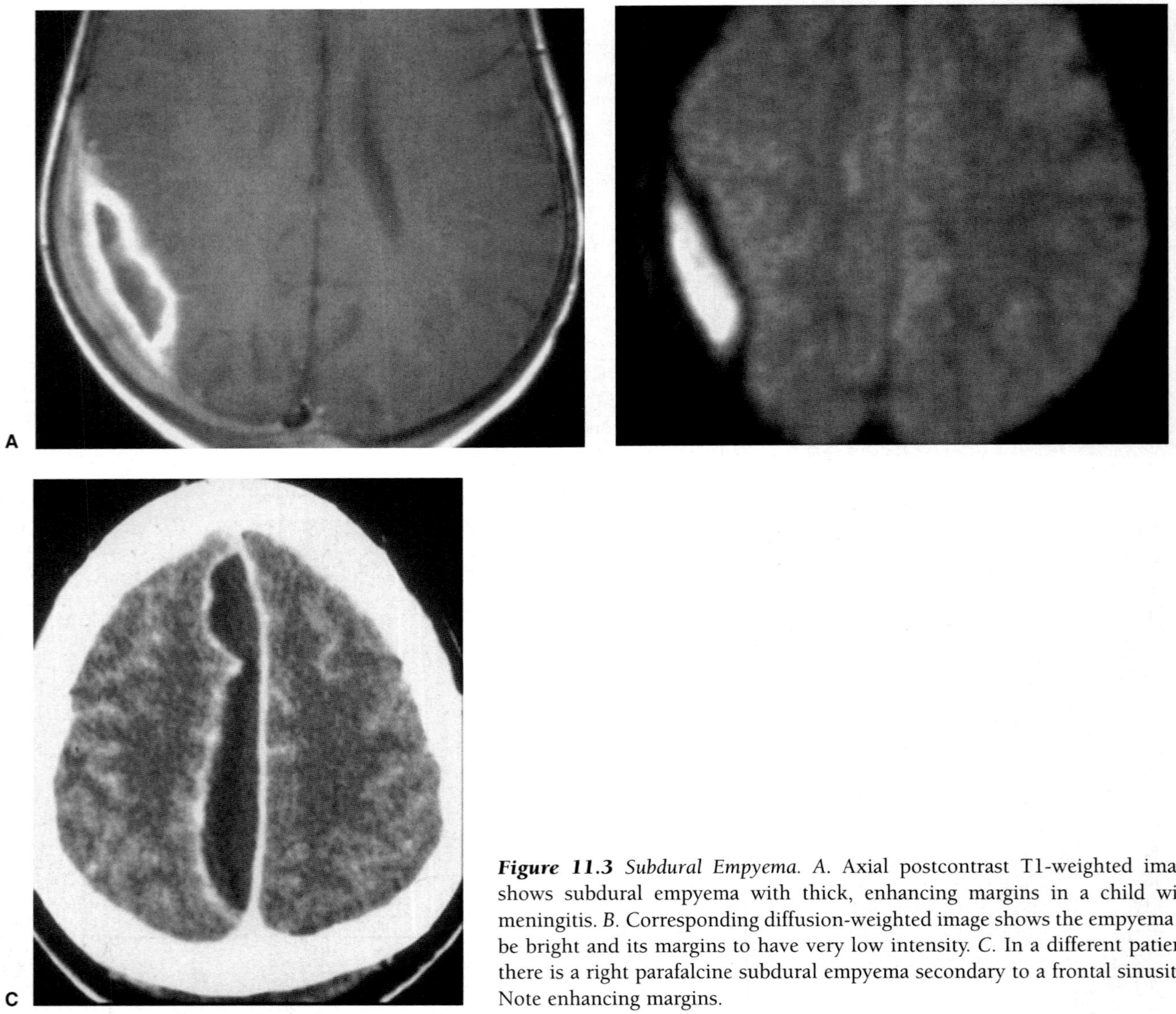

Figure 11.3 *Subdural Empyema. A.* Axial postcontrast T1-weighted image shows subdural empyema with thick, enhancing margins in a child with meningitis. *B.* Corresponding diffusion-weighted image shows the empyema to be bright and its margins to have very low intensity. *C.* In a different patient, there is a right parafalcine subdural empyema secondary to a frontal sinusitis. Note enhancing margins.

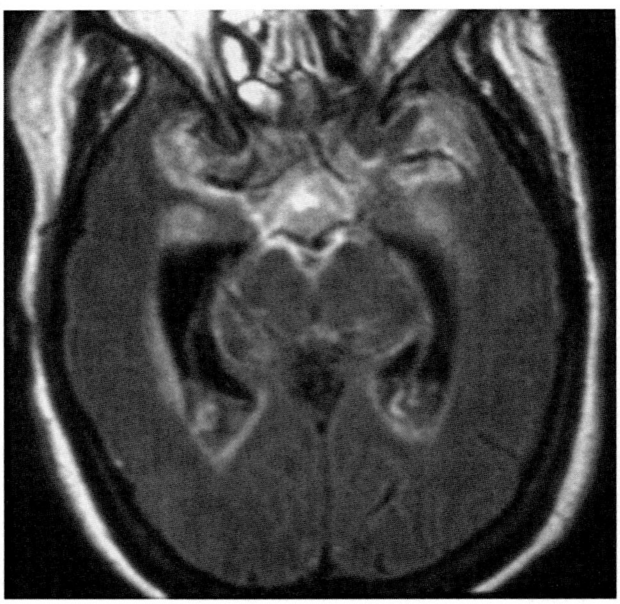

Figure 11.4 *Meningitis and Ventriculitis.* Axial postcontrast T1-weighted image shows enhancement of the ventricular ependyma and of the suprasellar and sylvian cisterns.

Table 11.3: Stages in the Formation of Cerebral Abscesses

Stage	*T2-Weighted Images*	*Enhancement*	*Diffusion-Weighted Images (Trace Images)*
Cerebritis (<1 wk)	Bright	None or mild	Somewhat bright
Early abscess (1–2 wk)	Bright	Incomplete rim	Somewhat bright
Late (mature) abscess (2–3 wk)	Bright center, rim of low signal	Ring enhancement	Bright centrally

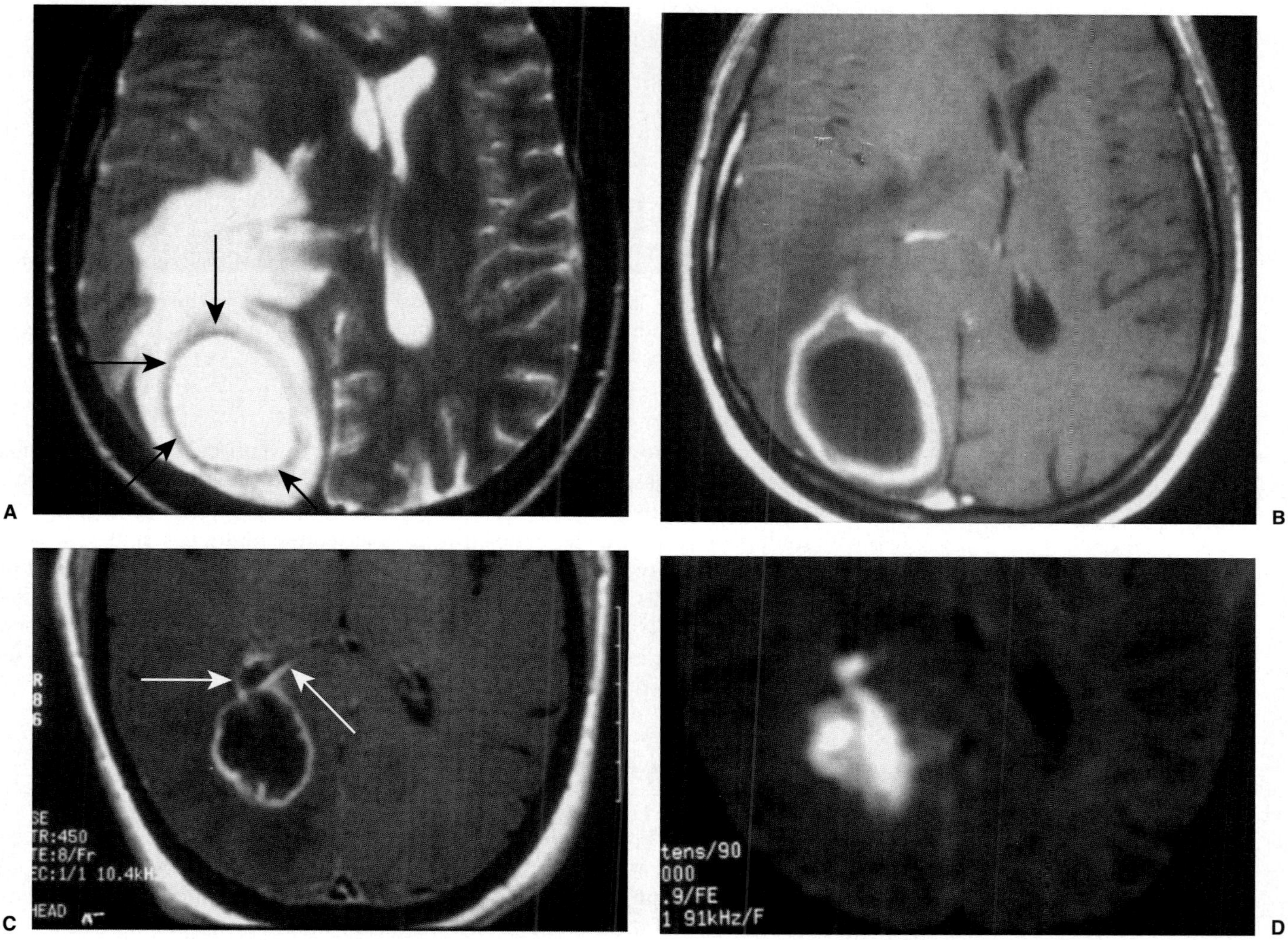

Figure 11.5 *Cerebral Abscesses. A.* Axial T2-weighted image shows large right parietooccipital abscess with a low-intensity capsule *(arrows)* and surrounding edema and mass effect. *B.* Corresponding postcontrast T1-weighted image shows typical thin and uniformly enhancing margin. The rim is slightly thicker close to gray matter. *C.* In a different patient, postcontrast axial T1-weighted image shows a right occipital abscess with a thin enhancing margin. Note extension of the infection into the right lateral ventricle, which shows ependymal enhancement *(arrows). D.* Corresponding diffusion-weighted image (DWI) shows the abscess and adjacent lateral ventricle to be bright. (Case courtesy of G. Fatterpekar, New York, NY.)

(continued on next page)

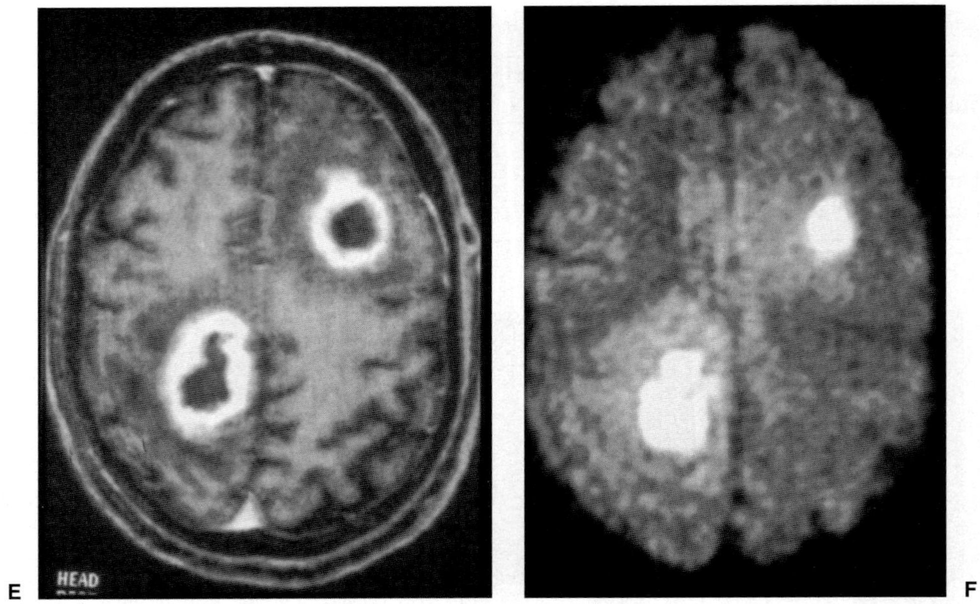

Figure 11.5 (continued) *E.* In a different patient, axial postcontrast T1-weighted image shows two right-sided abscesses with somewhat unusual thick enhancing margins. *F.* Corresponding DWI shows both lesions to be bright.

tis, is associated with a poor prognosis (Fig. 11.5C and D). In ventriculitis, the ependyma appears thick and enhances, and the ventricles may show fluid levels related to the presence of intraventricular pus. Chronically, hydrocephalus develops in all of these patients, often with multiple intraventricular compartments that require multiple shunts. The contents of an abscess are very bright on DWI, reflecting the complex internal structures of the pus (desquamated cells, hemorrhage, necrosis, inflammatory cells) that prevents the random motion of water (6) (Fig. 11.5C, E, and F). Occasionally, abscesses are dark on DWI, and I have seen this in *Toxoplasma* and tuberculous abscesses, but it also may occur in some abscesses of bacterial origin.

Human Immunodeficiency Virus Infection

Human immunodeficiency virus (HIV) infection probably is the most common viral disorder affecting the brain and spinal cord. HIV infects the brain in 30% to 80% of all patients with acquired immunodeficiency syndrome (AIDS), and clinical manifestations are seen in 10% to 30% of them (7). The virus results in subacute encephalitis and a syndrome of progressive dementia with cognitive, motor, and behavior abnormalities (called the *AIDS dementia complex*) (8). The pathologic hallmark of this infection is the presence of many microglial nodules and multinucleated giant cells in the white matter. This gives rise to patchy areas of confluent and somewhat diffuse high T2 signal intensity in the white matter. The increase in T2 signal intensity is only moderate; the disease tends to be bilateral and somewhat symmetric, and predominantly involves the frontal and parietal lobes (9–11) (Fig. 11.6A). There is no contrast enhancement. The presence of well defined white matter lesions is suggestive of disease other than HIV infection. Progressive brain atrophy occurs in all HIV-infected patients (12). In HIV-infected children, calcification of the basal ganglia and brain atrophy occur, particularly after the first year of life (Fig. 11.6B). Unfortunately, many brain sites affected by HIV also may harbor other infections, such as cytomegalovirus. Superimposed cytomegalovirus infection cannot be distinguished from HIV on imaging studies. Proton MR spectroscopy in patients with HIV shows initially low *N*-acetyl aspartate (NAA) and moderately elevated choline (13,14). This is followed by normalization of the choline level and an increase in the

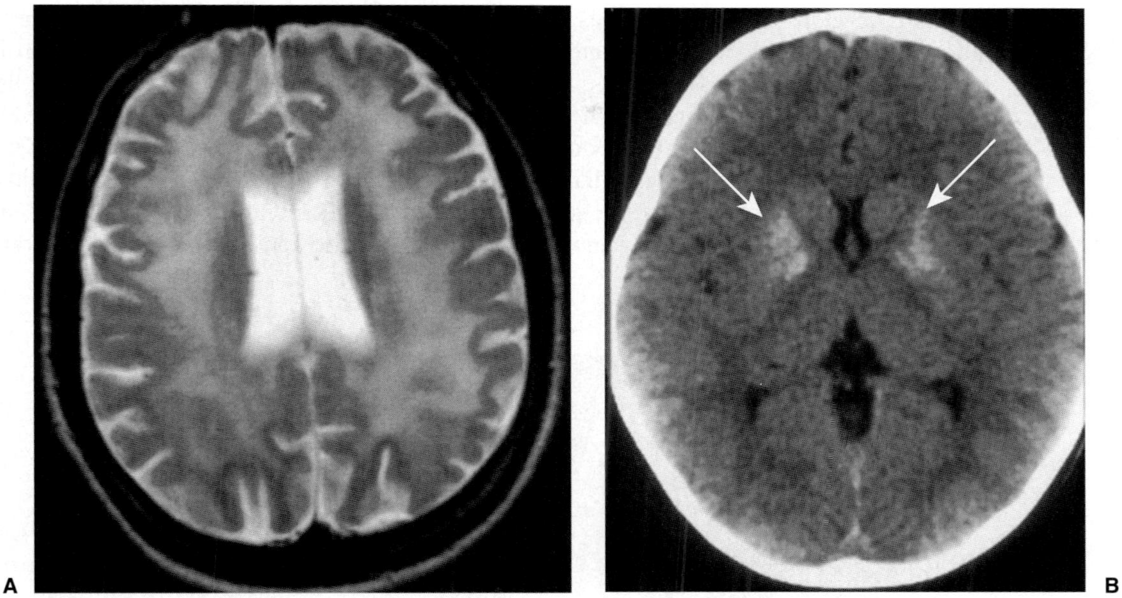

Figure 11.6 *Infection with Human Immunodeficiency Virus. A.* Axial T2-weighted image in an adult shows diffuse and homogeneous increased signal intensity in the white matter of both cerebral hemispheres and slight atrophy of the cortex and prominent lateral ventricles. *B.* Axial computed tomography in a child shows calcifications *(arrows)* in the basal ganglia.

NAA peak height that never returns to normal. As the disease progresses, the NAA becomes markedly reduced. Metabolite changes may be seen before results of imaging studies become abnormal. The low NAA implies neuronal death or dysfunction and correlates with the development of dementia. HIV in the spinal cord usually affects the posterior columns. The MRI abnormalities related to brain HIV infection may improve after treatment.

Progressive Multifocal Leukoencephalopathy

Progressive multifocal leukoencephalopathy (PML) is caused by a papovirus (called *JC virus* after the initials of the first patient with the disease) that commonly infects humans but produces no overt disease in immunocompetent individuals. The virus infects the oligodendrocytes, and normal myelin cannot be maintained (15). Groups of patients in which PML may occur are listed in Box 11.1 (7).

Box 11.1: Conditions Predisposing to Progressive Multifocal Leukoencephalopathy

Acquired immunodeficiency syndrome
Chronic leukemias
Lymphoma (particularly Hodgkin's disease)
Organ transplantation
Congenital immunodeficiency syndromes
Lupus erythematosus
Sarcoidosis
Chronic treatment with steroids

Progressive multifocal leukoencephalopathy may have atypical findings (e.g., involvement of gray matter and even contrast enhancement) in up to 50% of patients.

PML develops in >3% of patients with AIDS (7). The most common clinical manifestations are progressive neurologic deterioration, visual deficits, and ataxia without signs of increased intracranial pressure. Most PML affects the occipital and parietal regions, but it may involve the white matter anywhere. PML results in low computed tomography (CT) density and high T2 signal intensity on MRI (16) (Fig. 11.7). It produces no mass effect, and the abnormalities usually are bilateral but asymmetric. PML crosses the corpus callosum. In nearly 50% of patients, the gray matter also may be involved (17). This is seen most commonly as a bright T2 signal in the cortex, which also appears thin. The deep gray

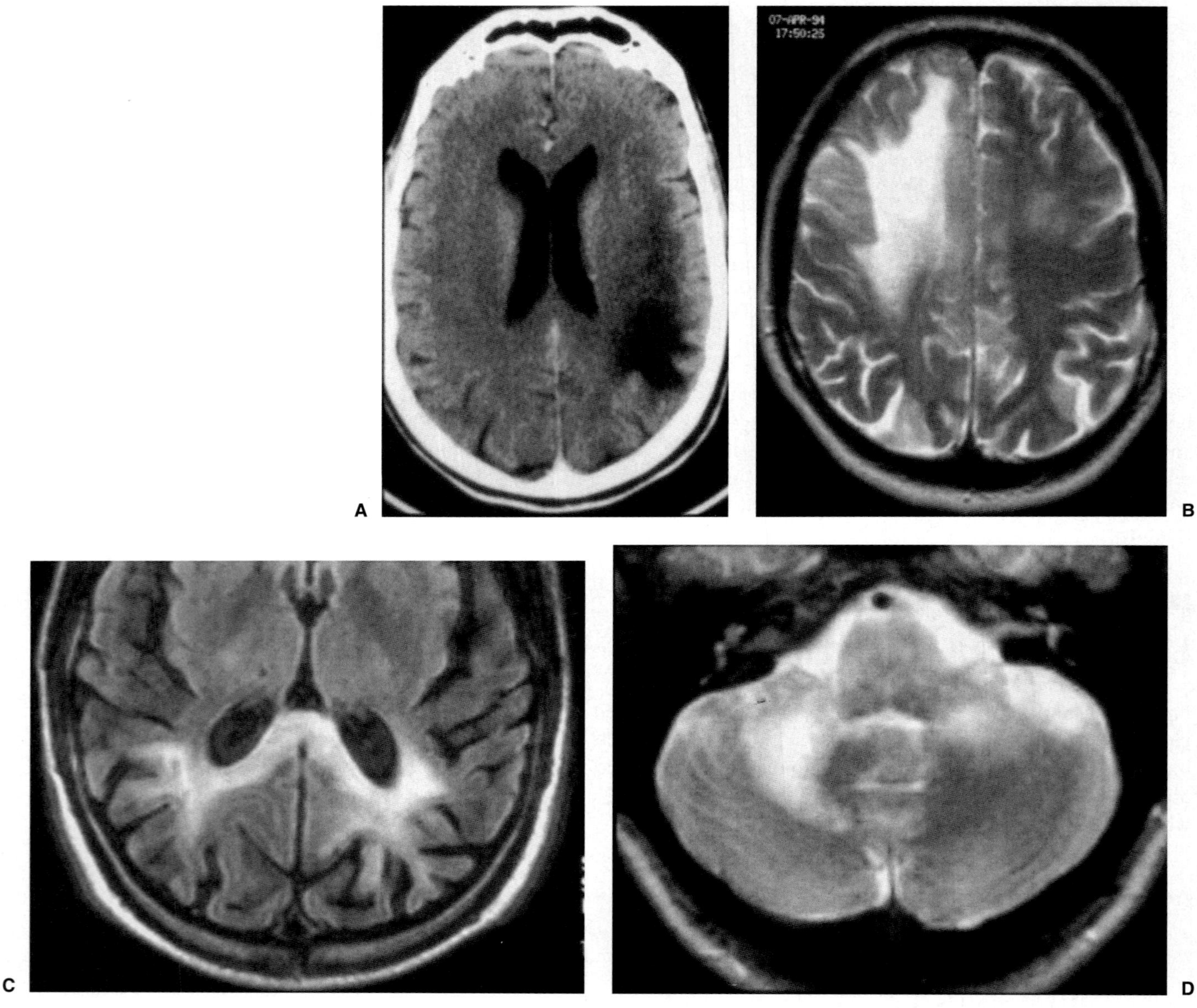

Figure 11.7 *Progressive Multifocal Leukoencephalopathy (PML). A.* Axial postcontrast computed tomography shows a low-density lesion in the left temporoparietal region. Note absence of mass effect. *B.* In a different patient, axial T2-weighted image shows large right frontal area of high signal intensity and a smaller one in the left centrum semiovale. Note lack of mass effect and of gray matter involvement. *C.* Axial fluid attenuation inversion recovery (FLAIR) image shows PML crossing the splenium of the corpus callosum and extending into the occipital white matter. *D.* In a different patient, axial T2-weighted image shows hyperintense lesions in both middle cerebellar peduncles (right greater than left) that produce no mass effect.

matter (basal ganglia and thalami) also may be affected. In most patients there is no contrast enhancement, reflecting the lack of inflammation that is typical of PML. Contrast enhancement in the periphery of the lesion does occur, however (18). The MRI abnormalities may improve after treatment (19).

Herpes Simplex Virus Infection

HSV type 1 infection is seen more commonly in adults, whereas HSV type 2 infection usually occurs in neonates.

Herpes simplex virus (HSV) type 1 is a common pathogen in children, usually acquired by the oral route (20). Most of these infections are asymptomatic. Most active infections occur after 30 years of age and represent reactivation of a dormant virus (20). The most common symptoms are speech difficulties, altered mental status, seizures (which occur in approximately 60% of patients), and coma. Without treatment, over 75% of patients die. Most HSV replicate in the peripheral nervous system and then travel and lodge in sensory ganglia, particularly spinal ganglia in the sacrum and the trigeminal nerve ganglia. The reactivation of the virus probably is induced by a variety of stresses. Although most (>60%) HSV encephalitis is considered to occur after reactivation, some arise *de novo*. Because there is no connection between the trigeminal nerve ganglia and the limbic system (the initially and most commonly affected region of the brain), the pathways for the spread of HSV encephalitis remain a matter of speculation. However, the frontal lobes may be affected by direct spread from the olfactory nerves. Viral antigens are present in the CSF in all persons with HSV encephalitis. Necrosis and inflammation are the typical histologic findings. The necrosis may be hemorrhagic. MRI is the imaging method of choice to evaluate patients with suspected HSV infection. T2-weighted images show high signal intensity in the mesial temporal lobes (Fig. 11.8A). The hippocampi may show contrast enhancement early in the course of the disease. The high T2 signal then spreads to the insular cortex, but commonly spares the basal ganglia. The basal and medial aspects of the frontal lobes also may show increased T2 signal intensity (Fig. 11.8B). In most patients, bilateral but asymmetric lesions eventually develop. The cortex may contain hemorrhage. Parenchymal enhancement occurs, but to a lesser degree than leptomeningeal enhancement (Fig. 11.8C). DWI may show the lesions to a better degree than conventional MRI (Fig. 11.8D and E). Proton MR spectroscopy shows elevation of the choline, reflecting the inflammatory response; low NAA, reflecting neuronal damage; and lipids and lactate secondary to necrosis (21). In some young children, HSV encephalitis results in a more disseminated disease that involves the gray and white matter of both cerebral hemispheres. Occasionally, HSV results in an infection of the brainstem. The sequelae of HSV infection include atrophy and cystic encephalomalacia of the affected regions (22). Treatment needs to be commenced immediately if HSV encephalitis is suspected because the mortality rate of untreated disease is over 70%.

Rasmussen's Encephalitis

Rasmussen's encephalitis is a rare syndrome that is presumed to be of viral etiology, although this has never been confirmed (23). The clinical signs are progressive seizures that are refractory to medications and unilateral neurologic deficits ultimately resulting in a hemiplegia. CSF usually is normal, but may show lymphocytosis. Histologically, there are perivascular inflammatory infiltrates, microglial nodules in the cortex, capillary proliferation, and meningeal thickening and inflammation (23). These changes lead to unilateral cerebral atrophy with dilatation of the ventricles. Occasionally the disease may be bilateral. MRI shows unilateral brain atrophy and, rarely, areas of increased T2 signal intensity in white or gray matter (20) (Fig. 11.9A). Proton MR spectroscopy may show low NAA even in a contralateral hemisphere that appears morphologically normal (23). Func-

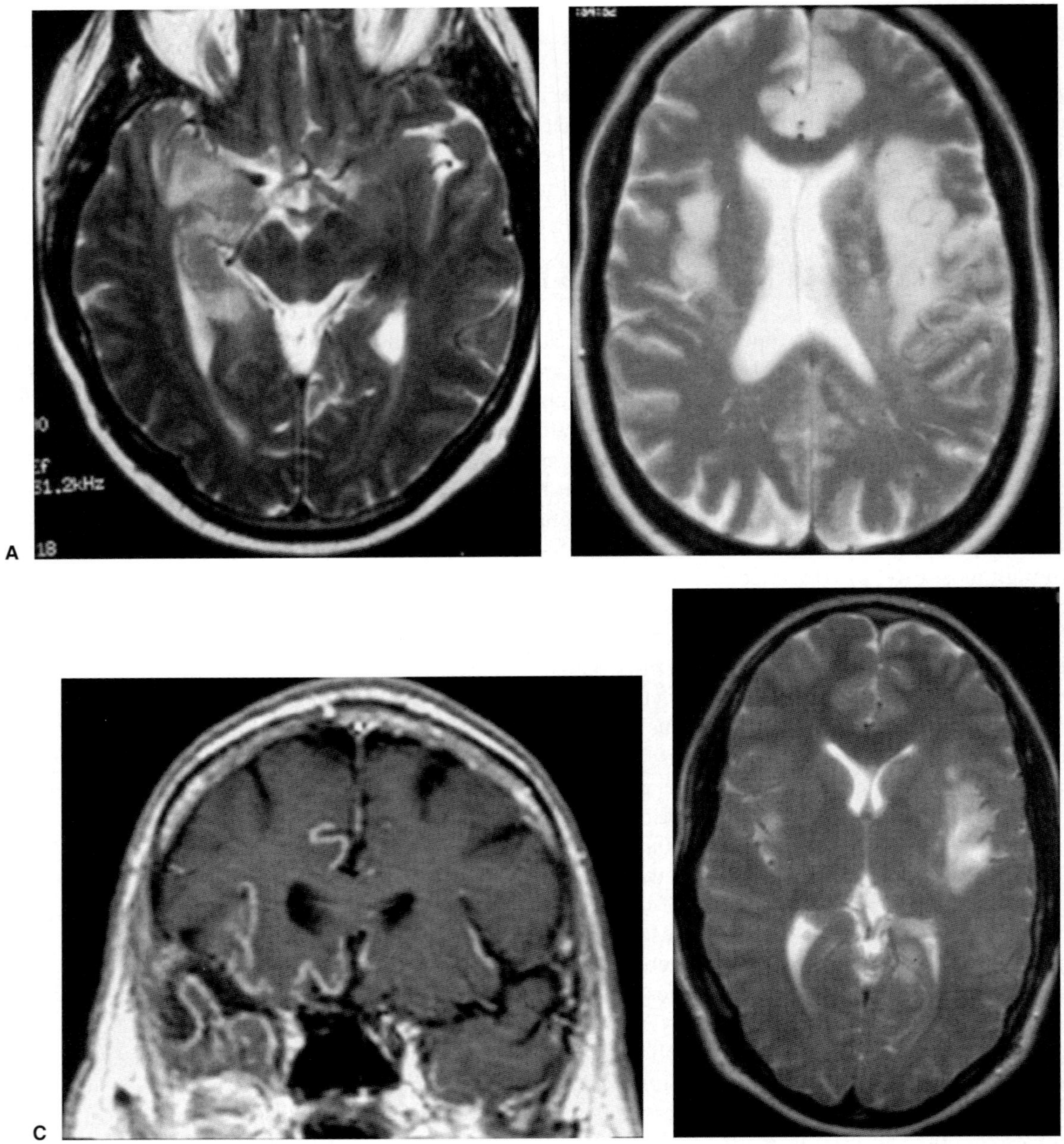

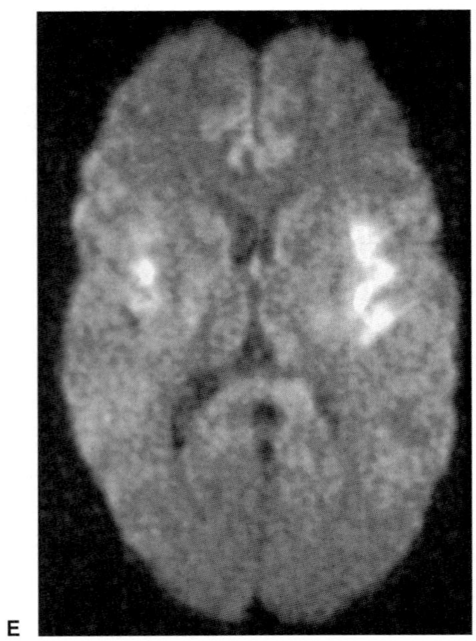

Figure 11.8 *Herpes Simplex Virus Type 1 Infection. A.* Axial fluid attenuation inversion recovery (FLAIR) image shows swollen and bright right hippocampus and amygdala. *B.* In a different patient, axial T2-weighted image shows swollen and hyperintense insular cortices (left greater than right) and along the medial surfaces of the frontal lobes. *C.* In a different patient, coronal postcontrast T1-weighted image shows gray matter enhancement in both temporal lobes (right greater than left) and medial right frontal lobe. *D.* Axial T2-weighted image shows bright left insular cortex. *E.* Corresponding diffusion-weighted image (DWI) shows left insular lesion as well as a right insular one. In some instances, DWI may show the extent of the lesions to better advantage than other sequences.

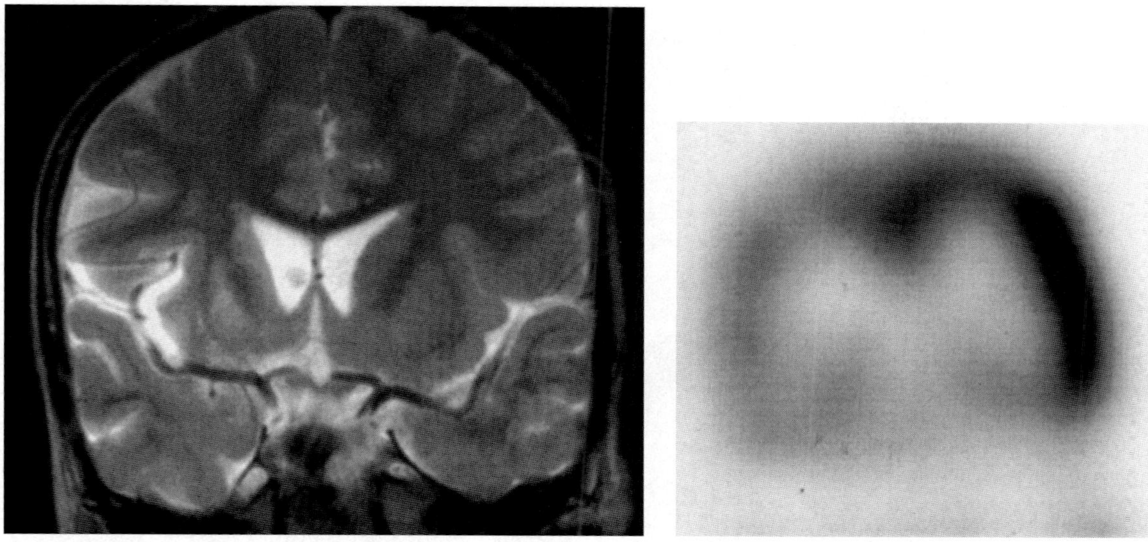

A B

Figure 11.9 *Rasmussen's Encephalitis. A.* Coronal T2-weighted image shows atrophy of the right hemisphere and perhaps mildly increased signal intensity in the cortex. *B.* Corresponding thallium-hexamethylenepropylene amine oxime (HM-PAO) single-photon emission computed tomography study shows decreased uptake of the radiotracer throughout the right cerebral hemisphere and left temporal lobe.

tional studies such as single-photon emission tomography, positron emission tomography, and proton MR spectroscopy may show bilateral abnormalities even when the imaging studies of those regions are unremarkable (Fig. 11.9B).

FUNGAL INFECTIONS

CRYPTOCOCCOSIS

Cryptococcus neoformans is the most common fungus to affect the brain (24). This yeast usually is found in the feces of birds. The yeasts have polysaccharide capsules that inhibit phagocytosis and may create or inhibit formation of antibodies depending on the immune status of the host. Most infections with *Cryptococcus* occur in patients with AIDS (25). The most common manifestation is meningitis, and in these patients most imaging studies are negative. Occasionally, thick meningeal contrast enhancement may be noted (26). A mild degree of hydrocephalus develops in approximately half of the patients with cryptococcal meningitis. Brain lesions develop in only 5% of patients infected with this organism. The type of parenchymal lesion depends on the immune status of the patient. Immunocompetent patients usually have solitary or multiple abscess-like lesions called *cryptococcomas* or *cryptococcal granulomas*. On imaging, these lesions show ring enhancement and some surrounding edema and are nonspecific in appearance. The most interesting manifestation of this disease is the infiltration of the perivascular spaces by the yeast. This commonly occurs in those spaces surrounding the arterioles supplying the basal ganglia and thalami. Once the yeasts have lodged in these spaces, they produce a mucoid material that expands the spaces and gives rise to "cystic" lesions (27) (Fig. 11.10). These lesions usually are multiple and are called *gelatinous pseudocysts*. These cystic lesions are of low T1 signal and bright on T2 and FLAIR images. They do not enhance after contrast is given. The most important differential diagnosis is that of multiple dilated perivascular spaces ("etat cribble"). Cryptococcosis also may involve the choroid plexus, resulting in a mass lesion that shows contrast enhancement (28).

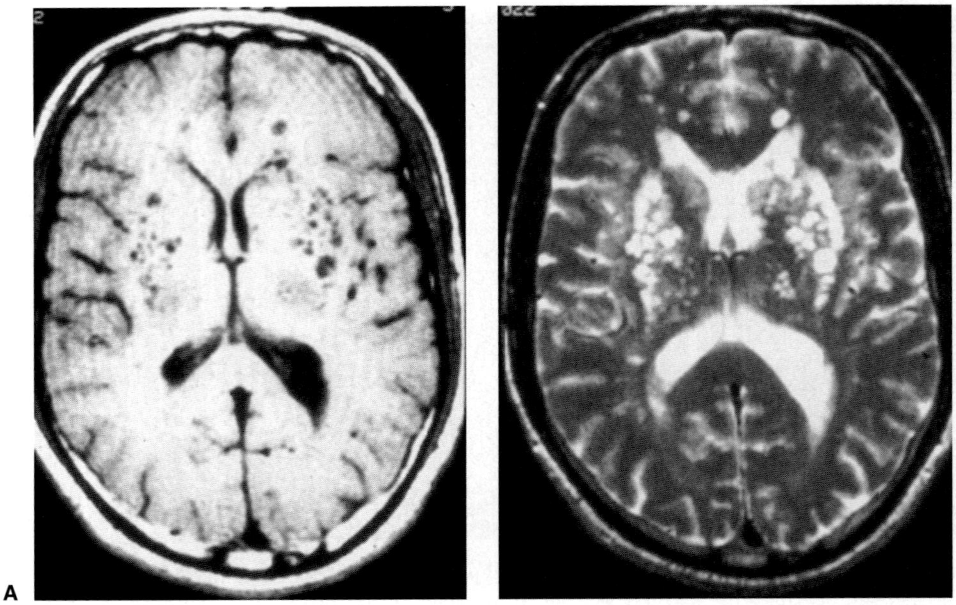

Figure 11.10 *Cryptococcosis. A.* Noncontrast axial T1-weighted image shows multiple cysts ("gelatinous pseudocysts") in the basal ganglia. *B.* In the same patient, axial T2-weighted image shows bright cysts in the basal ganglia and thalami. The lateral ventricles are slightly prominent.

Aspergillosis

Aspergillus is a family of fungi comprising over 350 species, of which the most common to infect humans is *Aspergillus fumigatus*. The disease typically is localized (lungs, paranasal sinuses), but the brain may be affected in up to 70% of patients with disseminated disease (29). *Aspergillus* is found in up to 10% of patients of patients with AIDS, cancer, and organ transplants (30). It is a disorder found mostly in adults. The forms of spread of the disease are direct (from the paranasal sinuses) or hematogenous (from pulmonary infection). *Aspergilllus* has an affinity for blood vessels (31). The fungus grows

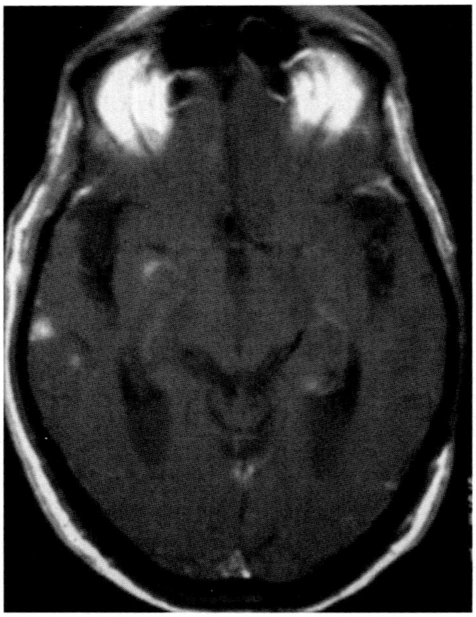

Figure 11.11 *Aspergillosis.* Axial postcontrast T1-weighted image shows multiple, nonspecific-appearing, enhancing lesions.

in their walls and leads to their occlusion and thrombosis. This fungus also may produce mycotic aneurysms. Indeed, aspergillosis is the most common fungal brain infection to produce mycotic aneurysms. Imaging studies usually show nonspecific, enhancing lesions with surrounding edema (Fig. 11.11). The imaging features usually are indistinguishable from those caused by pyogenic abscesses. In the paranasal sinuses, *Aspergillus* may produce secretions that are of very low T2 signal (32). This is due to magnetic susceptibility effects from iron, manganese, magnesium, and calcium deposited in mycetomas. Occasionally, paranasal sinus destruction and direct extension of the lesion into the brain may be found.

Mucormycosis

Similar to *Aspergillus*, the mucorales *zygomycosis* and *phycomycosis* have an affinity for brain and blood vessel invasion (29). Mucormycosis is being increasingly recognized and may be found in patients with the following disorders:

- Diabetes (70% of mucormycosis cases)
- Metabolic acidosis (chronic diarrhea, renal failure)
- Immunosuppression (AIDS, cancer, organ transplantation)
- Direct trauma
- Extensive burns

Invasion of the brain occurs through hematogenous dissemination or by direct invasion from disease in the paranasal sinuses (rhinocerebral form). Hematogenous dissemination of mucormycosis is less common and its imaging features are nonspecific. Once brain invasion has occurred, most patients die within 2 weeks. Fungi causing mucormycosis have an affinity for reproducing in blood vessel walls, leading to thrombosis and weakening and producing pseudoaneurysms. This results in a vasculitis and infarctions (Fig. 11.12). Destruction of the vessel walls leads to direct brain invasion with formation of abscesses. The intraaxial lesions may be hemorrhagic. When the disease arises in the paranasal sinuses, it results in mucosal thickening, and fluid levels are not common. Although the literature states that mucormycosis in the paranasal sinuses may be of low signal intensity (similar to aspergillosis), most of the cases that I have seen show only bright mucosal swelling on T2-weighted images. When mucormycosis affects the sphenoid sinus, the bone marrow in the clivus may be of abnormal low T1 signal intensity. A subtle but very important sign is that of signal intensity changes in the fat immediately outside of the walls of a sinus. The sinus walls usually are not destroyed because the fungus spreads through the vascular channels and the cranial nerves and their foramina (33). If abnormalities in the perisinus fat are noted in a patient who is predisposed to mucormycosis, a biopsy of the mucosa is indicated to confirm the diagnosis early and commence therapy. It is only at this stage that patients survive the disease. Mucormycosis also may spread through naturally occurring fissures and foramina (34). Invasion of the cavernous sinus, through the superior orbital fissure, leads to thrombosis and invasion of the internal carotid artery. After blood vessel destruction, the intraaxial findings are those of infection and infarction, and it is difficult to distinguish between these two abnormalities (DWI is useful in this setting). A less common but more indolent form of the disease is being increasingly recognized in immunocompetent patients (35). This less aggressive form may involve the subarachnoid spaces or the brain parenchyma.

Mucormycosis and aspergillosis have angiophillic properties and show a tendency to invade cerebral blood vessels, resulting in infarctions.

Other Less Common Fungi

Unfortunately, the less common fungi nearly always present with nonspecific imaging findings. Table 11.4 addresses the most common aspects of these rare infections.

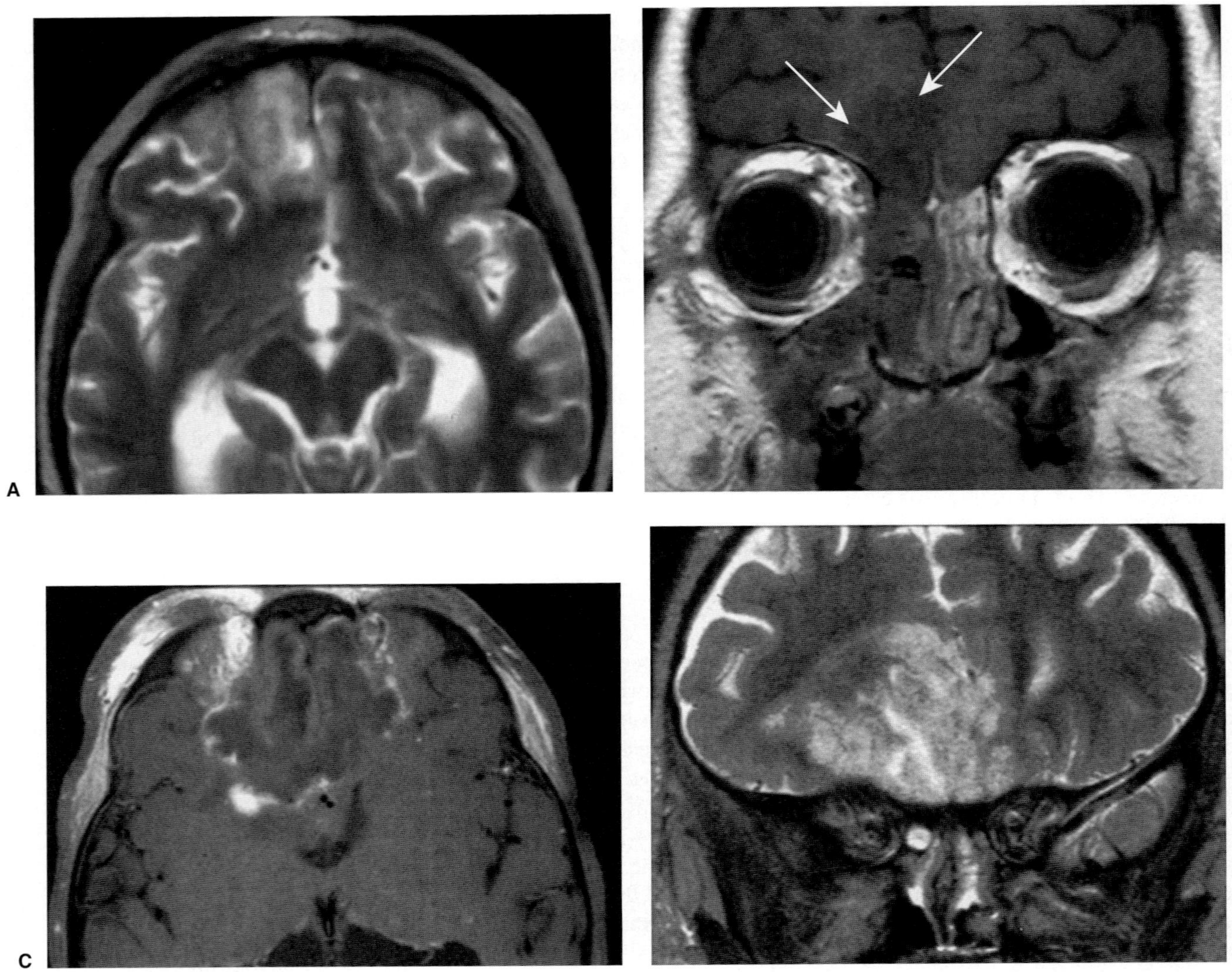

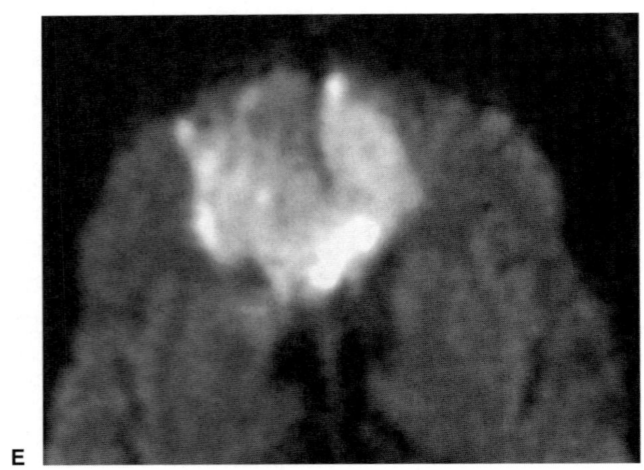

Figure 11.12 *Invasive Mucormycosis. A.* At presentation, an axial T2-weighted image shows high signal in both frontal lobes, right greater than left. *B.* Coronal postcontrast T1-weighted image in the same patient shows nonenhancing soft tissue in the right sinonasal cavities that has extended into the overlying frontal lobe *(arrows)* through erosion of the cribriform plate. *C.* One week later, axial postcontrast T1-weighted image shows a marked increase in the size of the lesion, which now has enhancement of its margins. *D.* Coronal T2-weighted image taken at the same time shows a large lesion in the right frontal lobe. *E.* Axial diffusion-weighted image shows bright infarction of both frontal lobes. The patient died soon after this study.

Table 11.4: Salient Aspects of Relatively Uncommon Fungal Infections of the Central Nervous System

Infection	*Clinical Features*	*Neuroimaging*
Coccidioidomycosis (36,37)	Southwestern U.S., Central and South America; most disease is in the lungs	Meningitis (most common), ventriculitis, vasculitis, infarctions, abscesses
Blastomycosis (38)	Midwestern U.S., southern Canada; mostly lungs, skin, and lymph nodes, but brain may be affected in up to 33% of patients	Meningitis, abscesses, granulomas (Fig. 11.13)
Histoplasmosis (39,40)	Ohio, Missisippi, St. Lawrence and Rio Grande River valleys, chicken farming; systems most affected are lungs, bones, lymph nodes, spleen, and liver, but brain involvement in up to 25% of patients	Meningitis, abscesses, miliary granulomas
Candidiasis (41)	Chronic antibiotics, steroids, cancer, diabetes, pregnancy, major surgery, organ transplantation, acquired immunodeficiency syndrome, burns, skin wounds; most commonly affects the kidneys, but brain disease seen in up to 20%–50% of patients	Multiple abscess-like lesions

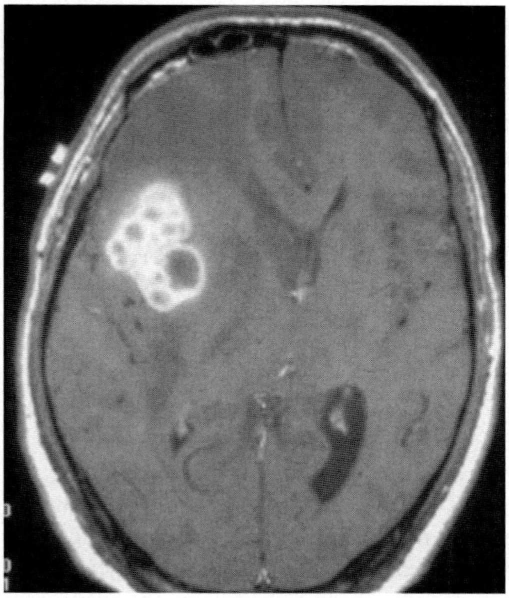

Figure 11.13 *Blastomycosis.* Axial postcontrast T1-weighted image shows unusual-appearing enhancing lesion in the right basal ganglia with mass effect, edema, and midline shift to the left. The appearance of the lesion is nonspecific.

Cysticercosis

Cysticercosis is the most common parasitic disease to affect the immunocompetent population, whereas toxoplasmosis is the most common parasitic disease to affect the immunocompromised population

This common parasitic disorder is caused by the pork worm (*Taenia solium*). There are two types of the disease (Table 11.5) (42).

When larvae are ingested, humans become the definitive host, whereas when eggs are ingested, humans are only the intermediate host for the disease. When eggs are ingested,

Table 11.5: Types of Human Cysticercosis

Type of Parasite Ingested	*Mode of Spread*	*End Result*
Larva	Ingestion of undercooked pork, released in stomach and duodenum and attached to jejunum	Intestinal disease
Eggs	Eggs mature and release larvae into the bloodstream	Central nervous system, eye, muscle, heart, and subcutaneous disease

Table 11.6: Common Sites in the Central Nervous System Infected by Cysticerosis

Location	Incidence
Brain	80%–100%
Ventricles	10%–15%
Subarachnoid space	10%
Spinal cord	<1%

the incidence of central nervous system (CNS) involvement reaches nearly 100% (42). Cysticercosis is endemic in Central and South America, India, and China. In the United States, most of the cases found are in California, Texas, Nevada, Florida, and North Carolina, although it may be found anywhere. Regardless of ethnicity, nearly 90% of cases occur in immigrants. The most common clinical features are headache and seizures. The sites of infection in the CNS are listed in Table 11.6 (43).

The parasites have a finite life, and the stages they undergo determine the clinical and imaging features of the disease (Table 11.7) (44).

The vesicle in the intraaxial lesions represents the dilated bladder of the parasite. The cystic lesions in the parenchyma contain a scolex, whereas those in the subarachnoid space ("racemose" type) do not (Fig. 11.14A). At the vesicular stage, there is a thin layer of chronic inflammatory tissues surrounding the parasite. After approximately 5 to 10 years, the cyst dies and swells as it looses its capacity for osmotic regulation. During this stage, antigens leak out and result in an inflammatory reaction, edema, and seizures (Fig. 11.14B and C). Once the inflammation subsides, calcification ensues, but the site may continue to be epileptogenic because of damage to the tissues (Fig. 11.14D). The second most common form of cysticercosis is the racemose type, in which the scolex does not form (42) (Fig. 11.14E). These parasites produce symptoms by virtue of their mass effect (commonly resulting in hydrocephalus) and an inflammatory reaction (producing meningitis and vasculitis). When these cysts die, they do not calcify.

Most patients are imaged during the symptomatic stages of the disease (colloidal and granular). Most patients, however, harbor parasites in all phases of evolution. During the acute phase, the human body produces immunoglobulin G (IgG) and IgM, which are detected in the serum in up 90% of patients. The cysts usually measure 3 to 20 mm in diameter and are located in the gray-white —matter junctions or deep gray matter, reflecting hematogenous spread (42). If many cysts die simultaneously, an encephalitis may result. Before the cysts die, MRI shows their contents to have the same signal intensity as CSF, without contrast enhancement and edema. When the cyst dies, enhancement and edema are seen. Similar findings may be induced by anticysticercal medications. In the eyes, most parasites are lodged in the choroid layer and the extraocular muscles, reflecting the increased vascularity of these structures. In the subarachnoid form of the disease, cysts commonly are encountered in the basal cisterns, sylvian fissures, and the interhemispheric fissure (45). The cysts in the subarachnoid spaces grow by proliferation of their walls. The cysts are of higher signal intensity than CSF on T1-weighted, proton density, and FLAIR images, but are isointense to CSF on heavily T2-weighted sequences (46). Care should be taken when interpreting the FLAIR images

Table 11.7: Stages of Cysticercosis

Stage	Clinical Features	Neuroimaging
Vesicular	Headaches	Small cystic lesions
Colloidal and granular	Seizures and headaches	Cystic lesions with surrounding edema and ring enhancement
Nodular	Headaches	Calcified lesions

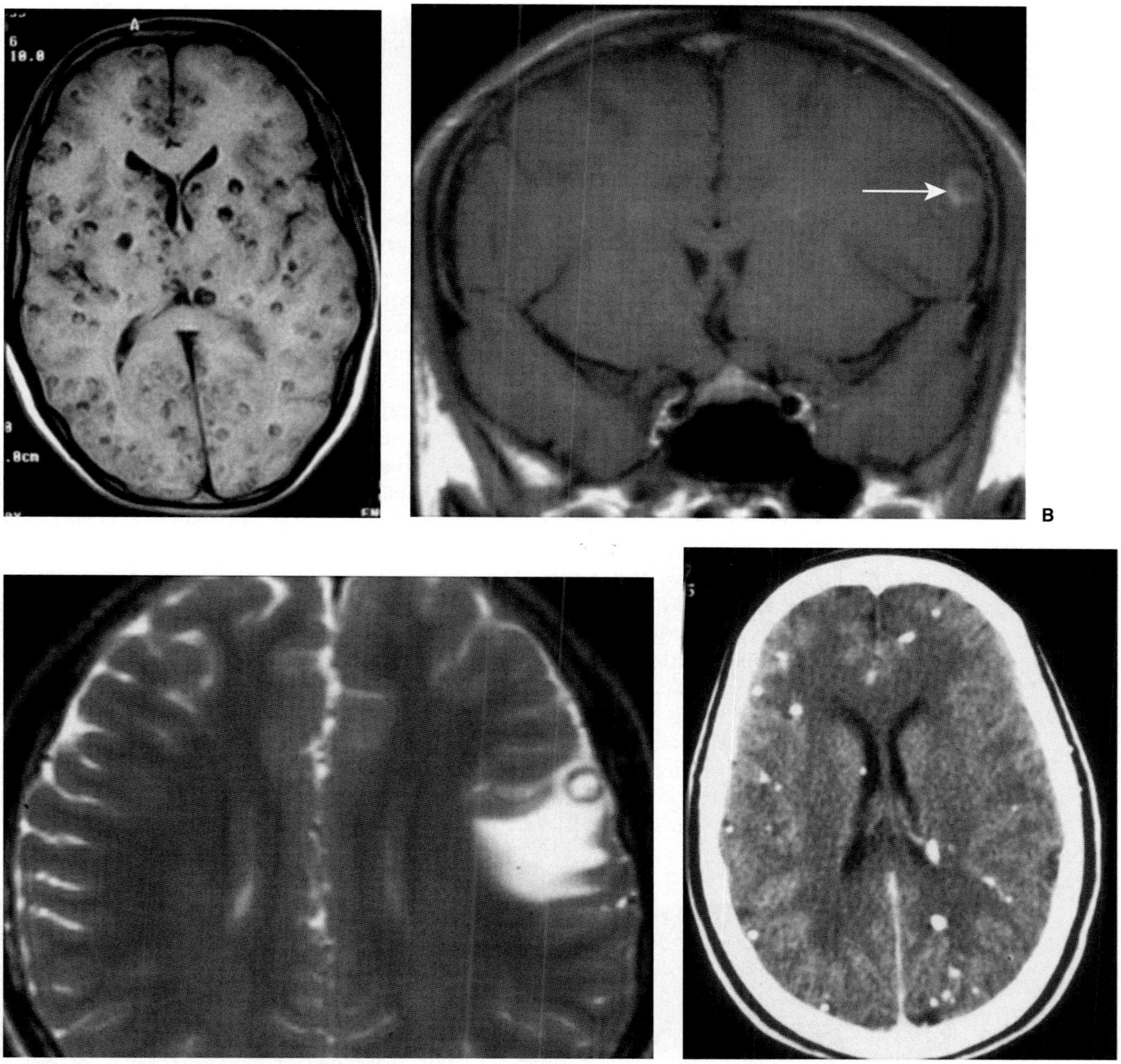

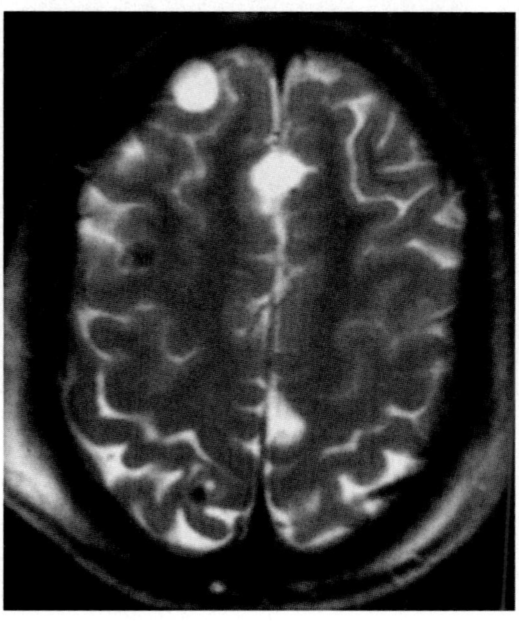

Figure 11.14 *Cysticercosis. A.* Axial noncontrast T1-weighted image shows a "miliary" distribution of cysticercosis with multiple cystic lesions, many of them containing a bright scolex. *B.* In a different patient presenting with new-onset seizures, coronal postcontrast T1-weighted image shows a small ring-enhancing lesion *(arrow)* close to the cortex of the left frontal operculum. *C.* Axial T2-weighted image in the same patient shows that the lesion's rim is hypointense and that there is considerable surrounding edema. *D.* Axial computed tomography shows multiple calcified lesions mostly at the gray–white matter junctions and in the ventricular ependyma and subarachnoid spaces. *E.* Axial T2-weighted image shows bright and cystic-appearing lesions in the subarachnoid spaces in the left frontal lobe, anterior midline, and left posterior parafalcine region. There are dark (calcified) lesions in the right frontal and parietal lobes.

because flow artifacts may simulate cysticercosis, particularly those seen in the region of the foramina of Monro and in the anterior third ventricle. Meningeal enhancement may occur with cysticercosis.

Toxoplasmosis

Toxoplasma gondii is responsible for the most common opportunistic brain infection in patients with AIDS (2). Up to 50% of the general population have antibodies against *Toxoplasma*. Many immunocompetent adults become infected with toxoplasmosis, and most remain asymptomatic or develop lymphadenopathy or a skin rash. Up to 50% of patients with AIDS contract toxoplasmosis during their life (2). When CNS infection occurs, the most common symptoms are headache, seizures, and fever. Toxoplasmosis may result in focal lesions (common) or disseminated encephalitis (uncommon). The most common sites affected by the parasite are the deep gray matter nuclei and the gray–white matter junctions, reflecting the hematogenous distribution of the disease, but the lesions may occur anywhere in the brain (Fig. 11.15). Histologically, there is an inflammatory infiltrate, gliosis, and necrosis. There may be blood vessel necrosis that leads to hemorrhage. On imaging studies, toxoplasmosis presents as ring-enhancing lesions with surrounding edema. Their rim is somewhat thicker than that seen in pyogenic abscesses. The lesions occasionally show hemorrhage at presentation, or hemorrhage develops during treatment. Some lesions may calcify after treatment, but more commonly the end result is a zone of malacia. Most lesions show improvement 2 to 4 weeks after initiation of treatment. The most important differential diagnosis is that of lymphoma, and this topic is addressed in Chapter 6. Briefly, differentiation between toxoplasmosis and lymphoma is highlighted in Table 11.8 (47).

I have seen cases of toxoplasmosis in which DWI showed low signal intensity, as well as cases in which the proton MR spectra were indistinguishable from those of lymphoma. There is no test to distinguish between toxoplasmosis and lymphoma that is correct at all

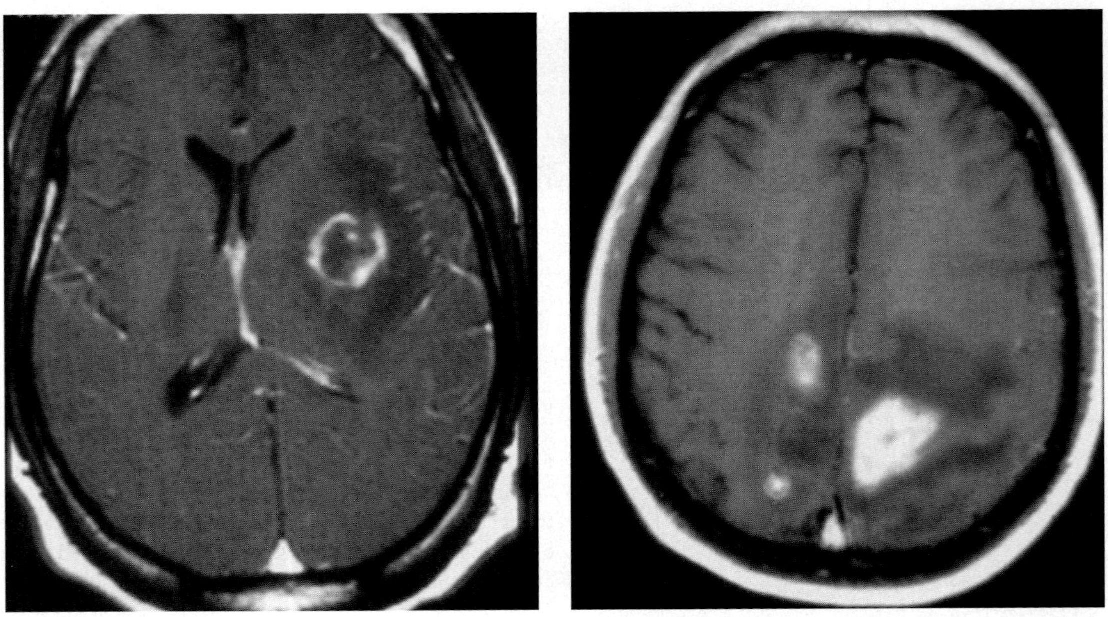

A B

Figure 11.15 *Toxoplasmosis. A.* In a patient with acquired immunodeficiency syndrome (AIDS), axial postcontrast T1-weighted image shows a nonspecific-appearing, ring-enhancing lesion in the left basal ganglia. *B.* In a different patient with AIDS, axial postcontrast T1-weighted image shows nonspecific, solid-enhancing lesions in the parietal lobes.

Table 11.8: *Different Features of Toxoplasmosis Versus Lymphoma*

Disease	*T1 Images*	*T2 Images*	*Contrast*	*DWI*	*Perfusion*	*Radionculide Studies (Thallium SPECT and FDG PET)*	*Proton MRS (Long and Short TE)*
Toxoplasmosis	Low signal	High signal	Ring enhancement	Bright	Relatively low	Relatively low uptake	Moderately high Cho, low NAA, high myoinositol
Lymphoma	Low signal	Isointense to hypointense	Ring enhancement	Dark or slightly bright	Relatively high	Relatively high uptake	High Cho, low NAA, low myoinositol

DWI, diffusion-weighted imaging; SPECT, single-photon emission computed tomography; FDG, fluorodeoxyglucose; PET, positron emission tomography; MRS, magnetic resonance spectroscopy; TE, echo time; Cho, choline; NAA, *N*-acetyl aspartate.

times, but a multimodality approach usually results in adequate characterization of a lesion in most patients.

Syphilis

This sexually transmitted disorder is caused by *Treponema pallidum*, and its incidence has increased recently, particularly in patients with AIDS (48). Most patients show a positive fluorescent treponemal absorption test result in the CSF. The disease occurs in three stages (Table 11.9).

Most patients with syphilis are imaged during the tertiary stage. The meninges are chronically inflamed and become thick, particularly at the base of the skull (49). Hydrocephalus and enhancement of the cranial nerves are not uncommon. The inflammatory process attacks the inner aspect of the blood vessels (Heubner's arteritis), leading to thrombosis and infarctions. This tends to involve the large arteries at the base of the skull, especially the basilar artery. Medium-sized arteries also may be affected. Cerebral gummas present as nonspecific-appearing, ring-enhancing lesions. Tabes dorsalis is characterized by degeneration of the dorsal root ganglia and wallerian degeneration of the posterior spinal cord columns, but has no obvious imaging findings. Rarely, findings compatible with a transverse myelitis (focal nonspecific areas of high T2 signal intensity) may be seen in the spinal cord. Congenital syphilis is very rare, and may occur at any time during pregnancy. Affected children are deaf and develop an interstitial keratitis, chorioretinitis, and hydrocephalus (50).

Table 11.9: *Clinical Stages of Syphilis*

Stages	*Clinical Findings*
Primary (early weeks)	Skin manifestations (local rash, primary chancre)
Secondary (weeks to months after latency period)	Maculopapular, vesicular, and bullous rash in skin and membranes that is highly contagious, meningitis, cranial neuropathies
Tertiary (develops in 10% of patients years after the first stages)	Meningovascular disease, parenchymal disease, congenital syphilis

Table 11.10: Clinical Stages of Lyme Borreliosis

Stage	Symptoms
First	Skin rash and general malaise
Second	Carditis, arthritis, meningitis, neuritis
Third	Chronic skin changes, arthritis, central nervous system symptoms (dementia, spasticity)

Lyme Disease

Cerebral Lyme disease is uncommon, and the lesions it produces are indistinguishable from multiple sclerosis, sarcoidosis, and vasculitis on imaging studies.

Lyme disease is a systemic disorder caused by the spirochete *Borrelia burgdorferi* (51). Only a small percentage of patients with Lyme disease have symptoms referable to the CNS. The disease is more common in the New England region of the United States and usually is transmitted by ticks. It is the most common tick-borne disease. The disease is characterized by the stages shown in Table 11.10 (51).

Most patients are imaged during the second and third stages of the disease. Unfortunately, there is a significant overlap among the different stages of the disease. CNS manifestations develop in only approximately 10% of patients infected. These patients all show lymphocytic meningitis. Most of the patients show areas of high T2 signal intensity in the white matter, reminiscent of those seen in multiple sclerosis (51). The lesions may enhance and occasionally affect the deep gray matter structures. Cerebral atrophy develops in the chronic stage of the disease. In many patients, an atypical facial nerve palsy (prolonged or bilateral) also develops. In these patients, the intracanalicular portion of the facial nerve(s) or the geniculate ganglion may enhance. Enhancement of the brain at the root entry zone of the facial nerves also occasionally is seen.

Creutzfeldt-Jakob Disease

If CJD is suspected, it is very important to inform the neurosurgeon performing the biopsy and the neuropathologist examining the specimen, because special handling of all instruments and the specimen is required owing to the inherent resistance and infectivity of prions.

Creutzfeldt-Jakob disease (CJD) is a rare disorder resulting in a "spongiform" degeneration of the brain (52). It is presumed to be caused by a prion (Table 11.11).

Prions are particles lacking DNA that are slow growing, resistant to inactivation by conventional methods (e.g., sterilization), and do not evoke an immune response. The following groups have a higher incidence of this very rare disorder: Libyan Jews, Slovakians, patients receiving human growth hormone, corneal transplant recipients, patients who have had cerebral electrodes implanted, meat handlers and butchers, patients after neurosurgery, and those with first-degree relatives who have had CJD. Patients usually are 40 to 80 years of age and develop a rapidly progressive dementia that leads to death in nearly all within 1 year. The histologic features are confined mostly to the gray matter and consist of neuronal loss and vacuolation (spongiform changes), gliosis, and a lack of inflammation. Imaging studies are negative or show only atrophy (particularly affecting the gray matter) in most patients. Increased T2 signal intensity in the cortex (particularly in the

Table 11.11: Disorders Caused by Prions

Disorder	Species
Creutzfeldt-Jakob disease	Humans
Gerstmann-Straussler syndrome	Humans
Kuru	Humans
Scrapie	Sheeps and goats
Mad cow disease	Bovines

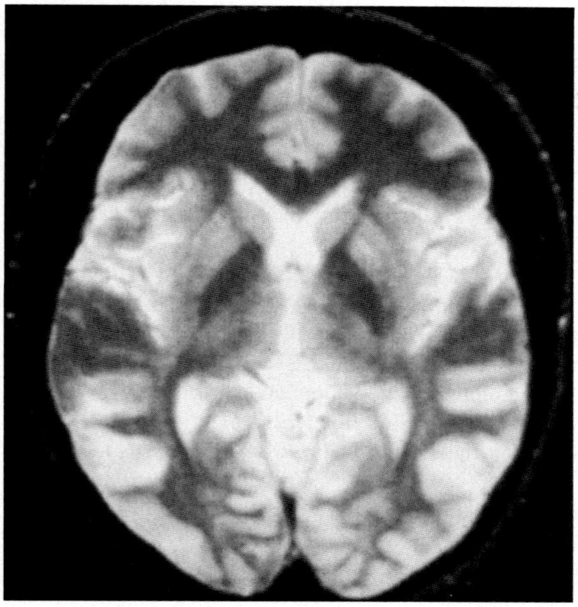

Figure 11.16 *Creutzfeldt-Jakob Disease.* Axial T2-weighted image shows high signal intensity in the cortex of the temporal and occipital lobes as well as the striatum and perhaps the thalami. (Case courtesy of T.P. Naidich, New York, NY.)

occipital lobes), thalami, and basal ganglia is typical (52,53) (Fig. 11.16). There is no contrast enhancement. The lesions usually are symmetric and accompanied by generalized atrophy (54). DWI may show the abnormalities earlier to a better advantage than conventional MRI.

SARCOIDOSIS

Sarcoidosis affects the CNS in only 5% of patients with the systemic form of the disease (55). CNS involvement usually occurs within 1 year of the diagnosis. Neurosarcoidosis may be monophasic or become a chronic, relapsing disease with symptoms that range from mild to severe, including death. Steroids are the treatment of choice, and most patients respond favorably to them (56). Nearly all patients complain of headaches, and cranial nerve palsies are found in 50% to 75% of patients. The most commonly affected cranial nerve is the facial (55). Neurosarcoidosis also may involve any part of the brain and spinal cord, as well as the meninges (Fig. 11.17). The globe, sclera, optic nerve, and lacrimal gland also commonly are affected (57). Meningeal disease is found in 20% of patients with neurosarcoidosis, and some degree of hydrocephalus is seen in 15% (58). When meningeal contrast enhancement occurs, it mostly involves the basilar cisterns, particularly the suprasellar one (Fig. 11.17A, C–E). The leptomeninges become thick and nodular and show marked contrast enhancement (59) (Fig. 11.17E). The disease may spread into the brain through the perivascular spaces. Many patients show areas of increased T2 signal intensity in the brain (affecting both gray and white matter) adjacent to the sites of the abnormal meninges. This is presumed to represent edema, probably secondary to compression of the draining veins. Rarely, the meningeal disease may appear identical to meningiomas. The disease along the perivascular spaces also enhances, but most of the areas of increased T2 signal do not. However, formation of enhancing intraaxial granulomas also may occur. Most granulomas are found in the areas supplied by perforating arterioles (basal ganglia, midbrain, and periventricular white matter). The granulomas enhance but otherwise have a nonspecific appearance. Granulomas also may involve the spinal cord. At times, the granulomas may appear identical to the lesions of multiple sclerosis. Infiltration of the pituitary gland stalk and the hypothalamus by sarcoidosis may result in hypopituitarism. When the cranial nerves are involved, the peripheries of the nerves and, rarely, the entire nerves enhance after contrast administration.

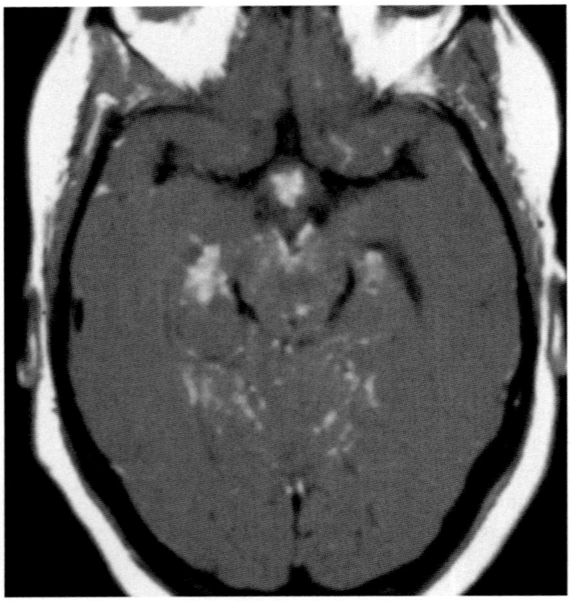

A

Figure 11.17 *Sarcoidosis. A.* Axial postcontrast T1-weighted image shows enhancement in the suprasellar cistern, around the midbrain, in the hippocampi, and on the surface of the cerebellum. *B.* In a different patient, mid-sagittal postcontrast T1-weighted image shows sarcoidosis involving the pituitary gland and along the medial parietal surfaces. *C.* Parasagittal postcontrast T1-weighted image in a different patient shows thick dural and pial enhancement in the frontal region. *D.* Coronal postcontrast T1-weighted image (different patient) shows enhancement in the suprasellar region, sylvian cisterns, and basal ganglia along the perivascular spaces. *E.* In a different patient, sagittal postcontrast T1-weighted image shows "plaquelike" sarcoidosis in the sella, clivus, foramen magnum, and upper cervical spinal canal.

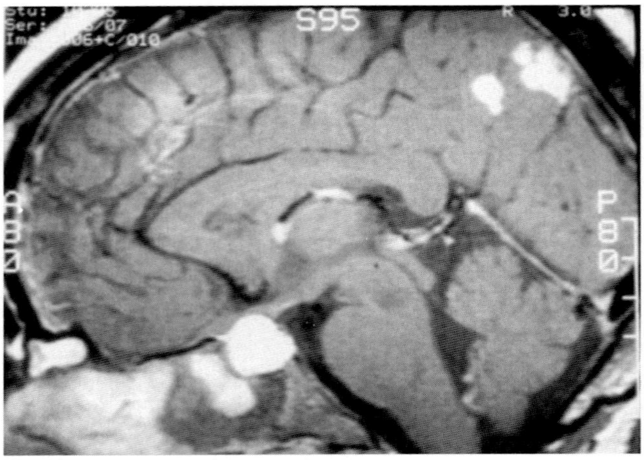

B

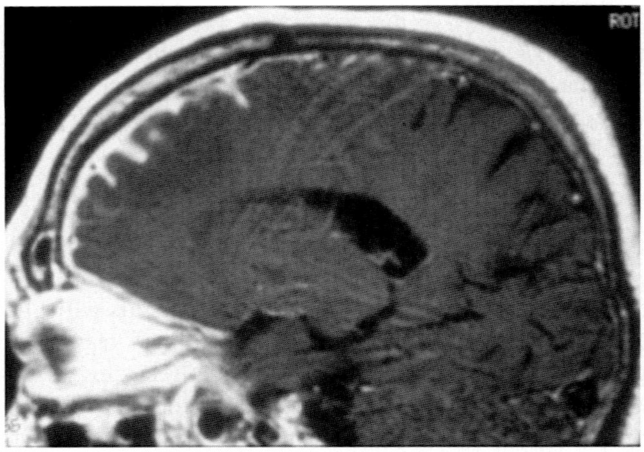

C

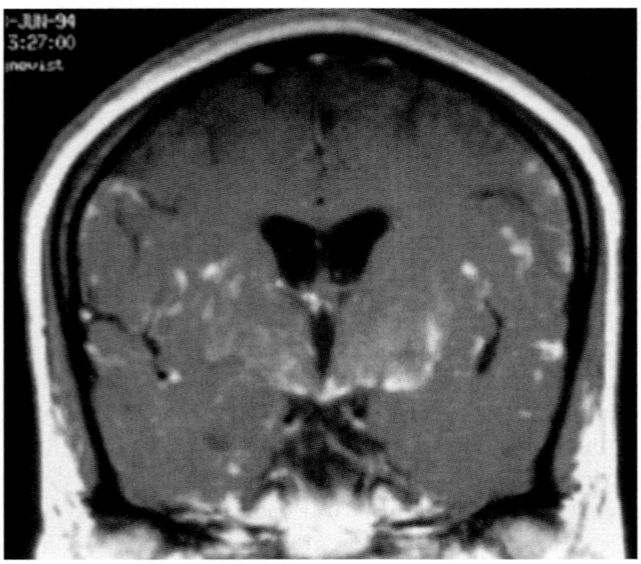

D

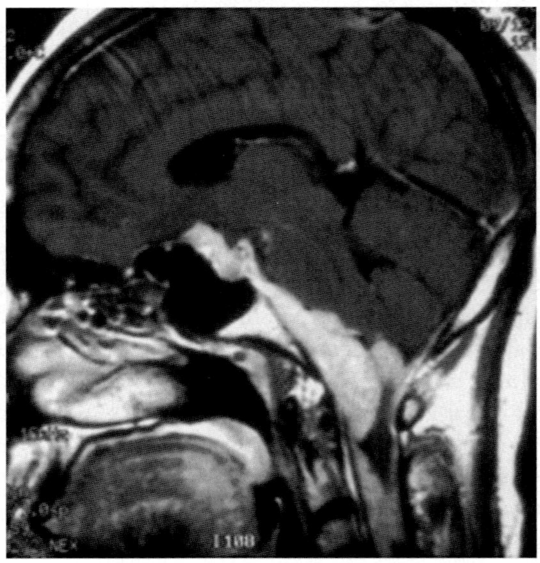

E

TUBERCULOSIS

Tuberculosis is a common disease worldwide, and its incidence is increasing because of a change in immigration patterns, AIDS, and the development of medically resistant strains. Most infections are caused by *Mycobacterium tuberculosis*, and atypical organisms (*Mycobacterium avium-intracellulare, Mycobacterium bovis*) usually are found in immunosuppressed patients (60). The most common manifestation of neurotuberculosis is meningitis followed by intraaxial lesions. The CNS becomes infected through hematogenous dissemination during the primary stage of the disease. Granulomas lodge in the brain and the meninges and produce meningitis when they rupture. The clinical symptoms are identical to those seen in bacterial meningitis, but the CSF shows lymphocytosis, increased proteins, and low glucose. Pathologically, there are thick, gelatinous exudates, particularly in the basal and sylvian cisterns. Hydrocephalus is common. CT shows that the cisterns are isodense or hyperdense with respect to the brain (61) (Fig. 11.18A). MRI shows increased signal intensity of the CSF on T1-weighted images and particularly on FLAIR images (62). There is prominent subarachnoid space enhancement after contrast administration (Fig.

Tuberculosis results in thick, regional subarachnoid and cisternal contrast-enhancing exudates on CT images. Sarcoidosis, metastases, lymphoma, and leukemia need to be included in the differential diagnosis.

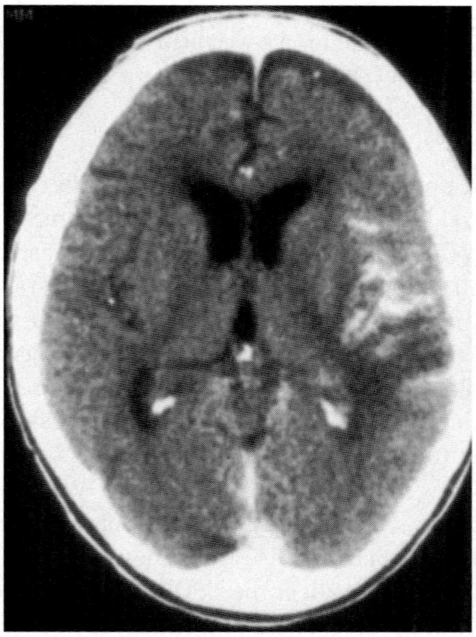
A

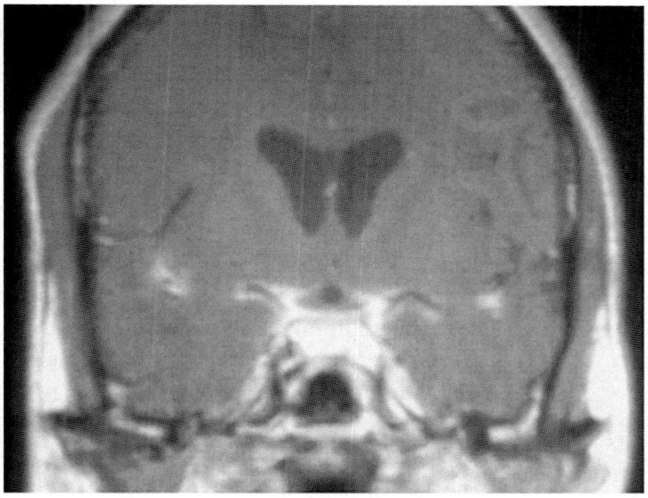
B

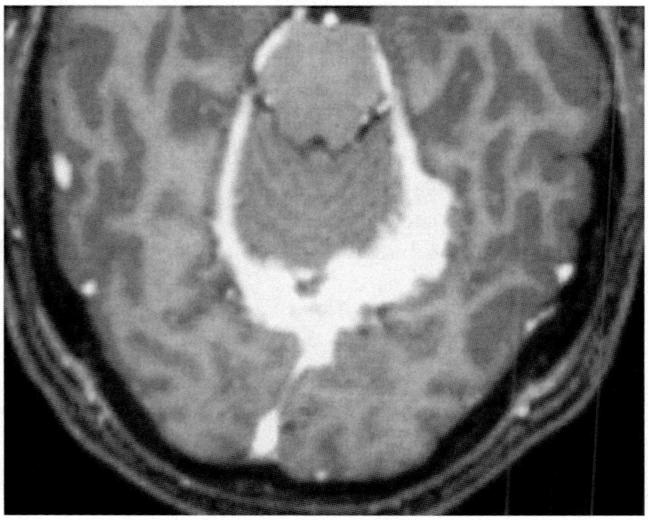
C

Figure 11.18 *Tuberculosis. A.* Axial postcontrast computed tomography shows thick pial enhancement in the left sylvian fissure. *B.* Coronal postcontrast T1-weighted image shows enhancement in the suprasellar and sylvian cisterns. *C.* Axial postcontrast T1-weighted image in a different patient shows plaquelike tuberculous involvement of the tentorium.

(continued on next page)

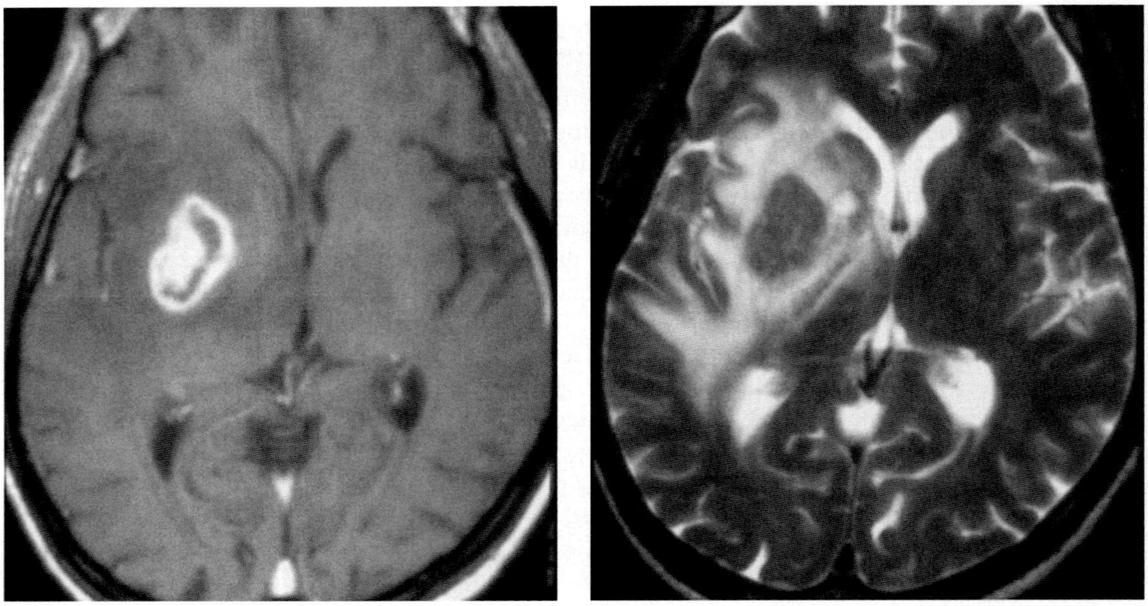

Figure 11.18 (continued) *D.* Axial postcontrast T1-weighted image shows enhancing tuberculoma (nonspecific appearance) in the right basal ganglia. *E.* Corresponding T2-weighted image shows that the tuberculoma is of low signal intensity and has significant surrounding edema.

11.18B). Occasionally, the dura may be affected predominantly (Fig. 11.18C). After treatment, calcification of the intraaxial and extraaxial lesions may occur. Similar findings may be seen inside the spinal canal, and syringomyelia may be a complication of intraspinal tuberculosis. When seizures develop in a patient known to have tuberculosis, intracranial tuberculomas become a diagnostic consideration. Tuberculomas may be solitary, but they usually are multiple. Tuberculomas are basically indistinguishable from pyogenic abscesses, but tuberculomas tend to have a slightly thicker and more nodular rim. The presence of peripheral or central ("target sign") calcifications is typical of tuberculosis. On MRI, tuberculomas may show somewhat low central T2 signal intensity, whereas pyogenic abscess are centrally bright most of the time (Fig. 11.18D and E). On trace DWI, many tuberculomas also show central low signal intensity. Occasionally, a true tubercular brain abscess may form, and these are larger than tuberculomas but also indistinguishable from abscesses of other etiologies by imaging. Tuberculosis may affect the skull. Calvarial tuberculosis is rare in the United States, but common in Latin America and India (63). It tends to affect children more often. The lesion may affect only a part of the skull, or both tables and marrow space. In calvarial tuberculosis, the underlying meninges are thick and an enhancing soft tissue mass may be present in the scalp. Some lesions are sclerotic, whereas others are lytic. Tuberculosis also may affect the middle ear and temporal bone (otomastoiditis). These patients present with what initially is mistaken for repeated bouts of bacterial middle ear infection. Unrecognized tuberculosis otomastoiditis often leads to complete and permanent hearing loss as well as facial nerve paralysis. The imaging findings are nonspecific, showing an enhancing and destructive mass involving the temporal bone. A definite diagnosis is reached by performing a biopsy. Tuberculous otomastoiditis also may result in thrombosis of the sigmoid sinus.

References

1. Sze G. Diseases of the intracranial meninges: MR imaging features. AJR Am J Roentgenol 1993; 160:727–733.
2. Castillo M. Magnetic resonance imaging of meningitis and its complications. Topics Magn Reson Imaging 1994;6:53–58.

3. Chang KH, Han MH, Roh JK, et al. Gd-DTPA-enhanced MR imaging of the brain in patients with meningitis: comparison with CT. AJNR Am J Neuroradiol 1990;11:69–76.
4. Zimmerman R, Leeds N, Danziger A. Subdural empyema: CT findings. Radiology 1984;150: 417–422.
5. Enzmann DR, Britt RR, Obana WG, et al. Experimental *Staphylococcus aureus* brain abscess. AJNR Am J Neuroradiol 1986;7:395–402.
6. Desprechins B, Stadnik T, Koerts G, et al. Use of diffusion-weighted MR imaging in differential diagnosis between intracerebral necrotic tumors and cerebral abscesses. AJNR Am J Neuroradiol 1999;20:1252–1257.
7. Castillo M. Brain infections in human immunodeficiency virus positive patients. Topics Magn Reson Imaging 1994;6:3–10.
8. Broderick D, Wippold F, Clifford D, et al. White matter lesions and cerebral atrophy on MR images in patients with and without AIDS dementia complex. AJR Am J Roentgenol 1993;161: 177–181.
9. Olsen W, Longo F, Mills C, et al. White matter disease in AIDS: findings at MR imaging. Radiology 1988;169:445–448.
10. Jensen M, Brant-Zawadzki M. MR imaging of the brain in patients with AIDS: value of routine use of IV gadopentetate dimeglumine. AJR Am J Roentgenol 1993;160:153–157.
11. Chrysikopoulos H, Press G, Grafe M, et al. Encephalitis caused by human immunodeficiency virus: CT and MR imaging manifestations with clinical and pathologic correlation. Radiology 1990;175:185–191.
12. Post M, Berger J, Quencer R. Asymptomatic and neurologically symptomatic HIV-seropositive individuals: prospective evaluation with cranial MR imaging. Radiology 1991;178:131–139.
13. Chong WK, Paley M, Wilkinson ID, et al. Localized cerebral proton MR spectroscopy in HIV infection and AIDS. AJNR Am J Neuroradiol 1994;15:21–25.
14. Meyerhoff DJ, Weiner MW, Fein G. Deep gray matter structures in HIV infection: a proton MR spectroscopic study. AJNR Am J Neuroradiol 1996;17:973–978.
15. Mark A, Atlas S. Progressive multifocal leukoencephalopathy in patients with AIDS: appearance on MR images. Radiology 1989;173:517–520.
16. Ernst T, Chang L, Witt M, et al. Progressive multifocal leukoencephalopathy and human immunodeficiency virus-associated white matter lesions in AIDS: magnetization transfer MR imaging. Radiology 1999;210:539–543.
17. Whiteman M, Post M, Berger J, et al. Progressive multifocal leukoencephalopathy in 47 HIV-seropositive patients: neuroimaging with clinical and pathologic correlation. Radiology 1993; 187:233–240.
18. Wheeler A, Truwit C, Kleinschmidt-DeMasters B, et al. Progressive multifocal leukoencephalopathy: contrast enhancement on CT scans and MR images. AJR Am J Roentgenol 1993;161:1049–1051.
19. Garrels K, Kucharczyk W, Wortzman G, et al. Progressive multifocal leukoencephalopathy: clinical and MR response to treatment. AJNR Am J Neuroradiol 1996;17:597–600.
20. Buff B, Mathews V, Elster A. Bacterial and viral parenchymal infections of the brain. Topics Magn Reson Imaging 1994;6:11–21.
21. Cecil K, Lenkinski R. Proton MR spectroscopy in inflammatory and infectious brain disorders. Neuroimaging Clin North Am 1998;8:863–880.
22. Herman TE, Cleveland RH, Kushner DC, et al. CT of neonatal herpes encephalitis. AJNR Am J Neuroradiol 1985;6:773–775.
23. Geller E, Faerber EN, Legido A, et al. Rasmussen encephalitis: complementary role of multitechnique neuroimaging. AJNR Am J Neuroradiol 1998;19:445–449.
24. Tien RD, Chu PK, Hesselink JR, et al. Intracranial cryptococcosis in immunocompromised patients: CT and MR findings in 29 cases. AJNR Am J Neuroradiol 1991;12:283–289.
25. Mathews VP, Alo PL, Glass JD, et al. AIDS-related CNS cryptococcosis: radiologic-pathologic correlation. AJNR Am J Neuroradiol 1992;13:1477–1486.
26. Arnder L, Castillo M, Heinz ER, et al. Unusual pattern of enhancement in cryptococcal meningitis: in vivo findings with postmortem correlation. J Comput Assist Tomogr 1996;20: 1023–1026.
27. Caldemeyer KS, Mathews WP, Edwards-Brown MK, et al. Central nervous system cryptococcosis: parenchymal calcification and large gelatinous pseudocysts. AJNR Am J Neuroradiol 1997; 18:107–109.
28. Vender JR, Miller DM, Roth T, et al. Intraventricular cryptococcal cysts. AJNR Am J Neuroradiol 1996;17:110–113.

29. Ostrow T, Hudgins P. Magnetic resonance imaging of intracranial fungal infections. Topics Magn Reson Imaging 1994;6:22–31.
30. Cox J, Murtagh FR, Wilfong A, et al. Cerebral aspergillosis: MR imaging and histopathologic correlation. AJNR Am J Neuroradiol 1992;13:1489–1492.
31. DeLone D, Goldstein R, Petermann G, et al. Disseminated aspergillosis involving the brain: distribution and imaging characteristics. AJNR Am J Neuroradiol 1999;20:1597–1604.
32. Fellows DW, King VD, Conturo T, et al. In vitro evaluation of MR hypointensity in *Aspergillus* colonies. AJNR Am J Neuroradiol 1994;15:1139–1144.
33. McLean FM, Ginsberg LE, Stanton CA. Perineural spread of rhinocerebral mucormycosis. AJNR Am J Neuroradiol 1996;17:114–116.
34. Chan L, Singh S, Jones D, et al. Imaging of mucormycosis skull base osteomyelitis. AJNR Am J Neuroradiol 2000;21:828–831.
35. Ginsberg F, Peyster RG, Hoover ED, et al. Isolated cerebral mucormycosis: case report with CT and pathologic correlation. AJNR Am J Neuroradiol 1987;8:558–560.
36. Wrobel CJ, Meyer S, Johnson RH, et al. MR findings in acute and chronic coccidioidomycosis meningitis. AJNR Am J Neuroradiol 1992;13:1241–1245.
37. Erly W, Bellon R, Seeger J, et al. MR imaging of acute coccidioidal meningitis. AJNR Am J Neuroradiol 1999;20:509–514.
38. Angtuaco EE, Angtuaco EJ, Glasier CM, et al. Nasopharyngeal and temporal bone blastomycosis: CT and MR findings. AJNR Am J Neuroradiol 1991;12:725–728.
39. Zalduondo F, Provenzale J, Hulette C, et al. Meningitis, vasculitis, and cerebritis caused by CNS histoplasmosis: radiologic-pathologic correlation. AJR Am J Roentgenol 1996;166:194–196.
40. Desai SP, Bazan C, Hummell W, et al. Disseminated CNS histoplasmosis. AJNR Am J Neuroradiol 1991;12:290–292.
41. Lai PH, Lin SM, Pan HB, et al. Disseminated military cerebral candidiasis. AJNR Am J Neuroradiol 1997;18:1303–1306.
42. Creasy J, Alarcon J. Magnetic resonance imaging of neurocysticercosis. Topics Magn Reson Imaging 1994;6:59–68.
43. Nourjaim SE, Rossi MD, Rao SK, et al. CT and MR imaging of neurocysticercosis. AJR Am J Roentgenol 1999;173:1485–1490.
44. Kramer L, Locke G, Byrd S, et al. Cerebral cysticercosis: documentation of natural history with CT. Radiology 1989;171:459–462.
45. Ginier BL, Poirier VC. MR imaging of intraventricular cysticercosis. AJNR Am J Neuroradiol 1992;13:1247–1248.
46. Tsuchiya K, Inaoka S, Mizutani Y, et al. Fast fluid-attenuated inversion-recovery MR of intracranial infections. AJNR Am J Neuroradiol 1997;18:909–913.
47. Ruiz A, Ganz WI, Post MJ, et al. Use of thallium-201 brain SPECT to differentiate cerebral lymphoma from toxoplasma encephalitis in AIDS patients. AJNR Am J Neuroradiol 1994;15: 1885–1894.
48. Brightbill TC, Ihmeidan IH, Post MJ, et al. Neurosyphilis in HIV-positive and HIV-negative patients: neuroimaging findings. AJNR Am J Neuroradiol 1995;16:703–711.
49. Holland B, Perrett L, Mills C. Meningovascular syphilis: CT and MR findings. Radiology 1986; 158:439–442.
50. Smith M, Anderson J. Neurosyphilis as a cause of facial and vestibulocochlear nerve dysfunction: MR imaging features. AJNR Am J Neuroradiol 2000;21:1673–1675.
51. Fernandez RE, Rothberg M, Ferencz G, et al. Lyme disease of the CNS: MR imaging findings in 14 cases. AJNR Am J Neuroradiol 1990;11:479–481.
52. Finkenstaedt M, Szudra A, Zerr I, et al. MR imaging of Creutzfeldt-Jakob disease. Radiology 1996;199:793–798.
53. Barboriak D, Provenzale J, Boyko O. MR diagnosis of Creutzfeldt-Jakob disease: significance of high signal intensity of the basal ganglia. AJR Am J Roentgenol 1994;162:137–140.
54. Falcone S, Quencer RM, Bowen B, et al. Creutzfeldt-Jakob disease: focal symmetrical cortical involvement demonstrated by MR imaging. AJNR Am J Neuroradiol 1992: 13:403–406.
55. Wilson J, Castillo M. Magnetic resonance imaging of granulomatous inflammations: sarcoidosis and tuberculosis. Topics Magn Reson Imaging 1994;6:32–40.
56. Lexa FJ, Grossman RI. MR of sarcoidosis in the head and spine: spectrum of manifestations and radiographic response to steroid therapy. AJNR Am J Neuroradiol 1994;15:973–982.
57. Simon EM, Zoarski GH, Rothman MI, et al. Systemic sarcoidosis with bilateral orbital involvement: MR findings. AJNR Am J Neuroradiol 1998;19:336–337.
58. Christoforidis G, Spickler EM, Recio MV, et al. MR of CNS sarcoidosis: correlation of imaging

features to clinical symptoms and response to treatment. AJNR Am J Neuroradiol 1999;20: 655–669.

59. Seltzer S, Mark AS, Atlas SW. CNS sarcoidosis: evaluation with contrast-enhances MR imaging. AJNR Am J Neuroradiol 1991;12:1227–1233.
60. Dastur D, Manghani D, Udani P. Pathology and pathogenetic mechanisms in neurotuberculosis. Radiol Clin North Am 1995;33:733–752.
61. Castro C, Barros N, Campos Z, et al. CT scans of cranial tuberculosis. Radiol Clin North Am 1995;33:753–769.
62. Jinkins J, Gupta R, Chang K, et al. MR imaging of central nervous system tuberculosis. Radiol Clin North Am 1995;33:771–786.
63. Patankar T, Varma R, Krishnan A, et al. Radiographic findings in tuberculosis of the calvarium. Neuroradiology 2000;42:518–521.

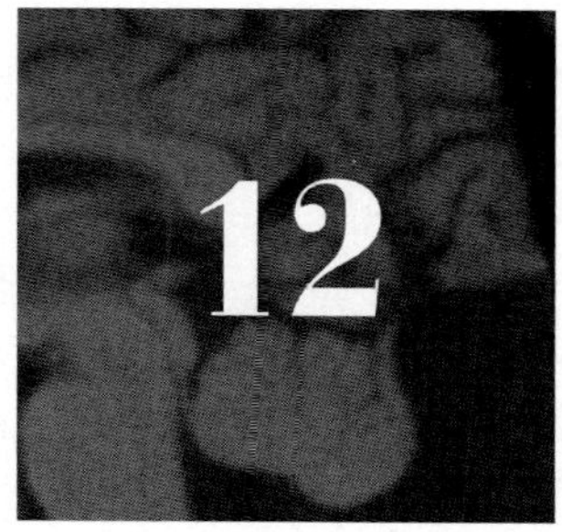

Effects of Therapy

- Irradiation and Its Effects
- Effects of Immunosuppressive Medications
- Effects of Chemotherapy Agents
- Graft-versus-Host Disease and Posttransplantation Lymphoproliferative Disorder
- Neoplasias Secondary to Transplantation Procedures
- Effects of Anticonvulsant Medications
- Effects of Total Parenteral Nutrition

Irradiation and Its Effects

Radiation injury to the brain is dose dependent. Doses higher than 70 Gy usually result in frank and acute necrosis. Doses between 50 and 70 Gy give rise to partial tissue necrosis. Overall, postirradiation changes manifest with doses above 24 Gy (1). The effects of radiation to the brain are augmented when a patient is receiving intrathecal or systemic chemotherapy as well. Children younger than 5 years of age are prone to development of brain complications, and radiation usually is avoided (if possible) until 7 to 8 years of age. The very young and girls are especially sensitive to irradiation because their brains experience the fastest and earliest growth (Fig. 12.1). The spinal cord is more sensitive to radiation than the brain. In addition, acute necrosis may develop quickly in patients undergoing stereotactic radiosurgery (Fig. 12.2). Histologically, radiation induces demyelination and occlusion of blood vessels. The effects of radiation on the brain may be divided into three types of reactions (2) (Table 12.1).

The effects of irradiation on the brain are more severe in very young children and girls, in whom the brain is experiencing fast growth.

A common sequela of brain irradiation is leukoencephalopathy. In patients with leukoencephalopathy, magnetic resonance imaging (MRI) shows increased T2 signal intensity [and hypodensity on computed tomography (CT)] that may be seen as early as 2 to 3 months after the radiation (Fig. 12.3). The abnormalities involve the deep and superficial (u-fibers) white matter. Brain atrophy is present and progressive, and there is no enhancement after contrast administration. Proton MR spectroscopy shows decreased metabolites, particularly the *N*-acetyl aspartate (NAA) peak, and the presence of a broad peak centered at 1.2 parts per million (ppm) that is thought to represent a combination of lactate and lipids due to cellular breakdown (3) (Fig. 12.2C). Remyelination and reversal of the vascular changes may occur, but the atrophy is permanent. A variation of this disease is progressive necrotizing leukoencephalopathy, an acute disorder that manifests a few weeks after the treatment. It is found almost exclusively in children. The clinical presentation is one of dementia, ataxia, and dysarthria rapidly progressing to spasticity, seizures, and coma. The brain shows acute reactive astrocytosis and demyelination. The imaging findings are those of diffuse and rapidly progressive increased T2 signal intensity in the white matter, initially affecting the u-fibers. The ventricles may be prominent.

To be considered radiation induced, a tumor needs to be of different histologic type than the original one, arise within the radiation field, and present several years (usually 10 years) after the therapy.

Acute and late radiation-induced necrosis appears identical to a tumor by conventional imaging (CT and MRI) (4). The lesion presents as an irregularly enhancing mass with central necrosis, surrounding edema, and considerable mass effect (Fig. 12.4). Unfortunately, in many cases in which the initial irradiation was given for a brain tumor, residual viable tumor is mixed with radiation necrosis. Because the brain is unable to remove detritus, radiation necrosis may need to be excised. Fortunately, once this is done, the prognosis for these

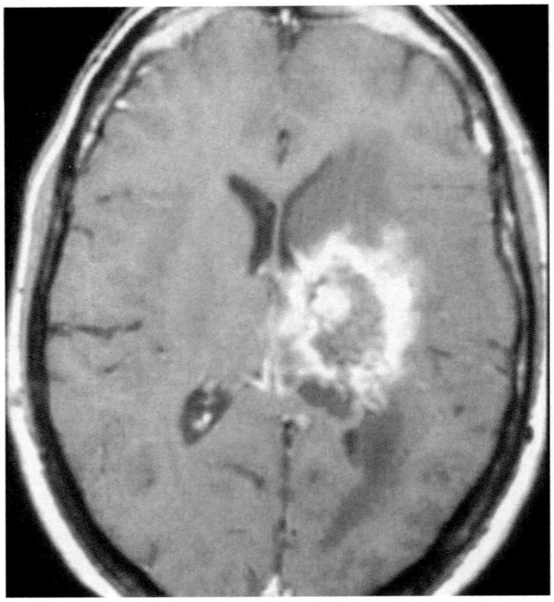

Figure 12.1 *Radiation- and Chemotherapy-Induced Necrosis after Treatment for Thalamic Astrocytoma.* Axial postcontrast T1-weighted image shows irregular enhancing mass in the left thalamus. There is mass effect and edema, and the lesion is indistinguishable from a primary malignant tumor.

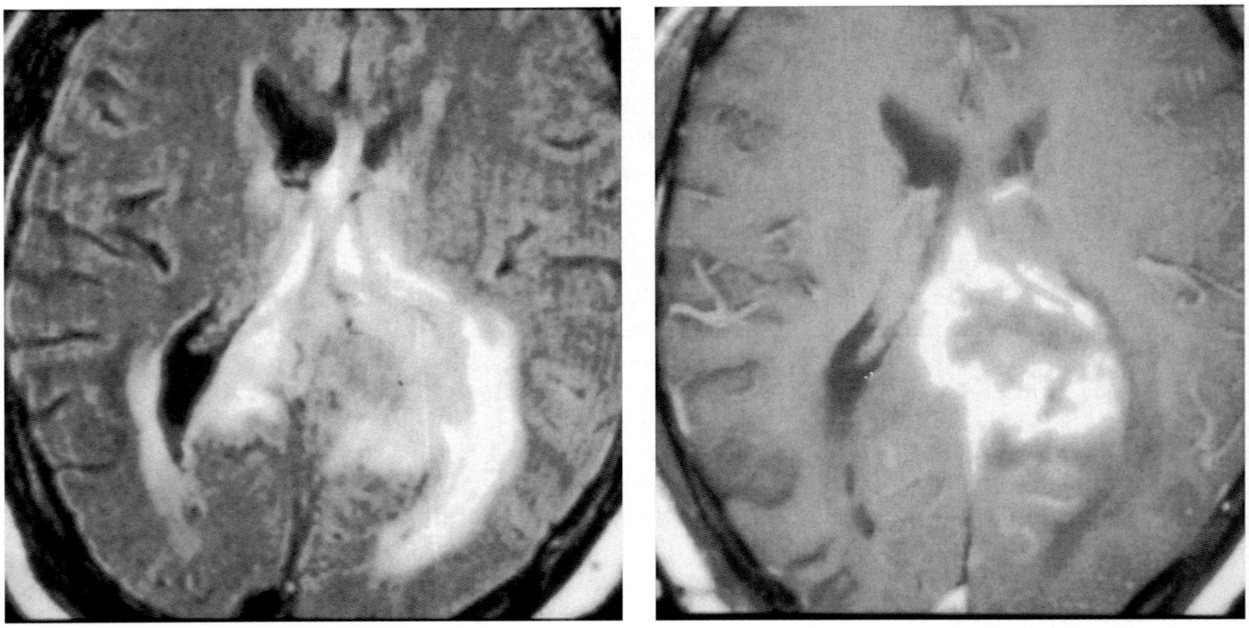

A B

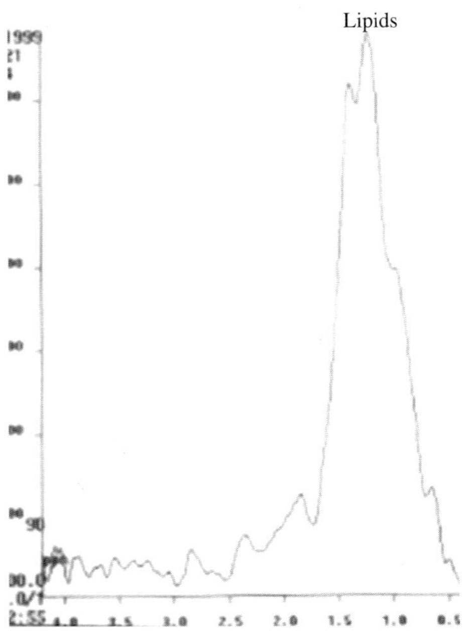

C

Figure 12.2 *Necrosis Induced by Stereotactic Radiosurgery. A.* Axial fluid attenuation inversion recovery (FLAIR) image shows large lesion with surrounding edema involving the posterior callosum. This occurred only 1 month after treatment of a recurrent pineal gland region meningioma. *B.* Corresponding postcontrast T1-weighted image shows irregular enhancement. *C.* In a different patient after treatment of a metastasis, proton magnetic resonance spectroscopy shows resonances only of macrolipids and lactate, and no choline to suggest tumor.

Table 12.1: Effects of Radiation on the Brain

Type of Reaction	*Pathology*
Acute	Edema and, rarely, acute necrosis
Early delayed (a few weeks after treatment)	Damage to neurons and axons, vascular hyalinization, no frank necrosis
Late delayed (years after treatment)	Coagulative necrosis, blood vessel hyalinization, perivascular fibrosis, gliosis

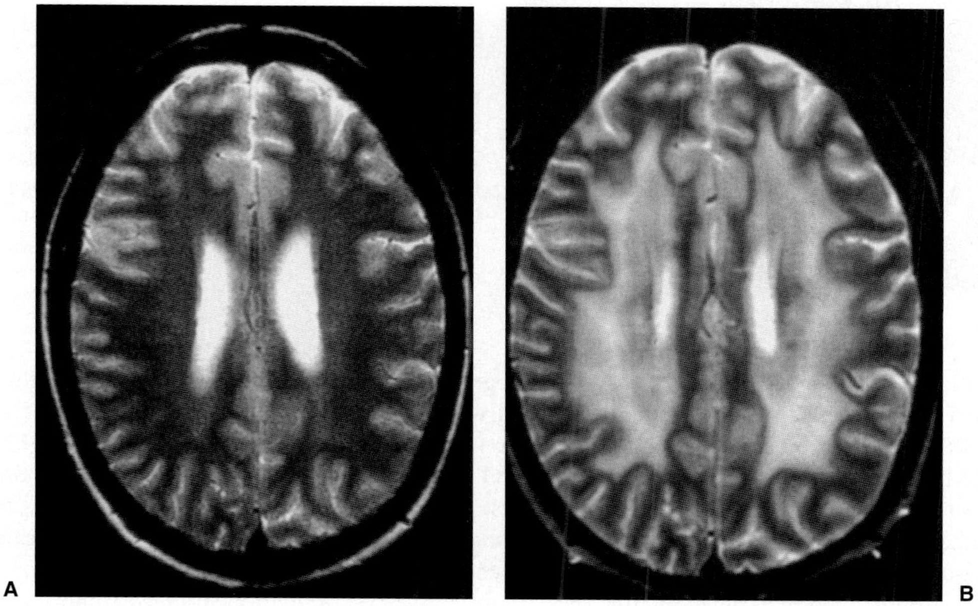

Figure 12.3 *Radiation-Induced Leukoencephalopathy. A.* Axial T2-weighted image in a patient with leptomeningeal lymphoma before whole-brain radiation shows no abnormality. *B.* Corresponding image 1 year after treatment shows diffuse white matter hyperintensity.

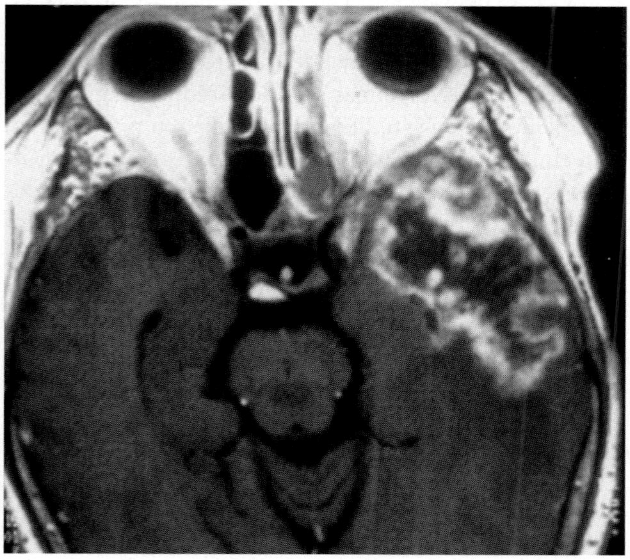

Figure 12.4 *Late Radiation-Induced Necrosis.* Axial postcontrast T1-weighted image in a patient treated for a left temporal lobe astrocytoma shows an irregular enhancing lesion in the tumor bed.

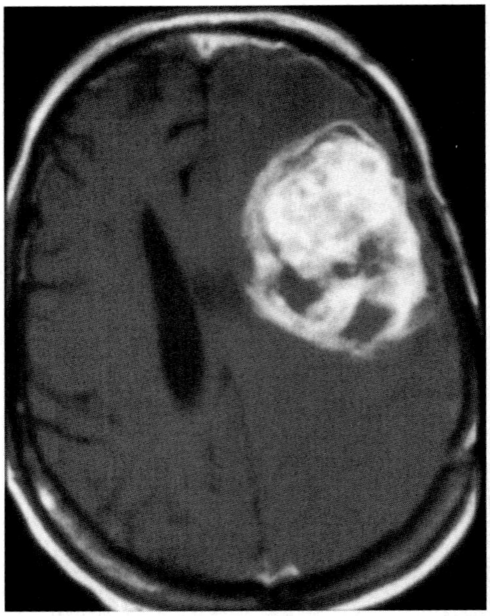

Figure 12.5 *Radiation-Induced Brain Tumor.* Axial postcontrast T1-weighted image obtained 20 years after treatment for a left frontal anaplastic astrocytoma shows a large mass with irregular but prominent contrast enhancement, surrounding edema, and mass effect. The mass was a osteosarcoma.

patients is favorable. Positron emission tomography shows low uptake of fluorodeoxyglucose in areas of radiation necrosis compared with tumor (5). Single-photon emission CT (SPECT) may show low uptake of thallium in radiation necrosis compared with tumor (6). MRI perfusion studies show low cerebral blood flow and cerebral blood volume in radiation necrosis relative to the normal cortex, whereas these parameters are high in tumors (7,8). In radiation necrosis, proton MR spectroscopy shows no viable metabolites and a broad peak centered at 1.2 to 1.4 ppm related to the presence of cellular breakdown products (4).

Tumors also may develop after irradiation (Fig. 12.5). Radiation-induced tumors are listed in Table 12.2.

Vascular lesions induced by radiation include arteritis, hemorrhage, and the formation of malformations. Cavernous hemangiomas, capillary telangiectasia, and venous angiomas may form many years after brain irradiation (9,10) (Fig. 12.6). This is seen mostly in younger patients with leukemia who received low doses of radiation. The vascular malformations usually are asymptomatic, but may produce seizures. It is unclear if the malformations arise *de novo* as a result of irradiation or become clinically overt only after the treatment. The imaging features of cavernous hemangiomas and venous angiomas are addressed in Chapter 9.

Even in the absence of changes visible by imaging studies, brain irradiation may result in significant abnormalities, particularly in children. These children show neurocognitive impairment, and 45% have a full-scale IQ of less than 90, with many of them requiring special education or institutionalization. These abnormalities may not become obvious until 3 years after the completion of radiation therapy. There are no histologic correlates, and the abnormalities are thought to be due to anomalies of dendritic arborization, axonal growth, and synaptogenesis. Full-brain radiation also may affect the pituitary gland (which in turns affects the thyroid gland), leading to developmental delay (11). Radiation to the spine affects growth by its effects

Table 12.2: Irradiation-Induced Brain Tumors

Type of Tumor	*Incidence*
High-grade astrocytoma	Relatively common
Medulloblastoma and other primitive neuroectodermal tumors	Relatively common
Meningioma	Relatively common
Low-grade astrocytoma	Relatively uncommon
Sarcomas	Relatively uncommon

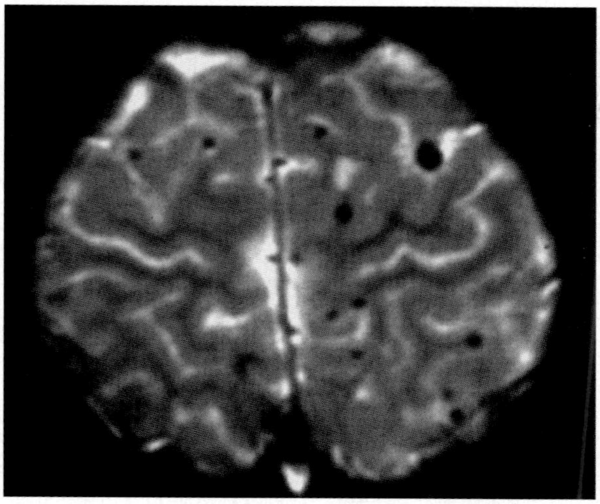

A

Figure 12.6 *Radiation-Induced "Cryptic" Vascular Malformations. A.* Axial T2-weighted image shows many small areas of signal void suggesting either capillary telangiectases or cavernous angiomas. *B.* In a different patient, axial proton density (left) and T2-weighted (right) images show presumed cavernous angiomas after low-dose whole-brain irradiation for leukemia. (Cases courtesy of B. Koch, Cincinnati, OH).

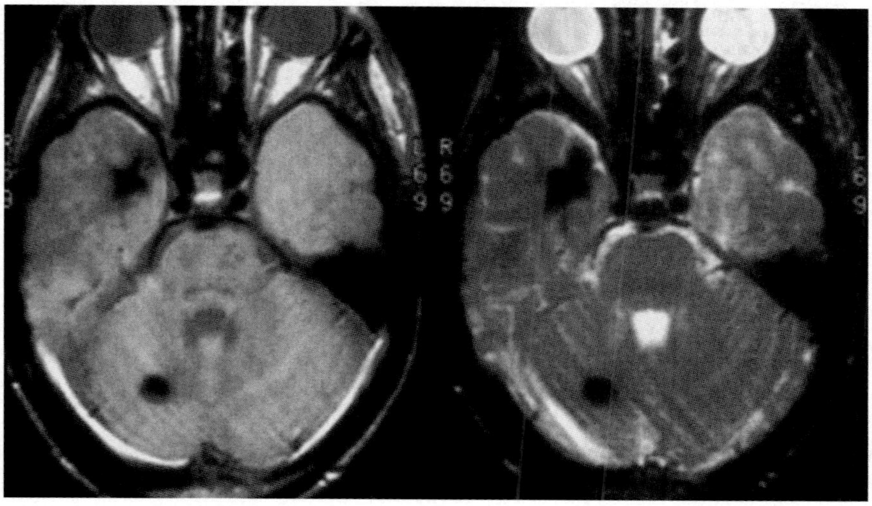

B

on the vertebral endplates. Radiation ports that include the face result in facial hypoplasia and anomalies of the teeth and mandible (12). Intraocular effusions due to radiation-induced retinitis may result in glaucoma and a painful eye and necessitate enucleation (Fig. 12.7). Vision loss also may be due to radiation-induced optic neuritis (13) (Fig. 12.8). Other cranial nerve palsies also may occur after brain irradiation. Shortly after brain radiation, many children become

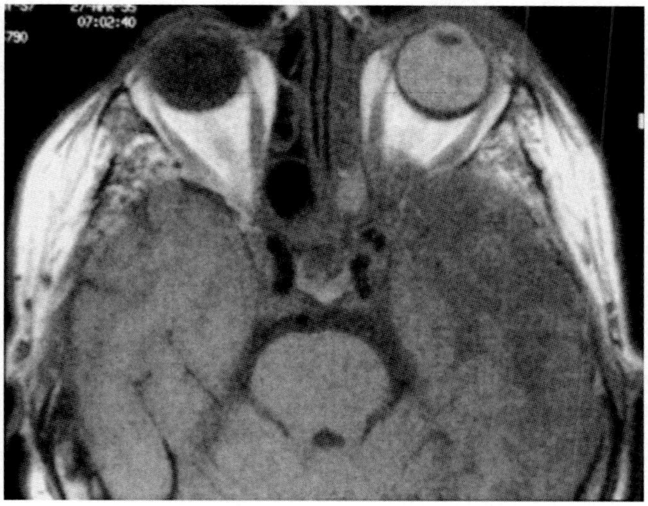

Figure 12.7 *Radiation-Induced Retinopathy.* Axial T1-weighted image obtained 1 year after radiation for a left temporal lobe astrocytoma and development of ipsilateral blindness and pain shows high signal in all chambers of the left globe.

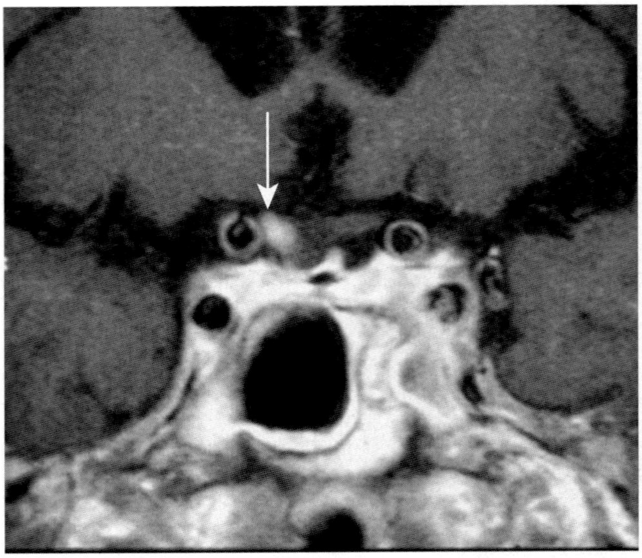

Figure 12.8 *Radiation-Induced Optic Neuritis.* Coronal postcontrast T1-weighted image shows a swollen and enhancing right optic nerve *(arrow).*

extremely sleepy ("somnolence syndrome"), and the reason for this remains uncertain. This sleepiness lasts for a few weeks and resolves spontaneously. Mineralizing angiopathy is a radiation-induced abnormality that is mostly asymptomatic, although many patients have significant headaches. This abnormality is better seen on CT and manifests as "brushlike" or stippled calcifications predominantly in the subcortical white matter (Fig.12.9).

Effects of Immunosuppressive Medications

Cyclosporine/tacrolimus toxicity probably is due to increased blood pressure and predominantly affects cerebral territories supplied by the posterior circulation.

Cyclosporine is a potent immunosuppressant used mostly in patients undergoing bone marrow and organ transplantation. Symptoms related to neurotoxicity are lethargy, headache, seizures, visual abnormalities, confusion, and coma. Cyclosporine toxicity affects both children and adults. Symptoms usually manifest during the first month of treatment. The relationship between serum drug levels and brain abnormalities is not clear, but in my experience, there is a correlation between the onset of MRI abnormalities and elevated

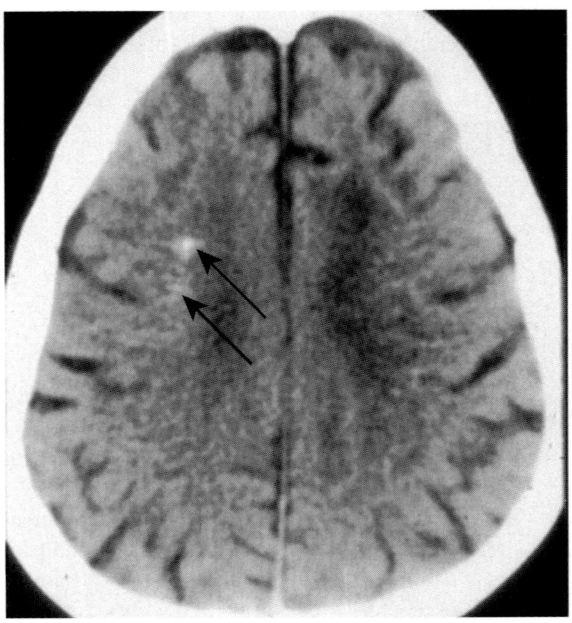

Figure 12.9 *Mineralizing Angiopathy.* Axial computed tomography after radiation and chemotherapy for medulloblastoma shows faint calcifications *(arrows)* at the gray–white matter junction of the right frontal lobe and diffuse atrophy.

drug levels (>300 ng/mL). Symptoms may be more common after liver transplantation (possibly due to hypocholesterolemia, which in turn results in larger amounts of unbound circulating drug). The possible mechanisms responsible for cyclosporine toxicity include neuropeptide-mediated ischemia and loss of autoregulation due to elevated blood pressure (14). The MRI findings are typical but nonspecific and are thought to be identical to those previously described for the posterior reversible encephalopathy syndrome (PRES; Chapter 8). T2-weighted images show areas of increased signal intensity involving gray and white matter in the occipital and parietal regions, but also occasionally involving the posterior temporal and frontal lobes (14,15) (Fig. 12.10). The cerebellum also may be

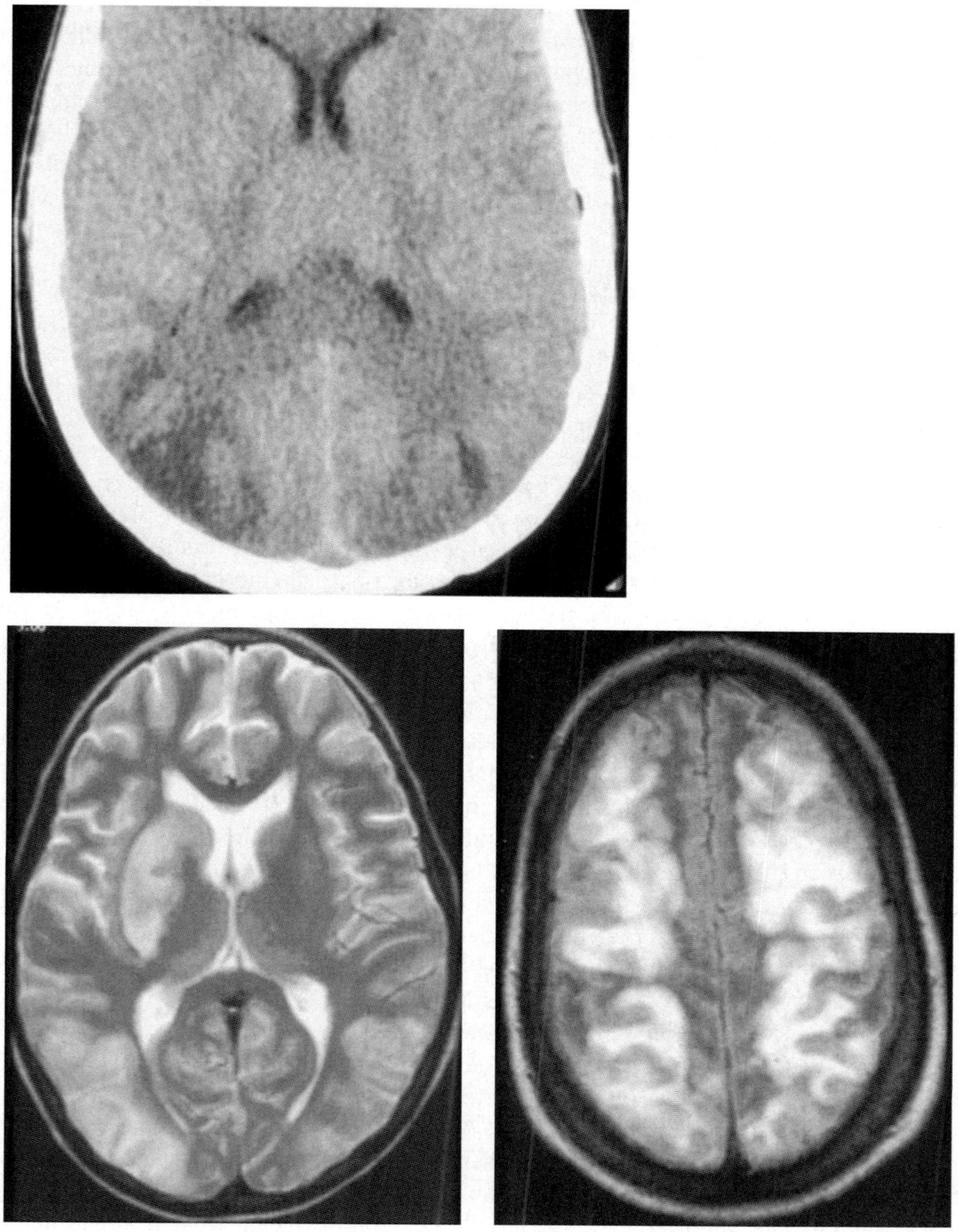

A

B

C

Figure 12.10 *CyclosporineTacrolimus–Induced Encephalopathy. A.* Axial computed tomography in a patient receiving cyclosporine shows low densities in the posterior brain (right greater than left) involving white and gray matter. *B.* Axial T2-weighted image after liver transplantation and administration of tacrolimus shows areas of hyperintensity in the posterior brain (right greater than left) involving both gray and white matter and also the right basal ganglia. *C.* In a different patient receiving cyclosporine, axial fluid attenuation inversion recovery (FLAIR) image shows diffuse hyperintensities in the white matter and involvement of the cortex posteriorly.

affected. The abnormal areas usually show no contrast enhancement, and most resolve spontaneously. Similar findings may be seen in patients taking tacrolimus (formerly FK-506). The underlying reason for the location of the abnormalities probably is related to the relative lack of sympathetic innervation of the vertebrobasilar system, making it poorly responsive to elevation of the blood pressure (16). On T2-weighted images, it is not possible to determine the etiology of the signal abnormality (vasogenic versus cytotoxic edema). Establishing the presence of cytotoxic edema conveys a worse prognosis because the lesions will be permanent. Diffusion-weighted imaging using apparent diffusion coefficient (ADC) maps may help with this issue. If the abnormal T2 regions show increased ADC, the mostly likely etiology is vasogenic edema, and the lesions will resolve (14). If the ADC values are low, the most likely etiology is cytotoxic edema and the lesions almost always will be permanent. SPECT also may be used to assess blood flow to the abnormal regions (17). Areas of vasogenic edema show no significant blood flow abnormalities. Similar observations have been made using gadolinium dynamic MR perfusion studies. Other drugs used for immunosuppressive purposes, such as vincristine, methotrexate, and prednisone, also may be neurotoxic alone or in combination with cyclosporine (18). The imaging findings produced by these agents are not well documented, with the exception of those caused by methotrexate (see later).

Effects of Chemotherapeutic Agents

Chemotherapy for the treatment of central nervous system (CNS) lesions may be given systemically, intrathecally, intraventricularly, intra-arterially, or in any combination of these routes (18). Regardless of the route of administration, CNS complications occur. In this section, I concentrate on the adverse effects of systemic chemotherapy on the CNS, but refer to complications associated with other routes of drug administration when pertinent. In addition, irradiation (alone or in combination with chemotherapy) may result in complications. Because irradiation (see earlier) is a local CNS treatment, it is mentioned in this section only to emphasize its synergistic effect with chemotherapy.

Methotrexate may produce headache, nuchal rigidity, aseptic meningitis, ataxia, paraplegia, and delirium when given systemically or intrathecally (19). In addition, scattered cerebral calcifications (related to mineralizing angiopathy) may be seen by CT. These calcifications have a brushlike appearance and usually are located in the subcortical regions (see earlier discussion). A unique and serious complication of methotrexate treatment is progressive leukoencephalopathy (20). This entity involves the white matter (including the u-fibers) and may be hemorrhagic or nonhemorrhagic. It usually manifests 3 to 9 months after the beginning of treatment and usually is seen as areas of increased T2 signal intensity in the white matter (Fig. 12.11). The lesions do not enhance. This leukoencephalopathy is seen more commonly as a result of intravenous methotrexate and irradiation, but also may occur after intrathecal methotrexate alone. Focal brain necrosis due to extravasation of methotrexate secondary to obstruction of the tip of a ventricular Ommaya reservoir catheter also is known to occur (Fig 12.12).

L-Asparaginase is a drug commonly used in the treatment of acute leukemias. CNS complications occur in approximately 2% of children receiving this drug (21). Symptoms of toxicity are altered mentation, somnolence, headache, and seizures. Intracranial venous thrombosis with subsequent hemorrhage also may occur. Vincristine also may induce neurologic complications, most of which present as cranial or peripheral neuropathies and have no specific imaging features. Platinum agents (particularly cisplatin) may result in CNS complications when given intraarterially (22). Optic neuritis may occur if the infusion is done with the catheter tip below the level of the ophthalmic artery. On postcontrast MRI studies, the optic nerves or optic chiasm are enlarged and show contrast enhancement. Cisplatin also results in reversible T2 signal intensity abnormalities in the posterior parietal, frontal, and occipital lobes. These abnormalities are identical to those in PRES (Chapter 8).

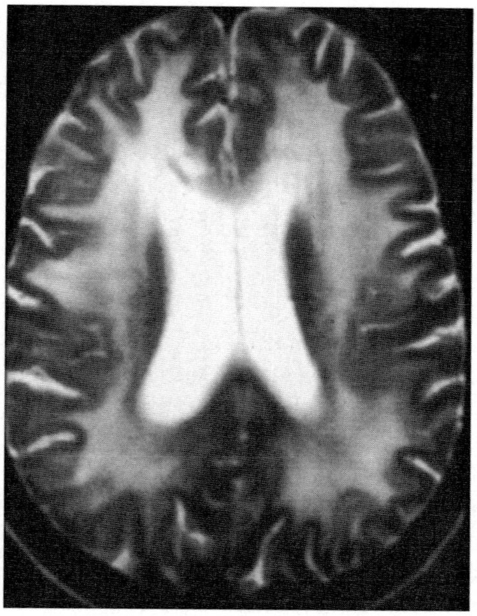

Figure 12.11 *Methotrexate-Induced Leukoencephalopathy.* Axial T2-weighted image demonstrates diffuse and symmetric hyperintensities in the white matter as well as diffuse brain atrophy.

The chronic and permanent effects of systemic chemotherapy on the CNS also have been studied. Approximately 86% of children treated for acute lymphoblastic leukemia exhibit permanent neuropsychological impairment (11,12). Although these children show only mild to moderate degrees of cerebral atrophy on MRI, brain perfusion studies using SPECT have shown cerebral blood flow defects in up to 44% of patients. It also is known that children who show either transient or permanent areas of high T2 signal intensity in the brain related to chemotherapy for acute lymphocytic leukemia show significant neuropsychological deficits (23). Proton MR spectroscopy also has been used to evaluate the

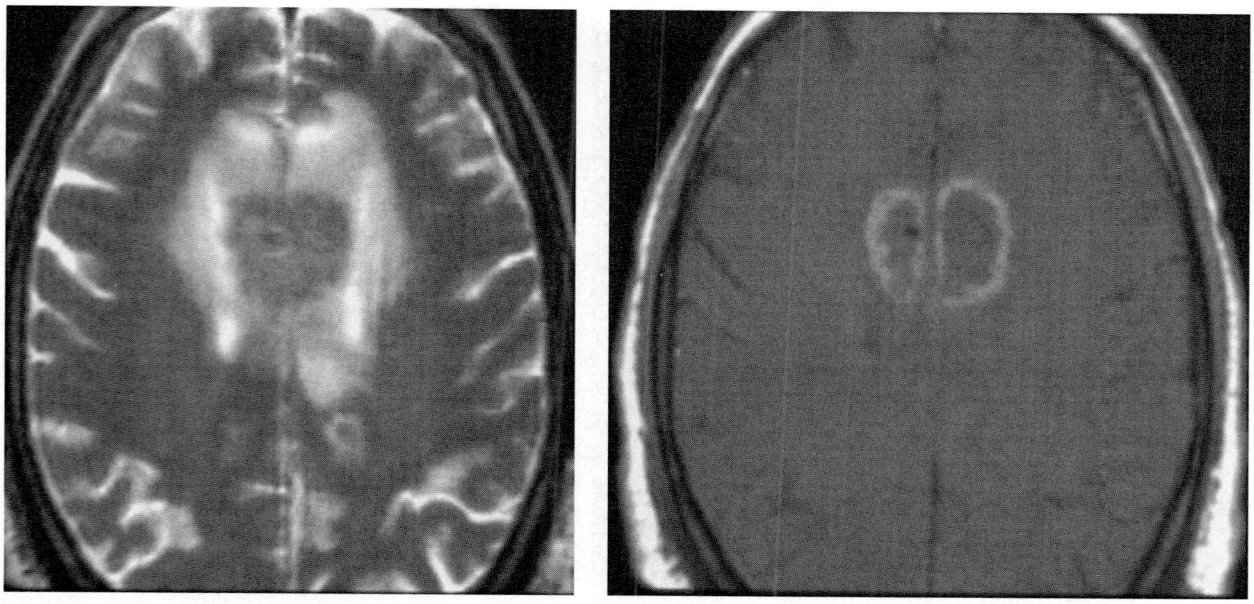

A B

Figure 12.12 *Methotrexate-Induced Focal Necrosis. A.* Axial T2-weighted image in a patient receiving the drug through a ventricular catheter. The catheter became obstructed and the drug leaked into its vicinity. Note hypointense lesion in the anterior callosum surrounded by edema. *B.* Corresponding postcontrast T1-weighted image shows marginal enhancement of the lesion. Note catheter amid the zone of necrosis.

brain sequelae of high-dose chemotherapy. In patients with good neurologic outcomes, the NAA is only minimally depressed, whereas it is markedly reduced in patients with poor outcomes.

Graft-versus-Host Disease and Posttransplantation Lymphoproliferative Disorder

Chronic graft-versus-host disease may present as cerebral mass lesions or areas of increased T2 signal, as well as a mass about the orbits.

In 25% to 75% of patients undergoing bone transplantation for leukemia, lymphoma, or anemia, some form of graft-versus-host disease (GVHD) develops (24). GVHD is secondary to a reaction of donor cells (especially CD4 helper cells) against the host cells. GVHD may be hyperacute, acute, or chronic. The organs primarily affected are the skin, thyroid gland, gastrointestinal tract, liver, and lymphatics. The brain and orbits rarely are affected, and mostly only in the chronic form of the disease (11%). Chronic GVHD may lead to the development of focal lesions. In the brain, chronic GVHD may present as basal ganglia mass lesions. The features of some lesions are similar to those of cerebral lymphoma on precontrast T1- and T2-weighted images. Contrast enhancement is minimal or absent, and this feature may serve to differentiate this rare disease from the more common cerebral lymphoma, which also may occur after bone marrow transplantation. Chronic GVHD also may present as nonspecific areas of abnormal high T2 signal intensity in the white matter accompanied by progressive atrophy. In the orbits, GVHD may result in periorbital swelling, subconjunctival fluid collections, and lacrimal gland involvement.

Posttransplantation lymphoproliferative disorder (PTLD) is due to chronic immunosuppression that leads to an upregulation and expansion of the volume of lymphoid cells, which may undergo malignant degeneration. PTLD is associated with infection by the Epstein-Barr virus. The lesions in the brain have a similar appearance to primary lymphoma (Fig. 12.13). As such, these brain lesions may require surgical resection or irradiation.

A

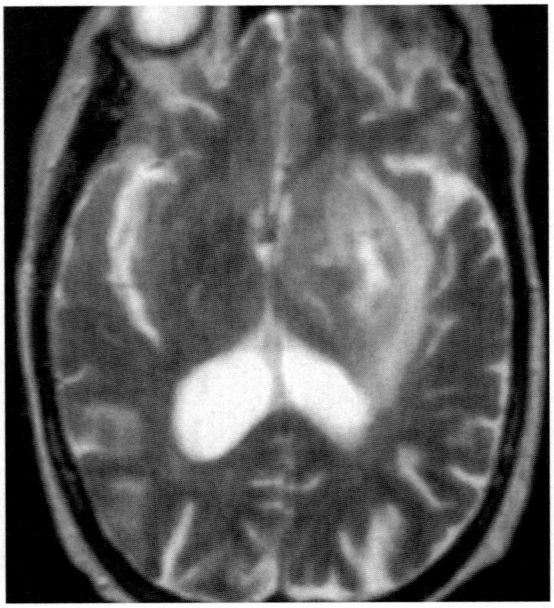

B

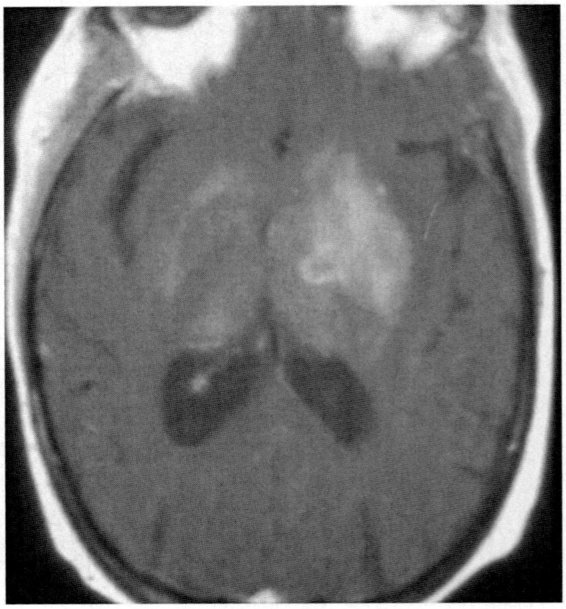

Figure 12.13 *Posttransplantation Lymphoproliferative Disorder. A.* Axial T2-weighted image shows a heterogeneous-appearing mass lesion in the left basal ganglia. *B.* Corresponding postcontrast T1-weighted image shows that the lesion enhances. The appearance of the lesion is similar to that of lymphoma.

Neoplasias Secondary to Transplantation Procedures

Secondary neoplasias also may occur after bone marrow transplantation (25). Solid tumors are particularly common if the bone transplantation occurred before 5 years of age (26). A secondary tumor develops in approximately 11% of transplant recipients. The most common secondary tumors involve the brain and the thyroid gland. Types of secondary tumors that are of interest to the neuroradiologist include squamous cell carcinomas of the buccal cavity and nasopharynx, nasopharyngeal neuroblastoma, cerebral astrocytoma, glioblastoma multiforme, primitive neuroectodermal tumors, and salivary gland tumors (mostly mucoepidermoid carcinoma). The genesis of these tumors probably is related to a combination of the effects of irradiation and chronic GVHD.

Effects of Anticonvulsant Medications

In patients with chronic seizures, the cerebellum may become atrophic secondary to phenytoin toxicity, or as a primary effect of seizures.

One of the most common antiepileptic drugs is phenytoin (Dilantin), and its adverse effects on the brain are well documented. Toxicity usually is seen with chronic phenytoin use and includes gingival hyperplasia and other dermatologic and hematologic complications. Neurologic symptoms related to its chronic use are ataxia, nystagmus, slurred speech, and a predominantly sensory peripheral neuropathy. Phenytoin induces axonal atrophy and loss of Purkinje cells in the cerebellar cortex (27) (Fig. 12.14A). It is not clear if the drug alone is responsible for the cerebellar abnormalities, or if chronic seizures also play a role in the development of cerebellar atrophy. In addition, phenytoin may induce a deficiency of folate that also has been linked to the development of cerebellar atrophy. The presence of a lesion in the splenium of the corpus callosum in patients taking either phenytoin or vigabatrin for seizures has been documented (28) (Fig. 12.14B). This area of abnormal increased T2 signal intensity does not enhance and is not hemorrhagic. Presumably it represents a response to high drug doses or an increased sensitivity to the

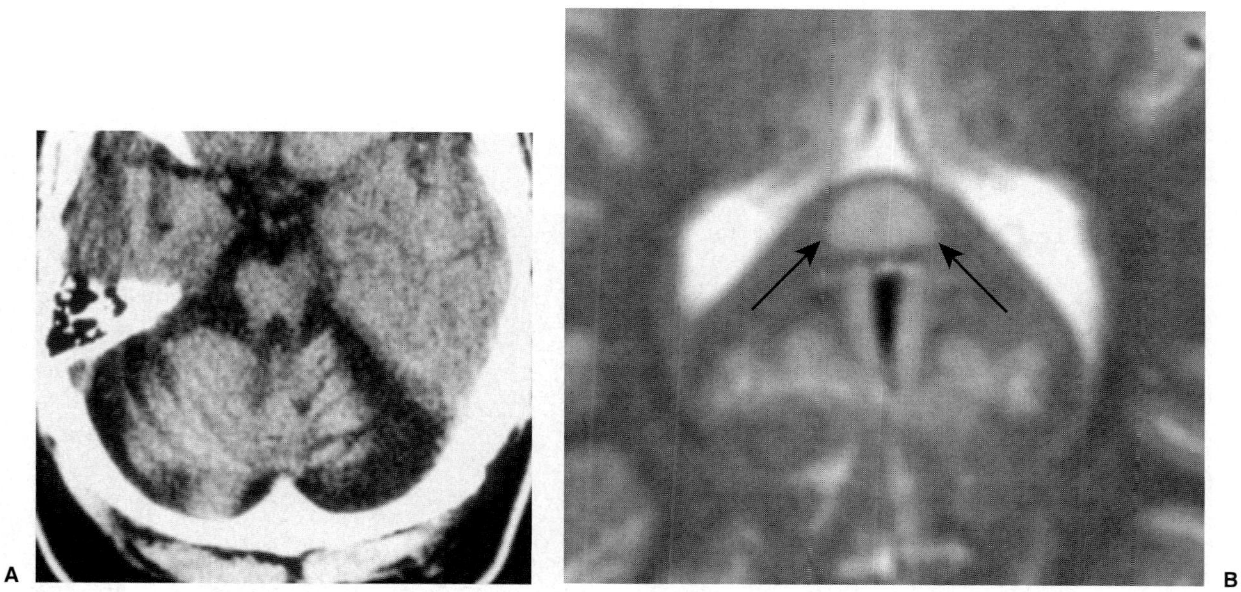

Figure 12.14 *Effects of Seizure Medications. A.* Axial computed tomography in a patient taking phenytoin for many years shows severe atrophy of the cerebellum and thickening of the skull. *B.* Axial T2-weighted image in a patient taking vigabatrin shows an area of increased signal intensity (*arrows*) in the splenium of the corpus callosum, presumably due to the drug.

drugs. Vigabatrin causes an irreversible inhibition of γ-aminobutyric acid that may result in damage to the white matter tracts, and this mechanism may result in a lesion in the posterior corpus callosum.

Effects of Total Parenteral Nutrition

Long-term total parenteral nutrition results in increased T1 signal intensity in the caudate nuclei, tectum (particularly the inferior colliculi), globi pallidi, putamina, subthalamic nuclei, red nuclei, adenohypophysis, and substantia nigra (29) (Fig. 12.15). The abnormalities are bilateral, symmetric, and of homogeneous signal intensity. There are no corresponding abnormalities on T2-weighted images, and CT scans are negative. The MRI findings are believed to be due to increased amounts of manganese and other factors leading to shortening of the T1 relaxation time (Box 12.1).

Manganese deposition results in increased T1 signal in the dorsal brainstem, basal ganglia, and anterior pituitary lobe, and may be reversible.

Increased plasma levels of Mn may be found in chronic liver failure and in patients receiving long-term parenteral nutrition, and as a consequence of occupational toxicity (30). Approximately 95% of Mn is excreted in bile. Mn is involved in some enzymatic cell cycles, including superoxide dismutase and glutamine synthetase. Mn reaches the brain by way of erythrocytes and plasma. Transferrin and albumin are its carriers in plasma. The half-life of blood Mn is 10 to 42 days, but when it reaches the brain it may remain there for prolonged periods (31). Astrocytes have specific transport systems for Mn. Mn is neurotoxic and results in striatal dopamine depletion, *N*-methyl-D-aspartate excitotoxicity, and oxidative stress. Thus, Mn may play a role in the development of an encephalopathy characterized by pyramidal and extrapyramidal dysfunction, brisk tendon reflexes, and tremors. Solutions that are rich in Mn lead to the development of neurologic symptoms. Once parenteral nutrition is discontinued, the MRI abnormalities may reverse to normal (32,33). The amount of time required for these abnormalities to resolve is not clear, but most do within 1 year after cessation of parenteral nutrition. Similar findings are noted in patients after liver transplantation and probably are due to a mild dysfunction of the transplanted organ.

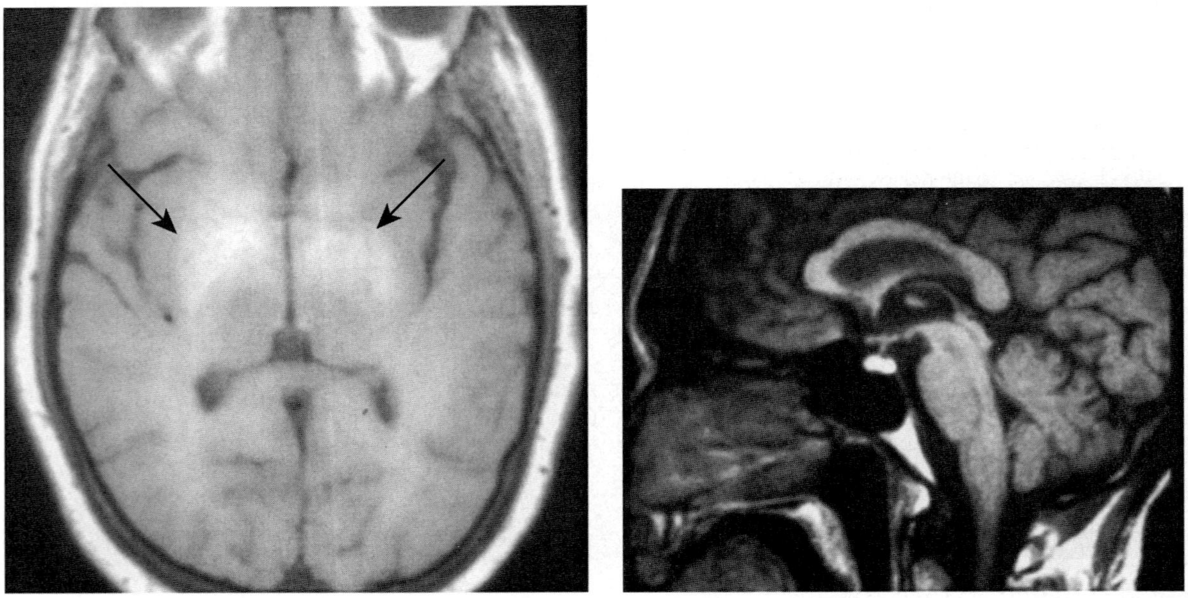

A B

Figure 12.15 *Effects of Chronic Liver Failure. A.* Axial T1-weighted image shows mildly increased signal intensity in the basal ganglia *(arrows)*. *B.* In a different patient, sagittal T1-weighted image shows increased signal in the dorsal brainstem and in the adenohypophysis.

Box 12.1: Conditions Resulting in Bright Basal Ganglia on T1-Weighted Images

Chronic liver failure
Total parenteral nutrition
Manganese poisoning
Normal calcifications
Neurofibromatosis type 1
Hyperglycemia

REFERENCES

1. Hecht-Leavitt C, Grossman RI, Curran WJ Jr, et al. MR of brain radiation injury: experimental studies in cats. AJNR Am J Neuroradiol 1987;8:427–430.
2. Valk PE, Dillon WP. Radiation injury of the brain. AJNR Am J Neuroradiol 1991;12:45–62.
3. Kinoshita K, Tada E, Matsumoto K, et al. Proton MR spectroscopy of delayed cerebral radiation in monkeys and humans after brachytherapy. AJNR Am J Neuroradiol 1997;18:1753–1761.
4. Castillo M, Kwock L. Proton MR spectroscopy of common brain tumors. Neuroimaging Clin North Am 1998;8:733–752.
5. Patronas NJ, Di Chiro G, Brooks RA, et al. Work in progress: [18F] fluorodeoxyglucose and positron emission tomography in the evaluation of radiation necrosis of the brain. Radiology 1982;144:885–889.
6. Yoshii Y, Moritake T, Suzuki K, et al. Cerebral radiation necrosis with accumulation of thallium 201 on single-photon emission CT. AJNR Am J Neuroradiol 1996;17:1773–1776.
7. Petrella JR, Provenzale JM. MR perfusion imaging of the brain: techniques and applications. AJR Am J Roentgenol 2000;175:207–219.
8. Wong JC, Provenzale JM, Petrella JR. Perfusion MR imaging of brain neoplasms. AJR Am J Roentgenol 2000;174:1147–1157.
9. Larson JJ, Ball WS, Bove KE, et al. Formation of intracerebral cavernous malformations after radiation treatment for central nervous system neoplasia in children. J Neurosurg 1998;88: 51–56.
10. Novelli PM, Reigel DH, Langham Gleason P, et al. Multiple cavernous angiomas after high-dose whole-brain radiation therapy. Pediatr Neurosurg 1997;26:322–325.
11. Chen CY, Zimmerman RA, Faro S, et al. Childhood leukemia: central nervous system abnormalities during and after treatment. AJNR Am J Neuroradiol 1996;17:295–310.
12. Parisi MT, Fahmy JL, Kaminsky JL, et al. Complications of cancer therapy in children: a radiologist's guide. Radiographics 1999;19:283–297.
13. Hudgins PA, Newman NJ, Dillon WP, et al. Radiation-induced optic neuropathy: characteristic appearances on gadolinium-enhanced MR. AJNR Am J Neuroradiol 1992;13:235–238.
14. Coley SC, Porter DA, Calamante F, et al. Quantitative MR diffusion mapping and cyclosporine-induced neurotoxicity. AJNR Am J Neuroradiol 1999;20:1507–1510.
15. Sheth TN, Ichise M, Kucharczyk W. Brain perfusion imaging in asymptomatic patients receiving cyclosporin. AJNR Am J Neuroradiol 1999;20:853–856.
16. Tweddle DA, Windebank KP, Hewson QC, et al. Drug points: cyclosporin neurotoxicity after chemotherapy. BMJ 1999;318:1113.
17. HarilaSaari AH, Ahonen AKA, Vainionpaa LK, et al. Brain perfusion after treatment of childhood acute lymphoblastic leukemia. J Nucl Med 1997;38:82–88.
18. Wilson DA, Nitschke R, Bowman ME, et al. Transient white matter changes on MR images in children undergoing chemotherapy for acute lymphocytic leukemia: correlation with neuropsychologic deficiencies. Radiology 1991;180:205–209.
19. Lovblad K, Kelkar P, Ozdoba C, et al. Pure methotrexate encephalopathy presenting with seizures: CT and MRI features. Pediatr Radiol 1998;28:86–91.
20. Fisher NC, Ruban E, Carey M, et al. Late-onset fatal acute leucoencephalopathy in liver transplant recipients. Lancet 1997;349:1884–1885.
21. Nicholson JC, Darmady JM, Kohler JA. Superior sagittal sinus thrombosis complicating maintenance treatment for acute lymphoblastic leukemia. Pediatr Hematol Oncol 1996;13:287–291.

22. Ito Y, Arahata Y, Goto Y, et al. Cisplatin neurotoxicity presenting as reversible posterior leukoencephalopathy syndrome. AJNR Am J Neuroradiol 1998;19:415–417.
23. Brown MS, Stemmer SM, Simon JH, et al. White matter disease induced by high-dose chemotherapy: longitudinal study with MR imaging and proton spectroscopy. AJNR Am J Neuroradiol 1998;19:217–221.
24. Cole JW, Quint DJ, Hutchinson RJ, et al. CT demonstration of periorbital graft-versus-host disease. AJNR Am J Neuroradiol 1997;18:730–732.
25. Socie G, Curtis RE, Deeg HJ, et al. New malignant diseases after allogeneic marrow transplantation for childhood acute leukemia. J Clin Oncol 2000;18:348–357.
26. Curtis RE, Rowlings PA, Deeg HJ, et al. Solid cancers after bone marrow transplantation. N Engl J Med 1997;336:897–904.
27. Verity MA. Toxic disorders. In: Graham DI, Lantos PD, eds. Greenfield's neuropathology, 6th ed. London: Arnold, 1997:788.
28. Kim SS, Change KH, Kim ST, et al. Focal lesion in the splenium of the corpus callosum in epileptic patients: antiepileptic drug toxicity. AJNR Am J Neuroradiol 1999;20:125–129.
29. Fell JME, Reynolds AP, Meadows N, et al. Manganese toxicity in children receiving long-term parenteral nutrition. Lancet 1996;347:1218–1221.
30. Krieger D, Krieger S, Jansen O, et al. Manganese and chronic hepatic encephalopathy. Lancet 1995;346:270–274.
31. Pomier-Layrargues G, Spahr L, Butterworth RF. Increased manganese concentrations in pallidum of cirrhotic patients. Lancet 1995;345:735.
32. Mirowitz SA, Westrich TJ. Basal ganglial signal intensity alterations: reversal after discontinuation of parenteral manganese administration. Radiology 1992;185:535–536.
33. Okamoto K, Ito J, Furusawa T, et al. Reversible hyperintensity of the anterior pituitary gland on T1-weighted MR images in a patient receiving temporary parenteral nutrition. AJNR Am J Neuroradiol 1998;19:1287–1289.

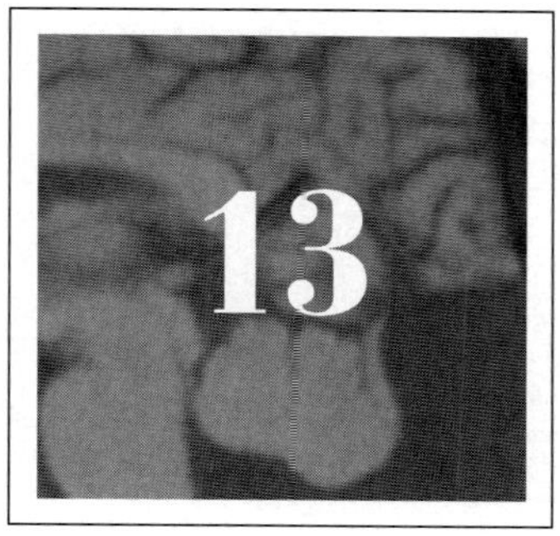

Congenital Spinal Anomalies

- Embryology and Classification
- Special Considerations in Magnetic Resonance Imaging of the Spine in Children
- Open Spinal Dysraphisms
- Closed Spinal Dysraphisms
- Dermal Sinus Tracts and Epidermoid/Dermoid Tumors
- Caudal Regression Syndrome
- Filar Lipoma
- Ventriculus Terminalis (Ventriculus Terminus)
- Tight Filum Terminale Syndrome
- Anterior Sacral Meningocele
- Sacrococcygeal Teratoma
- Terminal Myelocystocele
- Split Cord and Notochord Syndromes
- Scoliosis

Embryology and Classification

The spine begins to form by the process of neurulation. The primitive neural plate is located in the back of the embryo and extends from cephalad to caudal. Between the second and third weeks of life, the edges of the neural plate thicken and form the neural folds (1). These folds grow and approximate to each other in the midline, forming a tube (the neural tube). The closure probably begins in the middle to upper portions of the neural tube and then extends superiorly and inferiorly (this is debatable, but nicely explains many of the defects occurring at this stage; see later). The process of neural tube closure is called *neurulation*. Neurulation is affected and guided by the presence of the notochord (2). The notochord is a tube of mesodermal elements lying ventral to the neural tube. The notochord is traversed by the neuroenteric canal, which allows for a transient communication between the yolk sac and the amniotic cavity (see sections on split notochord and split cord malformations, later). Anomalies due to persistence of this communication are extremely rare and are termed the *split notochord* or *split cord syndrome*, and include intraspinal enteric cysts, dorsal enteric fistula, dorsal enteric diverticula, dorsal enteric sinus, diastematomyelia, and diplomyelia (3). A common factor seen in all of these defects is that the spinal column is split near its midline. The distal spine forms by a different process (called *canalization and retrogressive differentiation*) and is addressed later. Processes affecting neurulation prevent closure of the spine and give rise to a group of disorders termed *open dysraphisms*, in which the neural elements remain exposed and are clinically visible. The most important open dysraphisms are:

Most of the spine forms through a mechanism called neurulation; however, the distal spine forms by a different process called canalization and retrogressive differentiation.

- Myelocele
- Myelomeningocele (nearly always associated with the Chiari type 2 malformation)
- Hemimyelocele
- Myelocystocele

Once the neural tube has closed, it begins the process of separating itself from the overlying ectoderm (a mechanism called *disjunction*). Disjunction is abnormal if it occurs too early (premature disjunction) or is only partial (failure of disjunction). In premature disjunction, ectodermal elements are allowed to enter the neural tube before its closure. These ectopic cells usually become adipocytes and form intraspinal lipomas. The disorders of premature disjunction are covered by skin and are termed *closed* or *occult dysraphisms*. The most important closed dysraphisms are:

- Lipomyelocele
- Lipomyelomeningocele
- Intraspinal lipoma

Another group of disorders I discuss in this chapter are those secondary to an incomplete separation of the neural tube and the overlying ectoderm (failure of disjunction). The adherence between the closing neural tube and the ectoderm leads to the formation of a communicating tract between these two structures. The tract does not permit the closure of the tube and results in a spina bifida. These disorders have a skin defect accompanied by an intraspinal anomaly and include:

- Dermal sinus tract with or with out epidermoid/dermoid
- Midline spinal hamartoma

I now briefly address the formation of most of the vertebral column (except the sacrum, which is addressed later) and its most common defects. Early in life, the notochord separates from the primitive gut. As this is occurring, the mesenchyme located along the sides of the neural tube migrates into a gap located between the dorsal and ventral components of the notochord. The mesenchyme then divides into somites. Each somite will further subdivide into (1):

Myotomes giving rise to the paraspinal musculature
Dermatomes giving rise to the skin of the back
Sclerotomes giving rise to the vertebrae

Remnants of the notochord presumably are located in the nucleus pulposus, clivus, nasopharyngeal notochordal bursa, and sacrum.

The sclerotomes are separated ("segmented") by the course of veins (basivertebral veins) in their central aspect. Each sclerotome is formed by the lower part of a future vertebra and the upper part of the adjacent future vertebra. At this time, the spine is in a "membranous" stage. In between the lower and upper segments of each sclerotome is a residual part of the notochord (which eventually becomes the nucleus pulposus). The sclerotomes are then resegmented. That is, as the nerve roots exit the lower aspect of a sclerotome, the lower aspect fuses with its corresponding upper aspect (for example, the lower aspect of the C4 sclerotome fuses with the upper aspect of the C5 sclerotome to give rise to the C4 vertebra, leaving the nerve roots between them). This fusion results in the formation of vertebrae that contain the basivertebral veins in their middle, with the notochord remnant (nucleus pulposus) lying between them. Laterally, the neural foramina form to allow the nerve roots to exit. During this process, the spine is in its "chondrification" stage. Once resegmentation is completed, the upper and lower vertebrae fuse and the residual notochord becomes the intervertebral disk (particularly the nucleus pulposus). The most common anomaly due to incomplete reabsorption of the notochord is a butterfly vertebra. Incomplete resegmentation results in blocked vertebrae or fusion bars (the lateral aspects of two vertebrae are fused). The final stage of development occurring after resegmentation is that of ossification. Each vertebra normally contains three ossification centers, one for the body and one on each side that will form the neural arch. Anomalies in the midline ossification center may give rise to "wedge" vertebral bodies.

All of the aforementioned mechanisms are involved in the formation of the spine, with the exception of its distalmost region. The inferior aspect of the neural tube elongates inferiorly by a process called *canalization* (4). The neural tube elongates inferiorly and joins with the caudal cell mass, a group of undifferentiated cells located in the embryonic tail. The caudal cell mass is composed of notochordal and neural elements. Between the caudal cell mass and the notochord is the cloaca (which explains why anomalies of the distal genitourinary and gastrointestinal tracts commonly are associated with malformations of the sacrum and the distal spinal cord). The caudal cell mass forms multiple internal cavities, all of which eventually fuse into one canal that unites with the central aspect of the elongated neural tube (which will form the central spinal canal). Programmed cell death (apoptosis) results in a retrogressive differentiation by which the caudal cell mass and the distal neural tube jointly form the conus medullaris, cauda equina, and filum terminale. Disorders at this stage result in a rare group of anomalies called the *caudal regression syndrome*. Persistence of the central cavity in the conus medullaris gives rise to ventriculus terminus. The following are disorders arising from faulty canalization and retrogressive differentiation:

- Caudal regression syndrome
- Filar lipoma
- Terminal ventricle
- Tight filum terminale syndrome
- Anterior sacral meningocele
- Sacrococcygeal teratoma
- Terminal myelocystocele

The normal conus medullaris terminates at the T12 to L2 levels.

Canalization and retrogressive differentiation, as well as the differential growth between the spinal column and the spinal cord, determine the position of the conus medullaris. The normal conus medullaris is always above the level of the L2-L3 disk space. If the conus is located below this level, a search for an anomaly tethering it should be performed. A conus medullaris that terminates at the mid-L2 level is abnormal in patients who are symptomatic, and in those who are apparently asymptomatic, careful clinical follow-up is necessary. If the patient remains asymptomatic, a conus terminating at the mid-L2 level may be considered as a normal variant as long as a magnetic resonance imaging (MRI) study also is negative.

The genetic mechanisms that affect the formation of the spine are complex and beyond the scope of this book. I mention only three genes that are critical to the formation of the spine (1):

Hox genes. These genes are highly conserved (homeotic) from the lower species to humans. They presumably regulate the differentiation of the somites and help establish their cephalad and caudal portions by producing gradients of the substances for which they encode. Transitional vertebrae, occipitalization of C1 (and other craniocervical junction anomalies), and perhaps even the Chiari type 1 malformation result from anomalies of these genes.

Sonic hedgehog genes. These genes encode for a protein that may be produced in the notochord. This messenger protein appears to induce the formation of the sclerotomes.

Pax genes. These genes encode for transcription factors that bind to specific DNA sequences. These genes are important in segmentation and also help to establish the dorsal and ventral aspects of the neural tube. The notochord and the *sonic hedgehog* genes induce the expression of the *Pax* genes in the somites. Specific *Pax* genes guide the formation of the dorsal, intermediate, and ventral regions of the spinal cord. In animals, mutations of the *Pax* genes have been known to result in disorders of neural crest migration, anomalous vertebrae and disks, spina bifida, and exencephaly.

Special Considerations in Magnetic Resonance Imaging of the Spine in Children

The spine in children has a very different MRI appearance compared with the adult spine (5) (Table 13.1).

After contrast administration, the pediatric spine also enhances in a different fashion than the adult spine (6). Before 18 months of age, there is striking enhancement of the cartilage in the endplates. In patients younger than 2 years of age, there also is marked enhancement of the bone marrow, a finding that progressively diminishes (but never dis-

Table 13.1: Magnetic Resonance Imaging Features of the Spine in Children

Stage	*Age*	*T1 Images*	*T2 Images*
I	Birth to 1 mo	Ossification center: bright Endplate: bright Disk: isointense	Ossification center: dark Endplate: mildly bright Disk: bright
II	1–6 mo	Ossification center: centrally dark with bright edges Endplate: bright Disk: isointense	Ossification center: similar to T1 Endplate: mildly bright Disk: bright
III	>7 mo	Ossification center: bright Endplate: isointense Disk: isointense	Ossification center: mildly bright Endplate: mildly bright Disk: bright

appears) until 7 years of age. These prominent enhancement patterns should not be confused with a pathologic process. They are believed to be due to prominent vasculature in the structures mentioned.

In addition, the MRI protocols needed to evaluate the pediatric spine vary from those commonly used for adults. I recommend the following:

1. Suspected occult dysraphism: sagittal T1 and T2 images, coronal T1 images, axial T1 images through the abnormality. If an abnormality is found, add sagittal T1 images of the thoracic and cervical regions (to exclude syrinx). Contrast should be given in cases of infection (or suspected infection), and sagittal and axial T1 images repeated.
2. Repaired open dysraphism: sagittal T1 and T2 images of lumbosacral region, axial T1 images at level of repair, sagittal T1 of the thoracic and cervical regions.
3. Congenital vertebral anomalies: sagittal and axial T1 images of the lumbar region (check for position of the conus medullaris) and coronal and axial T1 images through the abnormal vertebra(e).
4. Scoliosis: sagittal T1 and T2 images of the entire spine, coronal T1 and axial T1 images at primary curvature; if contrast is given, repeat the coronal and axial T1 images at the primary curvature.

Open Spinal Dysraphisms

Nearly all patients with myelomeningoceles have a Chiari type 2 malformation.

This group of disorders comprises the myelocele, myelomeningocele, hemimyelocele, and myelocystocele. Only myelocele and myelomeningocele are discussed here in detail. Most affected patients are girls, and in industrialized countries the diagnosis usually is made *in utero* by sonography. Some patients now undergo *in utero* repair that prevents the formation of hydrocephalus and avoids placement of a shunt in up to 50% of patients. Most open dysraphisms are due to a localized lack of closure of the neural tube. The early prenatal administration of folate is known to reduce the incidence of open spinal dysraphisms (7). Most of these defects are closed immediately after birth, and the patients require no acute imaging. To exclude the presence of hydrocephalus, cranial sonography may be used and, if needed, a ventricular shunt may be inserted at the time of the spinal repair. The typical and main clinical feature of both myeloceles and myelomeningoceles is the exposed neural placode (unfolded neural tube) (8). On physical examination, the unfolded spinal cord is seen as a flat, reddish, moist structure in the middle of the skin defect. The portion of the placode that is visible is the inside of the spinal cord, with its outer surface lying ventral and projecting into the spinal canal. The skin approximates the edges of the placode and becomes thin and atrophic before it fuses with it. The dura also is fused at the edges of the placode. The laminae and spinous processes are missing and the pedicles are everted. The spinal canal may be wide, and segmentation anomalies of the vertebrae at the level of the dysraphism are common. Most open dysraphisms are in the lumbosacral junction, but they may be localized to any part of the lumbar spine, the lumbothoracic junction, and, rarely, isolated to the thoracic region. When the dysraphism involves the lumbar and thoracic regions, significant kyphoscoliosis is present in up to 35% of patients. However, kyphoscoliosis eventually develops in most patients with open dysraphisms because of a muscular imbalance. The spinal cord usually is tethered to the ectoderm at the level of the dysraphism, and cysts (syringohydromyelia) may be present in it. The basic difference between a myelocele and a myelomeningocele lies in the location of the neural placode. If the placode is flush with the level of the skin and does not project outward, the malformation is called a *myelocele* (9). If the placode is pushed outward and rises above the level of the skin, the malformation is called a *myelomeningocele*. In a myelomeningocele, the subarachnoid cystic space protruding from the spinal canal is prominent and nerves roots coursing through it are elongated (Fig. 13.1).

During surgery, the placode may be refolded and separated from the adjacent tissues. A dural patch usually is placed (or the edges of the dura are pulled toward the midline and sutured) and the skin defect is closed. This "neo" spinal cord remains tethered at the site of previous surgery in nearly all patients (Fig. 13.2). Most imaging studies in patients with open spinal dysraphisms are obtained after the initial closure and on the occurrence of new or progressive symptoms (8). The purpose of imaging in these children is not primarily to assess tethering of the cord at the level of the repair, but to detect new or previously unrecognized lesions. Many techniques have been tried to evaluate for retethering of the spinal cord at the repair level, including scanning the patient prone with MRI (if the distal spinal cord at the level of the repair does not move ventrally, it is assumed to the tethered). Cine-MRI also may be used to visualize pulsations of the cord at this level (absence of pulsations may indicate retethering). Unfortunately, I have found these tech-

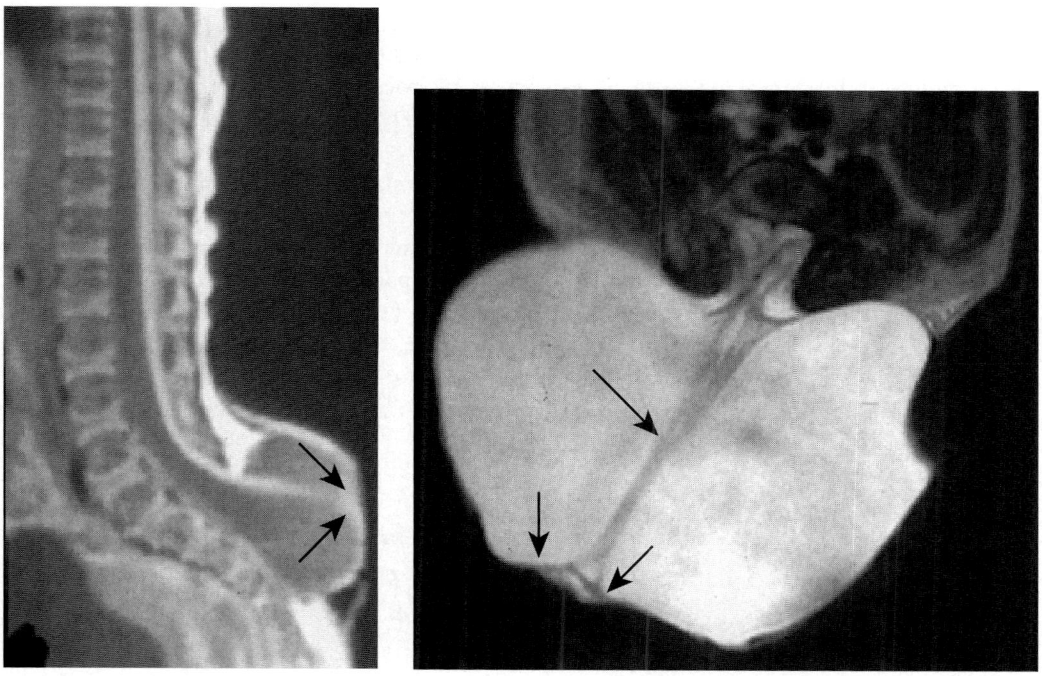

Figure 13.1 *Unrepaired Myelomeningocele. A.* Sagittal T1-weighted image shows open and fluid-filled posterior lumbosacral defect containing a dysplastic and tethered spinal cord. Note the placode *(arrows)*. (Case courtesy of P. Tortori, Genova, Italy.) *B.* In a different patient, axial T2-weighted image shows large meningocele containing markedly stretched nerve roots *(long arrow)* terminating in a midline placode *(short arrows)*.

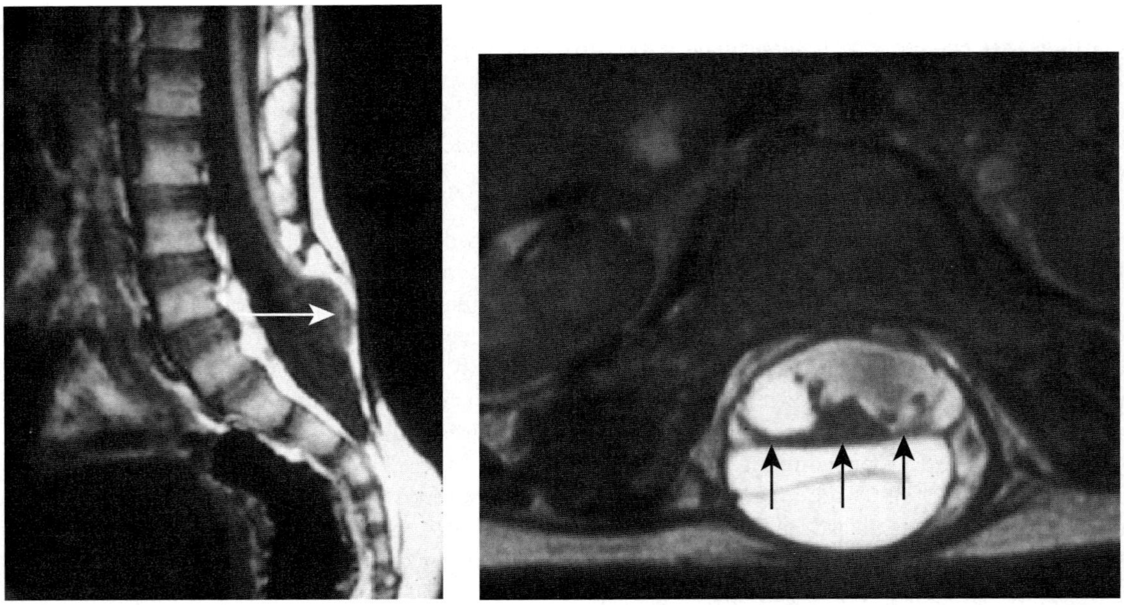

Figure 13.2 *Repaired Myelomeningocele. A.* Sagittal T1-weighted image shows that the placode *(arrow)* is now flush at the level of the bony defect and covered by a skin graft. The spinal cord remains dysplastic and inferiorly tethered. *B.* Axial T2-weighted image in a different patient. There is a skin graft covering the defect and a dural graft separated from the placode *(arrows)* by cerebrospinal fluid.

niques unrewarding in most patients. An important finding at the level of the repair is a focal narrowing of the cord. This usually is due to a dural ring created by pulling the dura too tightly at the time of the repair. The most important aspect of postoperative imaging is to assess for other complications (Box 13.1).

After surgical repair of myelomeningocele, imaging of the entire spine is mandatory.

Clinical deterioration in patients with repaired open spinal dysraphisms may be secondary to intracranial abnormalities such as hydrocephalus. In many patients presenting acutely, evaluation of the brain to rule out hydrocephalus is performed before the spine is imaged.

A myelocystocele is not an anomaly of neurulation because the neural tube closes completely (see later). It is included in this section (and also briefly addressed later) because it is a defect in which neural elements may be visible. In this very rare anomaly, there is a cyst in the spinal cord. The severely expanded spinal cord herniates through a spina bifida, presenting as a midline cystic mass (10). Myelocystoceles affect either the cervical or lumbosacral regions (in the latter case, they are called *terminal myelocystoceles*). The etiology of cervical myelocystoceles is not clear, but the terminal ones are considered by some to be anomalies of canalization and retrogressive differentiation (see later).

Box 13.1 Complications after Repair of Open Spinal Dysraphism

Dural ring with focal cord narrowing	Dermoid
Spinal cord cyst	Formation of arachnoid cyst(s)
Diastematomyelia	Spinal cord ischemia
Epidermoid	

For the sake of completeness, I briefly address the hemimyelocele (10). These are thought to represent approximately 10% of myelomeningoceles, but in my experience they are very rare. The spinal cord is split and a bar of bone resulting in two spinal canals may or may not be present. One of the hemicords lies in a myelomeningocele, whereas the other one remains inside of the native spinal canal. The former hemicord is smaller in diameter.

The incidence of open spinal dysraphisms in industrialized countries has significantly decreased during the last decade. This is due to the prenatal administration of folic acid and the use of sonography for early detection and therapeutic abortion.

Closed Spinal Dysraphisms

From a clinical standpoint, there are two types of closed neural tube defects. In the first and more common type, there is a soft (fatty), skin-covered mass over the defect, and in the second type there no mass is present (11). The types that have a subcutaneous mass are the lipomyelocele and the lipomyelomeningoceles, and they are more common than the type without a soft tissue mass in the back. All closed spinal dysraphisms are more common in girls, and although most are recognized before 6 months of age, some patients may present later in life, and sometimes they even may be completely asymptomatic throughout their life. Most symptoms are due to weakness and deformities of the lower extremities (club feet) and bowel and bladder problems (12,13). Some degree of kyphoscoliosis develops in many patients during their lifetime. In this anomaly, pluripotential ectodermal cells enter the neural tube before or as it is closing. The neural elements induce these cells to become lipomas (10). If the cells are completely separated from the overlying ectoderm, an intraspinal lipoma forms, but if they are in continuity with the overlying ectoderm, a lipomyelocele or lipomyelomeningocele forms. These lipomas increase in size with age and may become clinically evident or symptomatic only during periods of weight gain. Regardless of the size of the lipoma, the neural tube remains unfolded at that level. It is the location of the placode with respect to the dorsalmost aspect of the hypoplastic neural arch (equivalent to the level of the skin in patients with open dysraphism) that determines the name of the malformation (analogous to the open dysraphisms). If the placode lies at the level of the spina bifida and is covered by skin and subcutaneous fat, the malformation is called a *lipomyelocele* (analogous to the myelocele). If the subarachnoid space ventral to the placode is prominent and it pushes the placode above the level of the spina bifida, the malformation is called a *lipomyelomeningocele* (analogous to the myelomeningocele). In the lipomyelomeningocele, the placode is not horizontal but is oriented obliquely, with one or two meningoceles usually herniating laterally on one of side of placode (Fig. 13.3). The defect is covered by an asymmetric subcutaneous lipoma. Because one side of the placode lies closer to the spinal canal, the nerve roots on that side are shorter and create a "physiologic" tethering of the placode—that is, regardless of surgery, these short nerve roots keep the placode fixed at that level. At the level of the dysraphism, the vertebrae are abnormal and show butterfly-type deformities and segmentation anomalies in 40% to 50% of patients. Surgery for patients with lipomyelocele or lipomyelomeningocele is more complicated than that performed for those with open spinal dysraphisms. The lipoma needs to be resected and usually it is vaporized by laser as close as possible to the placode, trying not to damage it. It is difficult to find a plane between the lipoma and neural structures, so a small amount of lipoma nearly always is left behind. Once the lipoma has been grossly resected, the surgery continues in a fashion similar to that described previously for open spinal dysraphisms.

Patients with lipomyelocele and lipomyelomeningocele also may have associated anomalies (Box 13.2).

The term *intraspinal lipoma* refers to accumulations of fat usually restricted to the intradural space (10). However, many of these lipomas extend into the epidural fat and often into the subcutaneous fat. Because their precursor cells are trapped in the closing neural tube, the underlying spinal cord may be incompletely closed. Frequently, the spinal cord is normally closed but compressed by the lipoma. Intradural lipomas may present in childhood (25%), but because they may enlarge during periods of growth, most (>50%)

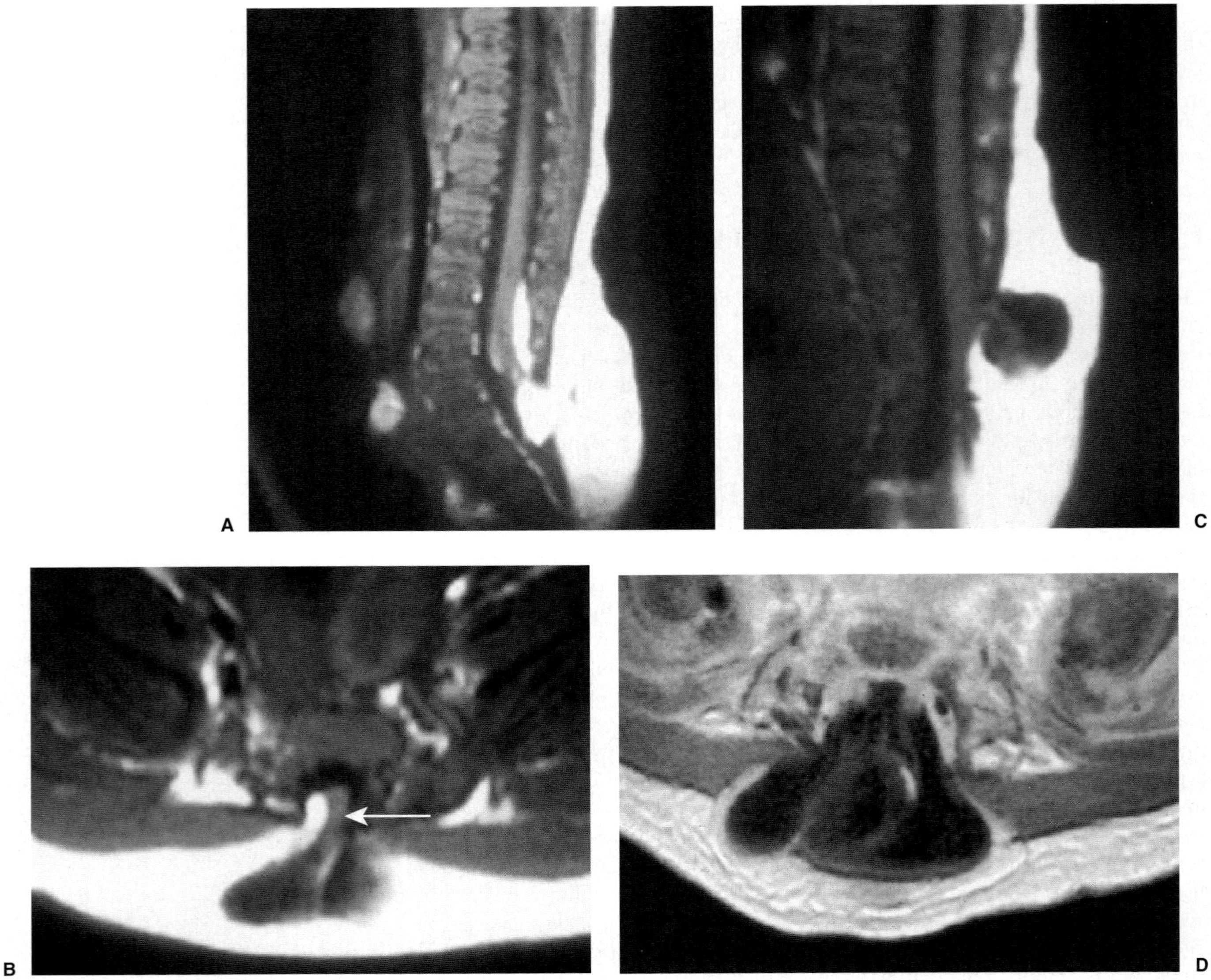

Figure 13.3 *Lipomyelomeningocele. A.* Sagittal T1-weighted image in a patient with a small lipomyelomeningocele shows extension of subcutaneous fat into the spinal canal through a posterior defect. The spinal cord is dysplastic and tethered at the level of the lipoma. *B.* Axial T1-weighted image in the same patient shows a small lipomyelomeningocele containing an obliquely oriented placode *(arrow)* adjacent to the fat. *C.* In a different patient, sagittal T1-weighted image shows a posterior meningocele containing a part of the tethered and dysplastic spinal cord that is contiguous with the subcutaneous fat. Nerve roots continue caudal to the defect, and the sacrum is dysplastic. *D.* In another patient, axial T1-weighted image shows a complex placode somewhat obliquely oriented and contiguous with the subcutaneous fat. Note meningocele projecting outward from the spina bifida defect.

Box 13.2 Associated Anomalies in Patients with Closed Spinal Dysraphism

- Spinal cord cysts
- Sacral hypogenesis
- Anorectal anomalies
- Lower genitourinary tract anomalies
- Epidermoids
- Dermal sinus tract
- Arachnoid cysts

A

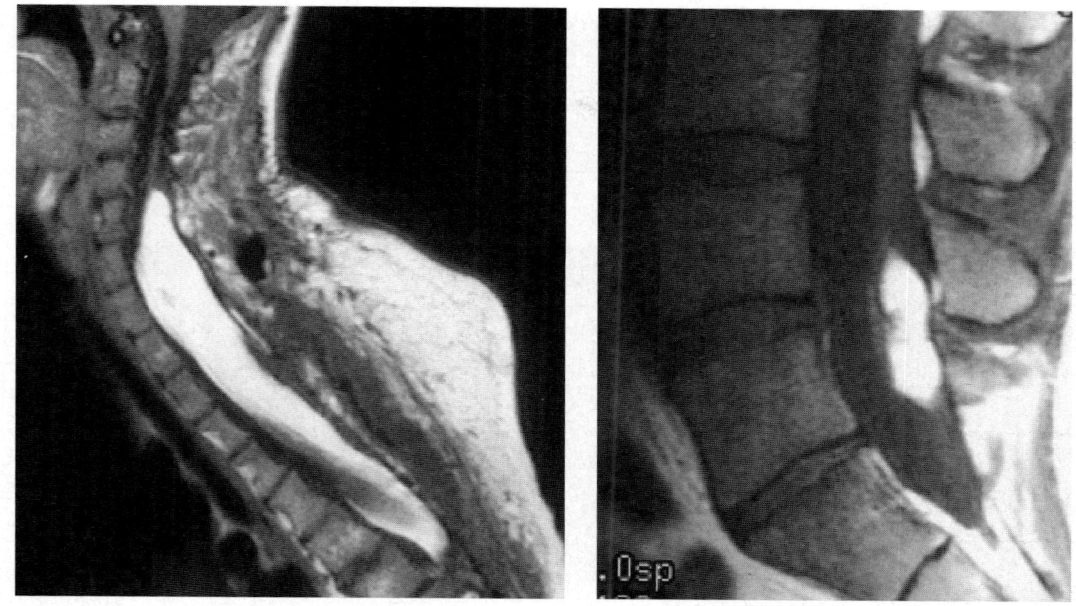

B

Figure 13.4 *Intraspinal Lipoma. A.* Sagittal T1-weighted image shows a large, bright lipoma in the cervicothoracic region compressing the spinal cord. This patient had undergone extensive posterior laminectomies in an unsuccessful attempt to resect the lipoma. *B.* In a different patient, sagittal T1-weighted image shows small, bright intraspinal lipoma at the L4 to L5 levels. Note dysplastic and tethered spinal cord terminating at the lipoma.

present during adolescence and early adulthood (10). Most patients with intraspinal lipomas present with a myelopathy. Intradural lipomas are found most commonly in the cervical region, followed by the thoracic spine, and are less common in the lumbar region (Fig. 13.4). As may be expected from their embryologic origin, most intraspinal lipomas lie dorsal to the spinal cord, but occasionally they may be lateral or even ventral in location (or in any combination). Chronic compression of the cord and its tethering by the lipoma may result in formation of an intramedullary cyst. In patients with large lipomas, the spinal canal may be enlarged, and although the vertebrae are normal in most patients, a spina bifida occulta may be found in some instances.

Unlike lipomyelomeningoceles and lipomyeloceles, which are more common in the lumbar region, isolated intraspinal lipomas are more common in the cervical region.

Dermal Sinus Tracts and Epidermoid/ Dermoid Tumors

As discussed earlier, an incomplete separation of the folding neural tube from the overlying ectoderm may result in the presence of a dermal-lined tract extending from the point of incomplete disjunction into the spinal canal (14). The tract usually continues superiorly and merges with the filum terminale, conus medullaris, or spinal cord. As the spinal cord experiences its normal differential growth with respect to the vertebral column, the tract ascends with the cord. At some point during this growth, the tract tethers the spinal cord. Based on the assumption that neural tube closure begins in the middle and occurs last in the most cephalad and caudal regions of the spine, the location of dermal sinus tracts may be easily explained—that is, most of these defects occur in the lumbosacral region, followed by the craniocervical junction. Approximately 50% to 70% of dermal sinus tracts extend into the spinal canal, and the rest end blindly (10). Dermal sinus tracts may be associated with epidermoid and dermoid tumors. These tumors are thought to arise from growth of trapped elements and may be classified as shown in Table 13.2.

Table 13.2: Contents of Epidermoid versus Dermoid

Epidermoid	*Dermoid*
Stratified squamous epithelium	Stratified squamous epithelium, sweat glands, sebaceous glands, hair follicles

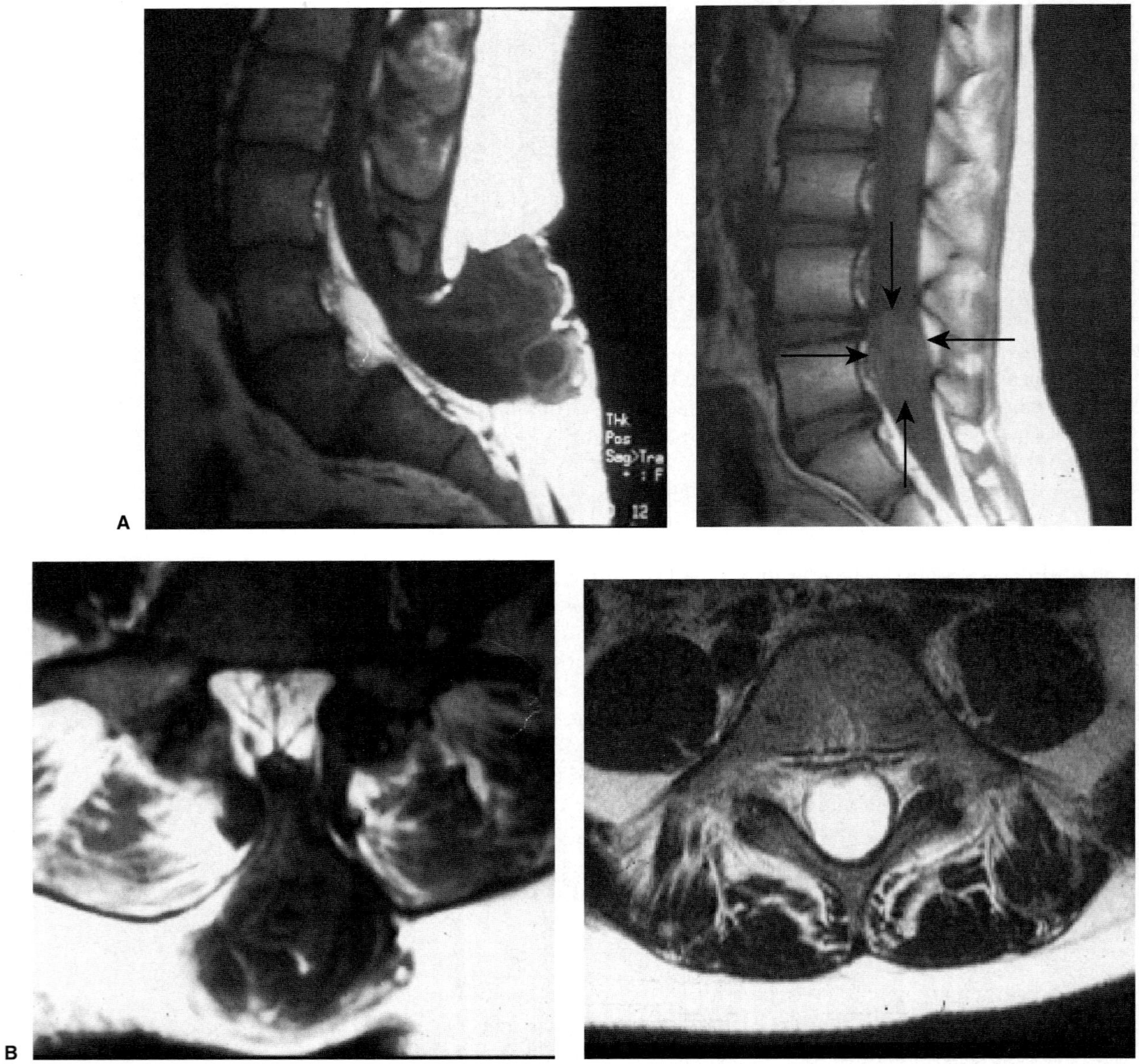

Figure 13.5 *Epidermoid. A.* Sagittal T1-weighted image shows subcutaneous epidermoid extending into the spinal canal through a spina bifida. The mass is not entirely cystic appearing but contains serpiginous areas of intermediate signal intensity. Note atrophic skin over the epidermoid and a thick filum terminale. *B.* Axial T1-weighted image in the same patient shows complex appearance of the epidermoid. *C.* In a different patient, sagittal T1-weighted image shows intraspinal epidermoid *(arrows)* at the L5 level that is slightly more intense than the cerebrospinal fluid (CSF). *D.* In the same patient, axial T2-weighted image through the epidermoid shows it to be as bright as CSF. Note that the nerve roots are compressed against the dural walls of the thecal sac.

Intraspinal epidermoids/dermoids may be congenital or acquired secondary to lumbar puncture or surgery.

Approximately 50% of dermal sinus tracts contain an epidermoid/dermoid. Conversely, approximately 30% of spinal epidermoid/dermoids are associated with a dermal sinus tract. Dermal sinus tracts usually manifest as a small opening in the skin. The opening usually is midline and located above the intergluteal fold (>2.5 cm above the anus) or below the occiput. These dimples are large (>5 mm in diameter) and usually have atrophic skin accompanied by tufts of hair, hemangioma, or the excrescence of caseous material. Defects located below the top of the intergluteal fold and slightly off midline probably are simple sacral dimples and are not associated with dermal sinus tracts. As the tract traverses the posterior vertebral bone elements, a spina bifida occulta is formed. Symptoms related to a dermal sinus tract include a myelopathy secondary to tethering of the spinal cord and septic or aseptic (due to rupture of an epidermoid/dermoid) meningitis (15). The goal of imaging is twofold: to identify the entire length of the tract and associated tumors, and to assess for the possibility of infection (including the presence of abscesses). Although contrast administration usually is not necessary for the evaluation of congenital spinal anomalies, I use it when a child is suspected of having dermal sinus tract. We usually mark the level of the skin opening with a vitamin E capsule. The tract is seen as a band of intermediate T1 and T2 signal intensity extending from the skin to the general region of the conus medullaris. Wide window settings are needed to visualize the tract and separate it from the adjacent bright fat. The conus medullaris may be abnormally low-lying (below the L2 to L3 level). If a mass is associated with a tract, it may be a lipoma, dermoid, or epidermoid. If the mass is of low T1 and high T2 signal intensity, the differential diagnosis is that of an epidermoid versus a dermoid (many dermoids in the spine do not have the typical brightness on T1 sequences that most intracranial dermoids do; Fig. 13.5). If the mass is fatty in appearance, the differential diagnosis is that of a lipoma versus a dermoid (Fig. 13.6). Epidermoids and dermoids do not enhance unless they are or have been previously infected. If peripheral enhancement is present, an abscess should be considered. Also, if the tract enhances, infection needs to be considered. Intraspinal epidermoids may be very difficult to identify because their signal characteristics may be similar to those of cerebrospinal fluid (CSF). Often, all that one can see is some slightly heterogenous signal intensity in the spinal canal at the level of the lesion.

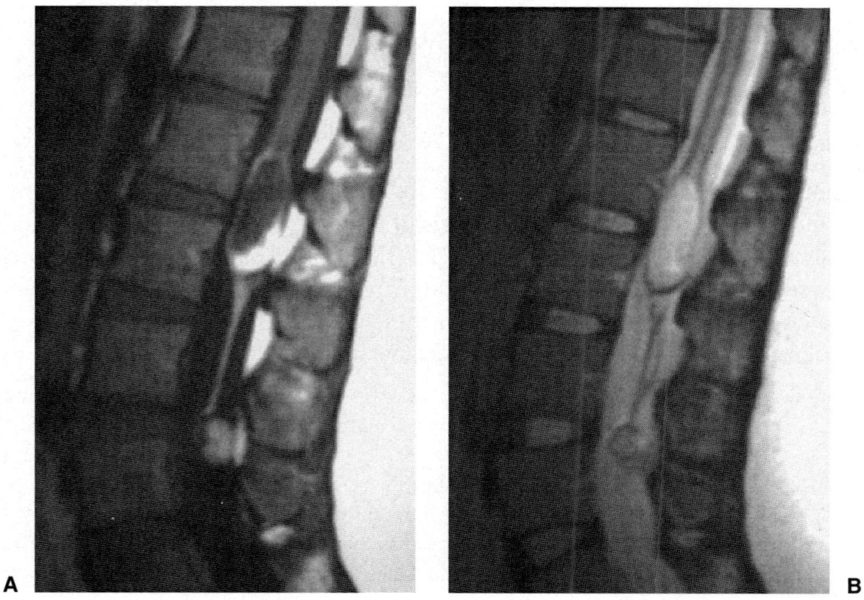

Figure 13.6 *Dermoid. A.* Sagittal T1-weighted image shows multifocal intraspinal dermoid involving the filum terminale and conus medullaris. Note that the signal from the dermoid is inhomogeneous, containing zones of high and low intensities. *B.* On a corresponding T2-weighted image, the masses are mostly bright.

Spinal epidermoids/dermoids also may occur in an isolated form (without a dermal sinus tract) (10). In this situation, they may be congenital or secondary to the iatrogenic introduction of skin elements and appendages by a needle (usually those without a stylet) used for a lumbar puncture or as a sequela of surgery. As such, most (>60%) isolated spinal epidermoid/dermoid tumors occur in the lumbar region. Their appearance is identical to that described for epidermoids/dermoids associated with dermal sinus tracts.

Last, I mention a newly recognized entity called *midline spinal hamartoma*, which I include here because in the past they have been mistaken for epidermoids/dermoids (16–18). These hamartomas usually affect the thoracic region and also may be accompanied by an overlying skin defect, a dermal sinus tract, and a spina bifida occulta. Most patients are asymptomatic and remain so for long periods. The lesions contain ectodermal, mesodermal, and neural elements and are not teratomas. They insinuate themselves into the spinal cord, are of similar signal intensity to the cord, do not enhance, and widen the spinal canal, and their borders are inseparable from the spinal cord (19). They occasionally produce symptoms by virtue of tethering or compressing the spinal cord. Surgery usually is performed to avoid tethering of the cord and its complications.

Caudal Regression Syndrome

Nearly one-third of patients with caudal regression syndrome are the offspring of diabetic mothers.

This is a spectrum of malformations that ranges from the clinically insignificant agenesis of the coccyx to a complete absence of the lower spine and lower limbs (sirenomyelia) (20). This group of disorders occurs equally in both boys and girls, unlike the other spinal dysraphisms, which are more common in girls. Many of these patients have a deletion located in chromosome 7, and caudal regression syndrome is seen with many systemic syndromes [e.g., OEIS, Potter's syndrome, and VACTERL (vertebral, anal, cardiac, tracheal, esophageal, renal, and limb deformities) syndrome]. All patients with the caudal regression syndrome have bowel and bladder problems as well as lower extremity weakness. Approximately one-third of patients with imperforate anus have some degree of the caudal regression syndrome. Overall, this syndrome represents a relatively rare malformation. The following are forms of caudal regression syndrome, from mild to severe:

- Agenesis of the coccyx
- Scimitar sacrum
- Sacral agenesis
- Lumbar or lower thoracic agenesis
- Sirenomyelia

Urinary anomalies such as ectopic, fused, or absent kidneys are not uncommon in patients with caudal regression syndrome. Agenesis of the coccyx may be an isolated and asymptomatic abnormality. In a scimitar sacrum, one-half of this bone is absent. Patients with scimitar sacrum present with difficulty walking, and the diagnosis is confirmed easily with plain radiographs. Scoliosis is common in these patients.

Vertebral column agenesis may occur at the various levels (10) (Table 13.3).

Table 13.3: Levels and Incidence of Caudal Regression Syndrome

Level	*Incidence*
T11–T12	35%
L1–L4	40%
Below L5	25%

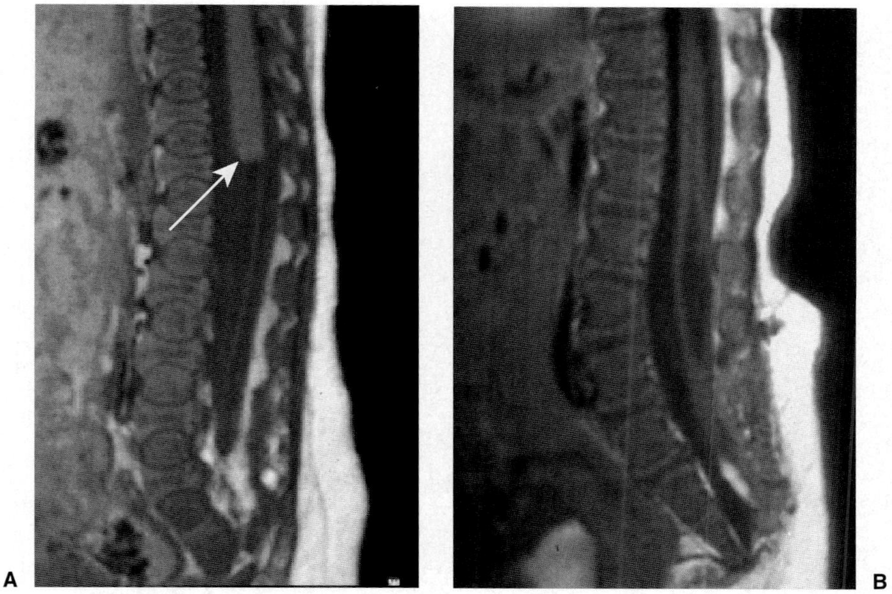

Figure 13.7 *Caudal Regression Syndrome. A.* Sagittal T1-weighted image in a patient with partial sacral agenesis shows a superiorly positioned truncated ("wedge shaped") conus medullaris *(arrow)* and a sparse cauda equina. *B.* In a different patient with distal sacral agenesis, sagittal T1-weighted image shows a dysplastic and tethered spinal cord terminating in a small intraspinal lipoma. The spinal cord contains a cyst.

Other anomalies seen in patients with caudal regression syndrome include spina bifida occulta (33%), segmentation anomalies of the vertebrae (20%), dermoid/epidermoid, and dermal sinus tracts. There are two types of caudal regression anomalies of interest to radiologists. In most patients with sacral agenesis, the tip of the conus medullaris is absent, and the distal cord assumes a "truncated" or wedge-shaped appearance on sagittal MRI (4) (Fig. 13.7A). This dysplastic cord usually terminates approximately at the L1 level. The cauda equina has a "sparse" appearance because many of the distal lumbar and sacral nerve roots do not form. In a smaller percentage of patients with sacral agenesis, the dysplastic cord extends down to the level of the agenesis and may be tethered by a distal lipoma (20,21) (Fig. 13.7B). In these patients, the sacral agenesis usually is below the S2 level, and the tethered cord may contain a cyst.

FILAR LIPOMA

The filum terminale normally is a pial-ependymal strand that extends from the tip of the conus medullaris to the coccyx. In its first few centimeters, it contains glial elements (explaining why astrocytomas and ependymomas may arise at this level). The presence of fat in the filum terminale may be explained by abnormal retrogressive differentiation of the pluripotential cells found in the distal caudal mass. The diameter of the normal filum terminale is 1 to 2 mm (my rule of thumb is that it normally is approximately the same size as or smaller than one of the adjacent nerve roots). Incidental lipomas of the filum terminale are found in approximately 5% of MRI examinations of the lumbar spine (10). Incidental filar lipomas are clearly separable from the adjacent nerve roots, and more important in these patients is the fact that the conus medullaris terminates at a normal level (above L2). Most incidental filar lipomas follow the expected location of the filum, but occasionally the fatty filum may be located centrally or in anterior aspects of the spinal canal. If the lipoma is thick, some patients may be

Rule of thumb: the diameter of the normal filum terminale should be no greater than that of the neighboring nerve roots.

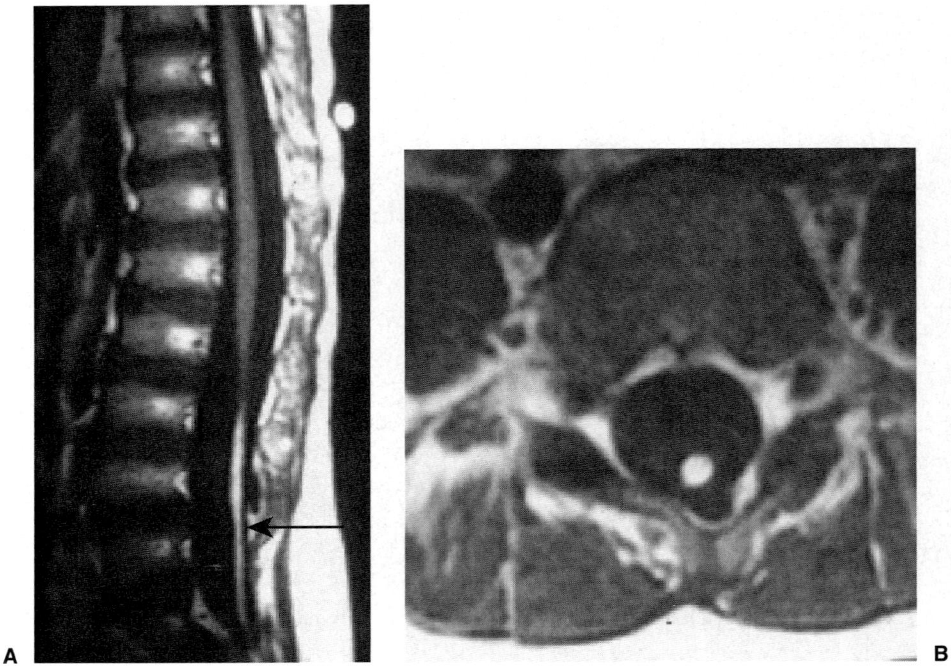

Figure 13.8 *Filar Lipoma. A.* Sagittal T1-weighted image shows a thick filar lipoma *(arrow)* and a conus medullaris located at a borderline position (L1 to L2 space). *B.* In the same patient, axial T1-weighted image shows a distal fatty filum that is much thicker than the adjacent nerve roots.

symptomatic and require a surgical division of it. In these patients, it is thought that the filar lipoma may cause tethering of the cord (Fig. 13.8). If the conus medullaris is low-lying and the patient is symptomatic, regardless of the width of the filar lipoma, surgical division is performed.

Ventriculus Terminalis (Ventriculus Terminus)

A terminal ventricle is a cavity located in the conus medullaris that may represent residual cavitation of the caudal cell mass (22). Others believe that it represents a dilated distal central spinal canal (this probably is correct because many of these ventricles are lined by ependyma). These fluid-containing spaces are found more commonly in premature than in term infants. A terminal ventricle is found in approximately 2% to 6% of spinal MRI studies obtained in infants, and commonly is seen in spinal sonograms (23) (Fig. 13.9). Most small cysts disappear with age. Like many of the spinal dysraphisms, the ventriculus terminus is more common in girls. This malformation nearly always is asymptomatic and incidentally found. Occasionally, the cyst may behave like a true hydromyelia and produce symptoms that include recurrent low back pain, sciatica, and bowel/bladder problems. The symptoms may manifest at any time in the patient's life. Regardless of its true nature, if the cyst is producing symptoms, its surgical decompression may be indicated. A terminal ventricle varies in shape (ovoid to oblong) and size (1 to 4 cm in length). Its walls may be thick or imperceptible. There is no contrast enhancement, and most of these anomalies remain stable in size and configuration on repeat MRI studies (24).

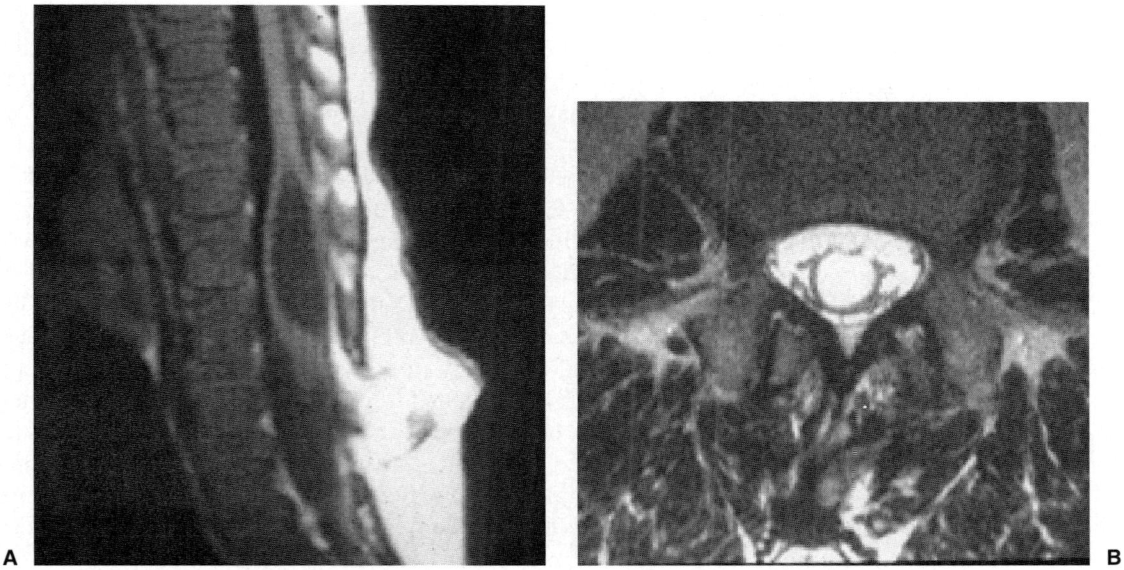

Figure 13.9 *Terminal Ventricle. A.* Sagittal T1-weighted image shows a large ventriculus terminus expanding a conus medullaris that is perhaps in a low position. *B.* In a different patient, axial T2-weighted image shows expansion of the distal conus medullaris by a presumed ventriculus terminus.

Tight Filum Terminale Syndrome

The tight filum terminale or short filum syndrome is characterized by a low-lying conus medullaris and a thick filum (25) (Fig. 13.10). Many patients are asymptomatic and remain so for their entire life. However, other patients become symptomatic early in life. Symptoms include back pain, bowel/bladder problems, lower extremity weakness and deformities, and spine deformities such as scoliosis and spina bifida occulta. The etiology for this controversial syndrome probably is an incomplete retrogressive differentiation resulting in a thick filum. This thick filum tethers the spinal cord and probably produces symptoms by virtue of stretching it and inducing ischemia (many patients are sympto-

In patients with tight filum terminale syndrome, prone MRI studies show that the conus does not move (Witkamp TD, Vandertop WP, Beek FJA, et al. Medullary cone movement in subjects with a normal spinal cord and in patients with a tethered spinal cord. Radiology 2001;220: 208–212).

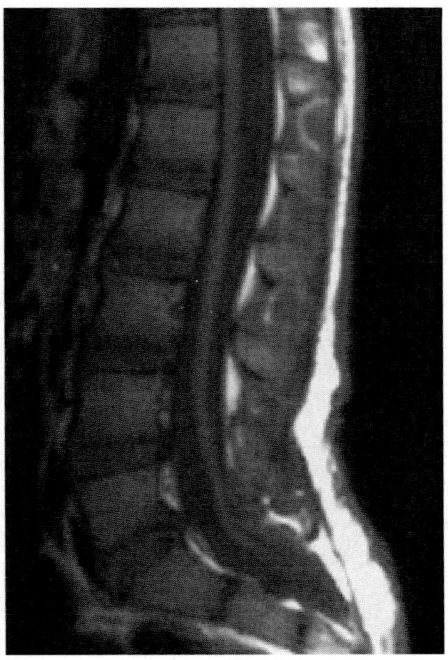

Figure 13.10 *Tight Filum Terminale Syndrome.* Sagittal T1-weighted image shows a thick filum terminale ending at the level of a spina bifida occulta. Note that the cord is dysplastic and a conus medullaris is not clearly identifiable.

matic only when flexing their spine) (26). Many symptomatic patients show increased signal intensity in the spinal cord in the region of the central canal, particularly at the level of the conus medullaris. This focal hyperintensity may be due to small cysts or myelomalacia. The conus medullaris always is low-lying and dysplastic. In many patients, it is difficult to see clearly where it ends. The filum is thick (>2 mm in diameter) and is seen clearly extending to the end of the thecal sac (Fig. 13.10). The filum may contain a lipoma (focal or generalized). The distal spinal canal may be slightly wide, especially if there is associated spina bifida occulta. Phase contrast MRI studies have been used in an attempt to visualize cord motion (the conus moves with heart pulsations if it is not tethered) in these patients. I have been disappointed with results of these studies and no longer use them. The patient may be placed prone in the magnet and if the conus does not move anteriorly, tethering may be suspected. In my opinion, it is the patient's symptoms that dictate his or her clinical management. If the patient is symptomatic, surgical division of the thick filum may be indicated. Although surgeons usually indicate that on sectioning the filum terminale, the conus "springs back" to a normal position, this usually is not evident on follow-up studies, which usually show the conus to be in the same position as before surgery. Because the cord is no longer tethered, the symptoms stabilize or improve. The success of the treatment needs to be judged on a clinical basis and not on the MRI results.

Anterior Sacral Meningocele

In these rare anomalies, a diverticulum (or sac) of dura herniates into the pelvis through a defect in the sacrum or coccyx. Both genders are affected equally, and most anterior sacral meningoceles are found either in infants or later in life, during the second and third decades. In both age groups, anterior sacral meningoceles present with a mass effect on the pelvic organs and low back pain. Compression of the nerve roots may result in sciatica. A very rare symptom is that of "shifting" headaches due to the sudden influx or egress of CSF from the sac into or out of the subarachnoid space. Anterior sacral meningoceles are associated with neurofibromatosis type 1, Marfan's syndrome, lower scoliosis, and distal genitourinary and anorectal anomalies (10). MRI is the best method to evaluate these malformations. Before ligation and decompression of the sac, the course of the nerve roots

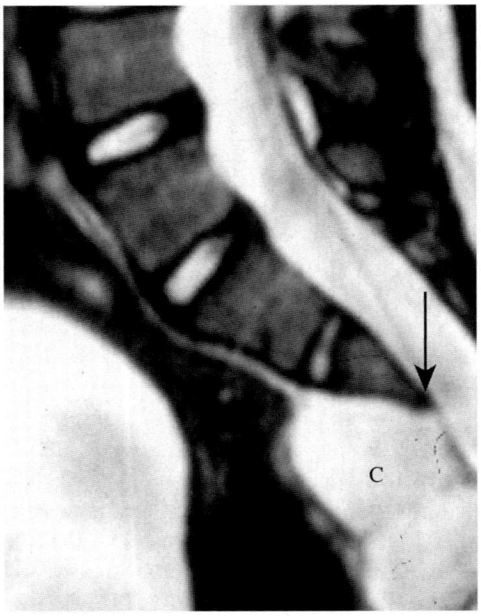

Figure 13.11 *Anterior Sacral Meningocele.* Sagittal T2-weighted image shows erosion *(arrow)* of the sacrum by a cystic mass *(C)* that is contiguous with the cerebrospinal fluid in the distal thecal sac.

needs to be established. Soft tissue strands inside the sac may be due to either nerve roots or pial septations. MRI clearly shows the neck of the malformation at the point of its communication with the spinal canal (Fig. 13.11). In some patients with anterior sacral meningoceles, the spinal cord may be low-lying. Obviously, this has surgical implications and needs to be assessed in patients before repair.

Sacrococcygeal Teratoma

Sacrococcygeal teratomas are very rare masses thought to arise from faulty development of the pluripotential cells in the distal cell mass. These teratomas may present as masses protruding through the back of the patient, as intrasacral/intraspinal masses, or as masses projecting into the pelvis. Approximately 75% of them are benign mature teratomas, whereas the rest contain immature and potentially malignant cells (10). A familiar form of sacrococcygeal teratoma is associated with distal spinal bone malformations and a low-lying spinal cord. These are familial, inherited as an autosomal dominant trait, and more common in girls. A classification of sacrococcygeal teratomas is given in Table 13.4.

Well differentiated tissues (fat, calcium) usually are found in mature teratomas, whereas immature teratomas have a more homogeneous appearance on imaging studies.

Extension of the tumor into the spinal canal is seen in less than 5% of cases (27). Both the sporadic and familial sacrococcygeal teratomas have an identical appearance by imaging. MRI is the imaging method of choice in these patient, although computed tomography (CT) is helpful in evaluation of the bones and establishing the presence of intratumoral calcifications. Sacrococcygeal teratomas are highly heterogenous in appearance (Fig. 13.12). Mature teratomas contain cysts, calcifications, and areas of fat. Approximately 5% of them are purely cystic in appearance. Immature teratomas have a more homogeneous and solid nature. In both types of teratomas, the solid components show contrast enhancement.

Terminal Myelocystocele

In my experience, terminal myelocystocele is perhaps the least common of the lesions related to abnormal canalization and retrogressive differentiation. In these cases, there is a wide spina bifida and a low-lying tethered cord. The cord has a distal and, at times, massively dilated syrinx that protrudes either posteriorly, inferiorly, or anteriorly through a bone defect. These anomalies (like all other ones due to abnormal canalization and retrogressive differentiation) can be considered "occult" because they are covered by skin (10). The patients, however, have a mass in their back. As with all other anomalies of this type, associated distal genitourinary and anorectal malformations are common. Imaging studies show a cystic mass arising in the distal spine. On sagittal views, the posterior wall of the mass is formed by the posterior aspect of the distended spinal cord. The fluid-filled center of the mass is a hydromyelia or syringomyelia. The ventral aspect of the mass is the anterior aspect of the spinal cord. Superior to the cystic mass, the spinal subarachnoid spaces may be wide and contain a tethered cord that also may harbor cysts.

Table 13.4: Types of Sacrococcygeal Teratomas

Type	*Incidence*	*Location*
1	47%	Posterior
2	35%	Posterior with extension into the pelvis
3	8%	Mainly in pelvis and abdomen
4	10%	Entirely presacral

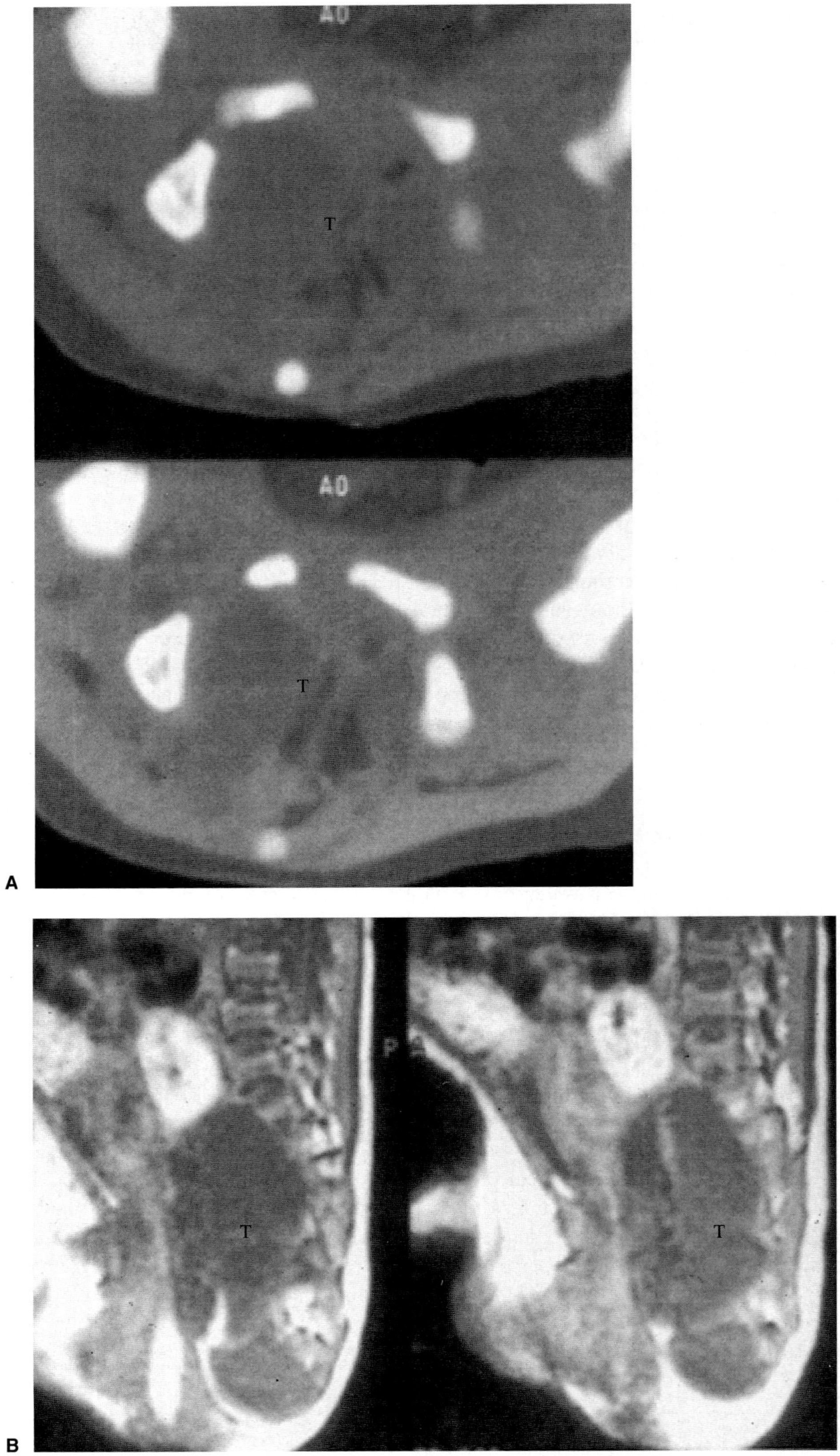

Figure 13.12 *Sacrococcygeal Teratoma. A.* Axial contiguous computed tomography sections show expansion of the distal sacrum by a complex mass *(T)* containing zones of soft tissue and fat. *B.* In a different patient, sagittal T1-weighted images show complex mass *(T)* located anterior to the sacrum.

Split Cord and Notochord Syndromes

This group of malformations includes those listed in Table 13.5 (3).

Table 13.5: Spinal Malformations Related to the Split Notochord and Split Cord Syndrome

Type	*Incidence*
Diastematomyelia	Relatively common
Diplomyelia	Very rare
Dorsal enteric sinus	Very rare
Dorsal enteric diverticulum	Extremely rare
Dorsal enteric fistula	Extremely rare

Split Spinal Cord Syndrome

Diastematomyelia may be isolated or found in patients with scoliosis and open spinal dysraphisms.

The term *diastema* refers to a space or cleft (28). In diastematomyelia, the spinal cord, the conus medullaris, or the filum terminale may be split in half. Each half is termed a *hemicord* and contains one set of anterior and posterior nerves. These hemicords each contain a central canal and often are asymmetric in size. This anomaly may be classified as a split cord syndrome. Diastematomyelia is found in approximately 5% of patients with scoliosis and in 30% to 45% of patients with open spinal dysraphisms (28). Approximately 50% of diastemata are found in the lumbar region, and the other 50% in the thoracic spine. Cervical diastemata are extremely rare and often associated with the Chiari type 2 malformation or Klippel-Feil syndrome. The possible etiology for diastematomyelia is persistence of one or more neuroenteric canals (primitive communications between the amniotic cavity and the yolk sac) or adhesions traversing the bilaminar germ cell disk that contains the notochord in its center (3). If the notochord is split, it induces the formation of two hemicords and results in vertebral body anomalies such as butterfly vertebrae (which commonly are associated with diastematomyelia). The persistence of primitive neuroenteric canals (termed the *canals of Kovalevsky*) or of adhesions induces the formation of mesodermal tissues. Although diastematomyelia is considered an "occult" defect because it is covered by skin, the overlying skin usually is abnormal and harbors a hemangioma, hairy patch, nevus, lipoma, or dimple (one of these anomalies is present in nearly 75% of such patients). Diastematomyelia is more common in girls. The most common presentation is deformity of the feet and lower extremity weakness. Most diastemata present during periods of growth spurts. Anomalies of vertebral segmentation are present in approximately 85% of patients, and scoliosis in over 50%. There are two types of diastematomyelia (Table 13.6).

In the external type of diastematomyelia, the hemicords are separated by a bar that may be composed of bone, cartilage, fat, or connective tissues (Fig. 13.13A–C). Identification of this bar is very important. This bar often tethers the spinal cord and needs to be surgically resected. The bar splits the dura into two sheaths (i.e., each hemicord is contained in its own dural sheath) (29). Constant traction on the spinal cord by the bar results in an ischemic myelopathy and symptoms. The bar usually extends from the posterior elements to the back of a vertebral body. The involved vertebra is deformed. The bar may traverse the entire width of the spinal canal or only a portion of it (complete versus incom-

Table 13.6: Types of Diastematomyelia

Type	*Incidence*	*Characteristics*
External	50%	Hemicords separated by a bar
Internal	50%	Hemicords without a bar

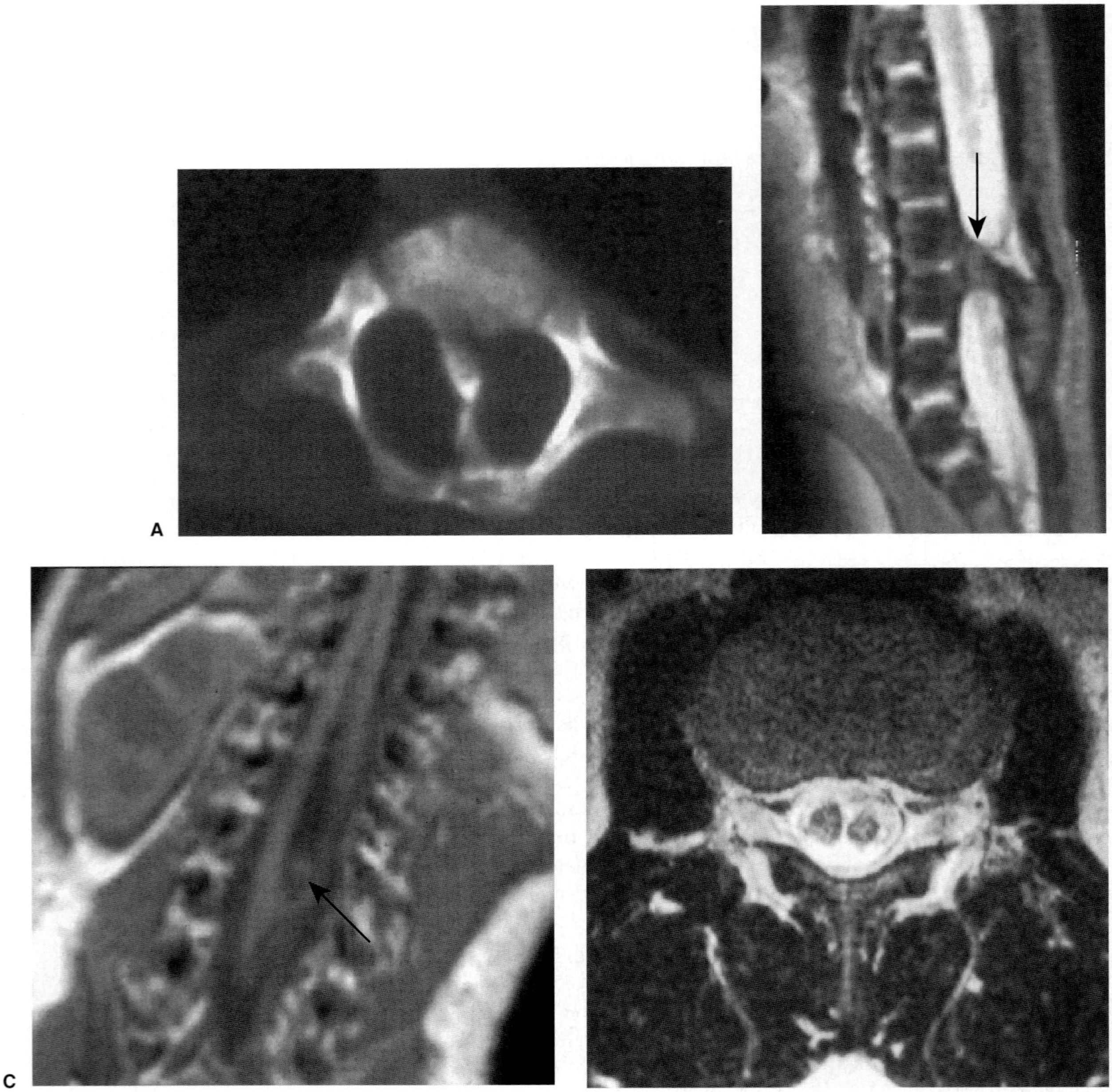

Figure 13.13 *Diastematomyelia. A.* Axial computed tomography shows a thick bone bar splitting the distal thoracic spinal canal into two nearly symmetric halves. *B.* Sagittal T1-weighted image (different patient) shows a midline thick bone bar *(arrow)* traversing the lumbar spinal canal. *C.* Coronal T1-weighted image (different patient) shows a diastema *(arrow)* that is isointense to the cord. Note that after splitting, the spinal cord reunites inferiorly. *D.* Axial T2-weighted image shows the internal type of diastematomyelia, in which the spinal cord is spilt into halves in the absence of a bar.

plete spur). Multiple spurs are rare and occur in less than 5% of patients with diastematomyelia. The spinal cord splits and reunites inferior to the spur in most patients. The spinal cord is low-lying and located below the L2 level in approximately 75% of cases (30). The filum terminale is thick in over half the cases.

In patients with the internal type of diastematomyelia, there is no spur (Fig. 13.13D). The hemicords lie close together, are asymmetric in size, and are contained in a single dural sheath. The cord splitting may be complete (traversing the cord) or incomplete (fissure-like). The most important MRI sequence to obtain when evaluating all patients with diastematomyelia is that of gradient-echo T2-weighted images. The purpose of this is to turn the CSF white and take advantage of a sequence that is sensitive to the magnetic susceptibility effects produced by the mesodermal tissues in the spur against the bright background of the CSF. Despite this, some thin spurs may be missed, and many neurosurgeons still prefer a conventional and CT myelogram before deciding if surgery is indicated. Both types of diastemata are associated with spinal cord cysts (31).

A very rare variation of the split cord syndrome is that of diplomyelia (32,33). In this syndrome, the spinal cord is entirely duplicated: Each half contains both sets of ventral and dorsal nerve roots, complete duplication of the gray matter horns, and a central spinal canal. In these patients, the dural sac and vertebral column also are duplicated.

Split Notochord Syndrome

The dorsal enteric fistula is the least severe anomaly pertaining to the split notochord syndrome. A persistent communication between the yolk sac and the amniotic cavity is produced by a canal that extends from the gastrointestinal tract and crosses the spine and the spinal cord (3). If this communication is in the form of tract that either ends blindly or opens into the skin of the back, it is termed a *fistula* (34). A part (or all) of this tract may contain cysts that are lined by enteric tissues. When this occurs, a dorsal enteric cyst is formed. These cysts most often are located anterior to the spinal cord and in the cervical and thoracic regions (Fig. 13.14). The cysts lie in the subarachnoid space and compress the spinal cord, often resulting in a myelopathy. They are smooth and unilocular and contain highly proteinaceous fluid that produces high signal intensity on T1-weighted images, low T2 signal intensity, and hyperdensity on CT. The spinal canal often is wide at the level of the cyst (10). Occasionally, the cyst may be located posterior to the spinal cord or in the paraspinal regions. A very rare variation of these anomalies is that of the dorsal enteric diverticulum. The diverticulum arises from the mesentery and often contains small or large bowel in it. A common denominator in all of the spilt notochord malformations is

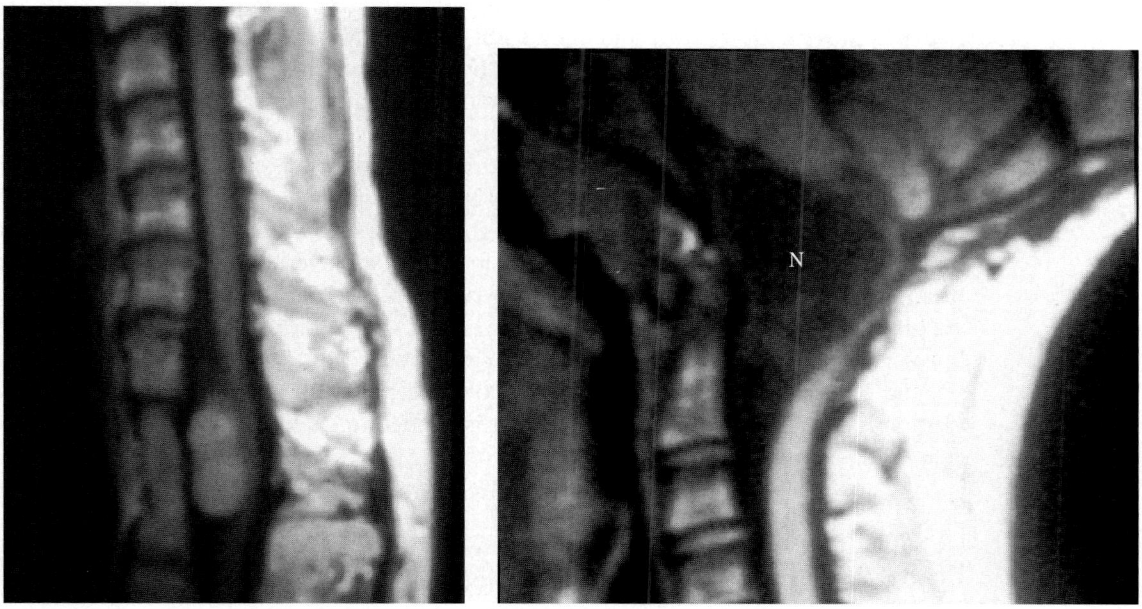

A B

Figure 13.14 *Neuroenteric Cyst. A.* Sagittal T1-weighted image shows a hyperintense neuroenteric cyst located in the ventral subarachnoid space in the cervicothoracic region. The cyst has a mass effect on the spinal cord. Note dysplastic vertebrae at the level of the cyst. *B.* In a different patient, sagittal T1-weighted image shows hypointense and multiseptate neuroenteric cyst *(N)* in the ventral perimedullary cistern resulting in significant mass effect on the brainstem.

that of severe vertebral body anomalies that usually are located at or slightly inferior to the site of the neuroenteric communication.

Scoliosis

Congenital scoliosis is common and, if not idiopathic, may be due to the following anomalies:

- Unilateral unsegmented bar
- Hemivertebra(e)
- Butterfly vertebra(e)
- Agenesis of a vertebra(e)
- Hypoplasia of the posterior arch
- Muscle imbalance due to underlying spinal dysraphism
- Block vertebrae

Scoliosis refers to a lateral spinal curvature, whereas kyphosis refers to an anterior curvature. In reality, most curvatures are a combination of both. Lordosis refers to a straightening of the vertebral column (it nearly always is muscular in nature, but occasionally it is due to fusion of the posterior elements). In cases of congenital or developmental scoliosis, an underlying reason usually is not found (35). Idiopathic scoliosis affects approximately 5% of the population. From a clinical standpoint, idiopathic scoliosis may be divided into three types (Table 13.7).

Like all congenital spinal deformities, scoliosis is more common in girls. It may be familial, and the parents and siblings also may be affected. When an underlying lesion is present, it is most likely in the form of a hemivertebra or wedge vertebra, or a segmentation anomaly. Segmentation anomalies resulting in scoliosis may be unilateral (unilateral unsegmented bar), anterior (anterior unsegmented bar), or posterior (laminar and facetal synostosis). When multiple anomalies are present, a hereditary factor usually is involved, whereas most solitary anomalies are sporadic. Scoliosis and kyphosis are also more common in girls. The earlier they become clinically evident, the worse their prognosis is. Progressive curvatures develop in over 85% of patients with congenital kyphoscoliosis (particularly those with juvenile and adolescent forms of the disease). In most patients with scoliosis, the primary curve is located in the lower thoracic region, with secondary and compensatory curvatures in the upper thoracic and lumbar regions (Fig 13.15). The most common symptom is back pain. Surgical fixation prevents the progression of the curvature but has minimal effects on axial growth. Evaluation of patients with scoliosis requires the use of radiographs and MRI (36). Radiographs are helpful in assessing the degree of the initial curvature and its progression. Using the Cobb method, one line is drawn tangent to the upper border of the most cephalad vertebra involved in the curvature. A similar line is drawn along the inferior border of the caudalmost vertebra. Lines are drawn perpendicular to the first two lines, and the inferior angle (between the second lines) is measured. An angle over 10 degrees is needed to make the diagnosis of scoliosis, and progression of this angle beyond 50 degrees indicates the need for surgical intervention. Before surgery is performed, MRI is needed to exclude the possibility of a tethered cord.

Table 13.7: Types of Idiopathic Scoliosis

Type	*Age*	*Incidence*
Infantile	0–3 yr	<10%
Juvenile	4–9 yr	12%–20%
Adolescent	>10 yr	70%–80%

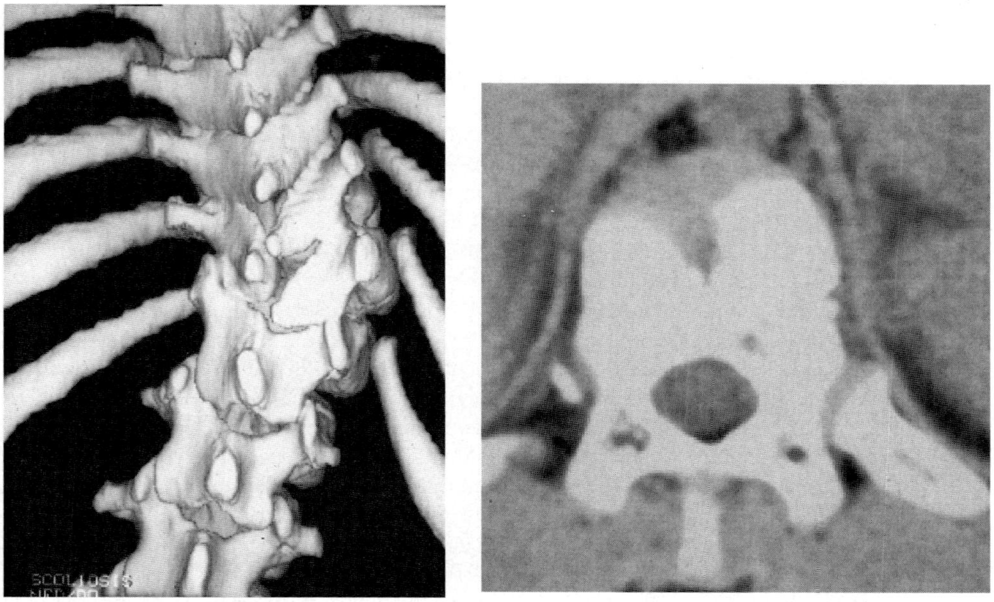

A B

Figure 13.15 *Scoliosis. A.* Posterior view of three-dimensional computed tomography (CT) reformation in a patient with scoliosis and a primary curve centered at the thoracolumbar region shows a T11 hemivertebra that is fused with T10 ("lateral unsegmented bar"). *B.* Axial CT shows midline defect in a butterfly-type vertebra.

References

1. Larsen WJ. Human embryology, 2nd ed. New York: Churchill Livingston, 1997:33–72.
2. Russ PD, Pretorius DH, Manco-Johnson ML, et al. The fetal spine. Neuroradiology 1986;28: 398–407.
3. Pang D, Dias MS, Ahab-Barmada M. Split cord malformation: part I. a unified theory of embryogenesis for double spinal cord malformations. Neurosurgery 1992;31:451–480.
4. Barkovich AJ, Raghavan N, Chuang S, et al. The wedge-shaped cord terminus: a radiographic sign of caudal regression. AJNR Am J Neuroradiol 1989;10:1223–1231.
5. Sze G, Baierl P, Brave S. Evolution of the infant spinal column: evaluation with MR imaging. Radiology 1991;181:819–827.
6. Sze G, Bravo S, Baierl P, et al. Developing spinal column: gadolinium-enhanced MR imaging. Radiology 1991;180:497–502.
7. Centers for Disease Control and Prevention. Recommendations for use of folic acid to reduce number of spina bifida cases and other neural tube defects. JAMA 1993;269:1233.
8. Nelson MD Jr, Bracchi M, Naidich TP, et al. The natural history of repaired myelomeningocele. Radiographics 1988;8:695–706.
9. Altman NR, Altman DH. MR imaging of spinal dysraphism. AJNR Am J Neuroradiol 1987;8: 533–538.
10. Barkovich AJ. Pediatric neuroimaging, 3rd ed. Philadelphia: Lippincott Williams & Wilkins, 2000:621–714.
11. Kriss VM, Desai NS. Occult spinal dysraphism in neonates: assessment of high-risk cutaneous stigmata on sonography. AJR Am J Roentgenol 1998;171:1687–1692.
12. Long FR, Hunter JV, Mahboubi S, et al. Tethered cord and associated vertebral anomalies in children and infants with imperforate anus: evaluation with MR imaging and plain radiography. Radiology 1996;200:377–382.
13. Appignani BA, Jaramillo D, Barnes PD, et al. Dysraphic myelodysplasias associated with urogenital and anorectal anomalies: prevalence and types seen with MR imaging. AJR Am J Roentgenol 1994;163:1199–1203.
14. Barkovich AJ, Edwards MS, Cogen PH. MR evaluation of spinal dermal sinus tracts in children. AJNR Am J Neuroradiol 1991;12:123–129.
15. Dev R, Husain M, Gupta A, et al. MR of multiple intraspinal abscesses associated with congenital dermal sinus. AJNR Am J Neuroradiol 1997;18:742–743.

16. Tibbs PA, James HE, Rorke LB, et al. Midline hamartomas masquerading as meningomyeloceles or teratomas in the newborn infant. J Pediatr 1976;89:928–933.
17. Morris GF, Murphy K, Rorke LB, et al. Spinal hamartomas: a distinct clinical entity. J Neurosurg 1998;88:954–961.
18. Tortori-Donati P, Fondelli MP, Rossi A, et al. MRI in an unusual case of congenital spinal mesenchymal proliferation. Neuroradiology 1996;38:S196–S199.
19. Castillo M, Smith MM, Armao D. Midline spinal cord hamartomas: MR imaging features of two patients. AJNR Am J Neuroradiol 1999;20:1169–1171.
20. Nievelstein RA, Valk J, Smit LM, et al. MR of the caudal-regression syndrome: embryologic implications. AJNR Am J Neuroradiol 1994;15:1021–1029.
21. Brooks BS, El Gammal T, Hartlage P, et al. Myelography of sacral agenesis. AJNR Am J Neuroradiol 1981;2:319–323.
22. Kriss VM, Kriss TC, Babcock DS. The ventriculus terminalis of the spinal cord in the neonate: a normal variant of sonography. AJR Am J Roentgenol 1995;165:1491–1493.
23. Coleman LT, Zimmerman RA, Rorke LB. Ventriculus terminalis of the conus medullaris: MR findings in children. AJNR Am J Neuroradiol 1995;16:1421–1426.
24. Sigal R, Denys A, Halimi P, et al. Ventriculus terminalis of the conus medullaris: MR imaging in four patients with congenital dilatation. AJNR Am J Neuroradiol 1991;12:733–737.
25. Baldwin HZ, Rekate HL, Sonntag VKH. Diagnosis, surgical management, and outcome of the adult tethered cord syndrome. BNI Q 1991;7:16–22.
26. Sarwar M, Virapongse C, Bhimani S. Primary tethered cord syndrome: a new hypothesis of its origin. AJNR Am J Neuroradiol 1984;5:235–242.
27. Smoker WR, Biller J, Moore SA, et al. Intradural spinal teratoma: case report and review of the literature. AJNR Am J Neuroradiol 1986;7:905–910.
28. Castillo M. MRI of diastematomyelia. MRI Decis 1991;5:12–16.
29. Naidich TP, Harwood-Nash DC. Diastematomyelia: hemicord and meningeal sheaths; single and double arachnoid and dural tubes. AJNR Am J Neuroradiol 1983;4:633–636.
30. Han JS, Benson JE, Kaufman B, et al. Demonstration of diastematomyelia and associated abnormalities with MR imaging. AJNR Am J Neuroradiol 1985;6:215–219.
31. Schlesinger AE, Naidich TP, Quencer RM. Concurrent hydromyelia and diastematomyelia. AJNR Am J Neuroradiol 1986;7:473–477.
32. Castillo M, Hankins L, Kramer L, et al. MR imaging of diplomyelia. Magn Reson Imaging 1992; 10:699–703.
33. Kelly A, Towbin R, Kaufman R, et al. Spine duplication. Spine 1985;10:15–18.
34. Hoffman CH, Dietrich RB, Pais MJ, et al. The split notchcord syndrome with dorsal enteric fistula. AJNR Am J Neuroradiol 1993;14:622–627.
35. Barnes PD, Brody JD, Jaramillo D, et al. Atypical idiopathic scoliosis: MR imaging evaluation. Radiology 1993;186:247–253.
36. Nokes SR, Murtagh FR, Jones JD III, et al. Childhood scoliosis: MR imaging. Radiology 1987; 164:791–797.

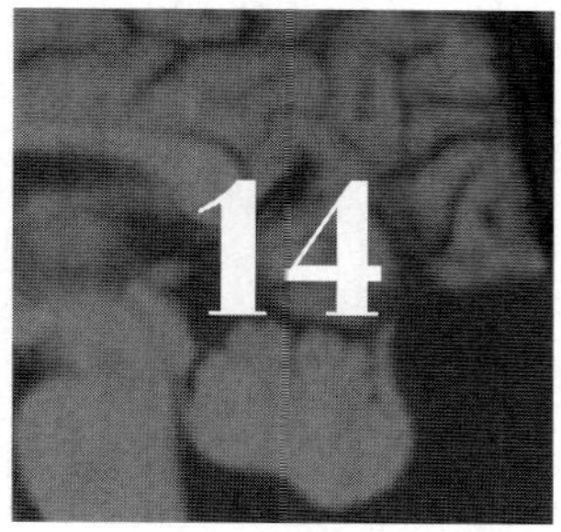

Spinal Trauma

- Current Concepts in the Diagnostic Evaluation of Spinal Trauma
- Specific Types of Spinal Injury

Current Concepts in the Diagnostic Evaluation of Spinal Trauma

Although radiographs and computed tomography (CT) continue to be of importance in the initial evaluation of spine trauma, magnetic resonance imaging (MRI) is gaining acceptance and is considered indispensable in many situations (1–15). At my hospital, all patients who have significant spine trauma with nondiagnostic radiographs or those who cannot have a complete physical examination are studied with CT. We initially obtain CT of the cervical spine in all patients who arrive to the emergency department with their head immobilized. This obviates the need for radiographs that are difficult to obtain and often nondiagnostic. If the CT is negative and there are no neurologic symptoms, no more studies are done. If CT is negative but neurologic symptoms are present, MRI is obtained. If radiography or CT shows a lesion in the absence of neurologic symptoms, MRI usually is not performed. Our CT protocol includes 2-mm spiral sections (pitch = 1) extending from the base of skull to the T1 vertebra. Sagittal reformations are performed in all patients. If needed, a focused additional study with 1-mm axial images is done. Our MRI protocol for the acutely injured spine includes sagittal T1-weighted images, fast spin-echo (FSE) T2-weighted images, fat-saturated T2-weighted images, and axial T1- and gradient-recalled echo (GRE or T2*) T2-weighted images. No contrast administration is needed. The sagittal FSE T2 images have high resolution but are less sensitive to susceptibility effects from blood than other T2 sequences. For this reason, the axial T2 images are obtained using a low flip angle gradient technique that is sensitive to susceptibility effects, making acute hemorrhage easier to see. Fat-saturated T2 images enhance the visibility of ligament and soft tissue injuries (14). Areas of edema in paraspinal soft tissue are seen clearly using this sequence.

Evaluation of Ligaments

Fat-suppressed T2-weighted images are best for evaluation of the posterior ligamentous complex, including the capsular ligaments.

Unlike CT, MRI permits visualization of the ligaments. In many cases, torn ligaments create instability and indicate the need for internal fixation (15–18) (Fig. 14.1).In the past, ligamentous injury only could be inferred from bone malalignment or abnormal mobility on flexion or extension radiographs. These techniques are not optimal because malalignment may be reduced by the time imaging is performed, and muscle spasm may limit abnormal mobility acutely (15). Important spinal ligaments that can be routinely assessed on MRI include the anterior longitudinal ligament (ALL), the posterior longitudinal ligament (PLL), and the posterior ligament complex (PLC). The PLC is composed of the

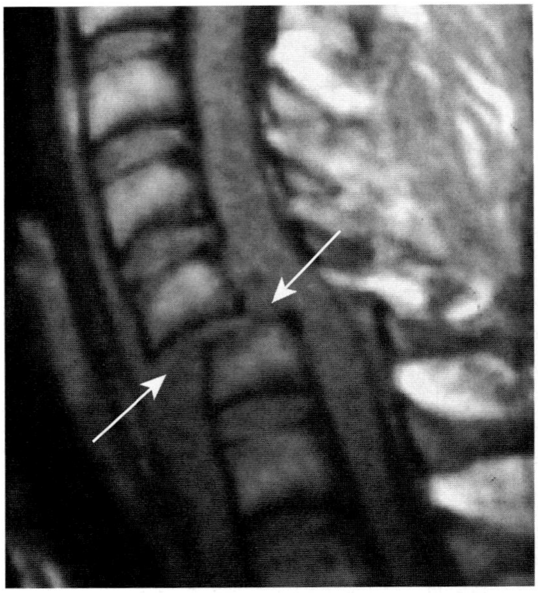

Figure 14.1 *Ligamentous Injury Depicted by Magnetic Resonance Imaging.* Sagittal T1-weighted image in a patient with a bilateral interfacetal dislocation shows torn anterior and posterior longitudinal ligaments *(arrows)* at the C5 to C6 level, making this an unstable injury that necessitates internal fixation. The spinal canal is slightly narrowed at the level of the injury.

supraspinous and intraspinous ligaments, capsular ligaments, and the ligamentum flavum (16). The ALL is best visualized on T1 and T2 sagittal images and appears as a homogeneous, linear low signal anteriorly that contrasts with the high signal from fat in the paravertebral and marrow spaces. This line consists of the ALL and cortical bone at the level of the vertebrae and the ALL and annulus fibrosus at the level of the disks. The PLL is best visualized on sagittal T2 images, where the high signal from the cerebrospinal fluid (CSF) provides contrast to the low-signal ligament. The line depicting the PLL is composed of the ligament itself, the dura, plus cortical bone (at the level of the vertebrae) or annulus fibrosus (at the level of the disks). The PLC is seen better on fat-saturated T2 images (14,18). This is because these ligaments are less well defined, and interspersed fat yields high signal intensity that is made more pronounced by proximity to the MRI spinal surface coil. Most ligamentous injuries are accompanied by edema in the perivertebral tissues that can be seen as areas of increased T2 signal intensity.

Evaluation of Disks

MRI allows for identification of disk abnormalities in acute spinal trauma (19–24). In severe trauma, disk herniations are present in 20% to 50% of cervical injuries (19). Most posttraumatic disk herniations occur in the cervical spine and at similar levels as degenerative disk herniations (C5 to C6, C6 to C7, and C4 to C5). This is due to a change in curvature resulting in redistribution of biomechanical forces and axial loading (20). Patients with acute anterior spinal cord syndrome have a nearly 100% incidence of disk herniations. The Brown-Sequard and central cord syndromes also are associated with a high incidence of herniated disks. These neurologic deficits usually correspond to the level of a disk herniation and may be clearly identified with MRI. With spine dislocations or fracture–dislocations, herniated disk fragments may become displaced into the spinal canal during reduction of the dislocation, leading to neurologic deterioration (4). For this reason, it has been recommended that patients with significant dislocations or fracture–dislocations be studied with MRI before surgery (19). The presence of a disk herniation may indicate the need for an anterior surgical approach with a diskectomy. Most acute posttrauma disk herniations are bright on T2 images, and some may be associated with ventral epidural hematoma. Acute intravertebral disk herniations (also called *Schmorl nodes*) may result in pain and show contrast enhancement (particularly in the vertebral endplates), but need no treatment. These are more common in the lumbar region and are rare in the cervical region. Acute Schmorl nodes may be difficult to differentiate from an acute fracture of an endplate. Many endplate fractures later show the development of a Schmorl node.

Evaluation of the Epidural, Subdural, and Subarachnoid Compartments

Most spinal epidural hematomas are spontaneous, with only 15% occurring as a consequence of trauma (25–29). Trauma-related extradural hematomas usually are found in the presence of severe trauma, but some are secondary to minor trauma (particularly in patients with a coagulopathy) or may be associated with acute disk herniations. Epidural hematoma also may follow lumbar puncture or spinal surgery, and most of these hematomas are located dorsally. Although most spontaneous epidural hematomas are venous, those following trauma are thought to be arterial in origin. Unlike the spontaneous spinal epidural hematomas that are located dorsally, posttraumatic ones are ventral and intimately related to the site of injury. Most posttraumatic spinal epidural hematomas are found in the thoracic, lumbar, and sacral regions and in the cervical spine. Spinal epidural hematomas have a biconvex shape (similar to intracranial ones) and tend to be short, whereas subdural hematomas conform to the shape of the spinal canal and tend to be long (Fig. 14.2A). Sometimes, epidural hematomas may be long and indistinguishable from a subdural hematoma (Fig. 14.2B).

With subdural hematomas, the fat normally located in the epidural space is preserved (Fig. 14.3). With spinal epidural hematomas, the clot dissects into the epidural fat, mixes with it, and effaces it. Unfortunately, as mentioned earlier, often it is not possible to differentiate a spinal epidural hematoma from one in the subdural space. From a clinical standpoint, this differentiation is important because in the presence of an epidural hematoma, the surgeon does not need to open the dura, and evacuation of the clot is a simpler procedure. In the presence of subdural hematoma, the dura needs to be opened

Most spontaneous epidural hematomas are located in the thoracic spine and in the dorsal epidural space, whereas most posttraumatic epidural hematomas are located in the lumbar and cervical spine in the ventral epidural space.

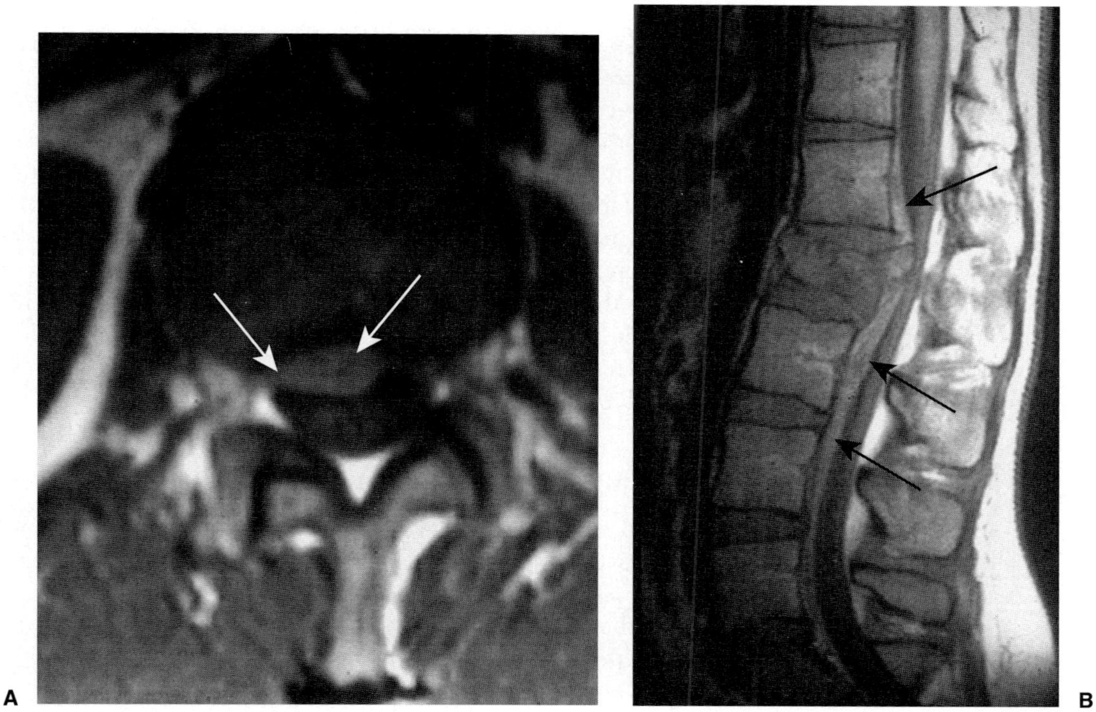

Figure 14.2 *Epidural Hematoma. A.* Axial T1-weighted image shows ventral biconvex epidural hematoma *(arrows)* compressing the thecal sac. *B.* In a different patient, sagittal T1-weighted image shows compression fracture of L2 and an extensive ventral bright epidural hematoma *(arrows)* above and below the fracture level compressing the thecal sac.

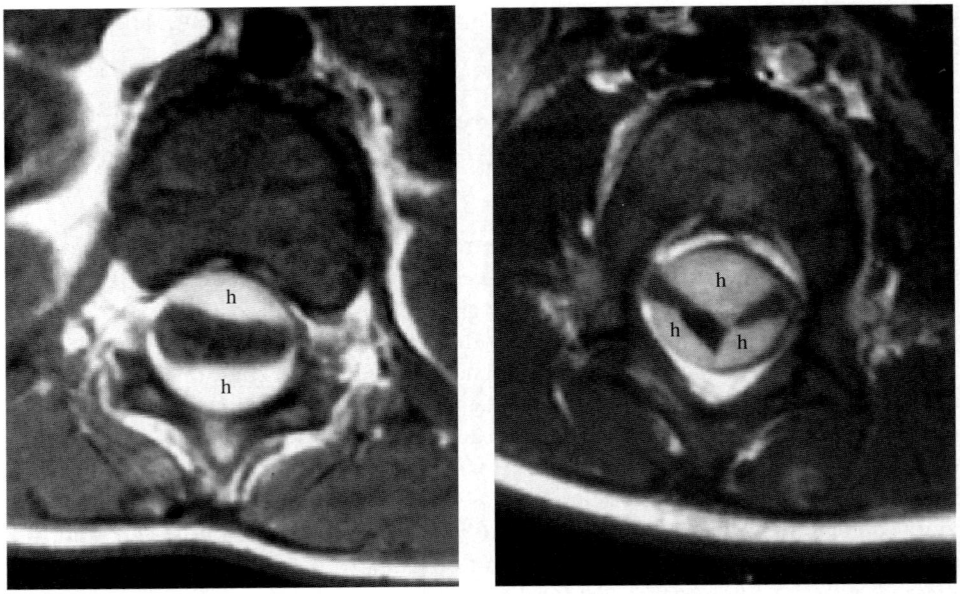

A B

Figure 14.3 *Subdural Hematoma. A.* Axial T1-weighted image shows bright hematoma *(h)* anterior and posterior to the thecal sac. *B.* Axial T1-weighted image obtained at a level below *A* shows typical "Mercedes Benz" configuration of the subdural hematoma *(h)* in the lower lumbar region. Note preservation of the bright epidural fat clearly separable from the subdural hematoma.

and then repaired. In addition, in many patients with spinal subdural hematoma, the dura is torn and a meningeal graft may be needed. If the dura is opened or torn, the incidence of complications, particularly a CSF leak, increases. Most spinal epidural and subdural hematomas are slightly bright on T1-weighted images, of moderate intensity on T2-weighted images, and dark on T2* images. Traditionally, spinal epidural hematomas have been considered surgical emergencies. Recently, several cases with improving or minimal neurologic deficits have been successfully managed conservatively (26).

An unusual complication of acute trauma is the formation of extramedullary CSF-filled cysts in either the epidural or subdural space. These probably are equivalent to subdural hygromas occurring intracranially, and also are seen in the presence of severe spine trauma. These cysts may compress the spinal cord, resulting in neurologic deficits (27,28). By MRI, they are collections of signal intensity equivalent to CSF in all sequences. They tend to be mostly dorsal in location and may be located anywhere in the spine, but I have seen them more commonly in the thoracic region. They occur at the fracture site and are more common in the face of spinal cord injury (which explains why most are found the thoracic region). They may compress the cord. Growth of these cysts on repeat studies may indicate the need for surgical decompression.

Evaluation of the Spinal Cord

Acute injuries to the spinal cord may be categorized as contusions (hemorrhagic and non-hemorrhagic), transection, and vascular injuries (30). Spinal cord contusions can be classified by their MRI appearance to assist in establishing a prognosis (Table 14.1).

In summary, type 1 injuries show inhomogeneous T1 signal, central dark T2 signal, and surrounding edema. They represent intramedullary hematoma, and these patients have a poor prognosis for any recovery of function. In type 2 injuries, there is homogeneous high signal on T2 images, reflecting edema in the spinal cord (Fig. 14.4A). These patients have a more favorable prognosis. Type 3 injuries show mottled signal abnormalities on all MRI sequences, which is related to edema and small hemorrhagic foci (Fig. 14.4B). These patients have an intermediate-to-poor prognosis. Chronically, there is atro-

Table 14.1: Magnetic Resonance Imaging Classification of Spinal Cord Injuries

Type of Injury	*T1 Signal*	*T2 Signal (Particularly on Gradient Echoes)*	*Prognosis*
Type 1 (hematoma)	Isointense	Low with rim of high signal related to edema	Poor
Type 2 (edema)	Low or isointense	High	Relatively good
Type 3 (mixture of edema and hematoma)	Low or isointense	Mottled	Poor to fair

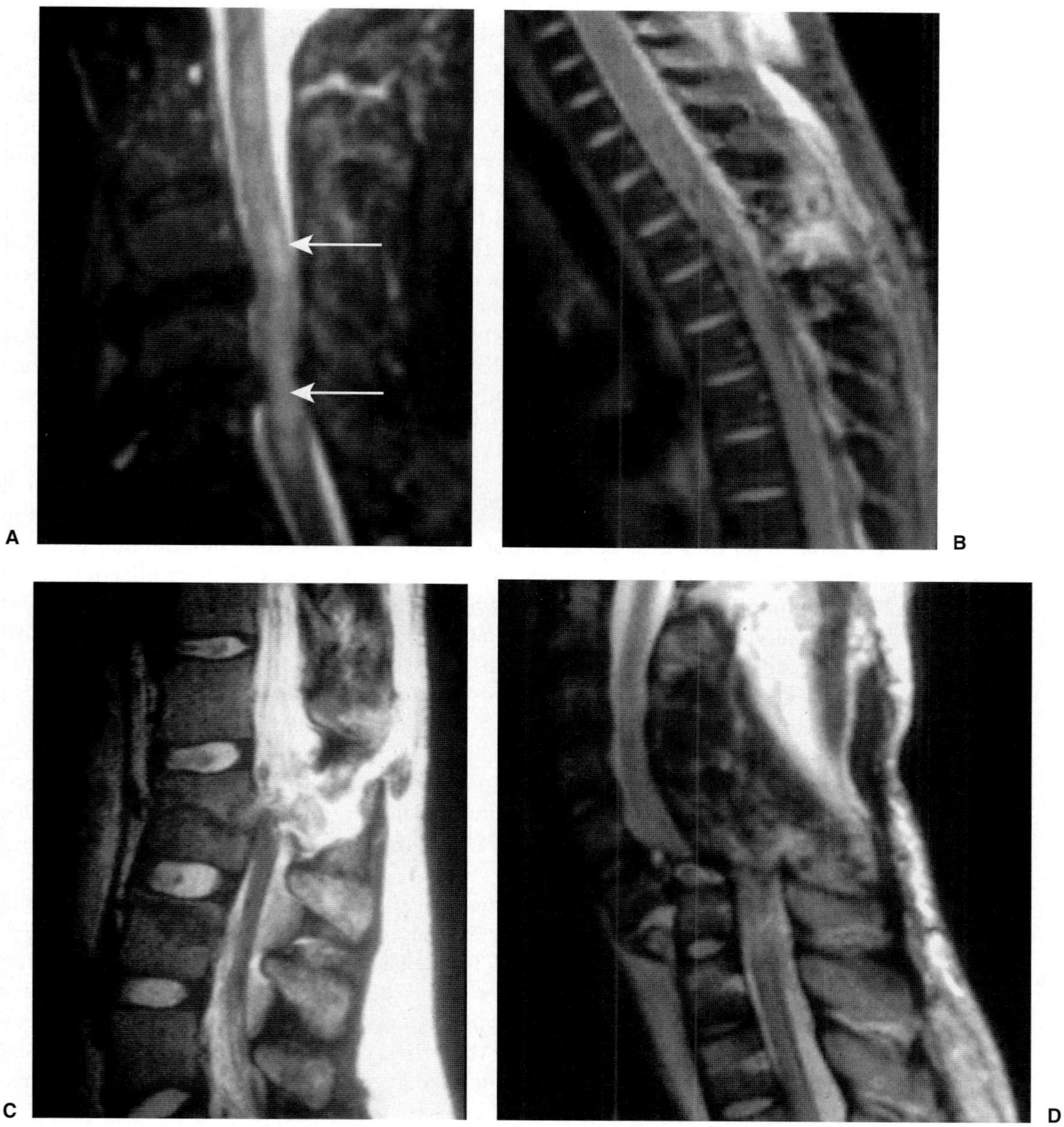

Figure 14.4 *Magnetic Resonance Imaging of Spinal Cord Injury. A.* Sagittal T2-weighted image after hyperextension injury shows focal abnormal increased signal *(arrows)* in the spinal cord in this patient with central spinal cord syndrome. *B.* Sagittal T2-weighted image in a child shows edema and hematoma in the midthoracic spinal cord. Note increased signal in the posterior interspinous region at the level of the injury, indicating ligamentous damage. No fractures were evident on radiographs in this patient. C. Sagittal T2-weighted image in a Chance injury at L3 shows complete transection of the cauda equina. Note fracture involving the posterior elements and body of L3. *D.* Sagittal T2-weighted image in a complete fracture–dislocation of C6 to C7 shows transection of the spinal cord.

phy of the cord and even development of intramedullary cysts in patients with types 1 and 3 injuries.

In children, spinal cord injury may occur in the absence of any bony or ligamentous lesions.

Spinal cord injury may occur in the absence of bone/ligamentous injury (30–34). This has been referred to as *s*pinal *c*ord *i*njury *w*ithout *r*adiographic *a*bnormality (SCIWORA; Fig. 14.4B). This type of injury is seen more commonly in children than in adults, and almost always occurs in the cervical spine, although the thoracic region also may be affected (33). This type of injury occurs mostly in children because although their bones and ligaments may be stretched, the cord cannot. In adults, degenerative disk disease, a congenitally narrow spinal canal, and ossification of the posterior longitudinal ligament predispose to acute spinal cord injury without bone abnormalities. This type of injury in adults most commonly involves the cervical region. A relatively common manifestation of cervical spinal cord injury without fractures in adults is the central cord syndrome (Fig. 14.4A). These patients present with significant upper extremity weakness and less weakness in the trunk and lower extremities. This is due to a vascular insult (probably ischemic) affecting the central aspect of the spinal cord supplied by the deep perforating arteries arising from the spinal circumflex arteries. Transient occlusion of the anterior spinal artery by spondylosis is considered the most likely mechanism. The corticospinal tract is organized in such a manner that the tracts for the upper extremities run in its deeper aspect, the ones for the trunk in the middle, and the ones for the lower extremities laterally. This "lamellar" arrangement of the corticospinal tract explains the symptoms of patients with the central cord syndrome. Although the main sequela of this syndrome was thought to be cord edema, many patients have a poor prognosis. It is possible that a hemorrhagic infarction of the spinal cord occurs in many patients with the central cord syndrome. Patients with neurologic deficits after trauma should be examined with MRI even in the face of negative radiographs or CT.

Spinal cord transection also is more common in children than in adults. When it occurs in adults, there usually is severe accompanying bone trauma. MRI reveals that the injured spinal cord may appear nearly transected (which has the same implications as a complete transection) or in shreds (Fig. 14.4C and D). MRI allows for identification of the level of the proximal spinal cord stump, which helps to establish the level of permanent clinical disability. Hemorrhage involving the entire transverse diameter of the spinal cord behaves clinically as a complete transection. Transection of the spinal cord also may occur in newborns during a difficult delivery. This is more common after difficult breech deliveries, but may occur in head presentations complicated by pelvic disproportion. In these children, the spinal cord may be directly injured or may be infarcted by stretching and compromise of its vascular supply. These infarctions are more common at the cervicothoracic junction because this area is the fulcrum of flexion during birth and because it is a watershed zone between vascular territories. This region of the spinal cord undergoes significant atrophy with time.

Most spinal cord infarctions occur in the distal thoracic and conus medullaris regions and are seen in patients after repair of abdominal aortic aneurysms.

Vascular injury to the spinal cord is rare after trauma or surgery. Initially, most spinal cord infarctions result in swelling of the gray matter, giving rise to the so-called owl-eye appearance on axial T2-weighted images. The edema then progresses to involve the white matter and, if the entire transverse diameter of the spinal cord is affected, the prognosis is poor. Most infarctions are secondary to involvement of the anterior spinal artery, but they also are known to occur after occlusion of the paired posterior spinal arteries. Most distal thoracic and conus medullaris infarcts occur during repair of abdominal aortic aneurysms. Spinal cord infarcts also may occur secondary to rib fractures (with occlusion of the intercostal arteries that supply the spinal cord).

Evaluation of the Vertebral Arteries

Approximately 20% of all patients with cervical spine fractures have either symptomatic or asymptomatic injuries to one or both vertebral arteries (35–39). In patients with fractures involving a foramen transversarium or with facet fracture–dislocations, the incidence of vertebral artery injury is as high as 50% to 75% (35) (Fig. 14.5A and B). A clinical finding that strongly suggests injury to a vertebral artery is that of ascending cord deficits. In such patients, 40% show injury to one or both vertebral arteries. Complete occlusion of a vertebral artery in the presence of a normal contralateral artery usually is asymptomatic and of little clinical significance (37). Dissection (and incomplete occlusion) of one vertebral artery (even if the contralateral one is normal) or bilateral occlusion may cause stroke or death, and may indicate the need for anticoagulation (35–39) (Fig. 14.5C). Unfortunately, many of these patients have other injuries that prevent anticoagulation, such as intracranial hemorrhage, spinal epidural and subdural hematomas, or a history of recent surgery.

The vertebral arteries may be occluded or dissected, or show pseudoaneurysm formation. Occluded and dissected vertebral arteries are well depicted by MRI and MR angiography, but suspected pseudoaneurysms need confirmation with catheter angiography. Evaluation of a possible dissection needs careful review of the source MR angiography images because the arteries may appear diffusely narrowed only on the maximum-intensity projection images. Because the intramural clot tends to be bright acutely, it may be difficult to separate it from the normal fat in the foramen transversarium without fat suppression techniques.

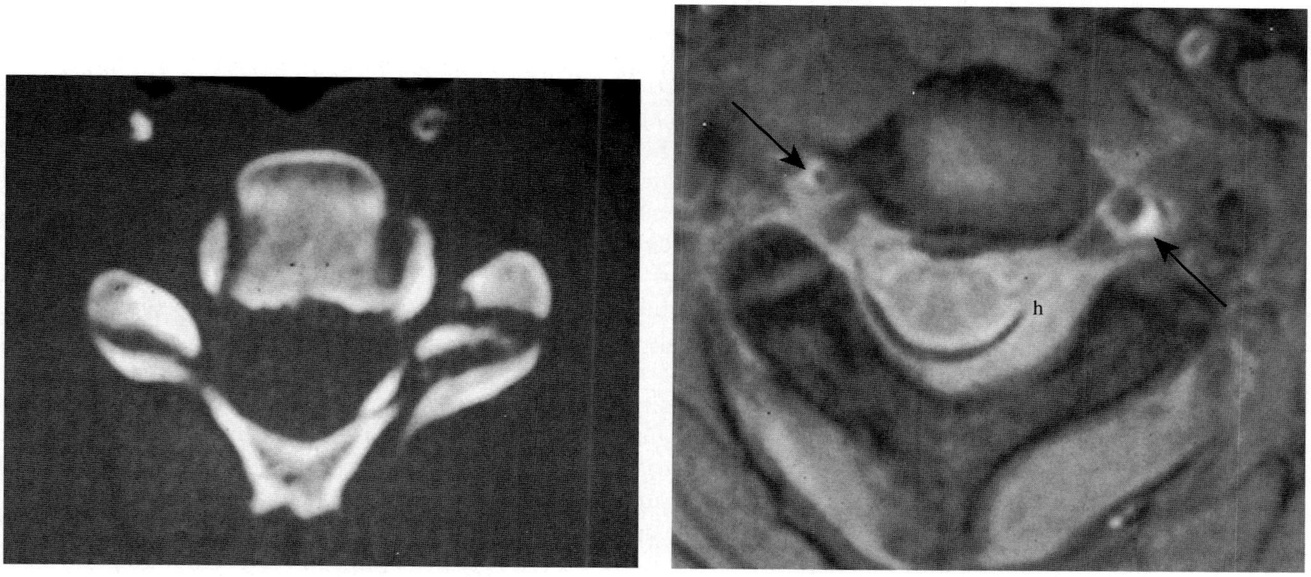

A

C

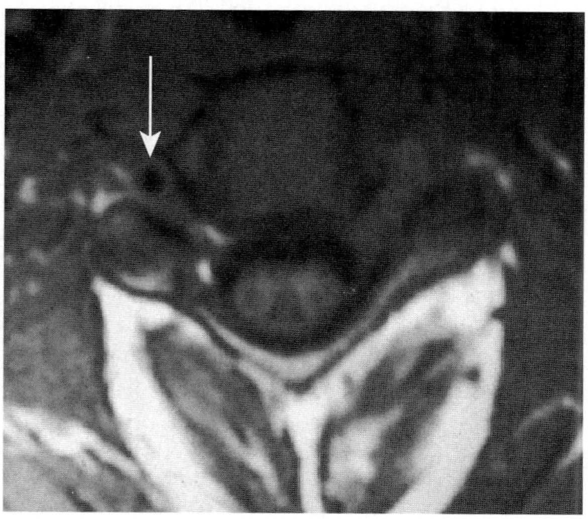

B

Figure 14.5 *Vertebral Artery Injury. A.* Axial computed tomography shows fractures of the left articular pillar. *B.* Corresponding axial T1-weighted image shows increased soft tissues in the left neural foramen and absence of flow void in the region of the vertebral artery. Note normal flow void in the patent right vertebral artery (*arrow*). *C.* In a different patient, axial T2-weighted image shows crescent-shaped hyperintensities (*arrows*) in the walls of both vertebral arteries compatible with mural clot secondary to dissections. There also is epidural hematoma (*h*).

Specific Types of Spinal Injury

Upper Cervical Spine

Biomechanically, the cervical spine may be divided into two segments:

Base of skull to C2 (upper segment)
C3 to C7 (lower segment)

The C3 vertebra represents a transitional segment and may behave as part of the upper or lower regions. The upper segment has considerable rotational and lateral motion, whereas the lower segment has mostly rotational and flexion motion. Each of these segments responds differently to trauma, and the mechanisms leading to fractures also are distinct for each region. The craniovertebral junction is well adapted to provide a remarkable range of motion, with approximately half of the neck rotation occurring at the C1 to C2 articulation. Because of the relatively large spinal canal diameter at this level (approximately twice the spinal cord diameter), neurologic deficits may be mild or absent in the face of trauma.

Occipitoatlantal Injuries

Occipitoatlantal injuries may be subluxations or dislocations. The term *occipitoatlantal dissociation* is nonspecific and refers to both types of injury. A dislocation at this level frequently is fatal and commonly accompanies other severe head and spinal trauma. The displacement may be anterior, posterior, or longitudinal (axial or vertical distraction; Fig. 14.6). Distraction is encountered more commonly in children than in adults. The Powers ratio probably is the most commonly used measurement to establish the diagnosis of anterior occipitoatlantal dislocation. This ratio is obtained by dividing the distance between the basion and the posterior lamina of C1 by the distance between the posterior cortex of the anterior tubercle of C1 and the opisthion. If the ratio is greater than 1, an anterior dislocation is present. This measurement is not useful for distraction (vertical) dislocations. I find the basion–dental interval measurement to be very useful in these instances. A line drawn from the tip of the dens to the basion normally should not measure more than 12 mm. This measurement is abnormal in anterior, posterior, and axial injuries. The initial diagnosis of this injury may be difficult because the numerical measurements are not perfect, and the dislocation might be reduced at the time of imaging. For this reason, MRI is recommended in suspected cases. MRI confirms the diagnosis by depicting disruption of the tectorial membrane, the superior band of the cruciate ligaments, the apical ligament, and the anterior and posterior atlantooccipital ligaments (40). Disruption of these ligaments indicates a severe injury. Less severe ligamentous and muscular injury also can be documented. Hematoma in the supradental space is common. The integrity of the tectorial membrane is critical in maintaining craniospinal stability (41).

Jefferson Fractures

The burst fracture of C1, or Jefferson burst fracture, is the result of axial loading, with bilateral or unilateral outward displacement of the lateral masses of C1 (Fig. 14.7A). This injury results in fractures in both the anterior and posterior arches of C1 (occasionally the fracture is unilateral). Usually there is no spinal cord injury because the canal becomes widened with the fractures. Some patients, however, may be symptomatic because of hematoma in the epidural space. Isolated fracture(s) of the posterior arch of C1 may result from hyperextension, with impaction of the posterior arch of C1 between the occiput and C2. This injury may be distinguished from the burst fracture of C1 by the involvement of only the posterior arch of C1. Isolated fracture of the anterior arch of C1 occurs less commonly. This injury also results from hyperextension, with avulsion of the attachment of

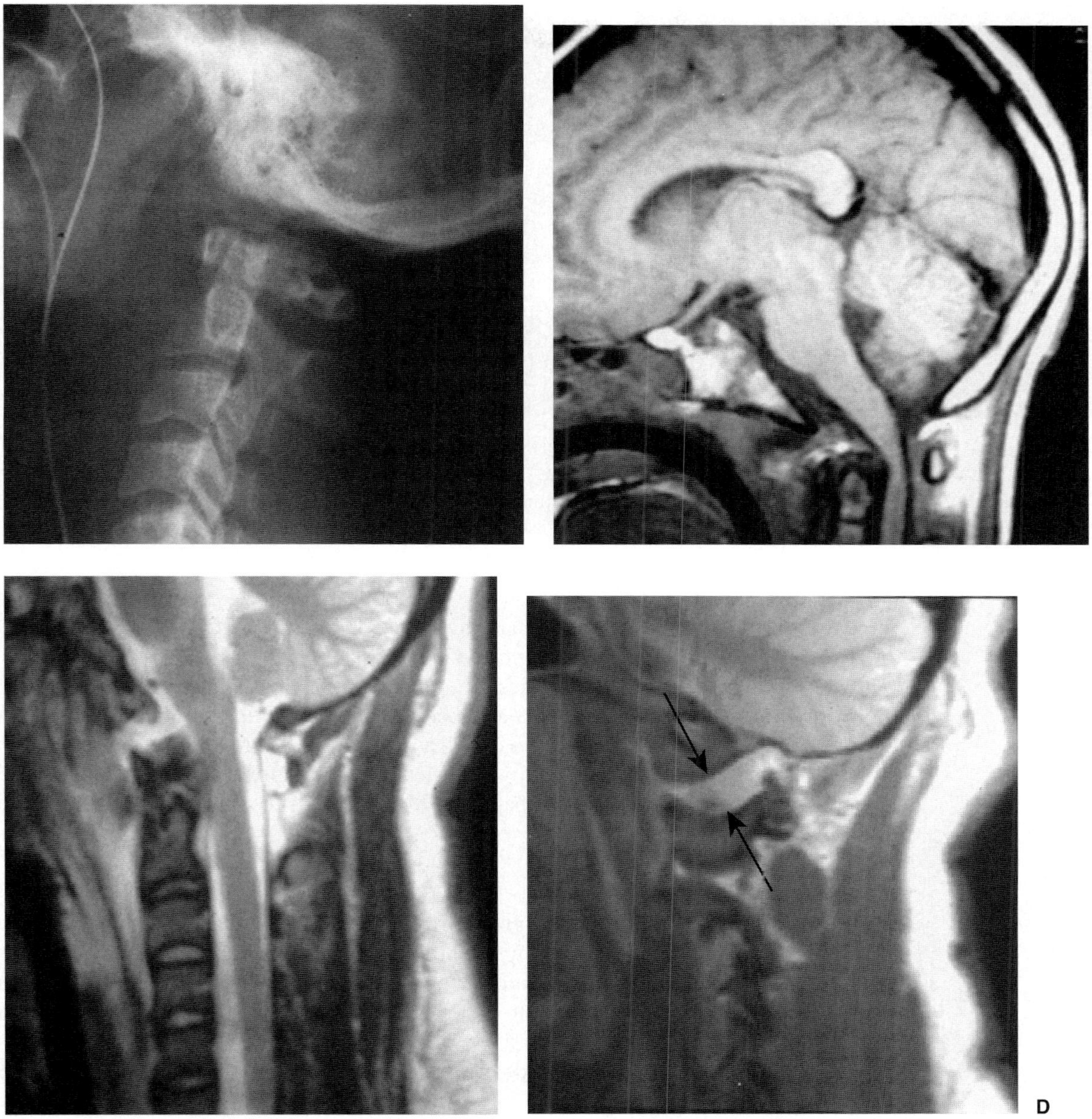

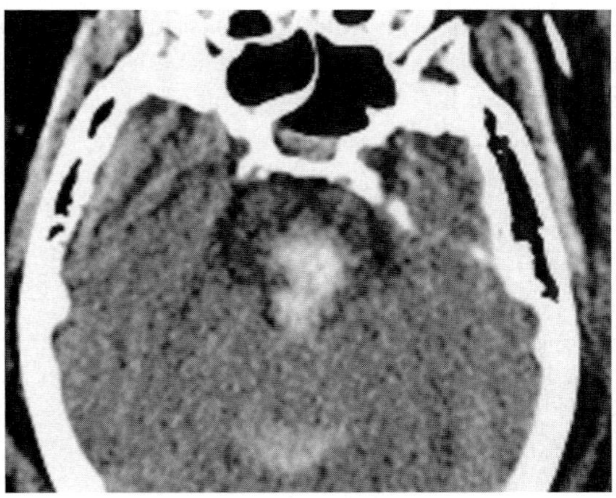

Figure 14.6 *Occipitoatlantal Injury*. *A*. Lateral radiograph shows increased distance between the tip of the dens and the basion. There is no significant anterior or posterior shift in this vertical injury. *B*. In a different patient, sagittal T1-weighted image shows anterior occipitoatlantal subluxation with supradental hematoma. *C*. Sagittal T2-weighted image (different patient) shows vertical injury with increased dens–basion distance and supradental hematoma. There is a large amount of precervical swelling. The tectorial membrane is disrupted and there is precervical hematoma and edema. *D*. In a different patient, parasagittal T2-weighted image shows increased distance (*arrows*) between the occipital condyle and the lateral mass of C1. *E*. In a different patient with an anterior occipitoatlantal subluxation, axial computed tomography shows a hematoma in the brainstem.

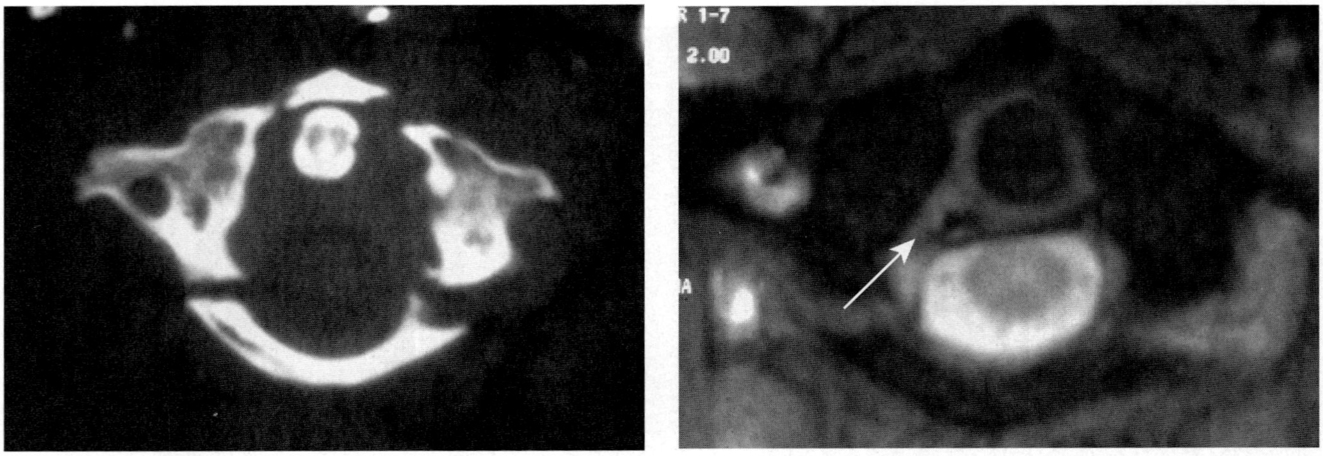

A B

Figure 14.7 *Jefferson Fracture. A.* Axial computed tomography shows bilateral fractures involving the anterior and posterior arches of C1. *B.* In a different patient, axial T2-weighted image shows avulsion *(arrow)* of the transverse ligament at the level of its insertion in the right tubercle.

the anterior spinal ligament. The small, avulsed bone fragment is visible ventral to the anterior arch of C1. The posterior arch of C1 remains intact.

MRI is helpful in a assessing these fractures. In the type 1 injury, the substance of the transverse ligament is disrupted and because ligaments do not heal, these patients require internal fixation. In the type 2 injury, the transverse ligament is avulsed at the level of its insertion and because this is basically a bone injury, healing occurs in 75% of patients (Fig. 14.7B). In other patients, MRI shows the transverse ligament to be intact.

Hangman's Fractures

Hangman's and hyperflexion teardrop fractures are the most severe bony injuries that the human cervical spine can sustain with preservation of life.

Traumatic spondylolysis of C2 (hangman's fracture) is the most common fracture of the axis. This injury usually is caused by hyperextension. It results in bilateral fractures of the pars interarticularis, the part of the vertebra between the superior and inferior facets. These fractures are graded from 1 to 3 depending on their severity (Table 14.2) (Fig. 14.8).

In addition, in the type 3 fracture, there is a wide gap between the pars interarticularis, bilateral interfacetal dislocation of C2 to C3, and injury to the corresponding intervertebral disk. Spinal cord injury is common with type 3 hangman's fractures but less common in type 1 and 2 fractures. The incidence of herniated disks and intraspinal hematomas is high with the type 3 fracture, which possibly is the most severe fracture that can be sustained by the spine with preservation of life.

Table 14.2: Grading of Hangman's Fractures of C2

Type	*Disk Space*	*Anterior Aspect of C2*
I	Near normal and minimal separation at the fracture sites (Fig. 14.8A)	Minimally or not displaced
II	Slightly opened anteriorly or posteriorly (Fig. 14.8B)	Slightly angled anteriorly or posteriorly
III	Frank splaying and angulation of the disk space (Fig. 14.8C,D)	Significant anterior or posterior angulation

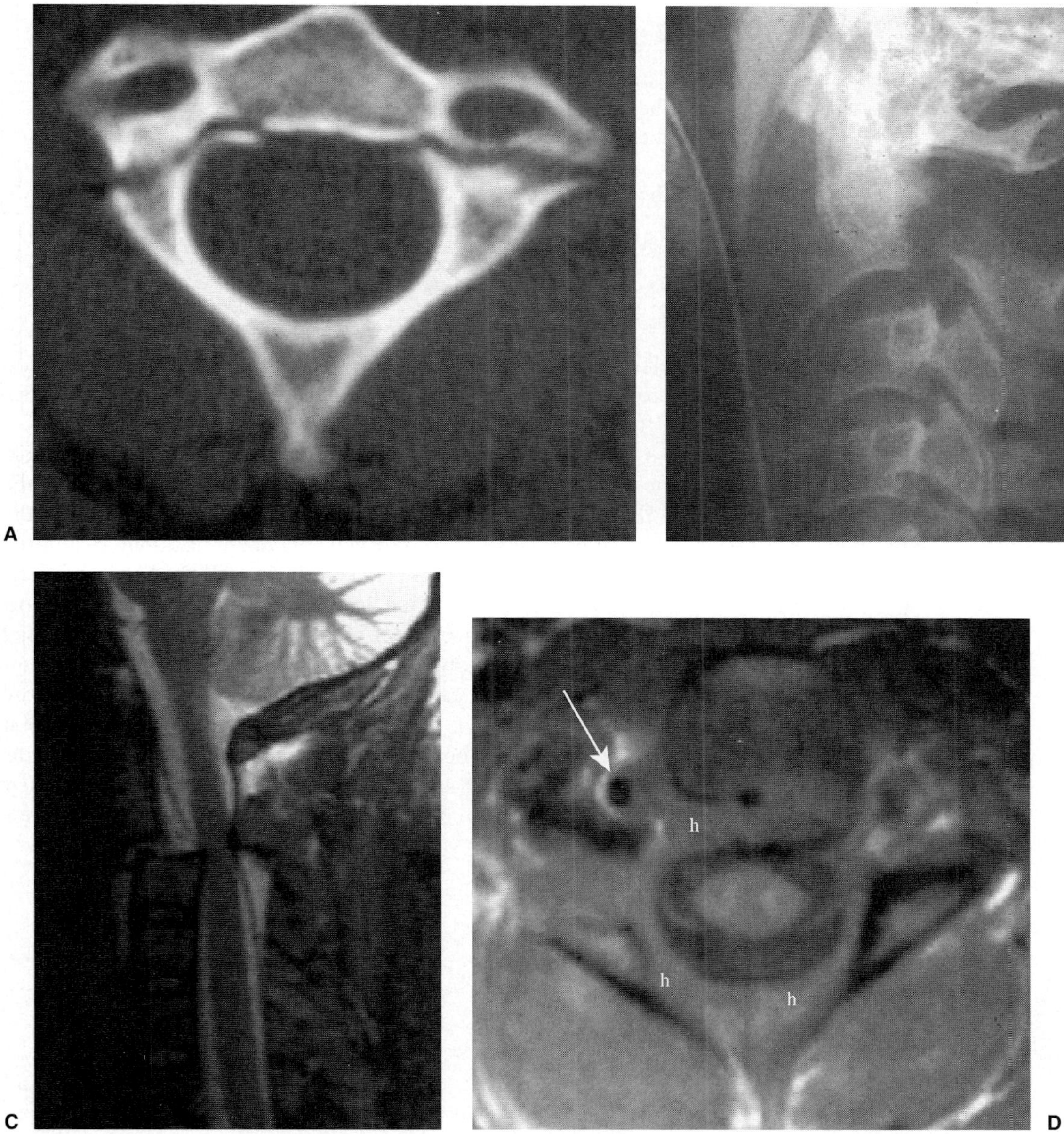

Figure 14.8 *Hangman's Fracture. A.* Axial computed tomography shows bilateral fractures through the pars interarticularis of C2, but no significant displacement. *B.* In a different patient, a lateral radiograph shows bilateral fractures through the pars interarticularis of C2. There is slight angulation and anterior subluxation of the C2 body. *C.* Sagittal T2-weighted image (different patient with a hangman's fracture) shows significant anterior subluxation of the C2 with compression of the spinal cord. *D.* In a different patient with a hangman's fracture, axial T1-weighted image shows significant epidural hematoma *(h)*, but no cord compression. The normal flow void in the left vertebral artery is not seen (compare with normal right vertebral artery, *arrow*).

Table 14.3: Traditional Classification of Dens Fractures

Type	*Features*	*Union Rate*
I	Through the tip of the dens	Low
II	Through the base of the dens	Varies according to status of transverse ligament (see below)
III	Through the body of C2	High

Type I dens fractures with preservation of the transverse ligament and the tectorial membrane are not clinically significant.

Dens Fractures

The mechanism responsible for dens fractures is poorly understood, but hyperextension is believed to play a major role (41–43). Fractures of the dens traditionally have been classified into types I, II, and III (42) (Table 14.3).

The type I fracture is an avulsion fracture of the tip of the dens. This is a rare injury. Type II fractures are the most common, and consist of a fracture through the base of the dens, at its junction with the C2 body (Fig. 14.9). If the fracture extends through the upper body of C2, it is classified as type III. The transverse ligament also may be injured in dens fractures. The transverse ligament extends between the medial portions of the lateral masses of C1, behind the odontoid process. This ligament provides the major support for the C1 to C2 articulation, allowing rotation of C1 about the dens, while maintaining their proximity. Transverse ligament injury can be inferred from widening of the atlanto-dental interval beyond 3 mm or lateral displacement of the lateral masses of C1 by more than 7 mm (45). Vertical fracture of the dens is a fourth and less common injury (44) that usually accompanies other spine fractures. They are seen better in axial images and sagittal reformations. They have a relatively high union rate. If fusion does not occur, their identification is important because they are a contraindication to the placement of a screw through the body of C2 into the dens.

A

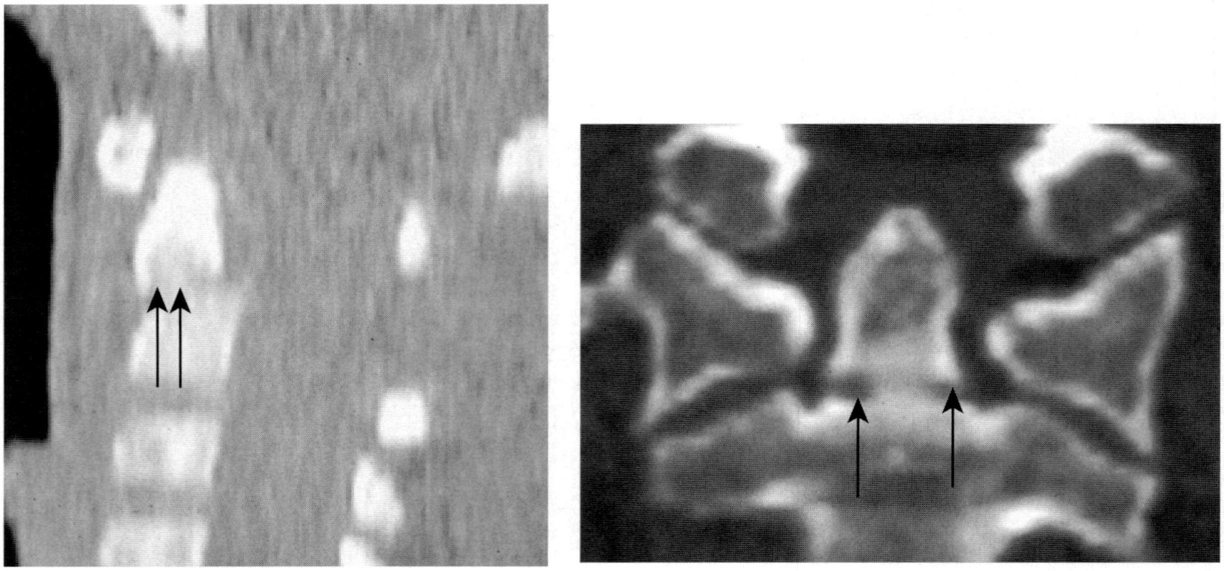

B

Figure 14.9 *Dens Fracture. A.* Sagittal computed tomography (CT) reformation shows type II fracture *(arrows)* through the base of the dens that is slightly angled anteriorly. *B.* In a different patient, coronal CT reformation shows type II fracture *(arrows)* at the base of the dens with slightly sclerotic margins, suggesting chronicity.

Lower Cervical Spine Fractures

Most fractures in adults occur in the lower cervical spine, predominantly at the C5 to C7 levels. The classification of these fractures traditionally has been based on the presumed mechanism of injury (i.e., hyperextension, hyperflexion, vertical compression, or mixed), and for convenience's sake I follow it here.

Hyperextension Injuries

Hyperextension injuries usually are secondary to an impact to the face or forehead. Injuries to the lower cervical spine caused by hyperextension include hyperextension dislocation and hyperextension teardrop fracture. Over one-half of hyperextension injuries may be associated with herniated disks, which may cause or worsen the associated spinal cord injury (17,20). Ligamentous disruption is the major pathologic process in these lesions, and MRI provides an excellent depiction of ligamentous injury.

Hyperextension dislocation is a disruption of the ligaments between adjacent vertebrae and of the annulus fibrosus. Severe cases show disruption of the posterior longitudinal ligament and facet capsular ligaments. Because the dislocation may be reduced at the time of imaging, and there may be no fracture, the appearance on radiographs may be near normal despite severe pain or neurologic deficits (Fig. 14.10). A key radiographic finding in many patients is that of diffuse thickening of the prevertebral soft tissues. MRI identifies the prevertebral hematoma and discontinuity of ligaments. Disruption of the anterior longitudinal ligament and separation of the disk from the vertebral body endplate may be associated with prolonged pain and delayed instability, and may require anterior fusion (17). This injury frequently is associated with severe spinal cord contusion, especially in patients with spondylosis. In approximately two-thirds of patients with hyperextension dislocation injury, the intact anterior annulus causes an avulsion fracture of the anterior inferior margin of the affected vertebral body. This fragment is larger in the transverse dimension than in height, with an almost horizontally oriented fracture line.

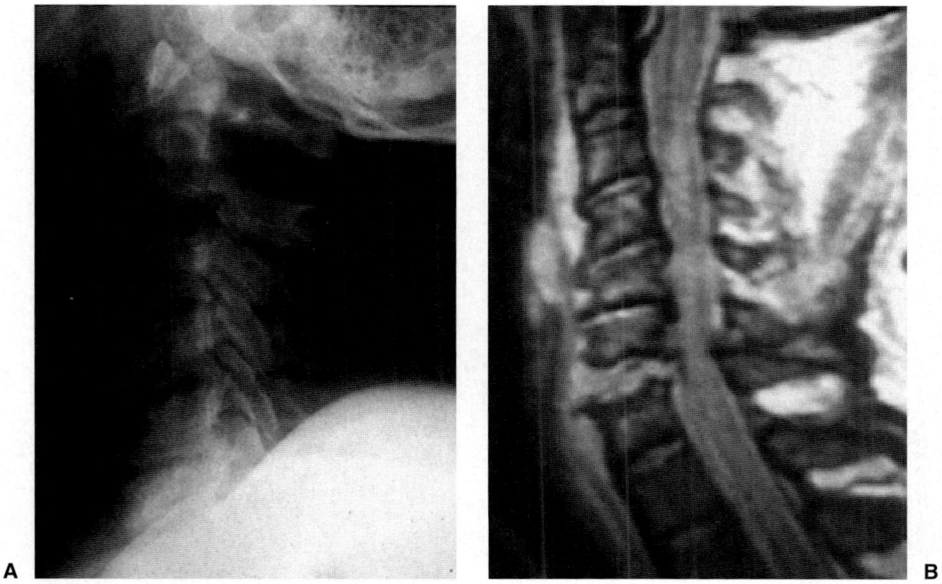

Figure 14.10 *Hyperextension Dislocation. A.* Limited portable lateral radiograph shows degenerative changes without any other obvious lesion. *B.* In the same patient, sagittal T2-weighted image shows ruptured anterior and posterior longitudinal ligaments and disruption of the disk at C6 to C7. There is prevertebral edema and patchy high signal intensity in the spinal cord.

A hyperextension teardrop fracture is an avulsion fracture of the anterior inferior margin of a vertebral body caused by traction from the anterior longitudinal ligament. This injury most commonly occurs at the C2 level and in older and osteoporotic individuals. Less commonly, it may occur at lower levels in nonosteoporotic patients. The fracture fragment can be distinguished from the avulsion fracture seen with hyperextension dislocation by the obliquity of the fracture line (approximately 45 degrees from vertical) and the relatively greater height of the fragment.

Hyperflexion Injuries

Hyperflexion injuries result from impact to the top or the back of the head with the neck in flexion (such as diving injuries). These injuries include hyperflexion sprain, wedge fractures, bilateral interfacetal joint dislocations, and hyperflexion teardrop fracture. A hyperflexion sprain refers to a disruption of the posterior ligament attachments between adjacent vertebrae. The disrupted ligaments include the nuchal ligament, interspinous ligaments, facet capsular ligaments, and the posterior longitudinal ligament. On radiographs, this injury may be recognized by an abnormal widening between adjacent posterior elements, and subtle, acute kyphotic angulation at the level of injury. On MRI, high–signal-intensity edema and hematoma in the posterior ligamentous structures on T2-weighted images (particularly fat-suppressed sequences) typically are seen. The diagnosis of this injury is important because it may be associated with chronic neck pain and a significant incidence of failure of ligamentous healing in patients managed nonsurgically.

Wedge Fractures. Wedge fractures share the posterior ligament disruption of a hyperflexion sprain, but in addition there is an impaction fracture of the superior endplate of a vertebral body. The inferior endplate remains intact (Fig. 14.11). There is greater loss of vertical height anteriorly, resulting in the typical wedge shape of a vertebral body seen in the lateral radiograph or sagittal CT reformations.

Bilateral Interfacetal Dislocations. With bilateral interfacetal joint dislocations, there is disruption of the posterior ligamentous structures, similar to hyperflexion sprain. In addi-

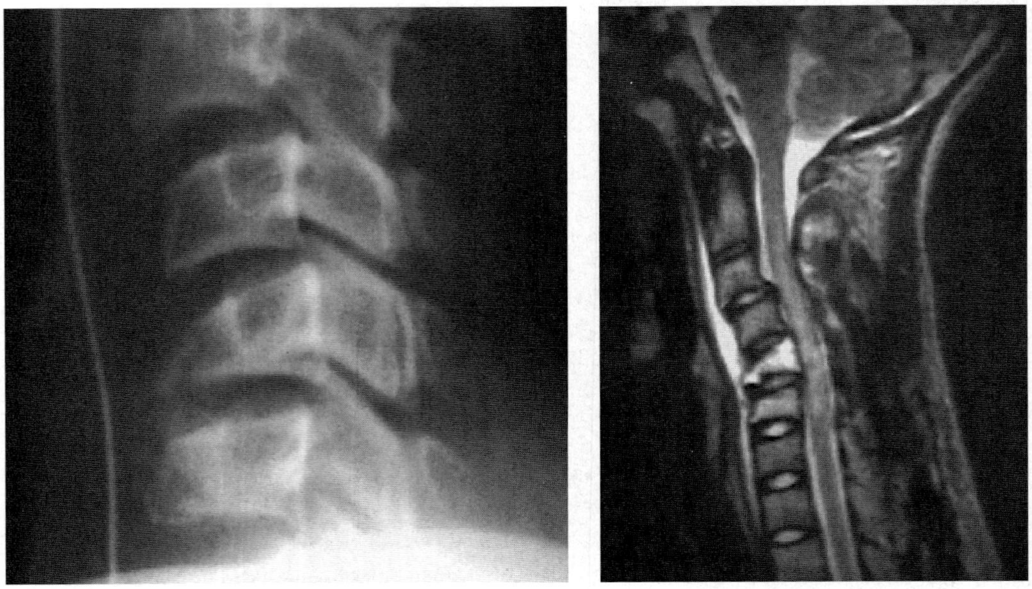

A B

Figure 14.11 *Cervical Wedge Fracture. A.* Lateral radiograph shows wedge-shaped compression fracture of C5. *B.* In the same patient, sagittal T2-weighted image shows the fracture and edema in the spinal cord above and below the level of the injury. Precervical edema also is seen.

tion, there is disruption of the annular fibers of the disk and of the ALL, and complete dislocations of the facet joints. The inferior articular processes of the upper vertebra become lodged in the neural foramina anterior to the superior articular process of the lower vertebra, preventing reduction. This injury is thus sometimes referred to as *bilaterally locked facets*, erroneously implying stability. On radiographs, this injury is diagnosed by the presence of anterior displacement of the upper vertebra by one-half or more of the width of the lower vertebral body. The "naked" articular surfaces of the dislocated facets also usually are visible, particularly on CT (Fig. 14.12A). MRI reveals these features, as well as detecting the presence of associated herniated disks, spinal cord injury, or epidural hematoma (Fig. 14.12B and C). In facet dislocations, 50% or more of patients may have significant disk herniations that necessitate anterior diskectomy and fusion to avoid additional compression of the spinal cord after reduction (4). More than half of these patients also have vertebral artery injuries that can be depicted on MR angiography (46). CT is helpful to assess for fractures of the articular masses, which may interfere with attempts at reduction.

Up to one-half of patients with bilateral interfacetal dislocations have significant herniated disks at the level of their injury.

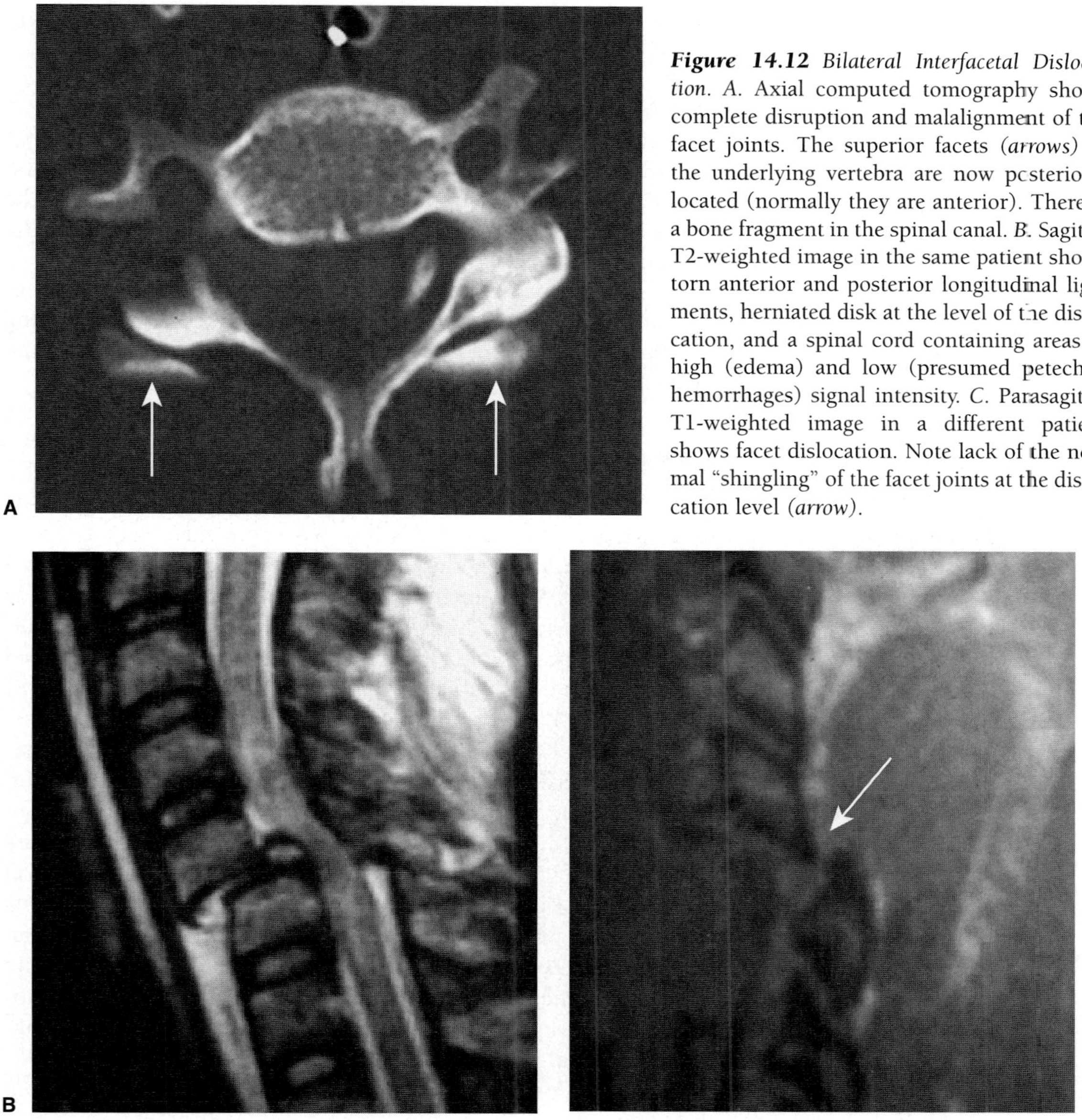

***Figure* 14.12** *Bilateral Interfacetal Dislocation. A.* Axial computed tomography shows complete disruption and malalignment of the facet joints. The superior facets *(arrows)* of the underlying vertebra are now posteriorly located (normally they are anterior). There is a bone fragment in the spinal canal. *B.* Sagittal T2-weighted image in the same patient shows torn anterior and posterior longitudinal ligaments, herniated disk at the level of the dislocation, and a spinal cord containing areas of high (edema) and low (presumed petechial hemorrhages) signal intensity. *C.* Parasagittal T1-weighted image in a different patient shows facet dislocation. Note lack of the normal "shingling" of the facet joints at the dislocation level *(arrow)*.

Hyperflexion Teardrop Fractures. A hyperflexion teardrop fracture occurs with forces of even greater magnitude. This injury shares the posterior ligamentous disruption of the other hyperflexion injuries, but in addition there is a large triangular fracture fragment of the anterior inferior margin of the upper vertebral body. There is associated severe narrowing of the spinal canal due to retropulsed bone fragments, with spinal cord injury in most patients. The larger size of the triangular fracture fragment and the presence of distraction of the posterior elements indicating the flexion mechanism serve to distinguish this fracture from the similarly named hyperextension teardrop fracture.

Vertical Compression Injuries

Vertical compression injuries occur with an impact to the top of the head while the spine is straight. These injuries include the Jefferson burst fracture of C1 (see earlier) and the burst fracture of the lower cervical spine. Burst fractures of a lower vertebral body are thought to occur when vertical compressive forces are transmitted through the intervertebral disks, with radial outward forces generated in one vertebral body. This results in a vertical fracture, with lateral dispersion of the vertebral body fragments. On radiographs, widening of the uncovertebral joints or identification of a vertical fracture makes the diagnosis. CT may aid in identifying the vertical fracture and the associated fractures of the pedicles or lamina(e). MRI is helpful in detecting herniated disks, which also are common (19).

Injuries Caused by Other Mechanisms

Less common mechanisms of injury also may lead to recognizable fracture patterns. The combination of flexion and rotational forces may result in unilateral interfacetal dislocation (Fig. 14.13). This injury may be distinguished from bilateral interfacetal dislocations by the presence of anterolisthesis of approximately 25% (versus 50% for the bilateral type). The features of unilateral and bilateral interfacetal dislocations are listed in Table 14.4.

Unilateral interfacetal dislocations also are associated with a high incidence of vertebral artery injury (35). Lateral force vectors also may result in isolated fractures of the uncinate processes. Combined extension and rotation forces may lead to fractures of the articular pillar or a pedicolaminar fracture.

Thoracic Spine Injuries

The normal thoracic spine is well stabilized by the rib cage, thoracic musculature, and its steeply oriented facet joints. Hence, fractures in this region are uncommon, except with severe trauma. Because of the normal fixed thoracic kyphosis, axial forces are transformed into flexion forces and most injuries are related to hyperflexion. These injuries include compression type fractures and flexion fracture–dislocations (47) (Fig. 14.14). Radiographs of the thoracic spine may be difficult to evaluate because of the superimposed shoulder girdle and ribs. In all cases, CT is valuable to assess the bony anatomy, and MRI depicts the status of the spinal cord.

Compression fractures are considered "simple" wedge fractures if there is involvement only of the anterior one-third of a vertebral body. Severe fractures involve the middle and posterior vertebral body with the potential for posterior displacement or retropulsion of bone fragments into the spinal canal. These fractures are considered unstable and are treated surgically. Disruption of the PLL may indicate the need for an anterior surgical approach to allow for the reduction of retropulsed bone fragments. In contrast, patients with an intact PLL may have a good prognosis with only a posterior fusion (48–51). Disruption of the ALL occurs in up to 25% of thoracolumbar fractures (48). MRI can identify disruptions of the ALL and PLC, which are seen in 30% to 40% of the more severe thoracic fractures (50). The presence of ligamentous disruption may result in delayed instability in patients managed without surgical fusion (51).

Fracture–dislocations occur with forces of larger magnitude. There is frequently a marked dislocation with accompanying severe spinal cord injury. MRI provides valuable

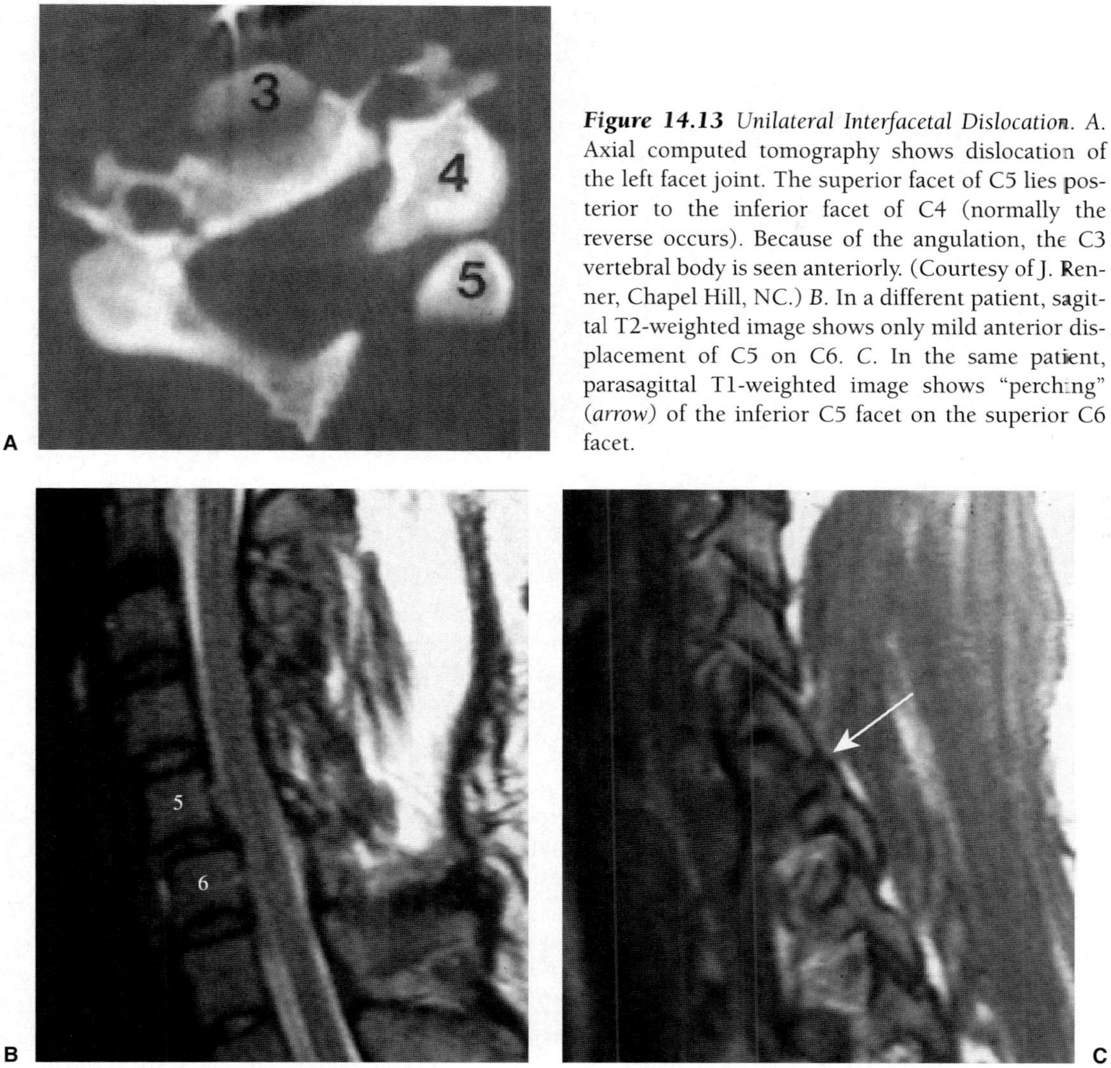

Figure 14.13 *Unilateral Interfacetal Dislocation. A.* Axial computed tomography shows dislocation of the left facet joint. The superior facet of C5 lies posterior to the inferior facet of C4 (normally the reverse occurs). Because of the angulation, the C3 vertebral body is seen anteriorly. (Courtesy of J. Renner, Chapel Hill, NC.) *B.* In a different patient, sagittal T2-weighted image shows only mild anterior displacement of C5 on C6. *C.* In the same patient, parasagittal T1-weighted image shows "perching" (*arrow*) of the inferior C5 facet on the superior C6 facet.

Table 14.4: Imaging Features of Interfacetal Dislocations

Type	*Mechanism*	*Facets Involved*	*Lack of Stability*	*Vertebral Body Displacement*	*Spinal Cord Injury*
Unilateral	Flexion, rotation	One	+	<50%	+
Bilateral	Hyperflexion	Two	+++	>50%	++

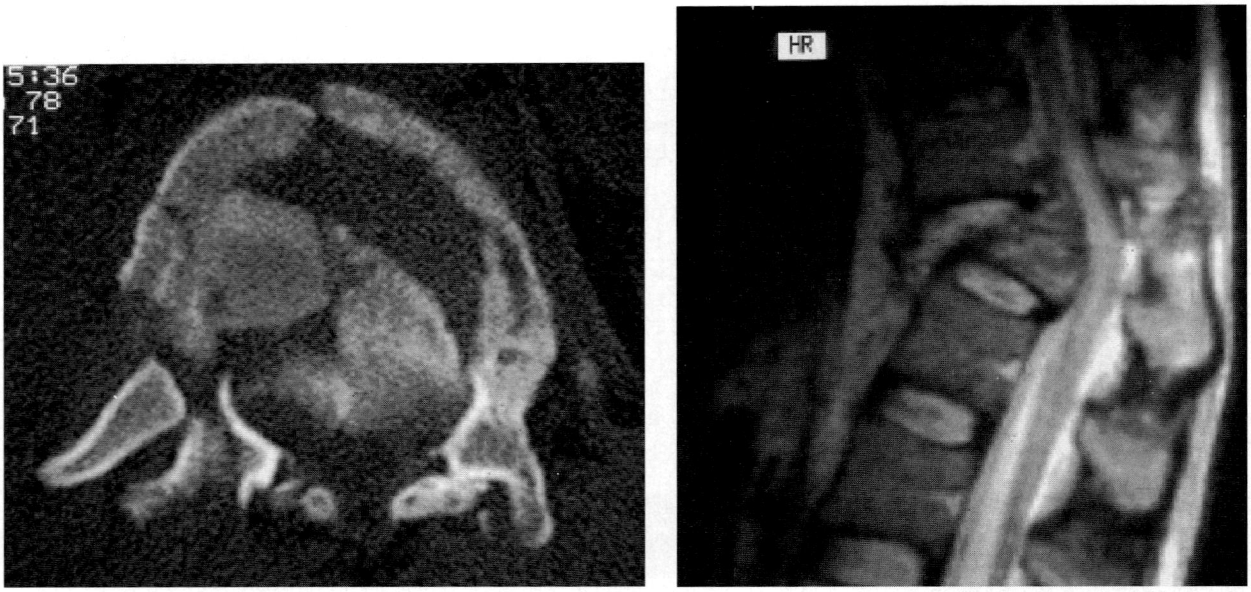

A B

Figure 14.14 *Thoracic Compression Fracture. A.* Axial computed tomography shows significant compression fracture of a lower thoracic vertebral body. The fracture extends into the posterior arch and narrows the canal. *B.* In the same patient, sagittal T2-weighted image shows marked compression of that vertebra, kyphosis, a narrowed canal, and edema in the conus medullaris.

information regarding spinal canal narrowing, cord injury, and the presence of associated epidural hematoma. Up to 50% of unstable thoracic spine fractures or dislocations may have an associated herniated disk (47).

Thoracolumbar Junction Injuries

The thoracolumbar junction (T12 to L2) is the next most common site of spinal fracture after the cervical spine. Most of the injuries to the lumbar spine and thoracolumbar junction are related to abnormal flexion or vertical compression forces. Common types of injuries include wedge, burst, and Chance fractures. Wedge fractures do not involve the posterior elements. Characteristically, there is greater loss of height in the anterior aspect of a vertebral body than in its posterior aspect. Radiographs are diagnostic in most cases. Classification into simple and severe wedge fractures is similar to that for the thoracic spine. If there is a question of posterior element fractures or posterior retropulsion of fragments, CT provides clarification and assessment of the residual spinal canal diameter. Burst fractures in the thoracolumbar spine are diagnosed when there is a vertically oriented fracture of the vertebral body with lateral dispersion of the fracture fragments. There usually are associated fractures in the posterior elements. This injury can be recognized on radiographs by identifying a vertical fracture or widening of the interpedicular distance on the frontal projection. CT is useful to characterize the associated posterior element fractures and assess spinal canal impingement. MRI permits assessment of the status of the conus medullaris and the spinal nerve roots in patients with neurologic deficits.

The thoracolumbar region is a biomechanically unique region of the spine and the only location where Chance fractures occur.

The Chance fracture is defined as a horizontally oriented fracture, which passes through the spinous process, laminae, vertebral body, or disk space (Fig. 14.15). This fracture occurs exclusively at the thoracolumbar junction. This unusual injury is thought to be the result of distractive forces generated when the spine is flexed about a fulcrum point, such as an automobile lap seatbelt. This has prompted the use of the term *seatbelt injury* to describe the fracture and its associated injuries. Injuries in which the horizontal plane of disruption passes through the intervertebral disk or posterior ligaments, rather than the vertebral body or posterior bony elements, can be considered as variations of the Chance

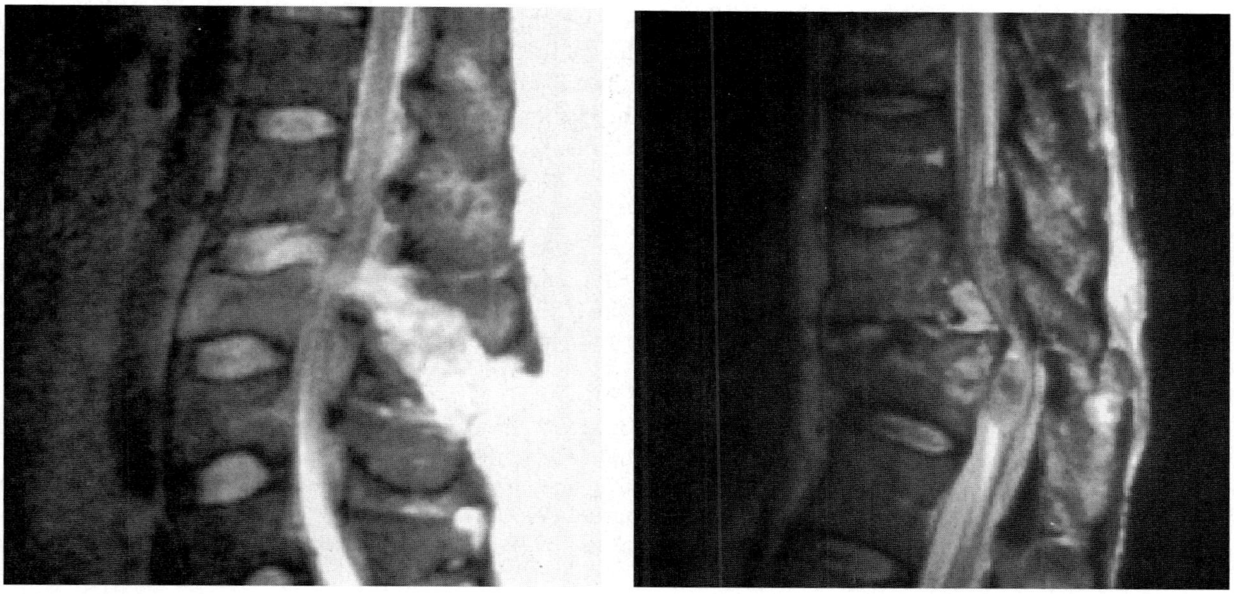
A B

Figure 14.15 *Chance Fracture. A.* Sagittal T2-weighted image shows disruption of the posterior elements at L1 to L2, edema of L2, and widening of the corresponding disk space. *B.* In a different patient, sagittal T2 shows Chance fracture involving the T11 to T12 level with compression fractures and edema of these two vertebrae. There also is edema and possibly petechial hemorrhage in the conus medullaris.

fracture. Usually, Chance fractures are visible on radiographs. MRI may demonstrate the ligamentous components of the variant forms of injury, along with any conus medullaris and cauda equina abnormalities. Significant intraperitoneal injuries are found in up to 50% of patients with Chance fractures, and this has prompted some authors to suggest routine CT scan of the abdomen in all patients with this type of injury.

Benign versus Malignant Vertebral Body Fractures

Distinguishing benign from malignant vertebral body fractures can be challenging. Conventional MRI can give valuable clues in making this distinction (52,53) (Table 14.5).

Recent studies using diffusion-weighted imaging may help establish the etiology of these fractures in uncertain cases. Benign fractures due to trauma or osteoporosis have

Table 14.5: Features of Benign versus Malignant Compression Fractures on Conventional Magnetic Resonance Imaging

Type of Fracture (Etiology)	*Imaging Features*
Benign (osteoporotic)	High signal intensity on T1, fracture line, retropulsed bone fragment, no or small soft tissue mass, intravertebral fluid or vacuum cleft, bandlike hyperintensity on T2
Malignant (underlying tumor)	Low signal intensity on T1, no fracture line, perivertebral soft tissue mass, soft tissue mass compressing spinal cord, no intravertebral gas or fluid, significant contrast enhancement of the collapsed vertebra and adjacent soft tissue mass, expansion of pedicle(s), low signal intensity in other vertebra(e)

high signal intensity on diffusion-weighted images, whereas those that are pathologic have low signal intensity (54,55). Most of these studies have been done using a reverse free-precession steady-state sequence. The B values used are relatively low, and this sequence is hampered by T2 shine-through. I have used this technique extensively and have found it helpful in many, but not all patients.

References

1. Quencer RM, Nunez D, Green BA. Controversies in imaging acute cervical spine trauma. AJNR Am J Neuroradiol 1997;18:1866–1868.
2. Lee RR. MR imaging and cervical spine injury. Radiology 1996;201:617–618.
3. Mirvis SE, Geisler FH, Jelinek JJ, et al. Acute cervical spine trauma: evaluation with 1.5-T MR imaging. Radiology 1988;166:807–816.
4. el-Khoury GY, Kathol MH, Daniel WW. Imaging of acute injuries of the cervical spine: value of plain radiography, CT, and MR imaging. AJR Am J Roentgenol 1995;64:43–50.
5. Bloom AI. Re: imaging of acute injuries of the cervical spine: value of plain radiography, CT, and MR imaging. AJR Am J Roentgenol 1996;166:218.
6. Williams RL, Hardman JA, Lyons K. MR imaging of suspected acute spinal instability. Injury 1998;29:109–113.
7. Katzberg RW, Benedetti PF, Drake CM, et al. Acute cervical spine injuries: prospective MR imaging assessment at a level 1 trauma center. Radiology 1999;213:203–212.
8. Corr P, Govender S. The role of magnetic resonance imaging on spinal trauma. Clin Radiol 1999; 54:629–635.
9. Lis E, Krol G, O'Malley B. Emergency magnetic resonance imaging of the spine. Top Magn Reson Imaging 1998;9:228–237.
10. Turgut M, Akpinar G, Akalan N, et al. Spinal injuries in the pediatric age group: a review of 82 cases of spinal cord and vertebral column injuries. Eur Spine J 1996;5:148–152.
11. Cornelius RS, Leach JL. Imaging evaluation of cervical spine trauma. Neuroimaging Clin North Am 1995;5:451–463.
12. White P, Seymour R, Powell N. MRI assessment of the pre-vertebral soft tissues in acute cervical spine trauma. Br J Radiol 1999;72:818–823.
13. Vaccaro AR, Kreidl KO, Pan W, et al. Usefulness of MRI in isolated upper cervical spine fractures in adults. J Spinal Disord 1998;11:289–293.
14. Keiper MD, Zimmerman RA, Bilaniuk LT. MRI in the assessment of the supportive soft tissues of the cervical spine in acute trauma in children. Neuroradiology 1998;40:359–363.
15. Halliday AL, Henderson BR, Hart BL, et al. The management of unilateral lateral mass/facet fractures of the subaxial cervical spine: the use of magnetic resonance imaging to predict instability. Spine 1997;22:2614–2621.
16. Kliewer MA, Gray L, Paver J, et al. Acute spinal ligament disruption: MR imaging with anatomic correlation. J Magn Reson Imaging 1993;3:855–861.
17. Davis SJ, Teresi LM, Bradley WG Jr, et al. Cervical spine hyperextension injuries: MR findings. Radiology 1991;180:245–251.
18. Terk MR, Hume-Neal M, Fraipont M, et al. Injury of the posterior ligament complex in patients with acute spinal trauma: evaluation by MR imaging. AJR Am J Roentgenol 1997;168:1481–1486.
19. Harrington JF, Likavec MJ, Smith AS. Disc herniation in cervical fracture subluxation. Neurosurgery 1991;29:374–379.
20. Pratt ES, Green DA, Spengler DM. Herniated intervertebral discs associated with unstable spinal injuries. Spine 1990;15:662–666.
21. Shiba K, El-Masry WS, Moraes AC, et al. Anterior dislocation and extruded disc of the lower cervical spine. Spinal Cord 1999;37:538–541.
22. Oner FC, v d Rijt RH, Ramos LM, et al. Correlation of MR images of disc injuries with anatomic sections in experimental thoracolumbar spine fractures. Eur Spine J 1999;8:194–198.
23. Knightly JJ, Greene KA, Marciano FF, et al. Locked facets and disc herniation. J Neurosurg 1994; 80:952–953.
24. Ando T, Mimatsu K. Traumatic lumbar disc herniation: a case report. Spine 1993;18:2355–2357.
25. Gupta SK, Dhir JS, Khosla VK. Traumatic spinal subarachnoid hematoma: report of a case with MRI. Surg Neurol 1997;48:189–192.
26. La Rosa G, d'Avella D, Conti A, et al. Magnetic resonance imaging-monitored conservative management of traumatic spinal epidural hematomas: report of four cases. J Neurosurg 1999;91: 128–132.

27. Fobe JL, Nishikuni K, Gianni MA. Evolving magnetic resonance spinal cord trauma in child: from hemorrhage to intradural arachnoid cyst. Spinal Cord 1998;36:864–866.
28. Chen HJ, Chen L. Traumatic interdural arachnoid cyst in the upper cervical spine: case report. J Neurosurg 1996;85:351–353.
29. Coffin CM, Weill A, Miaux Y, et al. Posttraumatic spinal subarachnoid cyst. Eur Radiol 1996;6: 523–525.
30. Kulkarni MV, Bondurant FJ, Rose SL, et al. 1.5 Tesla magnetic resonance imaging of acute spinal trauma. Radiographics 1988;8:1059–1082.
31. Murakami H, Tomita K, Baba H, et al. Central cord syndrome secondary to hyperflexion injury of the cervical spine in a child. J Spinal Disord 1995;8:494–498.
32. Wallace SK, Avellino AM. Predicting neurologic outcome with MR imaging in a patient in spinal shock. AJR Am J Roentgenol 1995;165:108.
33. Hirsh LF, Duarte L, Wolfson EH. Thoracic spinal cord injury without spine fracture in an adult: case report and literature review. Surg Neurol 1993;40:35–38.
34. Saleh J, Raycroft JF. Hyperflexion injury of cervical spine and central cord syndrome in a child. Spine 1992;17:234–237.
35. Friedman D, Flanders A, Thomas C, et al. Vertebral artery injury after acute cervical spine trauma: rate of occurrence as detected by MR angiography and assessment of clinical consequences. AJR Am J Roentgenol 1995;164:443–447.
36. Weller SJ, Rossitch E Jr, Malek AM. Detection of vertebral artery injury after cervical spine trauma using magnetic resonance angiography. J Trauma 1999;46:660–666.
37. Vaccaro AR, Klein GR, Flanders AE, et al. Long-term evaluation of vertebral artery injuries following cervical spine trauma using magnetic resonance angiography. Spine 1998;23:789–794.
38. Giacobetti FB, Vaccaro AR, Bos-Giacobetti MA, et al. Vertebral artery occlusion associated with cervical spine trauma: a prospective analysis. Spine 1997;22:188–192.
39. Wirbel R, Pistorius G, Braun C, et al. Bilateral vertebral artery lesion after dislocating cervical spine trauma: a case report. Spine 1996;21:1375–1379.
40. Grabb BC, Frye TA, Hedlund GL, et al. MRI diagnosis of suspected atlanto-occipital dissociation in childhood. Pediatr Radiol 1999;29:275–281.
41. Sun PP, Poffenbarger GJ, Durham S, et al. Spectrum of occipitoatlantal injury in young children. J Neurosurg (Spine) 2000;93:28–39.
42. Anderson D, D'Alonzo R. Fractures of the odontoid process of the axis. J Bone Joint Surg Am 1974;56:1663–1674.
43. Odent T, Langlais J, Glorion C, et al. Fractures of the odontoid process: a report of 15 cases in children younger than 6 years. J Pediatr Orthop 1999;19:51–54.
44. Castillo M, Mukherji SK. Vertical fractures of the dens. AJNR Am J Neuroradiol. 1996;17: 1627–1630.
45. Dickman CA, Greene KA, Sonntag VK. Injuries involving the transverse atlantal ligament: classification and treatment guidelines based upon experience with 39 injuries. Neurosurgery 1996; 38:44–50.
46. Leite CC, Escobar BE, Bazan C 3rd, et al. MRI of cervical facet dislocation. Neuroradiology 1997;39:583–588.
47. el-Khoury GY, Whitten CG. Trauma to the upper thoracic spine: anatomy, biomechanics, and unique imaging features. AJR Am J Roentgenol 1993;160:95–102.
48. Oner FC, van Gils AP, Dhert WJ, et al. MRI findings of thoracolumbar spine fractures: a categorisation based on MRI examinations of 100 fractures. Skeletal Radiol 1999;28:433–443.
49. Lund PJ, Ruth JT, Dzioba R, et al. Traumatic thoracolumbar facet instability: characteristic imaging findings. Skeletal Radiol 1997;26:360–365.
50. Petersilge CA, Pathria MN, Emery SE, et al. Thoracolumbar burst fractures: evaluation with MR imaging. Radiology 1995;194:49–54.
51. Brightman RP, Miller CA, Rea GL, et al. Magnetic resonance imaging of trauma to the thoracic and lumbar spine: the importance of the posterior longitudinal ligament. Spine 1992;17:541–550.
52. Moulopoulos LA, Yoshimitsu K, Johnston DA, et al. MR prediction of benign and malignant vertebral compression fractures. J Magn Reson Imaging 1996;6:667–674.
53. Shih TT, Huang KM, Li YWL. Solitary vertebral collapse: distinction between benign and malignant causes using MR patterns. J Magn Reson Imaging 1999;9:635–642.
54. Baur A, Stabler A, Bruning R, et al. Diffusion-weighted MR imaging of bone marrow: differentiation of benign versus pathologic compression fractures. Radiology 1998;207:349–356.
55. Le Bihan DJ. Differentiation of benign versus pathologic compression fractures with diffusion-weighted MR imaging: a closer step toward the "holy grail" of tissue characterization? Radiology 1998;207:305–307.

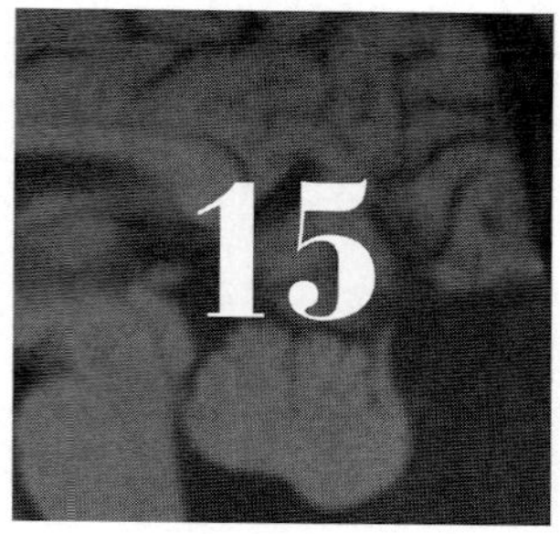

Inflammatory and Infectious Spinal Disorders

- Classification
- Disorders Predominantly Affecting the Spinal Cord
- Disorders Predominantly Affecting the Nerve Roots and the Meninges
- Disorders Predominantly Affecting the Vertebrae, Disks, and Epidural Space

Classification

Inflammatory and infectious disorders of the spine are more common in adults than in children. The most common infectious spinal disorder adult is pyogenic diskitis, and in children it is bacterial spinal meningitis. The latter does not require imaging studies because it is diagnosed and treated on the basis of clinical features and physical examination. In this chapter, I divide inflammatory and infectious spinal disorders as follows:

- Those predominantly affecting the spinal cord
- Those predominantly affecting the nerve roots and meninges
- Those predominantly affecting the vertebrae, disks, and epidural space

I believe that in all of these disorders, magnetic resonance imaging (MRI) is the imaging method of choice.

Disorders Predominantly Affecting the Spinal Cord

Acute Disseminated Encephalomyelitis and Transverse Myelitis

Approximately 30% of patients with acute disseminated encephalomyelitis (ADEM; Chapter 3) develop lesions in the spinal cord (1). Clinically, the most common presentation of ADEM is that of acute transverse myelitis. ADEM is monophasic, that is, it occurs only once in the life of the patient. Recurrent acute transverse myelitis is considered by some to be a variant of multiple sclerosis (MS) (2). Most cases are seen during the months of January to May. Most children with ADEM are 9 to 18 years of age. The most common symptoms of ADEM at presentation are seizures, headache, fever, signs of increased intracranial pressure, and a transverse myelitis (Box 15.1).

Box 15.1: Clinical Manifestations of Acute Transverse Myelitis Including Acute Disseminated Encephalomyelitis

Pain (often in the interscapular region)
Paresthesias (may progress rapidly)
Leg weakness (may progress rapidly)
Rectal and urinary sphincter dysfunction

The spinal cord is involved in approximately one-third of patients with acute disseminated encephalomyelitis.

The possible etiologies for ADEM include postviral, postinfectious, postvaccination, bacterial, and Lyme disease (1). ADEM commonly begins 1 to 2 weeks after a viral infection (most often of the respiratory tract) or a seemingly minor illness. Often, the initial illness may be subclinical. Once symptoms are present, they become more obvious 1 to 2 days after the diagnosis but may progress for up to 2 weeks. At this time, the clinical differential diagnosis includes Guillain-Barré syndrome (GB), disk disease, epidural abscess, trauma, tumor, MS, and poliomyelitis (3). Analysis of cerebrospinal fluid (CSF) is nonspecific and shows increased proteins and leukocytosis. The thoracic spinal cord is involved more often than the cervical region. Histologically, there is necrosis, inflammation, perivascular lymphocytic infiltration, and demyelination. Some authors believe that ischemia contributes to the pathology of the acute transverse myelitis. Once a well established myelopathy is present, the prognosis of patients with ADEM is poor. Treatment with steroids commonly is used, but its benefit is not certain. Some improvement may be evident in children during the first week of the disease regardless of the treatment.

MRI is the best method to assess patients suspected of having ADEM (4). T2-weighted images show multiple patchy areas of increased signal intensity in the cord. Some of these regions may be confined to the gray matter, whereas others are located in the white matter and some involve both white and gray matter. The borders of these lesions are somewhat fuzzy. Holocord involvement may be more common than segmental lesions (Fig. 15.1A). Seg-

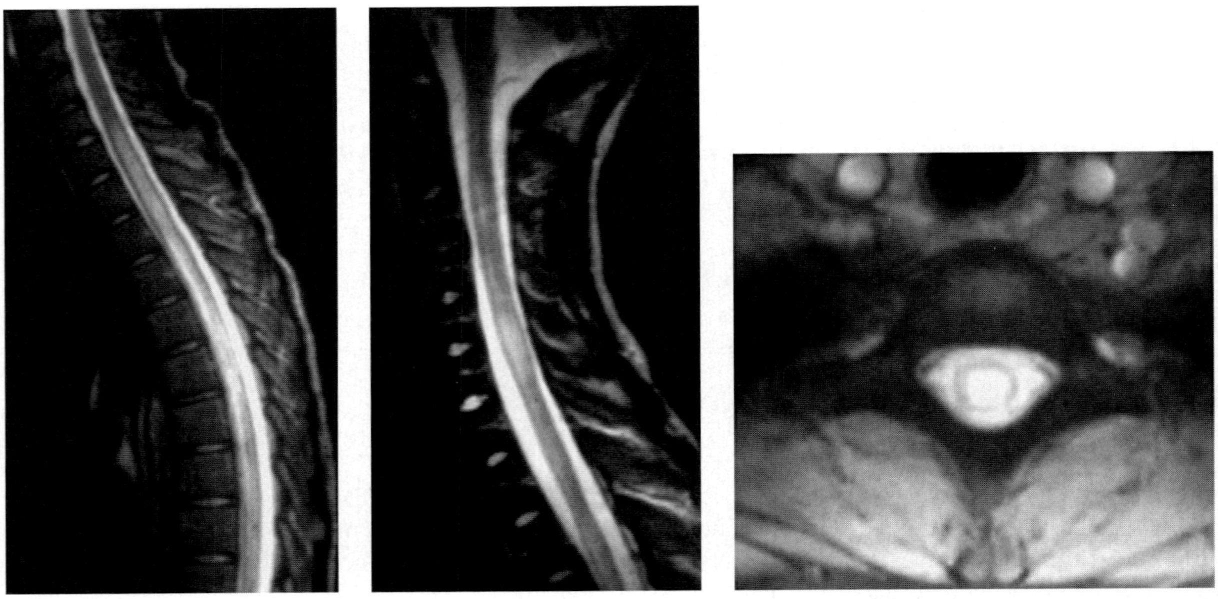

A,B C

Figure 15.1 *Acute Disseminated Encephalomyelitis. A.* Sagittal T2-weighted image shows a long, bright lesion in most of the thoracic spinal cord. *B.* In a different patient, sagittal T2-weighted image shows two bright skip lesions in the cervical spinal cord. The lesions expand the cord slightly. *C.* Axial T2-weighted image in a different patient shows nearly complete involvement by high signal intensity of the transverse diameter of the cord at the cervicothoracic junction.

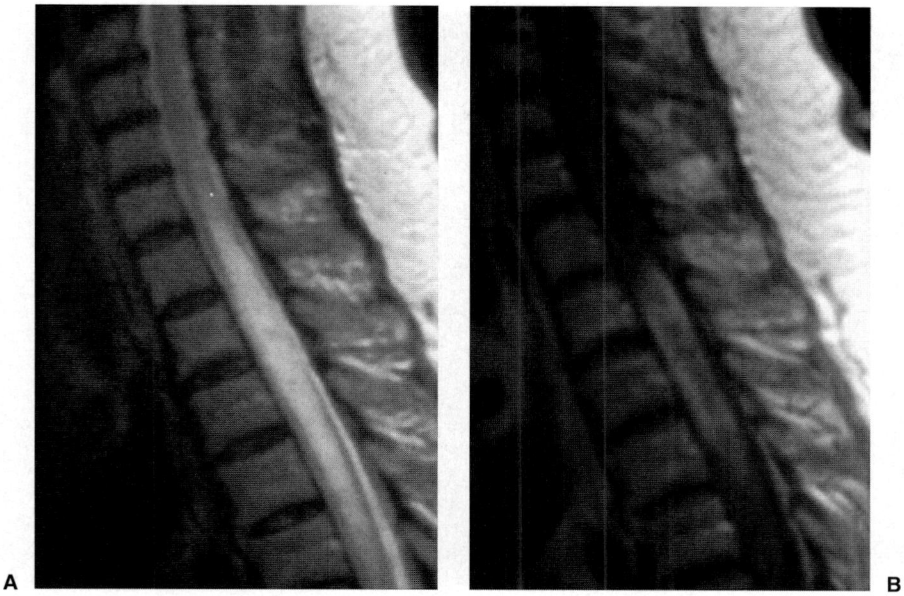

Figure 15.2 *Idiopathic Transverse Myelitis. A.* Sagittal T2-weighted image shows bright and expansile lesion involving the cord in the cervicothoracic junction. *B.* Corresponding postcontrast T1-weighted image shows that the central portion of the lesion enhances.

mental lesions usually involve two to three vertebral bodies in length and may expand the cord slightly (Fig. 15.1B and C). In ADEM, there usually is no enhancement after gadolinium administration, whereas in idiopathic transverse myelitis, some contrast enhancement is the rule (5). Some authors however, have found contrast enhancement in up 40% of spinal cord lesions presumably due to ADEM (3). Although ADEM is a disease of children, idiopathic transverse myelitis is more common in adults. In some patients there may be enhancement of the cauda equina, suggesting that transverse myelitis and GB have a similar etiology. The imaging findings of idiopathic transverse myelitis are similar to those seen in ADEM (Fig. 15.2).

Multiple Sclerosis

Devic's disease is a necrotizing myelitis and probably is not related to multiple sclerosis, as previously thought.

MS (Chapter 3) is predominantly a disorder of adults, although 4% to 5% of all cases are diagnosed in children (1). The onset of MS may occur before 10 years of age (childhood type), between 10 and 15 years of age (juvenile type), or after 15 years of age (adult type). MS is more common in women 20 to 40 years of age. The etiology of MS is not known. Most pediatric and adult MS is of the relapsing/remitting form. In this type of the disease, there are clearly defined relapses with full recovery between them, but the incidence of sequelae and residual deficits becomes greater with each episode. The symptoms in children and in adults are those of transverse myelitis (see earlier). Approximately 10% of all adults with MS present with an isolated myelopathy usually involving the cervical region (6) (Fig. 15.3A–C). Overall, involvement of the cervical spinal cord is twice as common as involvement of the thoracic region in MS. Approximately 30% of patients with MS eventually develop plaques in the spinal cord. CSF analysis shows that immunoglobulin G index and oligoclonal bands are positive in over 75% of patients with MS. Schilder's disease is an acute variant of MS that predominantly affects children; it affects the brain, not the spinal cord, and is not addressed further here. The MRI findings in all forms of childhood and adult MS are similar. Patients with juvenile MS have an increased incidence of lesions in the posterior fossa structures compared with adults.

MRI is the best imaging method in patients suspected of having spinal MS (6). The lesions are hyperintense on T2-weighted images and hypointense on T1 sequences, and may have either ill-defined or sharp borders and variable contrast enhancement (Fig.

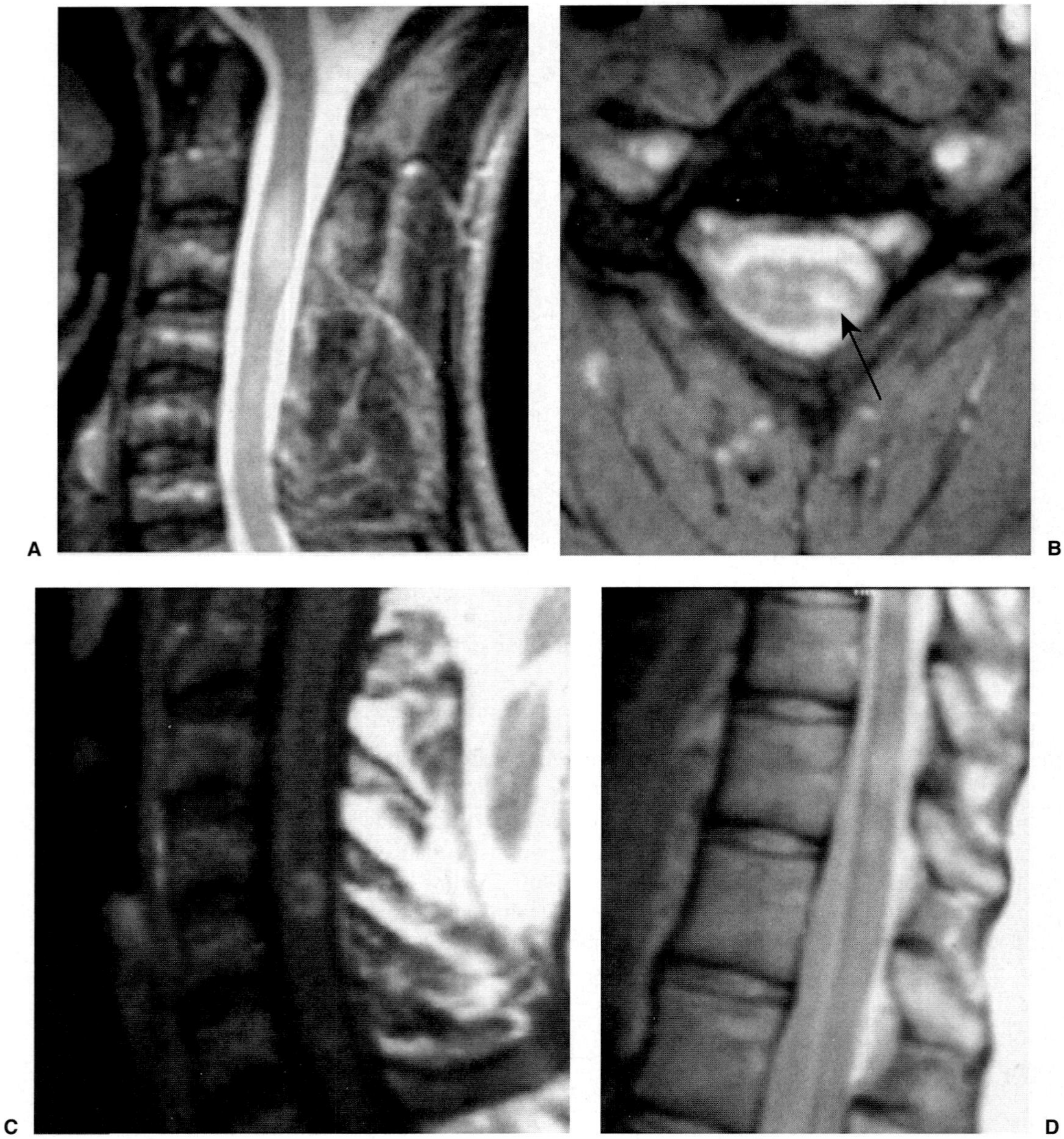

Figure 15.3 *Multiple Sclerosis. A.* Sagittal T2-weighted image shows bright and expansile lesion in the cord at the C2 to C3 levels and a smaller lesion at C4 to C5. *B.* Axial T2-weighted image in a different patient shows typical involvement of only the white matter tracts (in this case, the left lateral corticospinal tracts; *arrow*). *C.* Postcontrast T1-weighted image (different patient) shows ring-enhancing lesion at the C4 to C5 level and perhaps another small lesion at the C6 level. *D.* In a different patient, sagittal T2-weighted image shows patchy bright lesions in the distal thoracic cord and conus medullaris.

15.3A, C, and D). On axial images, the lesions may be noted to involve only the white matter tracts (especially the posterior columns and the lateral corticospinal tracts; Fig. 15.3B). In many cases, however, the plaques involve the entire transverse diameter of the cord. The lesions are short (one to two vertebrae in length), although occasionally they are extensive. The cord is mildly expanded at the level of the lesions, and many acute plaques show contrast enhancement. With chronic plaques, the cord may become slightly atrophic at that level and retains high T2 signal intensity. Rarely, the plaques have a rim of T2 hypointensity that is presumed to be due to iron deposition. A very important fact to remember is that a negative MRI study of the spine and the brain does not exclude the possibility of MS. Although fluid attenuation inversion recovery (FLAIR) images are very helpful in the evaluation of intracranial plaques, they should not be used in the evaluation of the spinal cord because they are known to be less sensitive than conventional and fast spin-echo T2 images (7). Acute plaques may enhance, reflecting alterations in the blood–spinal cord barrier. The pattern of enhancement varies from mild to significant, patchy to solid, or incomplete to ring enhancement (Fig. 15.3C).

POLIOMYELITIS

Poliomyelitis is very uncommon today. Most cases of polio and poliolike clusters are related to prior polio vaccination (particularly the live type of vaccine) (8). The risk for development of poliomyelitis after oral vaccination is approximately 1 in 2,500,000 doses. Only 7 to 10 cases per year are reported in the United States. Poliomyelitis also may be encountered in immunosuppressed patients. The spread of the disease usually is by the fecal–oral route. Most cases of poliovirus infection are asymptomatic and many present with only a nonspecific aseptic meningitis. I address here only the paralytic type of the disease, which is the most severe type. This type predominantly affects the motor neurons. Spinal cord involvement is seen in approximately 50% of patients with polio and is the most common variant of the disease encountered in children (9). The classic clinical presentation of poliomyelitis is that of fever, nuchal rigidity, and spasm of the paraspinal muscles. Rapid progression of the symptoms may occur and portrays a poor prognosis. Weakness usually is asymmetric and quadriplegia is common in patients younger than 1 year of age. CSF analysis shows slightly elevated proteins and mononuclear cells. Analysis for viral DNA (polymerase chain reaction test) in the CSF makes the diagnosis fast and reliable. Histologically, there is parenchymal and perivascular inflammation, gliosis, and destruction of the anterior horn cells, leading chronically to spinal cord atrophy. Treatment is supportive only.

MRI is the imaging method of choice when poliomyelitis is suspected. The spinal cord shows increased T2 signal intensity involving the ventral gray matter horns (9) (Figs. 15.4A and B). The cord may be mildly expanded at the level of the lesions. The lesions enhance after contrast administration. The anterior roots of the cauda equina also may enhance (Figs. 15.4C and D). Findings similar to those described for the lumbar region may be seen elsewhere in the spine cord. The brainstem also may be involved, and this involvement may be documented by MRI.

POSTVACCINATION MYELITIS

Most cases of postvaccination myelitis commonly manifest as either ADEM or an acute transverse myelitis, and those two entities were discussed previously. Vaccines known to induce myelitis include:

- Poliomyelitis
- Rabies
- Tetanus
- Smallpox
- Influenza
- Rubella
- Hepatitis B
- DPT (diphtheria–pertussis–tetanus; causes mostly a peripheral neuropathy)

In most patients, postvaccination myelitis is a presumptive diagnosis based on the temporal relationship between the vaccine administration and the onset of symptoms. Most reactions to the live poliovirus vaccine manifest as a cluster of GB-like illnesses (Fig. 15.4A and B). The myelitis usually occurs 40 to 50 days after the administration of the vaccine (8). The imaging findings are identical to those described for poliomyelitis (see earlier). Myelitis secondary to hepatitis B vaccination is rare but its incidence is increasing because of the widespread use of the vaccine in adults and children. Symptoms of transverse myelitis usually occur 1 to 3 weeks after vaccination. The MRI findings are nonspecific and show only focal intramedullary spinal cord high T2 signal intensity. Patterns of

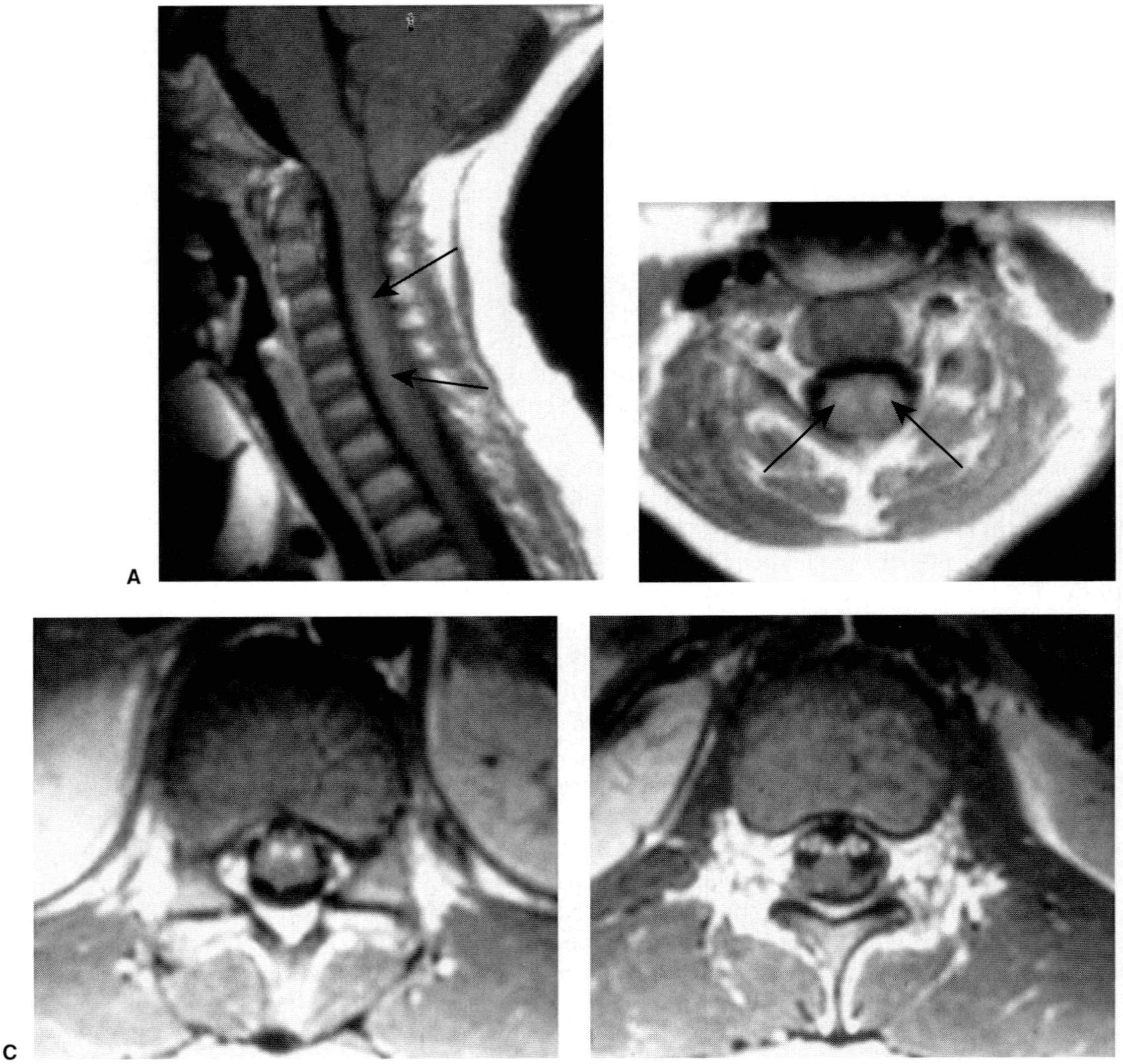

Figure 15.4 *Poliomyelitis. A.* Sagittal postcontrast T1-weighted image in a child after vaccination for poliomyelitis shows faint linear enhancement *(arrows)* in the anterior aspect of the cervical spinal cord. *B.* Axial postcontrast T1-weighted image in the same child shows enhancement of enlarged anterior gray matter horns *(arrows)*. *C.* In a different patient, axial postcontrast T1-weighted image shows enhancement of the anterior gray matter horns in the distal thoracic cord (presumed atypical poliomyelitis). *D.* In the same patient, the anterior roots of the cauda equina show contrast enhancement.

contrast enhancement are nonspecific and vary from diffuse to peripheral to nodular. The posterior columns may enhance (similar to MS). Transverse myelitis also may occur after vaccination for tetanus. Unlike other postvaccination reactions, transverse myelitis secondary to tetanus occurs acutely after the vaccine is given. Some vaccines, such as DPT and influenza, may result in a polyneuropathy in addition to spinal cord involvement.

Devic's Disease (Neuromyelitis Optica)

Until recently, this disease was thought to be a variant of MS, but Devic's disease now is considered a separate entity. Devic's disease affects the spinal and the optic nerves nearly simultaneously (10). Unlike MS, Devic's disease is rapidly progressive and CSF analysis shows the presence of neutrophils and markedly elevated protein. Oligoclonal bands in the CSF typically are absent (they typically are present in MS), and this finding is consid-

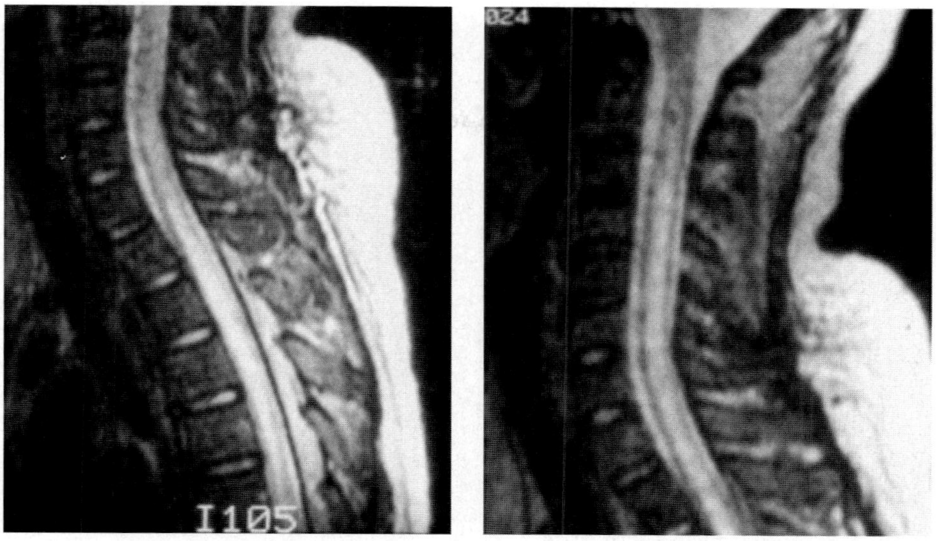

Figure 15.5 *Devic's Disease. A.* Slightly off-midline sagittal T1-weighted image shows bright lesion involving the lower thoracic spinal cord. *B.* In the same patient, an adjacent sagittal T1-weighted image shows that the bright intramedullary lesion continues cephalad to the C2 level.

ered to be highly suggestive for Devic's disease. In addition, in Devic's disease the lesions are confined to the spinal cord and the optic nerves and the brain is not affected. Histologically, there is demyelination and necrosis but little or no inflammation; thus, Devic's disease may be considered a necrotizing myelitis. Devic's disease affects women more often than men and it is mostly a disease of adults, although it occasionally is seen in children.

By MRI, the spinal cord lesions are of high T2 signal intensity (10). These lesions usually affect a section longer than two vertebral bodies and occasionally involve the entire span of the cord (Fig. 15.5). The lesions may show contrast enhancement after gadolinium is administered. The spinal cord may be expanded at the level of the lesion(s). Although the zones of necrosis may contain hemorrhage, this usually is not evident on MRI studies.

Other Inflammatory Disorders Affecting the Spinal Cord

Sarcoidosis affects the central nervous system (CNS) in less than 10% of patients, and involvement of the spinal cord is even less common. Occasionally, the vertebrae also may be affected by sarcoidosis. When the spinal cord is affected, approximately one-third of patients have disease confined to the spinal cord, one-third have intradural but extramedullary lesions, and one-third have both patterns of disease (11) (Fig. 15.6). The lesions are hyperintense on T2 images, may expand the cord, and show contrast enhancement. Pial and spinal cord enhancement is suggestive of sarcoidosis. The differential diagnosis of pial/cord enhancement most commonly includes tuberculosis (TB), toxoplasmosis, human immunodeficiency virus (HIV)–related myelitis, cytomegalovirus (CMV) myelitis, leptomeningeal metastases, lymphoma, leukemia, and exophytic primary tumors.

Radiation-induced myelitis is seen more commonly after treatment of head and neck and mediastinal tumors.

Radiation-induced myelitis is uncommon today (see Chapter 12 for a more complete discussion of radiation effects). It is seen more commonly in the cervical region after irradiation of head and neck cancers (affecting <10% of such patients). It also may be seen in the thoracic spine after treatment of mediastinal and lung tumors. In the abdomen and pelvis, irradiation may result in radiculitis. When the dose is less than 55 Gy, less than 5% of patients sustain spinal cord injury. If the dose is over 68 Gy, myelitis develops in over 50% of patients. Radiation-induced myelitis is seen 12 to 14 or 24 to 28 months after treatment. The disease basically is due to fibrosis and hyalinization of the blood vessels and predominantly results in damage to the white matter. Unfortunately, there is a poor

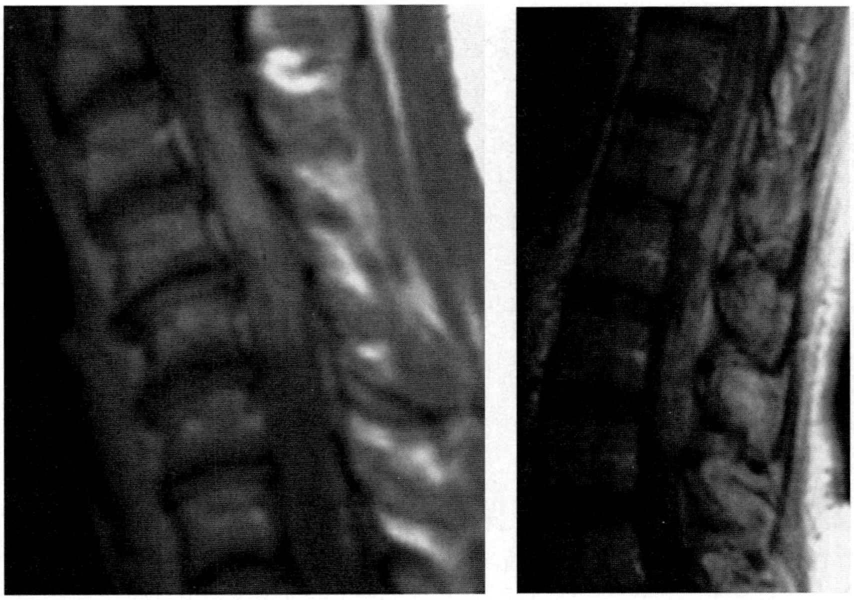

Figure 15.6 *Sarcoidosis. A.* Postcontrast sagittal T1-weighted image shows densely enhancing and nonspecific-appearing intramedullary lesion at the C3 to C5 levels. *B.* In a different patient, postcontrast sagittal T1-weighted image enhancement on the surfaces of the spinal cord and the nerve roots of the cauda equina.

correlation between the symptoms and the MRI findings. The area of abnormality always is within the radiation port limits. The lesion is T1 hypointense and T2 hyperintense. The cord is expanded and may enhance after contrast is given. At approximately 2 to 3 years after the therapy, the cord becomes significantly atrophic and remains T2 hyperintense. In the lumbar region, the nerve roots may be enlarged and show contrast enhancement (findings that may simulate arachnoiditis).

Spinal Cord Infections (Bacterial, Viral, and Fungal)

Bacterial spinal cord abscesses are extremely rare. They are more common in children than in adults. It is said that 20% to 50% of spinal cord abscesses occur in children (12). The most common organisms involved are streptococci, staphylococci, *Mycobacteria*, *Toxoplasma*, *Listeria*, fungi, viruses, and *Schistosoma*. The latter pathogen is particularly common in children. Abscesses in the spinal cord may be found in children with congenital heart disease and disorders of the immune system, in patients harboring long-term intravascular access lines, and in those with underlying spinal cord tumors or dermal sinus tracts. Dermal sinus tracts (Chapter 13) may give rise to intraspinal abscesses outside and inside the spinal cord (13). Multiple spinal cord abscesses also may occur in patients with dermal sinus tracts. Most patients with a spinal cord abscess have a history of infection elsewhere, and spinal cord involvement may be secondary to hematogenous or lymphatic spread. The process begins as myelitis and, if left untreated, may progress to frank abscess formation. MRI shows increased T2 signal intensity and expansion of the cord. After contrast administration there is ill- or well-defined marginal enhancement according to the stage of the inflammatory process (rim enhancement occurs with mature abscesses) (14). After initiation of antibiotic treatment the high signal on T2-weighted images decreases and ring enhancement becomes prominent. With adequate antibiotic therapy, the enhancement slowly resolves in 2 to 3 weeks.

Herpes zoster infection may result in myelitis (15). The symptoms and MRI findings usually correspond closely with the dermatomal distribution of the lesions. The presence of a sensory abnormality accompanied by the characteristic vesicular rash of herpes zoster should

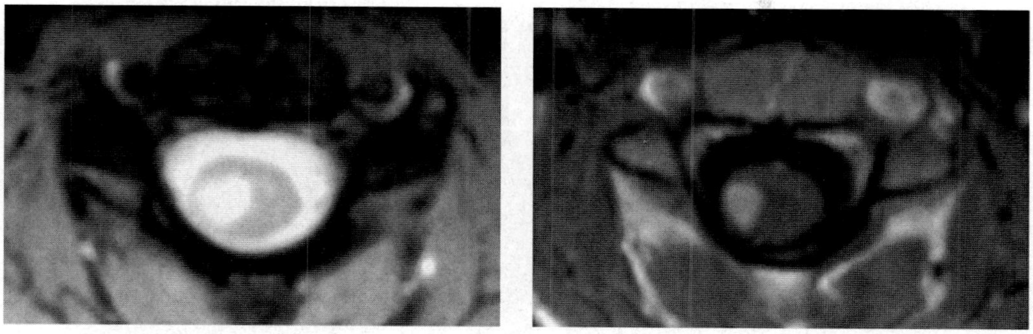

A B

Figure 15.7 *Herpes Simplex Virus Myelitis. A.* In a patient with shingles in the right C7 nerve root distribution, axial T2-weighted image shows focal and well demarcated hyperintense lesion in the ipsilateral aspect of the spinal cord. *B.* Corresponding postcontrast T1-weighted image shows that the lesion enhances.

lead the clinician to suspect a herpes-related myelitis. It is not clear if the herpes myelitis is due to an allergic reaction, autoimmune vasculitis, or demyelination, or is a result of direct viral infection. Viruses usually are absent in the CSF. These patients show fairly typical MRI characteristics. On T2 images, the spinal cord shows a focal, somewhat rounded, hypertense lesion involving one-half of the cord ipsilateral to the cutaneous rash (Fig. 15.7). With contrast administration, the lesion shows well defined margins and homogeneous enhancement.

CMV also may involve the spinal cord and nerve roots (16). Most affected patients are adults. MRI with gadolinium shows contrast enhancement in the posterior aspect of the cord, particularly in the lower thoracic segment. The enhancing lesions may extend to the pia and even the dura. The surface of the spinal cord may show a somewhat nodular pattern of enhancement. On T2-weighted images, the cord shows long segments of hyperintensity. The dorsal nerve roots of the cauda equina also may enhance. Most patients with CMV myelitis have acquired immunodeficiency syndrome (AIDS).

Patients with AIDS may present with a myelopathy, or one may develop in the course of their disease (16). This myelopathy is thought to be due to direct injury by HIV. Histologically, the virus induces vacuolar degeneration in the spinal cord. There is demyelination of the posterior columns and lateral tracts. MRI shows high T2 signal in the regions of myelopathy. These areas may enhance after gadolinium is given. The findings are nonspecific and seldom encountered in children with AIDS.

HIV and CMV are the most common spinal cord infections in patients with AIDS.

Fungal infections also may involve the spinal cord. I have seen these infections (mostly due to *Nocardia*, *Candida*, *Coccidioides*, and *Aspergillus*) almost exclusively in adults who are immunosuppressed (organ transplant recipients or patients with AIDS) (17). The lesions tend to be multiple and may be small, solid, or enhance in a ringlike pattern. They are accompanied by high T2 signal intensity extending beyond the area of enhancement. The imaging features are nonspecific

CYSTICERCOSIS

Cysticercosis is the most common parasitic disease affecting the CNS (18). The ova are ingested and their coverings are dissolved by gastric secretions. The oncospheres are then transported to the small bowel, where they penetrate the walls and gain access to the circulatory system (19). They become larvae once they lodge in the brain and other organs. The disease usually has a benign course, and the most common symptom is seizures. The diagnosis may be confirmed by positive complement fixation test, hemagglutination test, and enzyme-linked immunosorbent assay testing. Approximately 50% of patients with cerebral parenchymal disease have lesions in the subarachnoid space (19). Involvement of the spinal cord occurs in approximately 5% of patients with cerebral cysticercosis (20). Most cysticercosis in the spine actually occurs in the subarachnoid spaces. These lesions are cystic with or without areas of enhancement, similar to those found in the intracranial cisterns. Most parasites lodge

Cysticercosis is the most common parasitic disorder affecting the spinal cord.

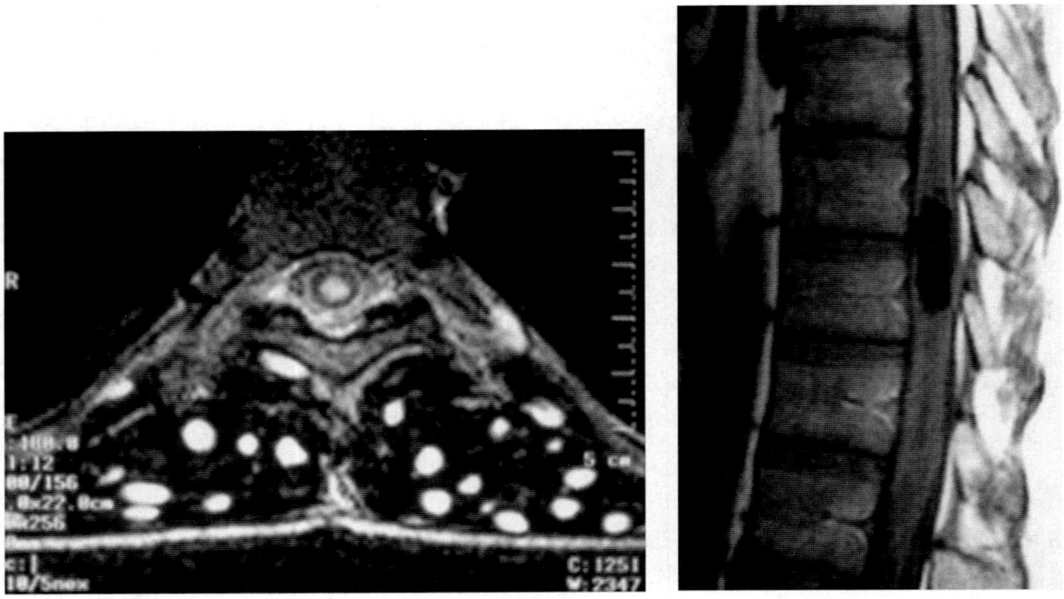

A B

Figure 15.8 *Cysticercosis. A.* Axial T2-weighted image shows an intramedullary cystic lesion as well as multiple cysts in the paraspinal musculature. *B.* Sagittal postcontrast T1-weighted image shows intramedullary nonenhancing cystic lesion in the distal thoracic spinal cord. There is a suggestion of the central scolex. (Case courtesy of T. P. Naidich, New York, NY.)

in the distal thecal sac. Classically, the cysts are known to move according to position of the patient (21). Because myelography no longer is commonly used for the evaluation of these patients, this feature seldom is seen. If intramedullary spinal cysticercosis is a consideration, the brain should be imaged to confirm the diagnosis because most patients have intracranial lesions. In some cases of spinal cord cysticercosis with severe neurologic deficits, surgery may be indicated. Myelotomy with delivery of the cysts is performed. With surgery, even patients with paraplegia may have a favorable outcome. Most intramedullary spinal cord lesions are either cystic with a peripheral nodule of contrast enhancement or appear as nonspecific, ring-enhancing lesions that also may have surrounding edema (22) (Fig. 15.8). Some lesions may simulate a syrinx. The preferred drug for the treatment of spinal cysticercosis is albendazole followed by praziquantel. The anticysticercal drugs may induce spinal seizures and progressive myelopathy when the parasite is dying, and some patients benefit from antiseizure medications and steroids during the administration of the antibiotic.

Disorders Predominantly Affecting the Nerve Roots and the Meninges

Acute Demyelinating Polyradiculopathy (Guillain-Barré Syndrome)

GB is an acute inflammatory disorder involving the spinal and peripheral nerves (23). GB presumably is caused by a prior viral disease and, as such, a prodromal illness may be identified in approximately 65% of patients. Most patients are younger that 18 years of age and most are male. Muscle pain is the earliest clinical symptom and is quickly followed by progressive weakness of the extremities, trunk, and even the face. Like poliomyelitis, GB progresses rapidly, then plateaus, and resolves/improves over a period of months. Symptoms of GB are as follows (Box 15.2):

Box 15.2: Symptoms of Guillain-Barré Syndrome

Onset of disease at approximately 7 years of age
Slightly more common in boys
Weakness in nearly 75% of patients
Pain in 55% of patients
Ataxia in 44% of patients
Paresthesias in 20% of patients
Shortness of breath is rare and may indicate bulbar involvement

Histologically there is demyelination and infiltration by acute mononuclear cells. The nerves (particularly of the cauda equina) become thick and swollen. CSF analysis shows elevation of proteins during the initial part of the disease and a lack of inflammatory cells. The treatment for these patients is mainly supportive. If the weakness becomes progressive and lasts for more than 2 months, the patients are said to have a chronic inflammatory demyelinating polyneuropathy. This type of polyneuropathy comprises approximately 10% of neuropathies. These patients benefit from the administration of intravenous immunoglobulins or plasmapheresis.

MRI findings reflect the pathologic process of the disease (24). The nerve roots of the cauda equina are thick but not overly hyperintense on T2-weighted images. After gadolinium administration, there is enhancement predominantly of the anterior roots, but sometimes, and to a lesser degree, in the posterior roots (Fig. 15.9). On some occasions, the anterior gray matter horns in the distal spinal cord and conus medullaris show contrast enhancement and hyperintensity on T2-weighted imaging. These findings are very similar to those seen (and previously described) in poliomyelitis.

A 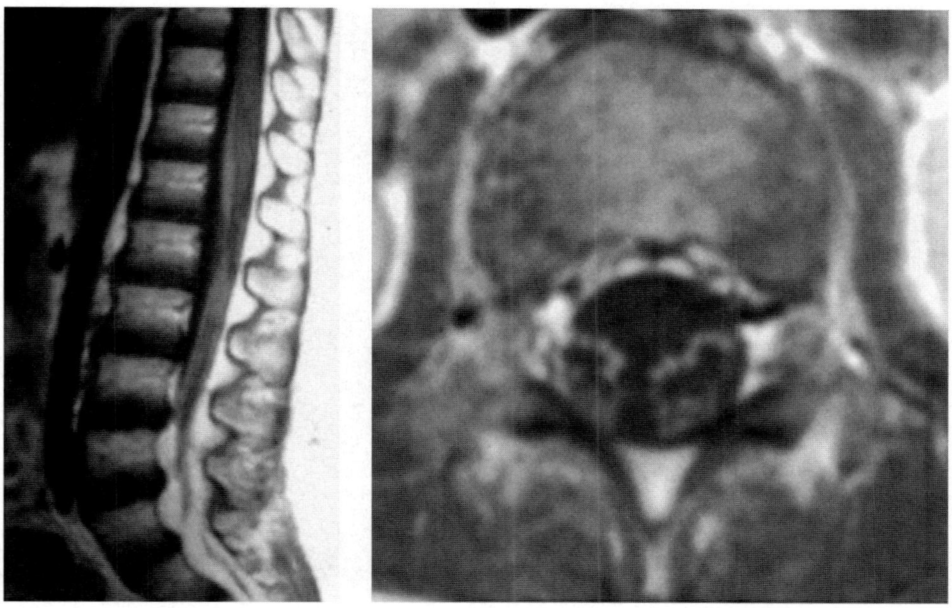 B

Figure 15.9 *Guillain-Barré Syndrome. A.* Sagittal postcontrast T1-weighted image shows enhancement of the ventral roots of the cauda equina. *B.* Axial postcontrast T1-weighted image confirms the enhancement of the ventral rootlets.

Hereditary Polyneuropathies

Approximately 70% of all childhood neuropathies fall into the category of hereditary polyneuropathies (25). The most common of these disorders probably is Charcot-Marie-Tooth disease (CMT). This worldwide disorder occurs in approximately 4 of every 10,000 individuals. Of the two types of CMT, type 1 is much more common.

The most common hereditary polyneuropathy is Charcot-Marie-Tooth disease.

Type 1 CMT is characterized by progressive motor and sensory symptoms. It usually becomes clinically evident during the first two decades of life, and a defect has been mapped to chromosomes 1 and 17. The defect on chromosome 17 leads to abnormal production of a specific myelin protein. The peripheral nerves typically are thick and easily palpated. Their thickening is secondary to proliferation of Schwann cells and fibroblasts, leading to the so-called onion-bulb configuration. This concentric layering reflects episodes of demyelination and remyelination. Eventually there is considerable loss of myelin. An early onset of the disease carries a poor prognosis. CMT presents with progressive distal lower extremity weakness that extends proximally. There is muscle wasting, loss of tendon reflexes, and loss of vibration sense. Spinal deformities develop in 10% of patients. The longevity of these patients is not altered. Treatment of this disease is supportive. MRI shows significant thickening of the nerve roots in both their intradural and extradural segments (26) (Fig. 15.10). This thickening is seen in the cervical, thoracic, and lumbar regions. The thick nerve roots show no contrast enhancement. The dorsal root ganglia also are thick.

Type 2 hereditary motor and sensory neuropathy corresponds to the classic description of CMT (20). It usually is inherited as an autosomal dominant trait. The autosomal recessive variant presents earlier in life and its symptoms are more severe. The clinical course of type 2 disease is similar to that of type 1, but the symptoms may present later in life. Contrary to type 1 disease, axonal degeneration is common and nerve thickening is rare in type 2 disease. No "onion-bulb" formation is present. Treatment is supportive. There are no specific imaging findings in type 2 CMT.

Type 3 hereditary polyneuropathy also is known as *Dejerine-Sottas disease* (DS) (27). This disease is one of the hypomyelinating neuropathies. In these disorders,

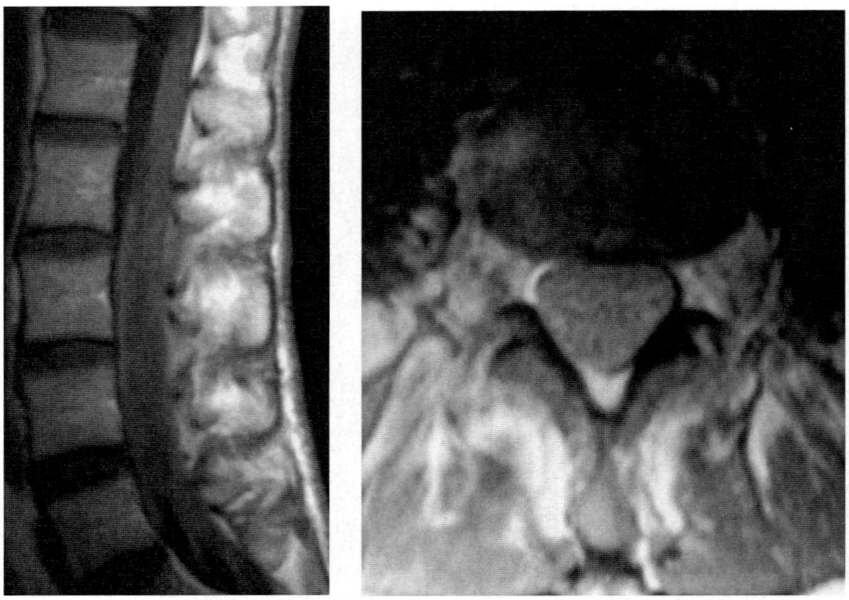

A B

Figure 15.10 *Charcot-Marie-Tooth Disease. A.* Sagittal postcontrast T1-weighted image shows enlargement and enhancement of all roots of the cauda equina that fill the thecal sac. *B.* Axial postcontrast T1-weighted image confirms enhancement and enlargement of all lumbosacral nerve roots.

myelin is not formed or is defective, and there is "onion-bulb" formation in response. There is evidence of abnormalities located in chromosome 17 leading to deficiencies in myelin proteins. In DS, the symptoms manifest during the first year of life. Hypotonia and delayed milestones are common and these children never learn to walk normally. With advancing age, proximal weakness ensues. Sensory abnormalities are uncommon. Treatment is supportive and the imaging findings are similar to those described previously for type 1 CMT.

Type 4 hereditary polyneuropathy is a term used by some for Refsum's disease (28). This disease is transmitted as an autosomal recessive trait and is characterized by a deficiency in phytanic acid oxidase activity. Typical symptoms include anorexia, ataxia, ichthyosis, facial dysmorphism, retinitis pigmentosa, hepatomegaly, growth retardation, and sensorineural hearing loss. There are three variations of the disease characterized by slightly different clinical manifestations. All patients eventually develop spastic quadriplegia and also have sensory abnormalities. The imaging findings in the spine are nonspecific, sometimes subtle, and similar to those previously described for type 1 CMT. Patients with Refsum's disease also show increased T2 signal intensity in the medial aspect of the cerebellum.

Other disorders that may give rise to neuropathies and those which are of interest to radiologists are Friedreich's ataxia and Krabbe's disease. Friedreich's ataxia is characterized by progressive ataxia and cardiomyopathy. There is degeneration of the posterior columns in the spinal cord and axonal degeneration and demyelination in the peripheral nerves. It is transmitted as an autosomal recessive trait linked to chromosome 9. Krabbe's disease is inherited as an autosomal recessive trait linked to an abnormality in chromosome 14 (Chapter 3). There is a deficiency of galactosylceramide β-galactosidase. This disorder is mentioned here because occasionally it may present as a neuropathy (29). Patients sometimes present with thickening of the cranial nerves (particularly cranial nerve II) or thickening of the nerve roots in the cauda equina.

Arachnoiditis

Arachnoiditis is an inflammatory process involving all three meningeal coverings (thus, *arachnoiditis* is a misnomer because more than just the arachnoid is affected). It may follow infections or aseptic inflammatory processes or, more commonly, spinal surgery or trauma. Arachnoiditis also may be idiopathic, or follow infectious meningitis, TB, neurofibromatosis type 1, irradiation, and syringomyelia (30,31). It is mostly a disorder of adults and affects men most commonly. The symptoms are secondary to adhesions in the cord and nerve roots to the meninges (Box 15.3).

The adhesions also may lead to the formation of the CSF-containing cysts in the subarachnoid space that may then compress the neural structures. Adhesions also may compromise the vascular supply to the spinal cord and nerves roots. Constant traction from spine movement worsens the symptoms. The most common symptoms are pain and pares-

The pain in arachnoiditis is caused by traction on the nerve roots by scars tethering them to the meninges.

Box 15.3: Clinical Manifestations of Arachnoiditis

- Chronic symptom progression
- Spotty or localized pain
- Migratory paresthesias
- Symptoms out of proportion to the findings on imaging studies
- Weakness that also may be progressive
- Eventual development of spastic paraparesis
- Rectal and urinary sphincter dysfunction

thesias. The symptoms usually are progressive but occasionally may resolve spontaneously. Antiinflammatory drugs and steroids usually are used to treat arachnoiditis. This treatment, however, is not satisfactory in most patients. Surgery usually is not indicated. Arachnoiditis occasionally may lead to the formation of syringomyelia.

The diagnosis of arachnoiditis is easily confirmed by myelography, but this diagnostic imaging method now is used less often (30). The findings on myelography are clumping and thickening of the nerve roots, adherence of the roots to the walls of the thecal sac (empty sac sign), loss of the normal configuration (blunting) of the nerve root sleeves and distal theca, and occasionally the formation of a mass (fibrosing or ossifying arachnoiditis). Because myelography is performed less frequently today, the radiologist almost never observes all of the aforementioned signs. By MRI, mild degrees of arachnoiditis may be difficult to identify (31). Signs of moderate to severe arachnoiditis are clearly seen on MRI and include clumping of the nerve roots, empty thecal sac sign, enhancement of the nerve roots, and, rarely, an intradural mass of low T2 signal intensity that also may enhance after gadolinium administration (Fig. 15.11). TB is a rare cause of arachnoiditis. Patients with tubercular arachnoiditis show increased T1 signal in the CSF, loss of the cord–CSF interface in all sequences, a "shaggy" cord

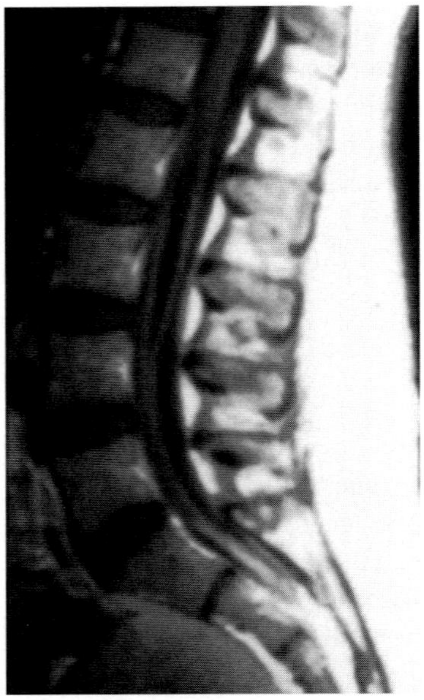
A

Figure 15.11 *Arachnoiditis. A.* Sagittal noncontrast T1-weighted image shows "clumping" of the roots of the cauda equina that appear adherent to the anterior and posterior walls of the thecal sac. *B.* Axial noncontrast T1-weighted image in the same patient confirms the clumped configuration of the nerve roots. *C.* In a different patient, axial T2-weighted image shows that all nerve roots are adhered laterally, giving the appearance of the "empty thecal sac."

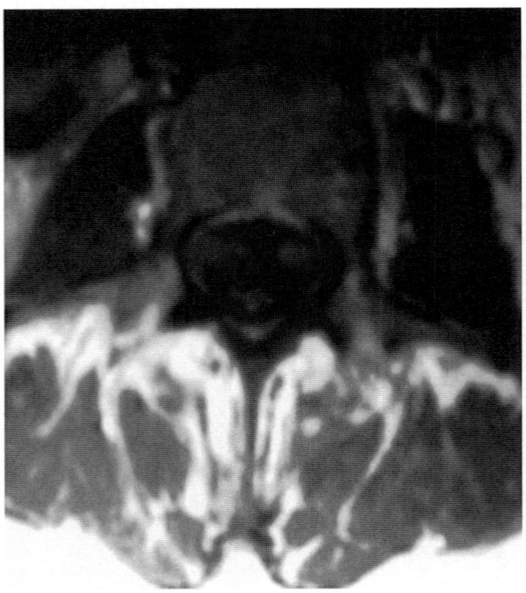
B

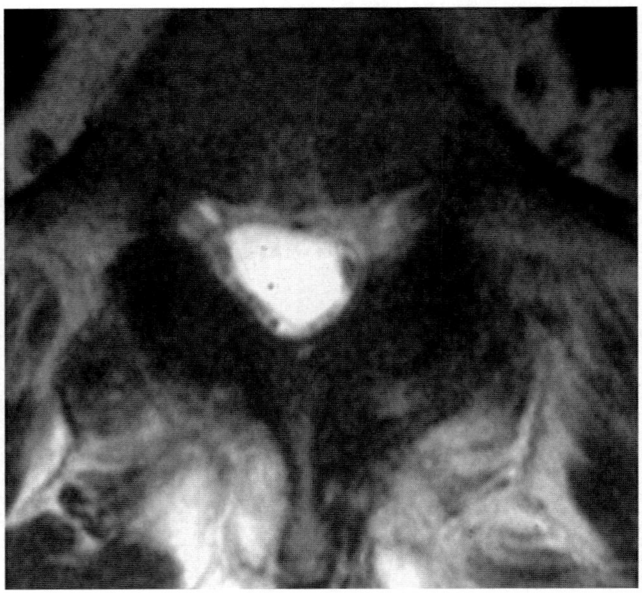
C

appearance, intramedullary cord high T2 signal intensity, meningeal enhancement, clumping of the nerve roots of the cauda equina, nerve root enhancement, and spinal cord enhancement.

Disorders Predominantly Affecting the Vertebrae, Disks, and Epidural Space

Rheumatoid Arthritis

Pannus due to rheumatoid arthritis is T1 hypointense, T2 hyperintense, and enhances after gadolinium administration.

The spine is second in involvement after the peripheral joints in patients with rheumatoid arthritis (RA). Spinal involvement occurs in 20% to 85% of all patients with RA (32), and occurs in the chronic phase of the disease (in general, 10 to 20 years after the diagnosis). The most commonly affected sites in the spine are the synovial joints at the C1 to C2 level. The most common symptom is cervical spine pain that may radiate to the suboccipital region. As the ligaments become lax, subluxations occur and may lead to myelopathy (33). Other symptoms are vertebrobasilar insufficiency and cranial neuropathies. The atlantodental subluxation usually is greater than 9 mm by the time these symptoms become manifest. With time, proliferation of the synovium occurs and pannus formation ensues. The pannus usually is hypointense on T1 and moderately to hyperintense on T2 images (34) (Fig. 15.12). It enhances after gadolinium administration. With proliferation of pannus, significant erosion of the dens occurs. Complete resorption of the dens or a fracture of the dens also may occur. Compression of the spinal cord by pannus (and skull base deformity) develops in nearly 50% of patients with cervical spine disease. The spinal cord may develop intrinsic high T2 signal, indicating myelomalacia. With time, basilar invagination (downward settling of the skull base) is seen. I usually use McGregor's line to measure basilar invagination. This line extends from the inferior aspect of the occipital bone at the level of the foramen magnum to the tip of the hard palate. The dens is considered to be "high" when it protrudes over 8 to 9 mm above this line. This vertical subluxation also is the cause of vertebrobasilar insufficiency. With progression of RA, subluxations also develop in the remainder of the cervical spine and may lead to multilevel spinal canal stenosis. Facet subluxations and resorption lead to hyperlordosis and a "stair step" appearance on sagittal MRI. Involvement of the uncovertebral joints leads to stenoses of the neural foramina. The disks become thin and eventually may be reabsorbed completely, resulting in fusion of the vertebral bodies at multiple levels. Occasionally these abnormal disks are of high T1 signal intensity. The rest of the spine eventually becomes affected in patients with RA.

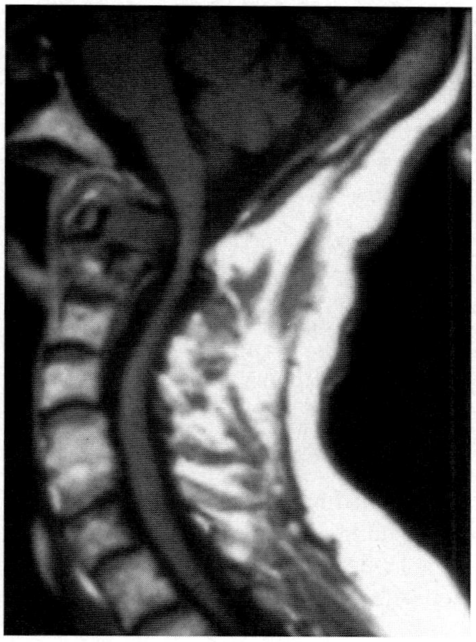

Figure 15.12 *Rheumatoid Arthritis.* Sagittal T1-weighted image shows destruction of the dens by pannus that compresses the spinal cord. The C5-6 vertebrae are fused.

Juvenile Rheumatoid Arthritis

Although juvenile rheumatoid arthritis (JRA) commonly involves the peripheral joints, it also may involve the spine, particularly in the cervical region. JRA usually is diagnosed before 16 years of age, particularly when joint symptoms persist for more than 6 weeks and an underlying infection has been excluded (32). JRA is more common in girls than in boys. JRA is a primary synovitis but results in secondary alterations of the vertebrae. The growth of the vertebrae and disks may be arrested and spinal deformities may ensue. Chronically, facet and uncovertebral joint ankylosis and vertebral body fusions are found. Symptoms of spine involvement are evident in approximately 60% of patients with JRA, whereas imaging abnormalities may be present (but clinically silent) in up 80% of cases. The earliest signs of spinal involvement occur in the cervical region and include stiffness and pain. The disease usually begins at the C2 to C3 level and then extends caudad or cephalad. The dens becomes eroded, first anteriorly and then posteriorly. Atlantodental subluxation is common. Unlike in adults, this subluxation in children seldom results in neurologic symptoms. Bone softening and basilar invagination also may occur (Fig. 15.13A). Calcifications in the paraspinal ligaments are said to be typical for JRA. The facet and uncovertebral joints may become completely fused (Fig. 15.13B). When the thoracic spine is involved, scoliosis, fusions, and degenerative disk disease may be found. Contrast-enhanced MRI may be used to discriminate between joint effusion and pannus because the latter shows contrast enhancement (27). In many patients, there is little relationship between symptoms and MRI findings.

Ankylosing Spondylitis

Ankylosing spondylitis (AS) is a seronegative arthritis that predominantly involves the axial skeleton and occurs most often in middle-aged men. Approximately 10% to 15% of cases begin during childhood (34). In the juvenile form of the disease, involvement of the sacroiliac joints occurs late in the course of the disease, whereas in older patients early

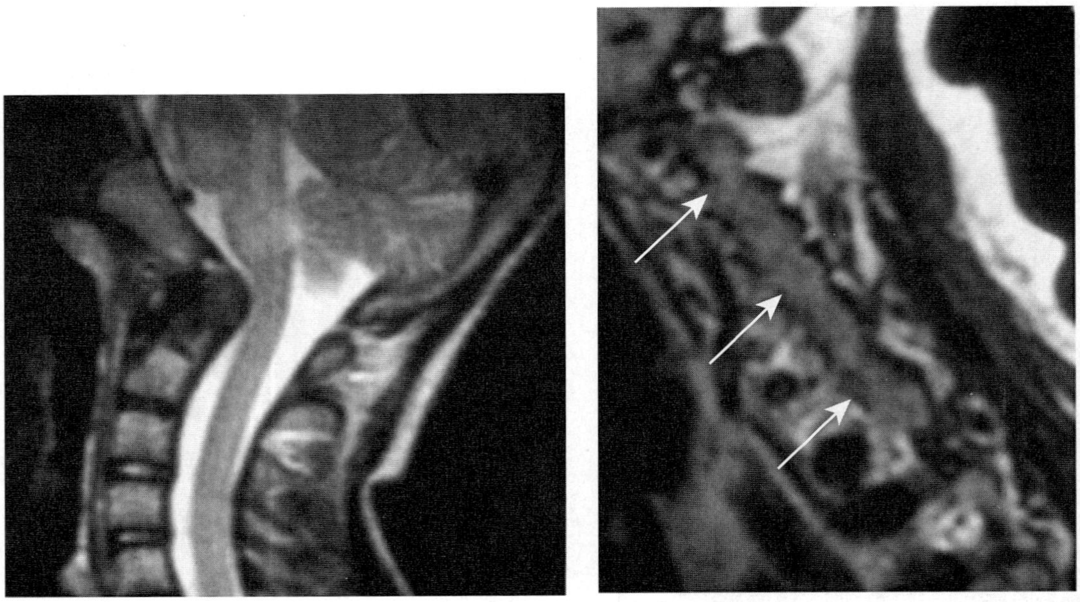

A B

Figure 15.13 *Juvenile Rheumatoid Arthritis. A.* Sagittal T2-weighted image shows a poorly defined dens that is superiorly displaced (basilar invagination), resulting in compression of the cervicomedullary junction. Note increased signal intensity in the brainstem. *B.* In a different patient, a parasagittal T2-weighted image shows fusion of all facet joints *(arrows)*.

sacroiliitis is the hallmark of the disease. Sacroiliac joint involvement first is unilateral but becomes bilateral in nearly all patients (35). From a clinical standpoint, the most important differential diagnosis is that of RA. AS occurs much more commonly in men. Unlike RA, AS begins in the lower axial skeleton and extends superiorly. Involvement of the cervical region early in the course of the disease is very rare. Radiographs may not be sensitive for early detection of sacroiliac joint disease, and computed tomography (CT) offers a better diagnostic imaging test. CT may show indistinct joint margins and subchondral sclerosis. In the spine, the earliest finding is sclerosis of the anterior margins of the vertebral endplates ("shiny corner" sign or Romanus lesions). Syndesmophyte formation leading to the so-called bamboo spine is rare in children but common in adults. These syndesmophytes bridge the disk spaces. Complications seen in adults with AS include "banana" fractures, epidural hematomas, atlantoaxial subluxation, erosive dural ectasia, spinal cord infarction, and aseptic bone destruction, and usually are not seen in children (Fig. 15.14).

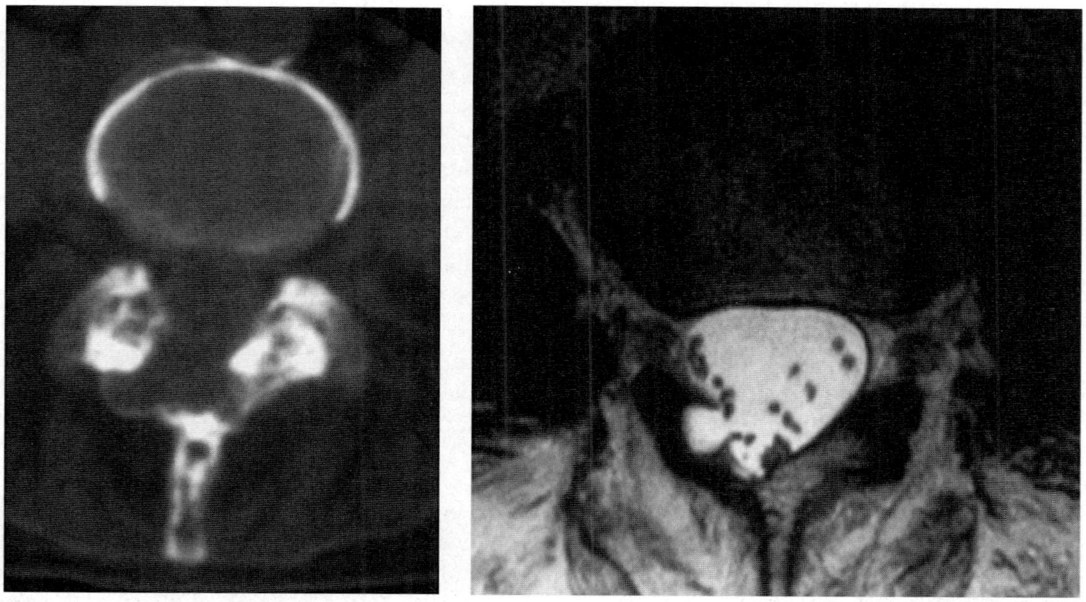
A B

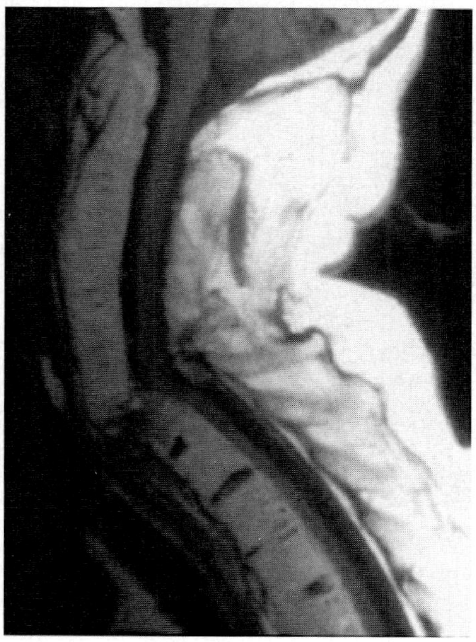
C

Figure 15.14 *Ankylosing Spondylitis. A.* Axial computed tomography shows ectatic dural walls that have eroded the spinal canal, especially posteriorly. Note dense syndesmophyte in the anterior and lateral margins of the vertebral body. *B.* In a different patient, axial T2-weighted image shows similar erosion of the posterior spinal canal by dural ectasia. Note multiple adherent nerve roots in the zone of ectasia. *C.* In a different patient, sagittal T1-weighted image shows fracture through a cervical disk, fusion of all disks, and increased bone marrow signal intensity. Fractures in patients with this disease may be very difficult to visualize on radiographs, and magnetic resonance imaging may play important role in their diagnosis.

Infectious Diskitis and Osteomyelitis

Factors predisposing to the development of spinal infections are diabetes, AIDS, intravenous drug use, immunosuppression, previous back surgery, and instrumentation of the genitourinary tract.

It usually is assumed that in children the disk is hypervascular and that infection begins inside it. There now is evidence that spine infection in children usually begins in the vertebral body adjacent to the endplate in the form of microabscesses (35). Because there are many perforating vascular channels extending into the endplate and the disk, the infection rapidly extends into these two structures. Once the disk is involved, the infection extends again superiorly and inferiorly to affect the adjacent vertebral bodies. This mechanism is similar to that occurring in adults. Most patients with diskitis and osteomyelitis are older men. Predisposing factors include diabetes, AIDS, intravenous drug use, immunosuppression, previous back surgery, and instrumentation of the genitourinary tract (36). The most common presentation is that of back pain (nearly 100% of patients) and fever. In half the patients, the back pain may be rapidly progressive. Although the clinical diagnosis is fairly straightforward in adults, many children present with nonspecific findings such as failure to walk, abdominal pain, and chronic back pain. The onset of diskitis may be gradual and subtle, progressing over the course of 2 to 4 weeks (37). The clinical differential diagnosis includes infection, Scheuermann's disease, TB, fungal infection, spinal epidural abscess, osteoid osteoma, tumor, and vertebra plana. In adults, *Staphylococcus aureus* is the most common causative organism (50% to 90% of cases). Other organisms include *Pseudomonas*, *Serratia*, *Escherichia coli*, *Streptococcus*, and *Salmonella*. Staphylococci and *Diplococcus pneumoniae* account for most cases of diskitis in children. In children with sickle cell disease, there is an increased incidence of salmonella diskitis and osteomyelitis. The earliest findings on radiographs (disk space narrowing and irregularities of the endplates) do not occur until 4 to 12 weeks into the infection, and thus radiographs are not helpful in the initial diagnosis. MRI is the best method to evaluate patients suspected of having spinal diskitis/osteomyelitis (37). The L3 to L4 and L4 to L5 interspaces are predominantly affected. The thoracic spine is involved in <35% of cases and the cervical region in <10% of patients. There is an increased incidence of infections at the thoracolumbar junction. Initially, there may be only narrowing of the disk space and slight hyperintensity on T2-weighted images compared with normal disks (Fig. 15.15). The endplates are irregular and not seen well. With advancing disease, the endplates and vertebrae become bright on T2-weighted sequences (Fig. 15.16). All of these abnormalities may show

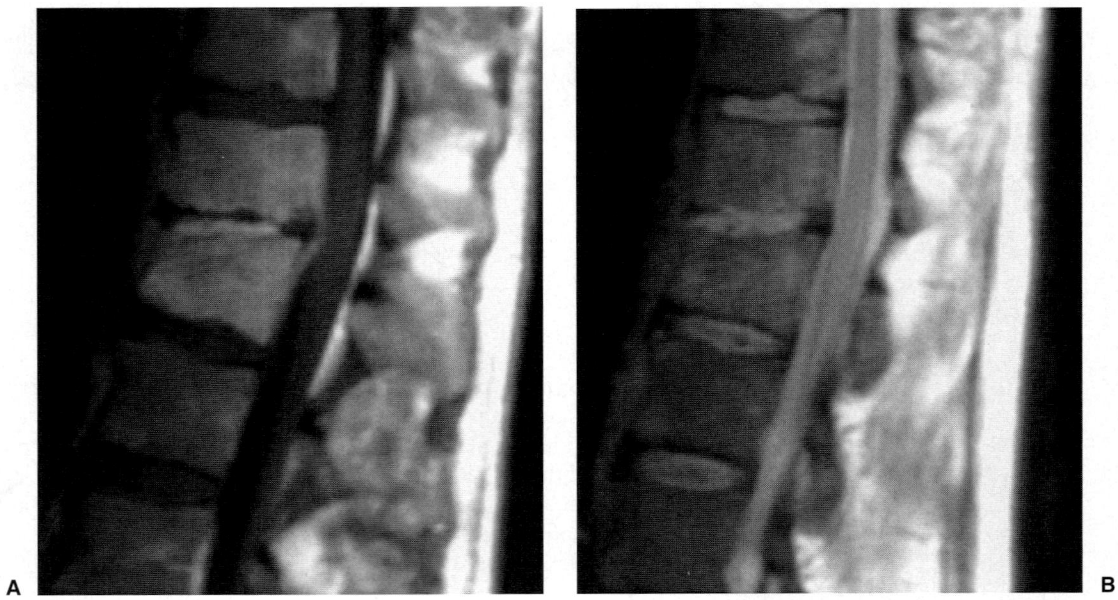

Figure 15.15 *Early Diskitis and Osteomyelitis in a Patient with Acquired Immunodeficiency Syndrome. A.* Sagittal postcontrast T1-weighted image (fat suppressed) shows enhancement of two adjacent vertebral bodies and of the disk between them. The disk space is narrowed and the endplates irregular. There also is some enhancement of the superiormost visualized vertebral body, particularly posteriorly. *B.* Corresponding T2-weighted image shows the involved vertebrae to be bright, as well as the disk. This proved to be a *Candida* infection.

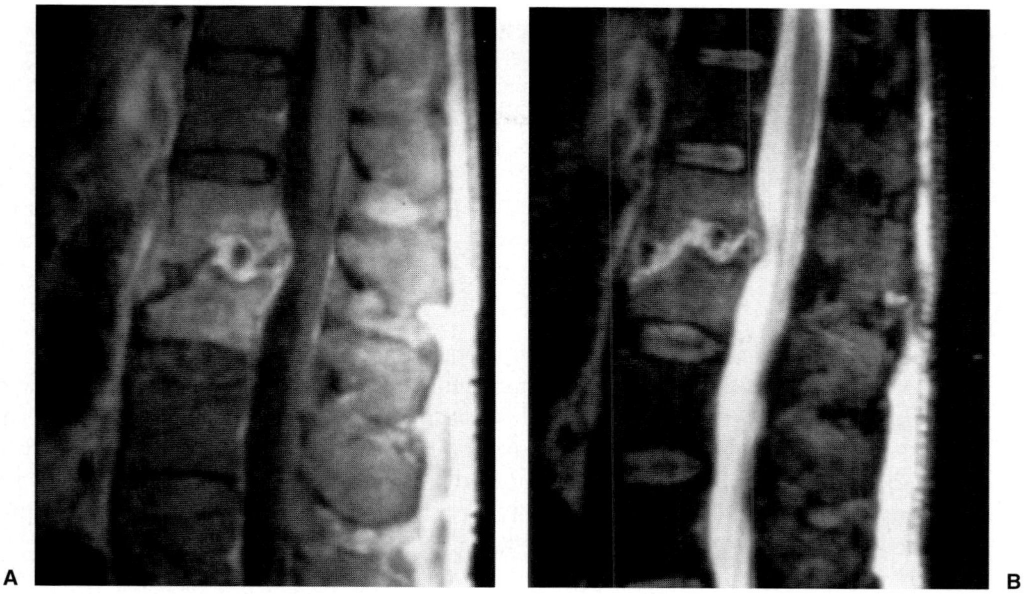

Figure 15.16 *Pyogenic Diskitis and Osteomyelitis. A.* Sagittal postcontrast T1-weighted image (fat suppressed) shows significant enhancement of two adjacent vertebral bodies and intervening disk. There is marked erosion of the endplates. *B.* Corresponding T2-weighted image shows that the involved disk is very bright. The affected vertebral bodies also are hyperintense.

gadolinium enhancement. Gas in a disk space is very rare with infection. Early on, the infection may spread into other vertebral bodies through the venous plexus. In this situation, adjacent vertebrae show abnormal signal intensity in the region of the canal for the basivertebral vein. Edema of the vertebral bodies and disk space is seen better in fat-suppressed T2-weighted images. Involvement of the posterior elements is rare in pyogenic infections but relatively common with TB. Extension into the paraspinal regions (including the epidural space) occurs in approximately 20% of patients with pyogenic infections (Fig. 15.17). The MRI find-

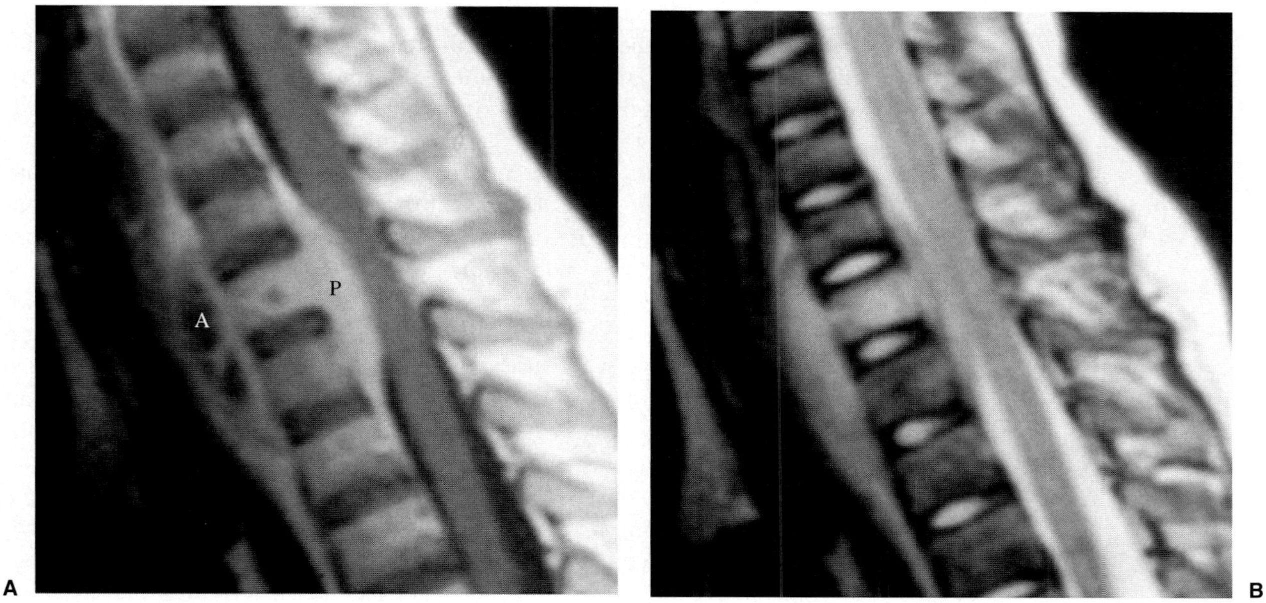

Figure 15.17 *Vertebral Osteomyelitis. A.* Sagittal postcontrast T1-weighted image shows enhancement of one vertebral body in absence of disk involvement. There is an anterior paraspinal abscess *(A)* and a ventral epidural space phlegmon *(P)* that compresses the spinal cord. *B.* Corresponding T2-weighted image shows the bright, abnormal vertebral body with normal-appearing adjacent disks and the extraspinal extension of the infection.

Table 15.1: Findings at Different Stages of Healing of Diskitis/Osteomyelitis by Magnetic

Early	*Late*
Reduction of enhancement in soft tissues, lack of progression of abnormalities	Recovery of high T1 signal in bone marrow, significant reduction of contrast enhancement, bone fusion at level of diskitis

Spinal coccidioidomycosis, similar to tuberculosis, tends to spread under the anterior longitudinal ligament [Wrobel CJ, Chappell ET, Taylor W. Clinical presentation, radiological findings, and treatment results of coccidioidomycosis involving the spine: report on 23 cases. J Neurosurg (Spine) 2001;95:33–39].

ings lag behind clinical improvement with adequate antibiotic treatment. When following these patients with MRI, the most important feature that predicts recovery is the absence of progression. The abnormalities may remain stable or improve slightly with time. Progression of disease indicates a failure of medical treatment. As healing progresses, the signal intensity of the disk space and vertebrae becomes normal and fusion may occur. The paraspinal soft tissue masses disappear. Improvement becomes evident 4 to 8 weeks after initiation of appropriate antibiotics. The stages of healing are listed in Table 15.1 (37).

I have seen several cases of fungal diskitis and vertebral osteomyelitis. In all patients, the infection was mainly in the disk space (Fig. 15.15). All patients were adults and immunosuppressed. The most common organisms in my experience are *Cryptococcus*, *Candida*, and *Aspergillus*. The imaging findings are nonspecific and the diagnosis requires biopsy.

TUBERCULOSIS

Isolated involvement of the posterior vertebral elements is more common with tuberculosis than with any other infection.

Spinal TB is common in children (mostly from 2 to 5 years of age) and adults (average age at presentation is 50 years), particularly in developing countries (38). As opposed to the adult form of the disease, childhood TB usually is more extensive and results in large abscess formation. Unlike adult TB, paraplegia seldom develops in children (39). In adults, the incidence of paraplegia at diagnosis varies from 4% to 35%. The disease is due to *Mycobacterium tuberculosis* and infection in the chest or genitourinary tract precedes spinal involvement in most patients. According to the location of the infection, three patterns of spinal involvement have been described: anterior, paradiskal, and central (40). In the anterior type, the infection begins in the anterior (and usually also inferior) aspect of a vertebral body and extends under the anterior longitudinal ligament to involve other vertebrae (Fig. 15.18). In the central type, the infection begins in the middle of the vertebral body, may produce a vertebra plana, and results in acute-angle kyphosis. In the paradiskal type, the infection begins in the lateral sides of the disk and results in narrowing of the disk space. Paradiskal disease is the least common form in children. TB also may involve the posterior elements in an isolated fashion (41). Before frank abscess formation, there is a stage characterized by development of masses of granulation tissues. These sites of infection reflect the fact that *M. tuberculosis* is an organism that has a proclivity for an environment with a high oxygen concentration (thus, mycobacteria usually do not infect the disk initially). Because mycobacteria also lack proteolytic enzymes, the infection tends to spread under the ligaments rather than by destruction of the disk space, as in bacterial infections. The disks initially are not involved in over 70% of patients with spinal TB.

The most frequent site for spinal TB is the thoracolumbar junction and the thoracic region (38). Pain and signs of chronic infection are common clinical manifestations. Low-grade fever and weight loss are typical. The symptoms usually are chronic and indolent and may be present for years before a diagnosis is established. Kyphosis may develop either chronically or acutely. Predisposing factors include AIDS, immunosuppression, alcoholism, malnutrition, and intravenous drug use. The diagnosis is difficult and may be

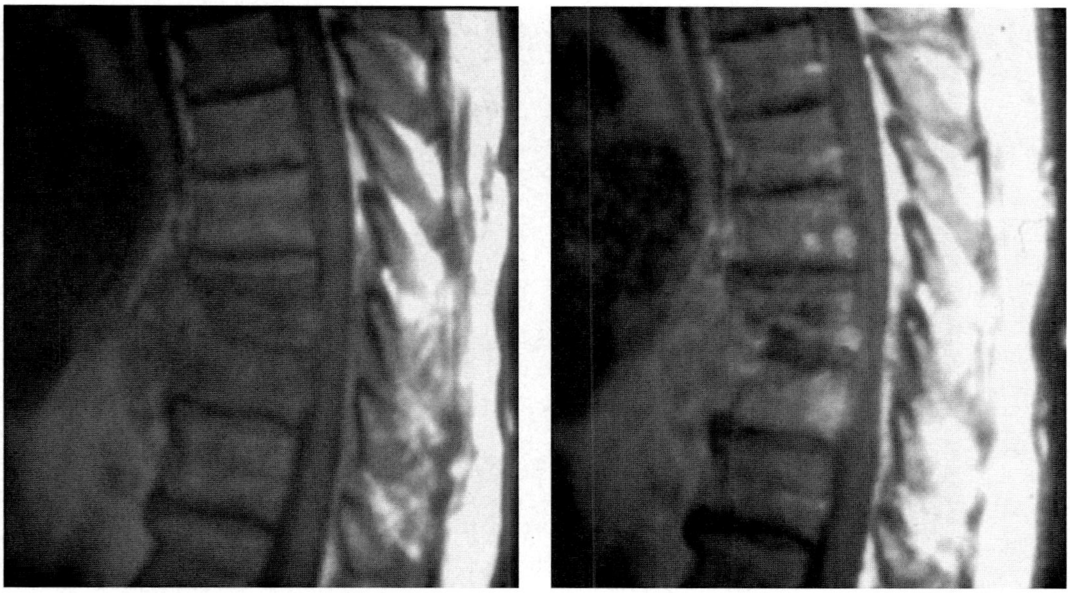

A B

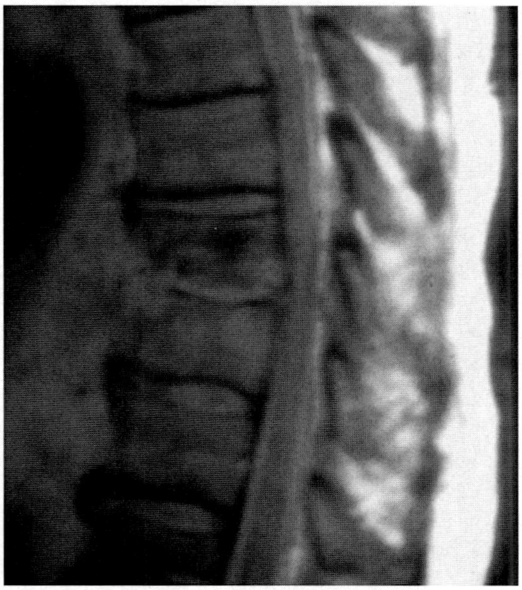

C

Figure 15.18 *Tuberculosis. A.* Sagittal noncontrast T1-weighted image shows erosion of the anterior aspects of the two contiguous vertebrae. There is edema (low signal) in the marrow of the involved vertebrae and an anterior spinal mass. *B.* Corresponding postcontrast T1-weighted image shows enhancement of the vertebral bodies and anterior spinal soft tissue mass, but not of the disk. *C.* Corresponding T2-weighted image clearly shows the anterior vertebral body erosion that is typical of tuberculosis.

confirmed by positive histology or culture. A primary site is found in only 20% of patients. Often, the diagnosis is based on clinical manifestations, radiographic findings, and the response to antibiotics. TB in the lumbosacral region is uncommon and other etiologies, such as brucellosis, should be considered when this area is primarily involved (42). Craniocervical involvement also may be seen and is accompanied by significant abscess formation. Cervical involvement almost always is accompanied by neighboring nodal disease. Two or more adjacent vertebrae are involved in over 50% of patients, and skip lesions are not uncommon. Paraspinal "cold" abscesses occur in 50% to 90% of patients (43). Spinal deformity (most often kyphosis) develops in approximately 60% of patients. TB also may affect the spinal cord and result in abscesses there (Fig. 15.19). This is seen mostly in developing countries. Brucellosis is a rare infection that may have identical findings to spinal TB (Fig. 15.20).

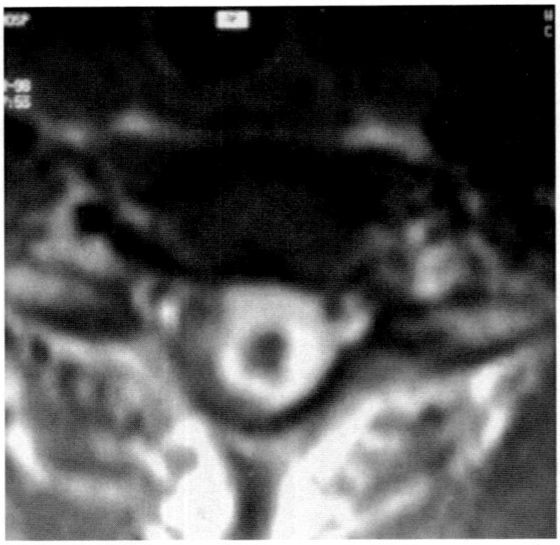

Figure 15.19 *Tuberculous Spinal Cord Abscess.* Axial postcontrast T1-weighted image shows a thick rim enhancement in this intramedullary abscess. (Case courtesy of T. Patankar, Mumbai, India.)

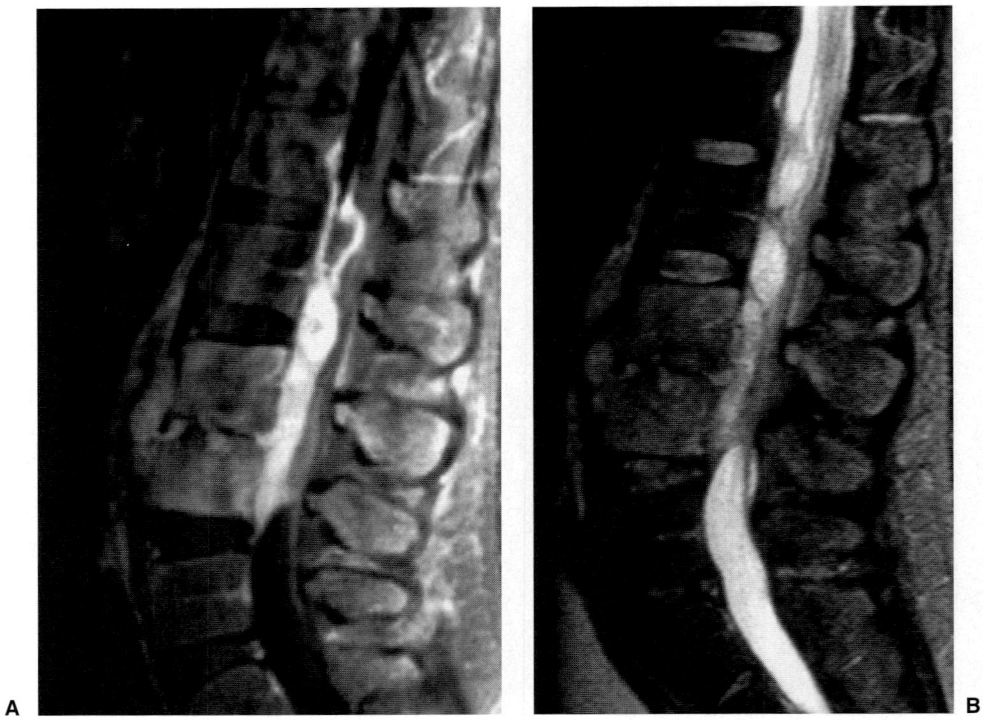

Figure 15.20 *Spinal Brucellosis. A.* Sagittal fat-suppressed postcontrast T1-weighted image shows involvement of L2 and L3 vertebrae and disk with an anterior paraspinal abscess and a ventral epidural abscess as well. *B.* Corresponding T2-weighted image shows similar findings. Note that findings are very similar to those seen with tuberculosis.

EPIDURAL ABSCESS

An epidural abscess is a collection of pus between the bone and the dura mater (35). When they occur in children, they are more common in girls, whereas in adults, men are affected more often. Epidural abscesses commonly are secondary to pyogenic or tuberculous diskitis and osteomyelitis (44). In the absence of disk/vertebra involvement, the infection usually is due to hematogenous spread from primary foci in the urinary tract, skin, lungs, and teeth. Patients with AIDS and long-term vascular access catheters also are prone to development of spinal epidural abscesses. Rarely, epidural abscesses are a complication of spinal needle puncture. Other predisposing factors for spinal epidural abscesses include diabetes, advanced age, prior surgery, a history of cancer, degenerative spinal disease, intravenous drug use, endocarditis, intrauterine contraception devices, septic arthritis, and pharyngitis. The most common clinical signs of spinal epidural abscesses are pain, fever, and rapidly progressing neurologic symptoms. Neurologic abnormalities are present in 40% to 45% of patients with epidural abscesses at the time of diagnosis. The symptoms of spinal epidural abscesses are shown in Box 15.4.

Most spinal epidural abscesses are secondary and adjacent to a diskitis/osteomyelitis.

In children, neurologic signs may be absent or masked by the common prior administration of antibiotics. From the clinical viewpoint, the differential diagnosis mainly includes acute transverse myelitis, tumor, trauma, TB, and herniated disk. Approximately one-third of patients with spinal epidural abscesses show no signs of an inflammatory process on laboratory studies. The most common causative organisms for spinal epidural abscesses include staphylococci, gram-negative rods, and streptococci (45). *Pseudomonas* infection is common in postsurgical abscesses, whereas *E. coli* is more common when the source of infection is the genitourinary tract. Epidural abscesses have a poor prognosis and high mortality rate. Rapid progression usually is an indication for surgical decompression, and most patients remain with deficits after surgery. Children tend to recover more completely than adults. Lumbar puncture is contraindicated in patients suspected of having an epidural abscess, and imaging is the diagnostic method of choice in such instances. Early on, MRI may show a prominent epidural space and is of intermediate signal intensity on both T1- and T2-weighted images (46). Most epidural abscesses affect the lumbar region, but approximately 10% to 15% are located in the cervical region (Fig. 15.21). When the cervical spine is affected, the course of the disease is more aggressive (47). The epidural abnormality enhances homogeneously after gadolinium administration and most often is a phlegmon initially. Surgery is not indicated in these patients, and they improve considerably after appropriate antibiotic therapy. In cases of frank abscess formation, there is a rim-enhancing abnormality in the epidural space with a nonenhancing area centrally (35). Most epidural abscesses are located ventrally, but up to 40% may be located in the dorsal epidural compartment (Fig. 15.21). An important finding in an epidural abscess is that of adjacent diskitis and osteomyelitis. The nonenhancing center usually corresponds to pus, and surgical

Box 15.4: Symptoms of Spinal Epidural Abscesses

- Rapid progression of signs and symptoms
- Localized or radicular pain
- Headache and fever
- Rapidly progressing or acute-onset paresis
- Back swelling, tenderness, and other local signs of infection
- Rectal and urinary sphincter dysfunction
- Sensory level that may change and progress rapidly

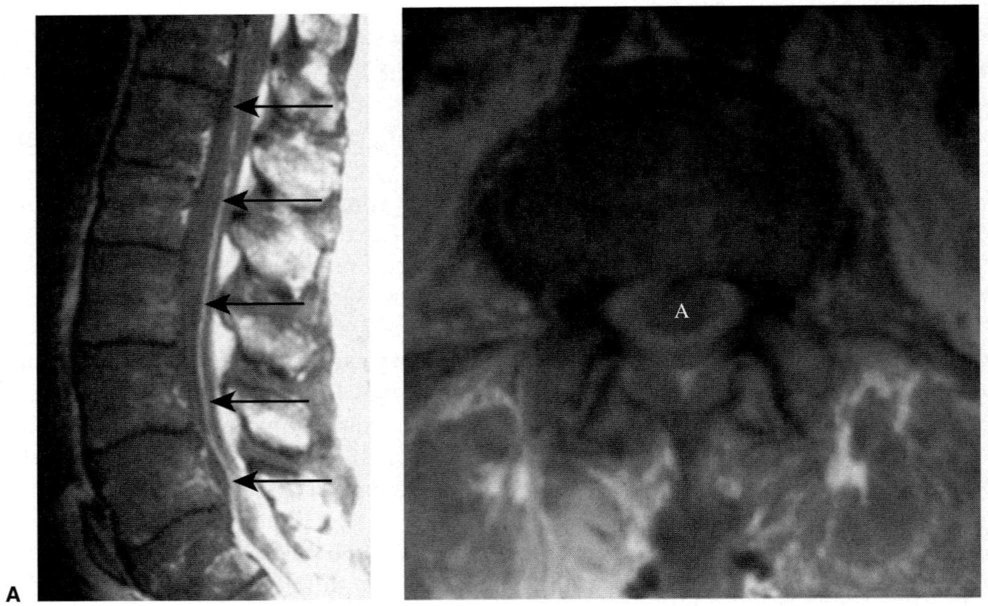

Figure 15.21 *Epidural Abscess. A.* Sagittal postcontrast T1-weighted image in a patient with acquired immunodeficiency syndrome (note low signal intensity from the vertebral bone marrow) shows a ventral epidural abscess extending from T12 to L5. Note that the contents of the abscess are hypointense and that it has an enhancing wall *(arrows)* separating it from the posteriorly located thecal sac. There is no diskitis or osteomyelitis in this abscess, presumed to be from hematogenous spread. *B.* Axial postcontrast T1-weighted image in the same patient shows that the ventrally located abscess *(A)* has very thick walls and virtually effaces the thecal sac.

drainage is indicated in nearly all patients showing this type of abnormality. The findings in epidural abscess on postcontrast MRI are as follows:

- Enhancement of disk and adjacent bone
- Diffuse enhancement of disk/vertebra complex
- Peripheral enhancement around pus collection
- Dural enhancement
- Prominence of epidural venous plexus

The abscesses usually are two to four vertebral bodies in length. In many patients with epidural abscesses, the spinal cord shows increased T2 signal intensity above, below, and at the level of the abscess. This finding is presumed to be cord edema secondary to compromise of the venous drainage from involvement of Batson's plexus. Occasionally, arterial compromise with subsequent cord ischemia may occur. The sensitivity of MRI for the detection of epidural abscesses is said to be over 90%.

References

1. Barkovick AJ. Pediatric neuroimaging, 3rd ed. Philadelphia: Lippincott Williams & Wilkins, 2000:102–106.
2. Tartaglino LM, Croul ES, Flanders AE, et al. Idiopathic acute transverse myelitis: MR imaging features. Radiology 1996;201:661–669.
3. Mark AS. MRI of infectious and inflammatory diseases of the spine. MRI Decis 1991;1:12–26.
4. Tartaglino LM, Croul SE, Flanders AE, et al. Idiopathic acute transverse myelitis: MR imaging findings. Radiology 1996;201:661–669.
5. Campi A, Filippi M, Comi V, et al. Acute transverse myelopathy: spinal and cranial MR study and clinical follow-up. AJNR Am J Neuroradiol 1995;16:115–123.
6. Tartaglino LM, Friedman DP, Flanders AE, et al. Multiple sclerosis in the spinal cord: MR appearance and correlation with clinical parameters. Radiology 1995;195:752–732.

7. Hittmair K, Mallek R, Prayer D, et al. Spinal cord lesions in patients with multiple sclerosis: comparison of MR pulse sequences. AJNR Am J Neuroradiol 1996;17:1555–1565.
8. Tartaglino LM, Heiman-Patterson T, Friedman DP, et al. MR imaging in a case of postvaccination myelitis. AJNR Am J Neuroradiol 1995;16:581–582.
9. Malzberg MS, Rogg JM, Tate CA, et al. Poliomyelitis: hyperintensity of the anterior horn cells on MR images of the spinal cord. AJR Am J Roentgenol 1993;161:863–865.
10. DeLara F, Tartaglino LM, Friedman D. Spinal cord multiple sclerosis and Devic neuromyelitis optica in children. AJNR Am J Neuroradiol 1995;16:1557–1558.
11. Seltzer S, Mark AS, Atlas SW. CNS sarcoidosis: evaluation with contrast-enhanced MR imaging. AJNR Am J Neuroradiol 1991;12:1227–1233.
12. Murphy KJ, Brunberg DJ, Quint DJ, et al. Spinal cord infection: myelitis and abscess formation. AJNR Am J Neuroradiol 1998;19:341–348.
13. Dev R, Husain M, Gupta A, et al. MR of multiple intraspinal abscesses associated with congenital dermal sinus. AJNR Am J Neuroradiol 1997;18:742–743.
14. Friess HM, Wasenko JJ. MR of staphylococcal myelitis of the cervical spinal cord. AJNR Am J Neuroradiol 1997;18:455–458.
15. Friedman DP. Herpes zoster myelitis: MR appearance. AJNR Am J Neuroradiol 1992;13:1404–1406.
16. Rovira MJ, Donovan Post J, Bowen BC. Central nervous system infections in HIV-positive persons. Neuroimaging Clin North Am 1991;1:179–200.
17. Olson EM, Duberg AC, Herron LD, et al. Coccidioidal spondylitis: MR findings in 15 patients. AJR Am J Roentgenol 1998;171:785–789.
18. Mohanty A, Venkatrama SK, Das S, et al. Spinal intramedullary cysticercosis. Neurosurgery 1997;40:82–87.
19. Chang KH, Cho SY, Hesselink JR, et al. Parasitic diseases of the central nervous system. Neuroimaging Clin North Am 1991;1:159–178.
20. Natarajan M, Ramasubramanian KR, Muthu AK. Intramedullary cysticercosis of spinal cord. Surg Neurol 1976;6:157–158.
21. Savoiardo M, Cimino C, Passerini A, et al. Mobile myelographic filling defects: spinal cysticercosis. Neuroradiology 1986;28:166–169.
22. Castillo M, Quencer RM, Donovan Post J. MR of intramedullary spinal cysticercosis. AJNR Am J Neuroradiol 1988;9:393–395.
23. Sladky JT, Ashwal S. Inflammatory neuropathies in childhood. In: Swaiman KF, Ahswal S, eds. Pediatric neurology: principles and practice, 3rd ed. St. Louis: Mosby, 1999:1202–1215.
24. Georgy BA, Chong B, Chamberlain M, et al. MR of the spine in Guillain-Barre syndrome. AJNR Am J Neuroradiol 1994;15:300–301.
25. Smith SA, Ouvrier R. Peripheral neuropathies in children. In: Swaiman KF, Aswal S, eds. Pediatric neurology: principles and practice, 3rd ed. St. Louis: Mosby, 1999:1178–1201.
26. Castillo M, Mukherji SK. MRI of enlarged dorsal ganglia, lumbar nerve roots, and cranial nerves in polyradiculoneuropathies. Neuroradiology 1996;38:516–520.
27. Maki DD, Yousem DM, Corcoran C, et al. MR imaging of Dejerine-Sottas disease. AJNR Am J Neuroradiol 1999;20:378–380.
28. Naidu S, Moser H. Infantile Refsum disease. AJNR Am J Neuroradiol 1991;12:1162–1163.
29. Kaye EM. Disorders primarily affecting white matter. In: Swaiman KF, Ahswal S, eds. Pediatric neurology: principles and practice, 3rd ed. St. Louis: Mosby, 1999:849–852.
30. Snyder R. Inflammatory diseases of the spinal cord, leptomeninges, and dura. In: The pediatric spine: principles and practice. New York: Raven Press, 1994:871–888.
31. Sharma A, Goyal M, Mishra NK, et al. MR imaging of tubercular spinal arachnoiditis. AJR Am J Roentgenol 1997;168:807–812.
32. Tucker LB, Miller LC, Schaller JG. Rheumatic diseases. In: The pediatric spine: principles and practice. New York: Raven Press, 1994:851–870.
33. Stiskal MA, Neuhold A, Szolar DH, et al. Rheumatoid arthritis of the craniocervical region by MR imaging: detection and characterization. AJR Am J Roentgenol 1995;165:585–592.
34. Bates DJ. Inflammatory diseases of the spine. Neuroimaging Clin North Am 1991;1:231–250.
35. Wenger DR, Davids JR, Ring D. Discitis and osteomyelitis. In: The pediatric spine: principles and practice. New York: Raven Press, 1994:813–836.
36. Boden SD, Davis DO, Dina TS, et al. Postoperative diskitis: distinguishing early MR imaging findings from normal postoperative disk space changes. Radiology 1992;184:765–771.
37. Gillams AR, Chaddha B, Carter AP. MR appearances of the temporal evolution and resolution of infectious spondylitis. AJR Am J Roentgenol 1996;166:903–907.

38. Shanley D. Tuberculosis of the spine: imaging features. AJR Am J Roentgenol 1995;164: 659–664.
39. Ho EKW, Leong JCY. Tuberculosis of the spine. In: The pediatric spine: principles and practice. New York: Raven Press, 1994:837–850.
40. Weaver P, Lifeso RM. The radiological diagnosis of tuberculosis of the adult spine. Skeletal Radiol 1984;12:178–186.
41. Ahmadi J, Bajaj A, Destian S, et al. Spinal tuberculosis: atypical observations at MR imaging. Radiology 1993;189:489–493.
42. Al-Shahed MS, Sharif HS, Haddad MC, et al. Imaging features of musculoskeletal brucellosis. Radiographics 1994;14:333–348.
43. Sharif HS, Morgan JL, Al Shahed MS, et al. Role of CT and MR imaging in the management of tuberculous spondylitis. Radiol Clin North Am 1995;33:787–804.
44. Ruiz A, Donovan Post J, Ganz WI. Inflammatory and infectious processes of the cervical spine. Neuroimaging Clin North Am 1995;5:401–426.
45. Numaguchi Y, Rigamonti D, Rothman MI, et al. Spinal epidural abscess: evaluation with gadolinium-enhanced MR imaging. Radiographics 1993;13:545–559.
46. Sandhu FS, Dillon WP. Spinal epidural abscess: evaluation with contrast-enhanced MR imaging. AJNR Am J Neuroradiol 1991;12:1087–1093.
47. Friedman DP, Hills JR. Cervical epidural spinal infection: MR imaging characteristics. AJR Am J Roentgenol 1994;163:699–704.

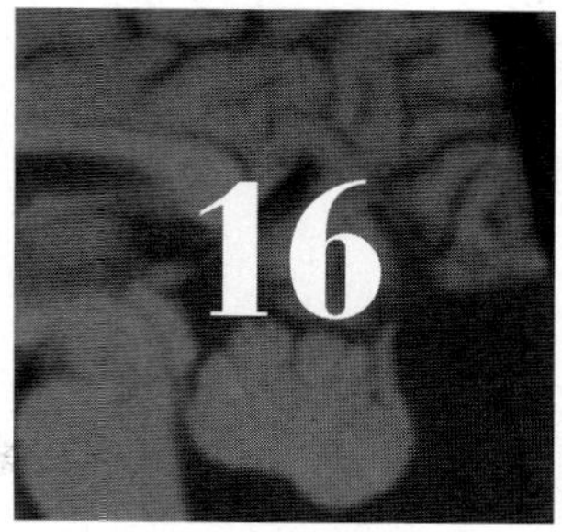

Spinal Tumors and Masses

- Classification of Lesions
- Extradural Lesions
- Intradural Extramedullary Lesions
- Intramedullary Lesions

Classification of Lesions

For the purposes of this review, I have divided this chapter into three sections. First, I address extradural (located in the vertebrae or epidural space) masses, as follows:

- Multiple vertebral lesions: metastases, myeloma, hemangioma
- Solitary vertebral lesions: eosinophilic granuloma, aneurysmal bone cyst, giant cell tumor, osteoid osteoma/osteoblastoma, chordoma (note that metastases, myeloma, and hemangioma also may be included in this group)
- Lesions in the epidural space: metastases, lymphoma, leukemia, angiolipoma, lipomatosis (infections also may occur here and be masslike; these are addressed in Chapter 15).

Intradural (in the subarachnoid space) and extramedullary (outside of the spinal cord) lesions may be divided into:

- Multiple: metastases, lymphoma/leukemia, nerve sheath tumors, meningiomas, cerebrospinal fluid (CSF)–filled cysts
- Single: any of the preceding (lipomas and teratomas are addressed in Chapter 13 and cysticercosis in Chapter 15, and are not addressed here).

Intramedullary (inside of the spinal cord) tumors and masses are rare and may be divided as follows:

- Single lesions: ependymoma, astrocytoma, hemangioblastoma, ganglioglioma, metastasis, paraganglioma, syringomyelia (and hydromyelia; both of which may be multiseptate)
- Multiple lesions: hemangioblastomas, metastases, lymphoma (the most common multiple spinal cord lesions probably are inflammatory in nature and are addressed in Chapter 15).

This classification also may be helpful in formulating a differential diagnosis for the most common tumors and masses affecting the spine.

Extradural Lesions

Multiple Lesions

Rule of thumb: the intervertebral disks always are darker than the normal bone marrow on T1-weighted images, if the reverse is seen, the bone marrow probably is abnormal.

Metastases

Metastases are the most common tumor affecting the spinal column (1). They are more common in adults, and the most common sites of primary tumors are breast, lung, prostate, and kidney. In children, most vertebral metastases arise from neuroblastoma and Ewing's sarcoma. The most commonly affected regions are the thoracic, lumbar, and, last, the cervical spine. Metastatic disease to the spine develops in approximately 10% of all patients with cancer (1). Spinal metastases are multiple in 90% of patients. The most common symptom at presentation is pain, but spinal cord compression is the initial symptom in 5% of patients with metastases to the spine. Compression fractures are common and extension of tumor into the epidural space may occur with or without

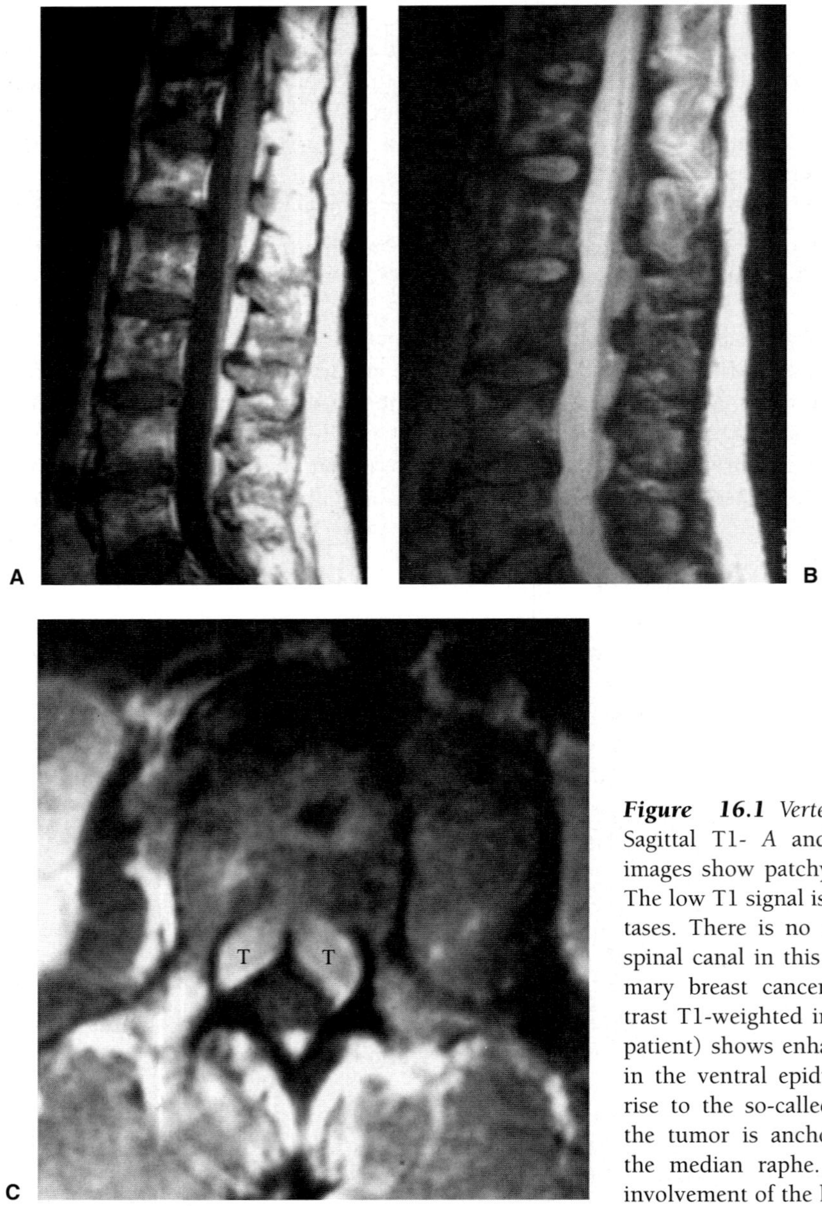

Figure 16.1 *Vertebral Metastases.* Sagittal T1- *A* and T2-weighted *B* images show patchy signal intensity. The low T1 signal is typical of metastases. There is no narrowing of the spinal canal in this patient with primary breast cancer. Axial postcontrast T1-weighted image *C* (different patient) shows enhancing tumor *(T)* in the ventral epidural space giving rise to the so-called curtain sign as the tumor is anchored centrally by the median raphe. There is tumor involvement of the left psoas muscle.

compression of neural and bone structures. It traditionally has been taught that metastases first involve the pedicles, whereas myeloma first involves the vertebral body. This observation was based on plain radiographic findings and perhaps is no longer true (basically, any tumor may initially involve any part of the vertebra). Most spinal metastases are lytic, and densely sclerotic metastases are typical (but not pathognomonic) for prostate and rare cancers such as carcinoid tumors. Although nuclear medicine studies are very sensitive, uptake of most radiotracers requires destruction of cortical bone, and thus metastases limited to the bone marrow may be missed. Because of this reason, I consider magnetic resonance imaging (MRI) as the imaging method of choice in these patients. Not only does MRI provide information regarding bone, it demonstrates overt or impending compression of the spinal cord. The most helpful sequence are the precontrast T1-weighted images (2). Metastases appear as nonspecific foci of low T1 signal (Fig. 16.1A). Most metastases are bright on T2 images (Fig. 16.1B). After contrast is given, most metastases enhance. Because metastases may enhance to the same degree as the normal bone marrow, they may become isointense in this sequence and difficult to see. It is important to understand that if only postcontrast imaging of the spine is obtained in these patients, the tumors may be difficult to identify and may be missed. Fat-suppressed postcontrast images do, however, clearly show the tumors. Occasionally, the entire spine is involved by tumor and its distribution may be so homogeneous as to cause the vertebrae to appear normal at first glance (this is particularly true of prostate metastases) (3). A clue that this is happening is the fact the intervertebral disks appear brighter than the bone marrow on T1 images (this is the reverse of normal, where the disks always are darker than the vertebral body bone marrow on T1 images). By the time of diagnosis, many vertebral metastases have epidural extension. The typical pattern of epidural extension is a soft tissue mass located behind a collapsed vertebra or adjacent to the canal for the basivertebral vein (tumor extrudes through this natural opening). On axial images, enhancing tumor extends along the epidural space along the sides of the median ligament of Trolard, which joins the dura mater with the periosteum/posterior longitudinal ligament. This gives rise to the so-called curtain sign (4) (Fig. 16.1C). This sign is not present in epidural abscess because the median ligament is lysed by proteolytic enzymes produced by bacteria. Evaluation of the suspected tumor in the epidural space is optimally accomplished with the use of MRI contrast material. Diffusion-weighted imaging may be helpful in differentiating benign osteoporotic vertebral body fractures (which have low signal intensity) from malignant ones (which have relatively high signal intensity) (5).

Myeloma

Multiple myeloma is a rare neoplasm arising from proliferation of plasma cells (6). Nearly always, the disease is systemic, but occasionally it may be isolated (plasmacytoma). In most patients, plasmacytoma is the initial manifestation of the disease, and multiple myeloma develops in most 5 to 10 years after the initial diagnosis. Although myeloma accounts for less than 1% of all cancers, it is the most common primary bone malignancy. Most patients are men, 60 years of age or older. The most commonly affected bones are the spine, central flat bones (pelvis, skull), and ribs. As such, the most common presentation is that of back pain with or without vertebral fractures. The diagnosis is made by finding Bence Jones proteins (excessive free light chains) in urine or by confirming the presence of a monoclonal gammopathy (usually of the immunoglobulin G type) in serum (7). Anemia and diffuse osteopenia are present at diagnosis in most patients. Of interest to neuroradiologists is the fact that a peripheral neuropathy develops in approximately 3% of patients with multiple myeloma, and this phenomenon is most likely to occur when sclerotic bone lesions are present. By MRI, multiple myeloma may be difficult to distinguish from the normal patchy-appearing bone marrow that some older adults harbor. Myeloma may be focal, diffuse, or patchy in appearance. The lesions show nonspecific low T1 and high T2 signal intensity (similar to metastases, from which they are indistinguishable) (6) (Fig. 16.2). Most of the lesions

Multiple myeloma is the most common malignant primary bone tumor in adults, whereas vertebral body hemangiomas are overall the most common primary bone tumors of adults.

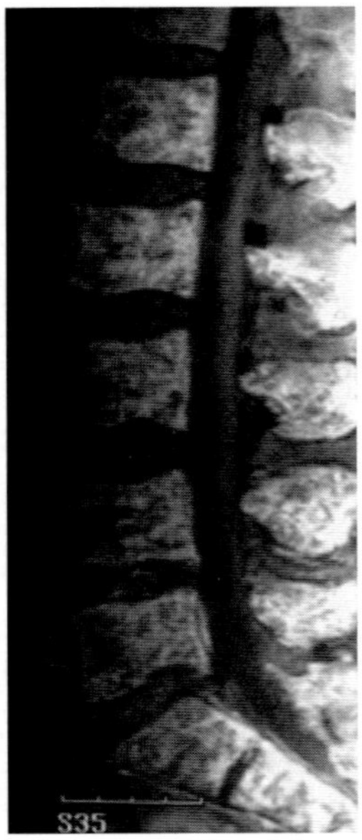

Figure 16.2 *Myeloma.* Sagittal T1-weighted image shows multiple, tiny, hypointense foci in all vertebral bodies.

show gadolinium enhancement. Once the lesions are treated, their T2 signal and contrast enhancement decreases (8). Compression fractures are common in multiple myeloma.

Lymphoma

Spinal lymphoma is found most often between the fifth and seventh decades of life (7). Most patients have underlying non-Hodgkin's lymphoma. Spinal involvement develops in approximately 2% of these patients and affects mostly the epidural space. Bony lesions also occur, and they are either sclerotic or lytic. On MRI, lymphoma appears as a nonspecific soft tissue mass that is hypointense on T1 images, hypointense or bright on T2 images, and enhances after contrast is given (Fig. 16.3).

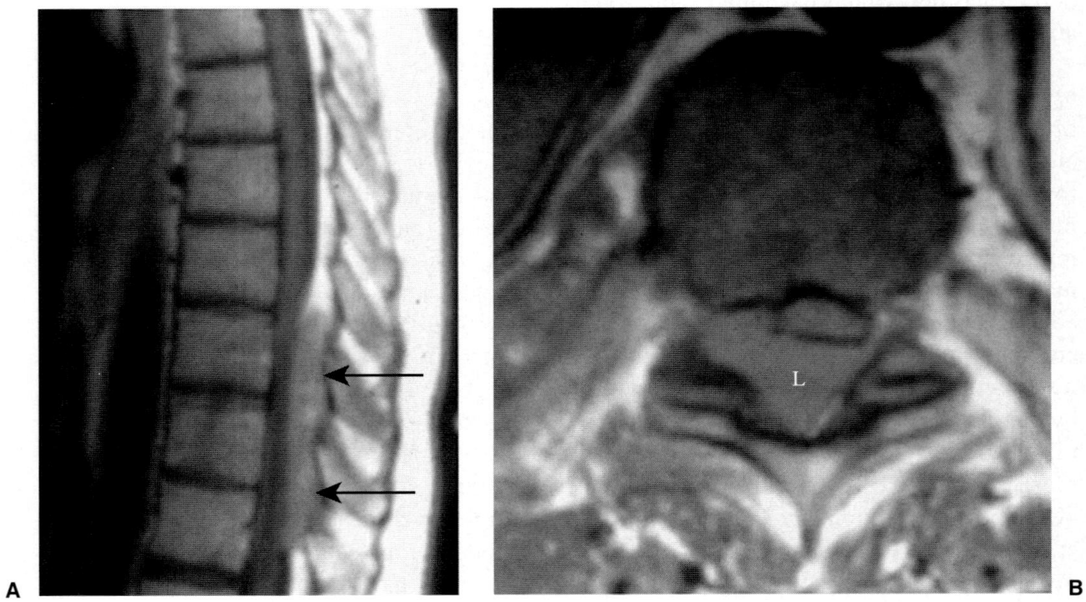

Figure 16.3 *Lymphoma. A.* Sagittal noncontrast T1-weighted image shows lymphoma *(arrows)* in the mid-thoracic posterior epidural space, resulting in compression of the spinal cord. *B.* Postcontrast axial T1-weighted image clearly shows the posterior location of the tumor *(L)* and the cord compression.

Hemangioma

Vertebral body hemangiomas are the most common primary bone tumor and are found in over 10% of the population (9). Most of these lesions occur in women. They may be solitary (70%) or multiple (30%). The most common locations are the thoracic, lumbar, and cervical regions. Most hemangiomas arise in the body of the vertebra, but also may involve the pedicles. These lesions almost always are asymptomatic and incidentally found, but occasionally they may present as large and aggressive masses destroying a vertebra and producing pain and even compression of the spinal cord (10). Some hemangiomas enlarge and become symptomatic during pregnancy. Radiographs and computed tomography (CT) show a lucent lesion that contains thickened secondary trabeculae (on lateral radiographs this is called a *corduroy* pattern and on axial CT images a *coarse* appearance. The MRI appearance reflects their histology (enlarged, slow-flowing vascular channels that may be partially thrombosed, fatty involution, and thick trabeculae). Vertebral hemangiomas are bright on T1 images, and this appearance is fairly typical (the other lesion that may be bright on T1 is metastatic melanotic melanoma, Fig. 16.4A and B). On T2 images,

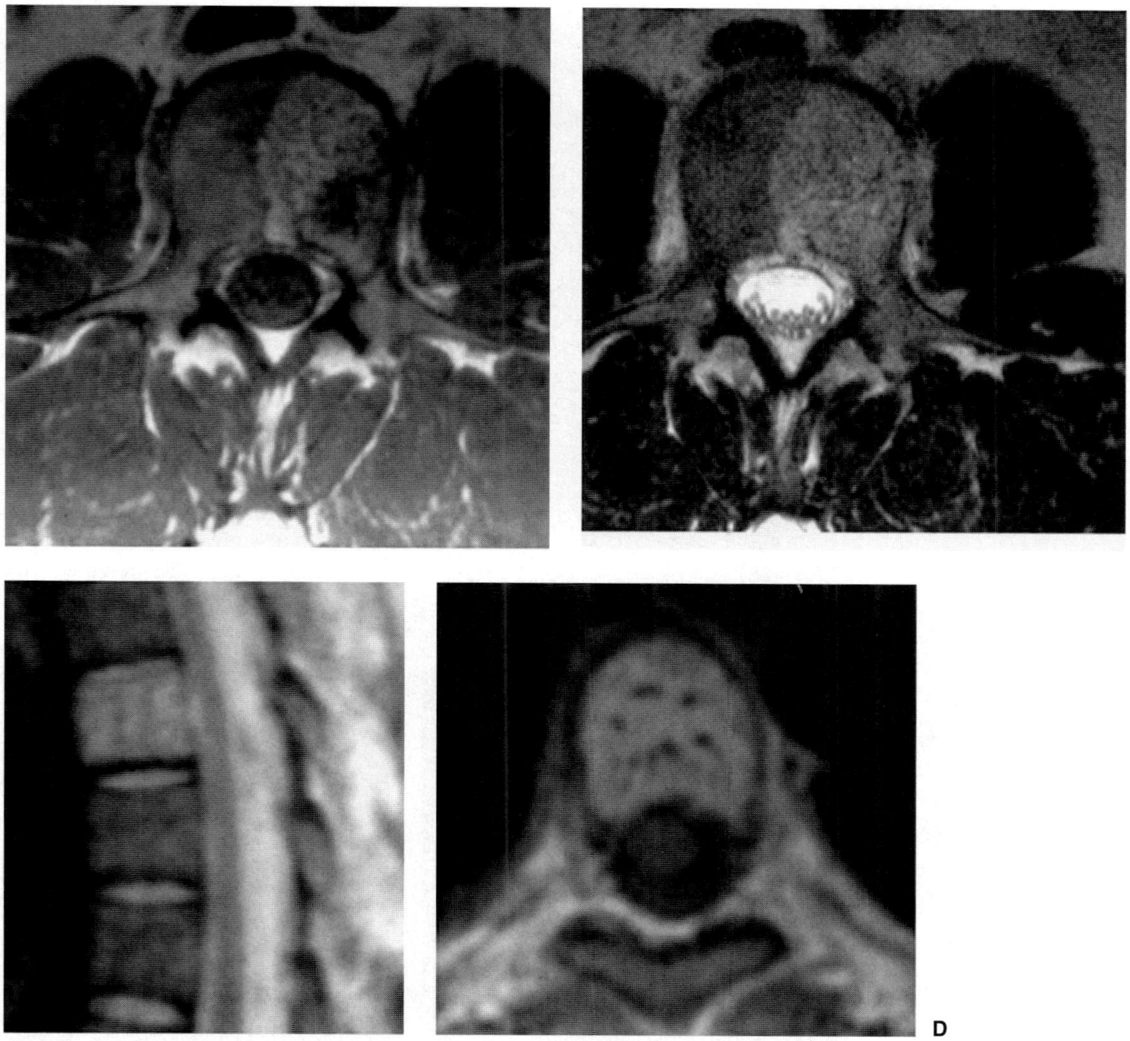

Figure 16.4 *Vertebral Hemangioma. A.* Axial noncontrast T1-weighted image shows a mostly hyperintense incidental hemangioma involving the left half of a lumbar vertebral body. Note slightly accentuated hypointense trabeculae in the lesion. *B.* Corresponding T2-weighted image shows that the lesion is bright. *C.* In a different patient, mid-sagittal T2-weighted image shows a bright hemangioma containing a subtle "corduroy" pattern due to hypertrophied secondary trabeculae. *D.* In the same patient, axial postcontrast T1-weighted image shows the lesion to enhance, and the hypertrophied trabeculae are clearly seen ("polka dot" pattern).

they may remain slightly hyperintense or become isointense with the rest of the bone marrow (Fig. 16.4C). They enhance after contrast administration (Fig. 16.4D). Aggressive hemangiomas have a nonspecific appearance and may simulate metastases (these specific lesions are not bright on T1 images) (10).

Eosinophilic Granuloma

In a vertebra plana due to eosinophilic granuloma, the disk is preserved and there is no or very little soft tissue density accompanying the abnormality.

Eosinophilic granuloma (EG) is the solitary lesion of a group of disorders belonging to the Langerhans cell histiocytoses (the others are Hand-Schüller-Christian and Letterer-Siwe diseases). EG comprises approximately 1% of all bone tumors and approximately 70% of all the histiocytoses (11). Most patients are approximately 5 to 15 years of age at the time of diagnosis, and pain is the most common clinical symptom. When EG affects the spinal column, other symptoms include muscle spasm, stiffness, scoliosis, and neurologic deficits due to compression of the spinal cord or nerve roots. The spine is not a common site for EG, but when it is affected, the thoracic region often is involved. Nearly all EG lesions are limited to the vertebral body and do not spread into the posterior arch.

The most striking feature on radiographs is that of vertebra plana (7) (Fig. 16.5A). After what may be seemingly minor trauma, the vertebra may completely collapse, assum-

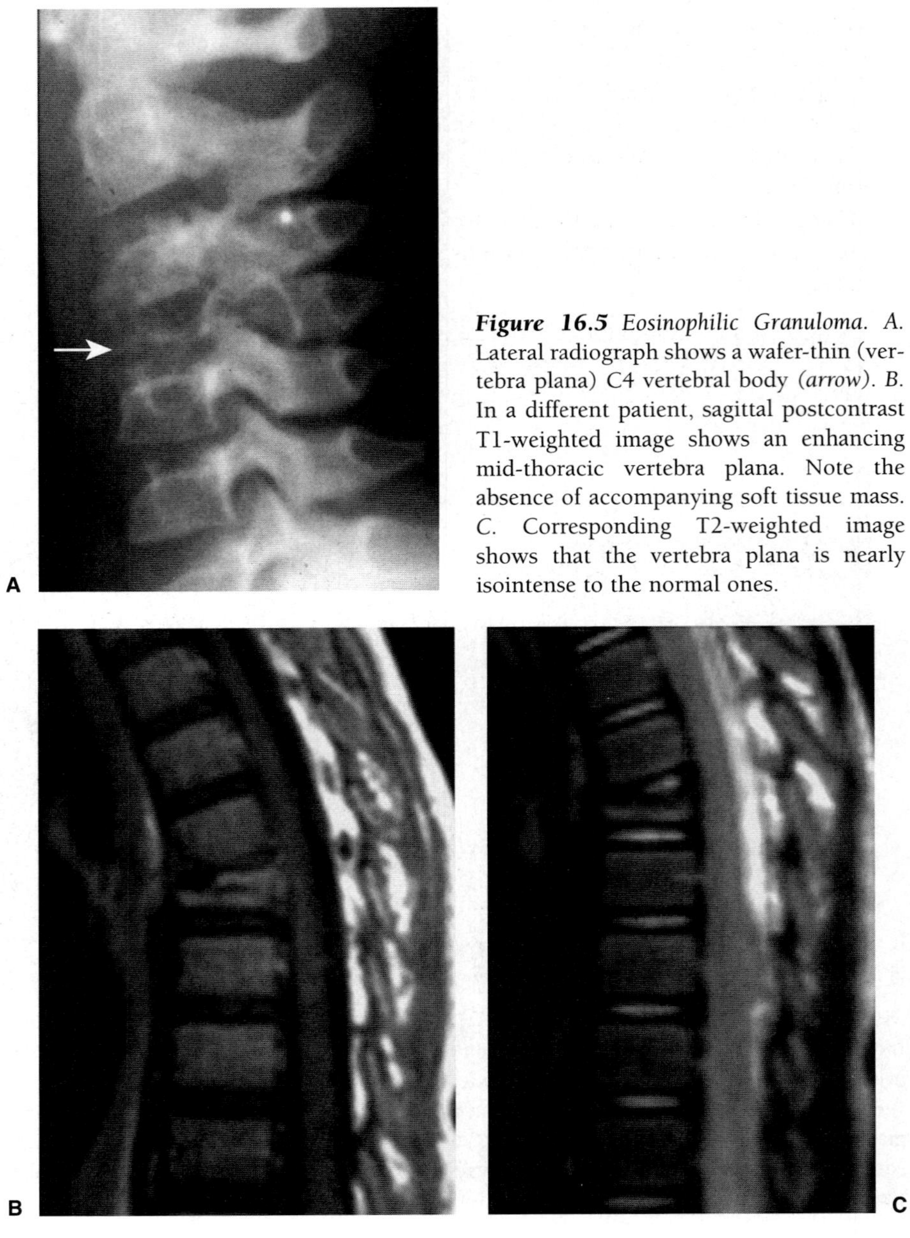

Figure 16.5 *Eosinophilic Granuloma. A.* Lateral radiograph shows a wafer-thin (vertebra plana) C4 vertebral body *(arrow). B.* In a different patient, sagittal postcontrast T1-weighted image shows an enhancing mid-thoracic vertebra plana. Note the absence of accompanying soft tissue mass. *C.* Corresponding T2-weighted image shows that the vertebra plana is nearly isointense to the normal ones.

ing a wafer-like configuration. This also is clearly seen on sagittal CT reformations. Axial CT shows the involved vertebra to be osteopenic. Typically, there is no or very little associated soft tissue mass around the vertebra plana (in contrast to metastases and other tumors, in which there is considerable associated soft tissue mass). MRI shows the affected vertebra to have low T1 and intermediate to high T2 signal intensity (Fig. 16.5B and C). The adjacent disks always are normal. Posterior protrusion of the fracture fragments may result in compression of the spinal cord. The differential diagnosis of a vertebra plana is as follows:

- Eosinophilic granuloma
- Leukemia
- Metastatic neuroblastoma

Solitary Lesions

Aneurysmal Bone Cyst

Aneurysmal bone cyst (ABC) represents less than 3% of all primary bone tumors. ABC may be primary (these arise *de novo*) or secondary (these are associated with other underlying bone lesions) (11). Secondary ABC may be associated with the following lesions:

Giant cell tumor
Chondroblastoma
Chondromyxoid fibroma
Fibrous dysplasia and other fibroosseous lesions
Giant cell reparative granuloma
Fibromyxoma
Osteosarcoma and other primary bone sarcomas
Brown tumors of hyperparathyroidism
Metastases

Most ABCs contain large, blood-filled spaces (hence, layering occurs if the patient is supine for a short while before the scan; Fig. 16.6). Unfortunately, some ABCs are completely solid and have a nonspecific appearance. Most ABCs are found before 20 years of

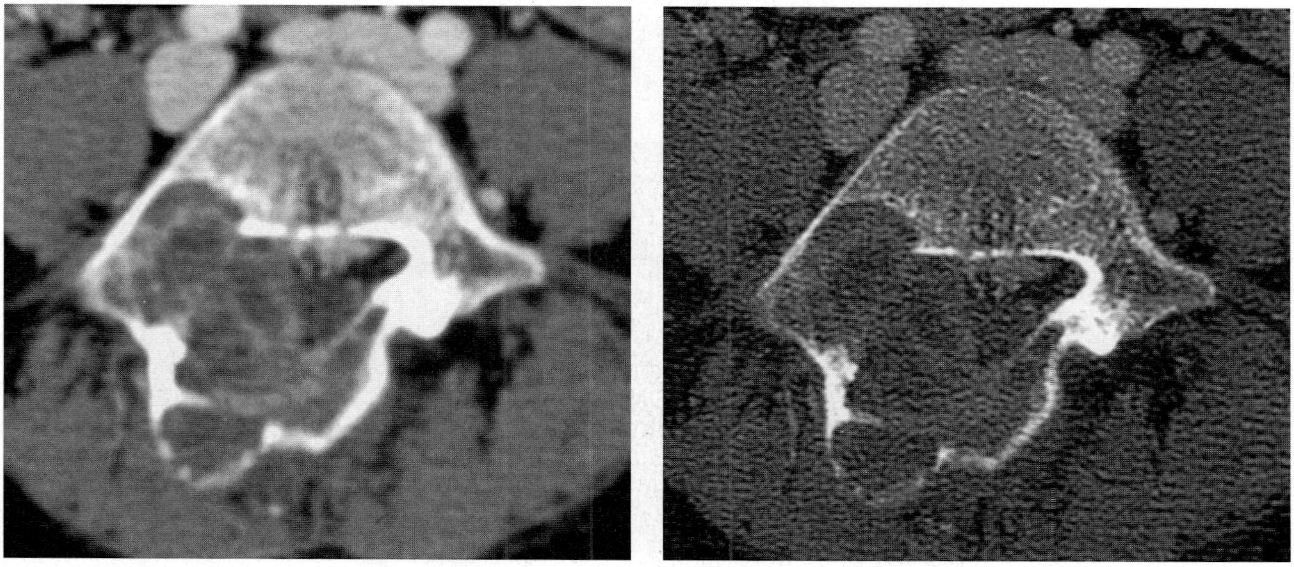

Figure 16.6 *Aneurysmal Bone Cyst. A.* Axial computed tomography scan (soft tissue window settings) shows a multicystic expansile mass involving the posterior arch and right pedicle of L5. The mass contains enhancing septa but no well defined fluid levels. There is intraspinal extension with compression of the distal thecal sac. *B.* Corresponding bone window settings shows the thin rim of bone marginating the mass.

age, and they are slightly more common in women (12). Approximately 20% of all ABCs arise in the spine (with an equal distribution between the cervical, thoracic, and lumbar spine). Less than 10% of all ABCs originate in the sacrum. Chronic local pain and radiculopathies are the most common symptoms. Their typical appearance is that of a "bubbly" expansile lesion surrounded by a thin shell of bone (which may be discontinuous). The mass may contain thin septa and usually shows multiple fluid–blood levels. These features are well seen on MRI and CT. The differential diagnosis for spinal bone lesions containing fluid levels is:

- Aneurysmal bone cyst
- Telangiectatic osteosarcoma and classic osteosarcoma
- Chondroblastoma
- Fractured simple cyst
- Fibrous dysplasia
- Malignant fibrous histiocytoma

By angiography, ABCs are hypervascular masses that may benefit from preoperative embolization. ABCs tend to involve the posterior elements (60%) and are one of the few tumors that cross the intervertebral space and extend into contiguous vertebrae.

Aneurysmal bone cysts, giant cell tumors, and osteoblastomas are the most likely tumors to involve several adjacent vertebrae.

Giant Cell Tumor

Giant cell tumor (GCT; also known as *osteoclastoma*) accounts for less than 5% of all primary bone tumors (7). Approximately 15% of GCTs affect the spine, and most are located in the cervical and upper thoracic regions and in the sacrum (GCT is the most common primary bone tumor of the sacrum, followed by chordoma and, in children, teratoma). GCTs are found predominantly in men during the third decade of life. In most instances, the vertebral body is involved, but the tumor may extend into the posterior elements and even adjacent vertebrae (11) (Fig. 16.7). GCT may occur in combination with ABC. Approximately 7% of GCTs show frankly malignant features at microscopy, and these are the ones that may metastasize (particularly to the lungs). GCT appears as an expansile mass that may or may not be surrounded by a thin shell of bone. On MRI, the mass has a nonspecific appearance with variable signal on T1- and T2-weighted images. Occasionally, hemorrhage may be present in the tumor (13). The soft tissue component of the mass usually enhances after contrast administration. On angiography, these tumors tend to be hypervascular, and preoperative embolization may be beneficial in some.

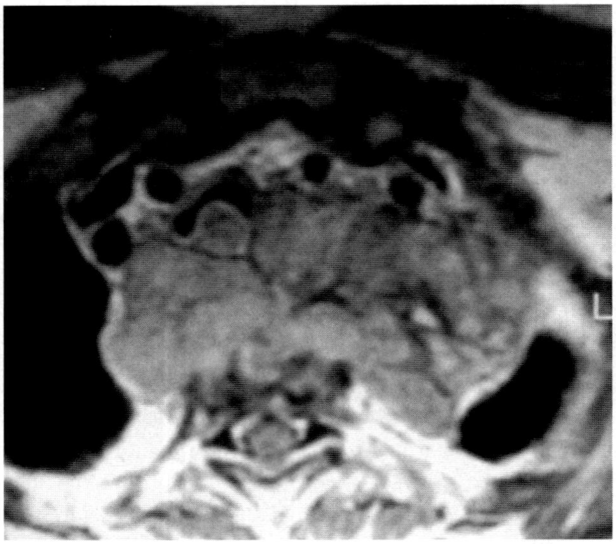

Figure 16.7 *Giant Cell Tumor.* Axial postcontrast T1-weighted image shows a large and complex mass arising from an upper thoracic vertebral body and projecting into the superior mediastinum with compression of the structures located there.

Osteoid Osteoma/Osteoblastoma

It is not clear if an osteoid osteoma is a tumor, an infection, or related to an unusual type of healing process (4). Osteoid osteomas account for approximately 10% of primary bone tumors, and 10% of them are found in the spine (7). Most are found the cervical and thoracic regions. In over 90% of instances, the posterior elements are affected (7). Osteoid osteomas arising in the vertebral body are very rare. Most osteoid osteomas are found in men younger than 30 years of age. The lesion may be classified according to its location in the bone as follows:

Cortical (arising in the cortex)
Cancellous (arising in the medullary cavity)
Subperiosteal (arising at the edge of the outer cortex)

Of these, only the cortical and cancellous types affect the spine. The tumor is a lucent lesion measuring only a few millimeters in diameter and surrounded by sclerosis (Fig. 16.8). The nidus is hypervascular. The tumor is presumed to produce prostaglandins that are thought to be responsible for pain (and it is their production that is blocked by the administration of salicylates). Pain is the most common symptom, occurring in approximately 80% of patients. The pain is more pronounced at night. The osteoid osteoma may irritate the adjacent tissues, and when this occurs in the spine a radiculopathy may develop in up to 50% of patients. Scoliosis also may ensue when the lesion arises in the thoracic region, and torticollis may develop when the lesion arises in the cervical spine. Other neurologic symptoms may be present in up to 20% of patients.

By imaging, the nidus of the osteoid osteoma is lucent on radiographs and CT, of low signal on T1, and variably bright on T2 images (14). The area surrounding the nidus is sclerotic on radiographs and CT and dark on T1 and T2 images. The nidus may enhance prominently after gadolinium administration. The differential diagnosis of osteoid osteoma includes bone island, Brodie's abscess, metastasis, and osteoblastoma. All osteoid osteomas show radionuclide uptake.

Osteoblastomas are included here because they also are called *giant osteoid osteomas* (7). They comprise less than 1% of primary bone tumors, and the spine is affected in 30% to 40% of cases. Nearly all regions of the spine are involved with similar frequency, and they almost always arise in the posterior elements. They occasionally may extend into the vertebral body or cross the intervertebral space to involve adjacent vertebrae. Most are found in young (<30 years of age) men. They are relatively large masses (usually >3 cm in diameter) and commonly encroach on the neural foramina and epidural space, resulting in neurologic symptoms. The common complaints are local pain, radicular pain, and a

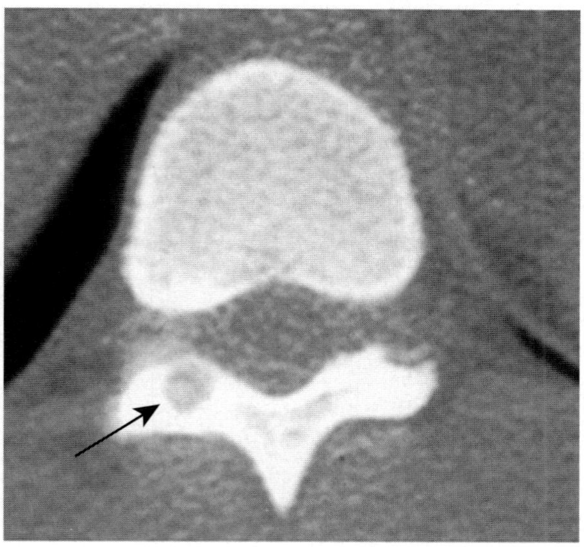

Figure 16.8 *Osteoid Osteoma.* Axial computed tomography shows typical rounded lucency *(arrow)* in the right lamina of a lower thoracic vertebra. The lucency contains faintly calcified central nidus.

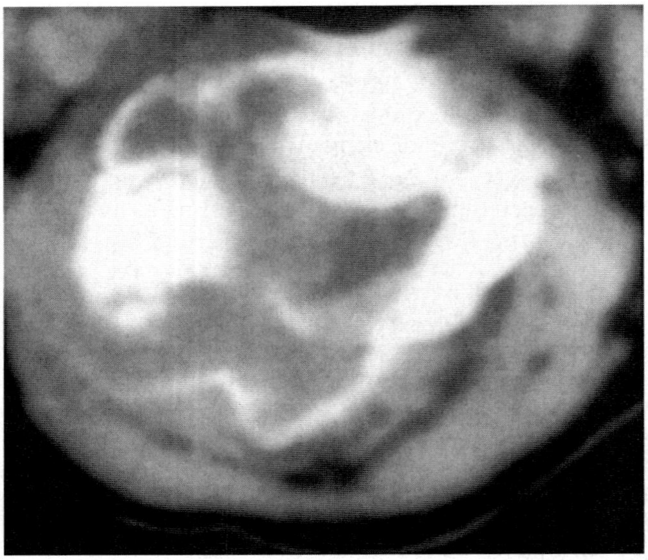

***Figure* 16.9** *Osteoblastoma.* Axial computed tomography shows large expansile mass involving the posterior elements of C3. The mass extends to involve the anterior aspect of the vertebra, narrows the spinal canal, and is marginated by a thin bone rim.

myelopathy. Their appearance is that of an expansile mass surrounded by thin bone walls and containing bone septa (15) (Fig. 16.9). On CT, they are of intermediate density, and on MRI they are of low T1 and variably high T2 signal intensities. The mass enhances after gadolinium administration. Occasionally, CT shows spinal osteoblastomas to be sclerotic.

Chordoma

Chordomas account for approximately 4% of primary bone tumors (7). They are thought to arise from remnants of the notochord and as such nearly all chordomas arise in the spine (rare notochordal ectopias may give rise to extraspinal chordomas). The most common sites for chordomas are listed in Table 16.1.

Chordomas are more common in men and generally present between 40 and 70 years of age. The symptoms are related to their site of origin, and are shown in Box 16.1

Cystic remnants from chordoma may occur in the clivus, where they are called *ecchordosis physaliphora.*

The histology of these tumors deserves to be mentioned here. They contain the so-called physaliphorous (bubbly) cells arranged in sheets. A variant of chordoma called a *chondroid chordoma* tends to arise at the level of the sphenooccipital synchondrosis, and this tumor actually may be a low-grade chondrosarcoma. By imaging, chordomas are destructive and somewhat expansile masses arising in the midline of the spine (Fig. 16.10). They may have a large soft tissue component that contains calcifications in nearly one-half of the tumors (18). This soft tissue mass also may contain cystlike areas. CT shows most of the lesions to be lytic, but occasionally they may be sclerotic. By the time of presentation, involvement of more than one vertebra generally is the rule. By MRI, chordomas have a heterogeneous appearance, with low to intermediate T1 signal intensity and occasionally areas of hemorrhage (high T1 signal) (19). On T2-weighted images, chordomas also have a variable appearance, but some tumors tend to be of relatively low signal on this sequence. After gadolinium administration, the soft tissue portion of the tumor enhances. MRI is the best method to evaluate extension of the tumor into the neural axis.

Table 16.1: Location of Spinal Chordomas

Location	*Incidence*
Sacrococcygeal	65%
Clivus	35%
Vertebrae (particularly cervical region)	10%

Box 16.1: Chordomas Symptoms Related to their Site of Origin

Sacrococcygeal: pain, leg numbness, bowel/bladder incontinence, constipation (16)
Clivus: pain, headache, cranial neuropathies, pituitary dysfunction
Vertebrae: pain, radiculopathies, myelopathy, dysphagia (17)

A

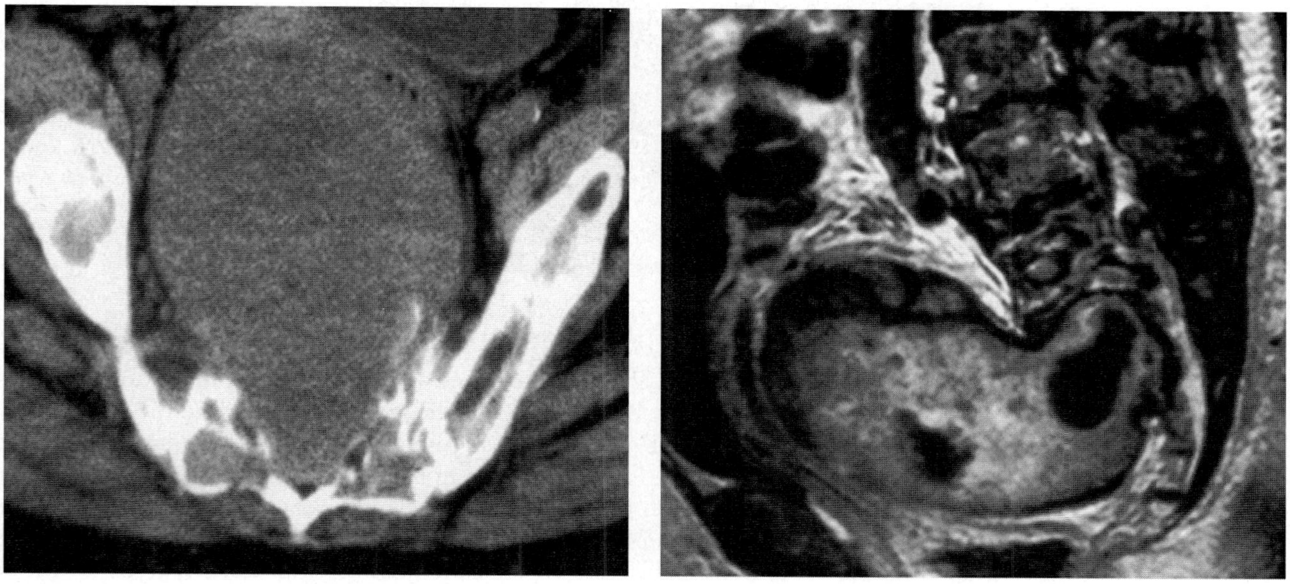

B

C

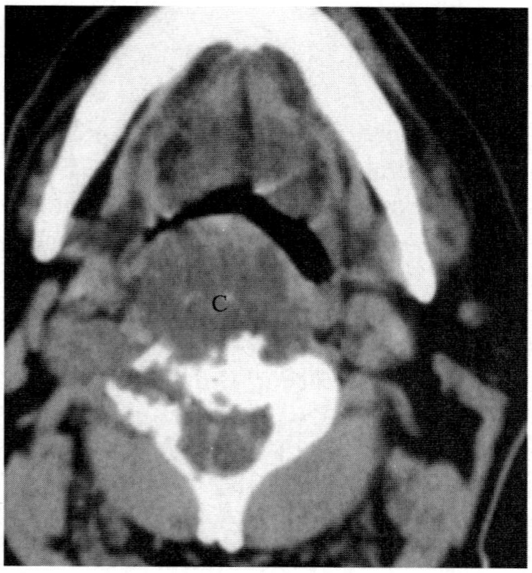

Figure 16.10 *Chordoma. A.* Axial computed tomography (CT) shows a large pelvic mass arising from the middle aspect of the sacrum. *B.* In the same patient, sagittal postcontrast T1-weighted image shows that most of the mass enhances, but that it also contains some cystic spaces. Its origin from the sacrum is clearly seen on this image. *C* In a different patient, axial CT shows a chordoma (C) arising from an upper cervical vertebra, destroying its body and right lateral aspect and extending into the epidural space. There is compression of the spinal cord. The mass contains a few flecks of calcium.

Epidural Lesions

Angiolipoma and Angiomyolipoma

These are very rare masses (but receiving increasing attention in the literature) arising from primitive mesenchymal elements contained in the epidural space. When an extradural lipoma also contains vascular elements, it is called an *angiolipoma* (20). When in addition to these elements the mass contains proliferative smooth muscle, it

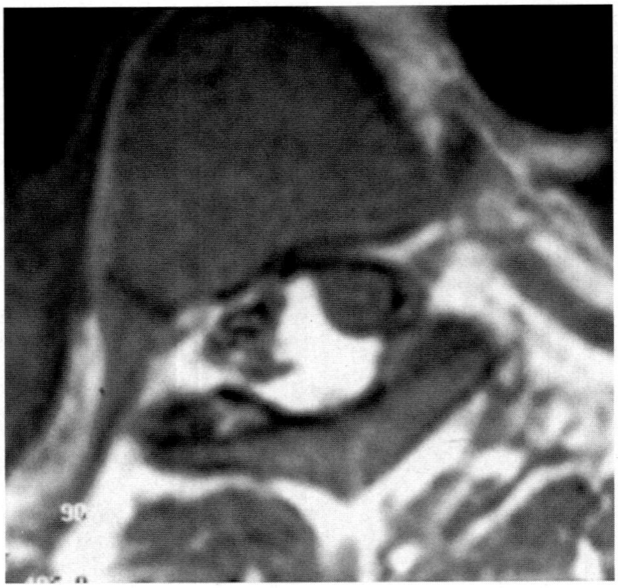

Figure 16.11 *Angiomyolipoma.* Axial T1-weighted image shows a mostly fatty mass in the dorsal and right lateral epidural space in the mid-thoracic region. The mass contains areas of very low signal and some of intermediate signal. There is compression of the spinal cord.

is called an *angiomyolipoma* (21). Most of these lesions are found in adults and in the thoracic region. Occasionally they are infiltrative and may extend into the adjacent tissues, including the vertebrae. Most of these tumors involve the posterior and lateral aspects of the epidural space (22). They tend to be somewhat spindle shaped and usually are no longer that two to three vertebral segments. They are of high signal intensity on T1- and fast spin-echo T2-weighted images. They contain areas of very low signal presumably related to blood flow in large vessels (Fig. 16.11). They show no significant contrast enhancement. The larger tumors may result in compression of the spinal cord.

The normal width of the spinal epidural fat is 3 to 5 mm.

Epidural Lipomatosis

This entity, although not a tumor, may behave as one and result in compression of neural elements, and thus is discussed here. Epidural lipomatosis was first noted in patients receiving long-term exogenous steroid therapy (7). Conversely, symptomatic epidural lipomatosis is very rare in patients with excessive production of endogenous steroids. Epidural lipomatosis also may be seen in morbidly obese patients. In this rare entity, there is hypertrophy of normal epidural fat, particularly in the dorsal aspects of the thoracic spine and less commonly in the lumbar region. The most common symptom is back pain, but compression of the spinal cord may occur. If the fat grows at the level of neural foramina, radiculopathies also occur. The typical MRI appearance of epidural lipomatosis is that of excessive bright T1 fat (>5 to 6 mm) in the posterior aspect of the canal on sagittal images (23) (Figs. 16.12A and B). The subarachnoid spaces are narrowed and the thoracic spinal cord appears thin. The superior and inferior aspects of the lipomatosis taper smoothly and usually extend at least six vertebral segments in length. On axial images, excessive fat is noted in the posterior aspect of the canal and extending laterally. This normal fat does not enhance after contrast administration. On sagittal MRI, the width of the normal posterior epidural fat is less than 3 to 5 mm. On CT, the abnormal fat is of low density, and on myelography the fat may compress the canal and result in complete blockage of the passage of contrast. Similar findings are noted when epidural lipomatosis develops in the lumbar region. When this occurs, the fat is particularly prominent in the distal aspect of the canal, where it may completely surround the nerve roots (Figs. 16.12C and D). The treatment for this rare disease consists of discontinuation of steroid therapy, control of endogenous steroid secretion, diet, and occasionally posterior unroofing of the spinal canal and resection of the fat to alleviate severe neurologic symptoms.

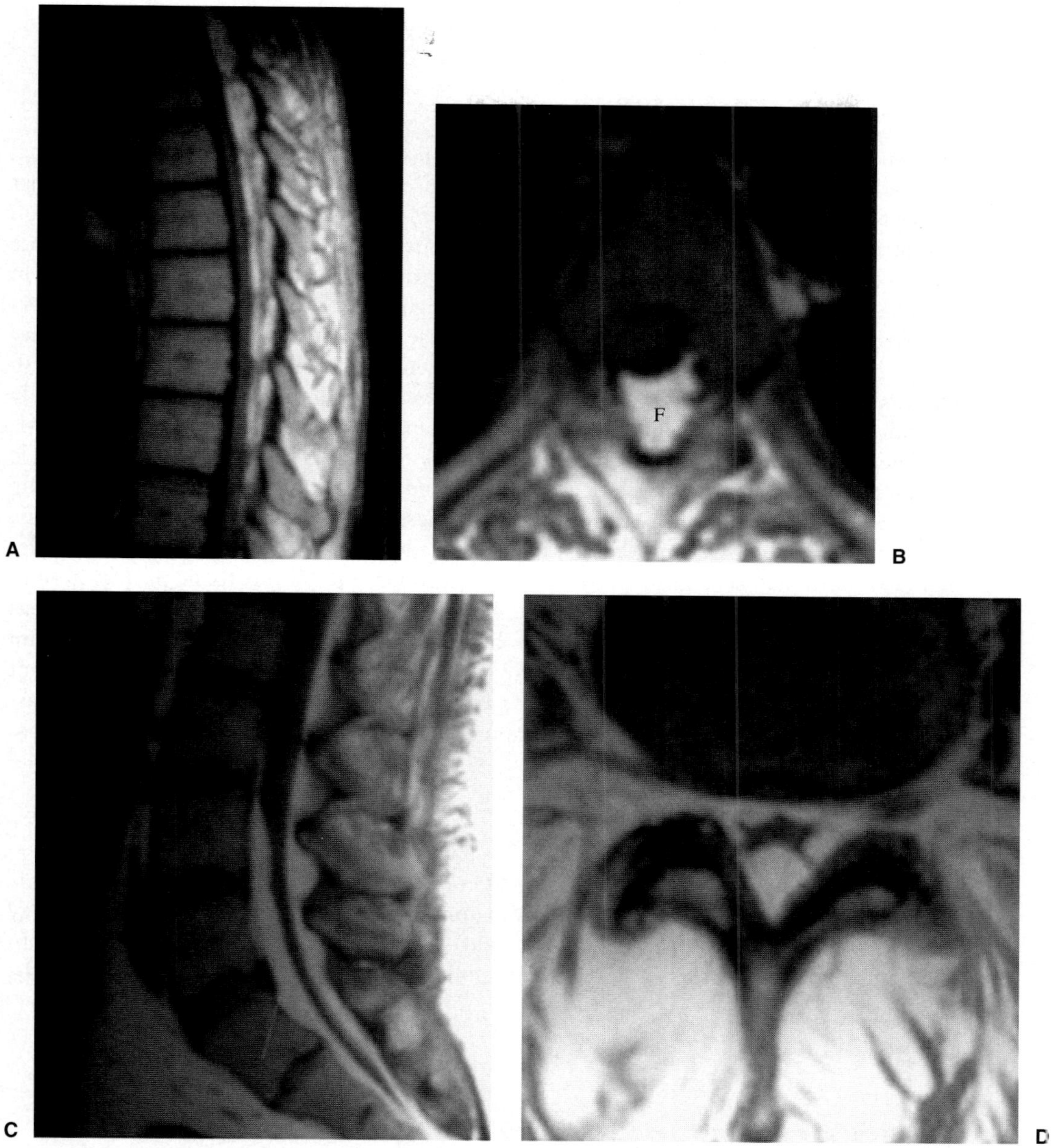

Figure 16.12 *Epidural Lipomatosis. A.* Sagittal T1-weighted image shows prominent thoracic posterior epidural fat resulting in compression of the spinal cord. *B.* Axial image confirms the markedly increased volume of the dorsal epidural fat *(F)* and the cord compression. *C.* In a different patient, sagittal T1-weighted image shows prominent ventral and dorsal epidural fat in the lumbosacral region. *D.* Axial image in the same patient shows the marked compression of the distal thecal sac by the epidural lipomatosis.

Lymphoma

Both Hodgkin's and non-Hodgkin's lymphoma may affect the bones and were addressed previously. Up to 50% of patients with Hodgkin's lymphoma have bone lesions, and many of them are located in the spine. Lymphoma may invade the spine from adjacent masses and adenopathy, involve the proper bone, may be located in the epidurally or leptomeningeally, or involve the spinal cord directly (24). Without the appropriate clinical history, distinguishing lymphoma from metastases (and distinguishing between the different types of lymphoma) or myeloma is not feasible. By MRI, lymphoma is of low to intermediate T1 and variably high T2 signal. All untreated lymphomas show gadolinium enhancement (Fig. 16.3). Occasionally, an affected vertebral body is dark on T1 and T2 images because of sclerosis, which can be seen on radiographs or CT.

INTRADURAL EXTRAMEDULLARY LESIONS

NERVE SHEATH TUMORS

In this category, most authors include neurofibromas and schwannomas. Strictly speaking, only schwannomas are nerve sheath tumors because neurofibromas arise from the proper nerve fascicles. Regardless of this distinction, nerve sheath tumors are the most common spinal tumor (30%) and account for most (70%) intraspinal tumors (7). Schwannomas are most common, whereas neurofibromas (particularly of the plexiform type) are seen in patients with neurofibromatosis type 1 (NF-1; Chapter 2). Like all nerve sheath tumors (in the absence of NF-1), these tumors tend to arise from sensory (posterior in the spine) nerves. They are more common in middle-aged men. Approximately 50% of nerve sheath tumors are intradural–extradural (dumb-bell shaped) in location and 50% are purely extradural. Malignant degeneration of neurofibromas may occur in patients with NF-1, but degeneration of schwannomas is extremely rare. Although many authors have attempted to distinguish between neurofibroma and schwannoma based on their imaging features, I do not believe this is possible. Both masses are slow growing and cause bone remodeling (e.g., expansion of neural foramina), and both show low T1 and high T2 signal (25). Both may be slightly T2 hypointense secondary to fibrous tissue proliferation in the mass. Cystic spaces and hemorrhage, however, are more common in schwannomas than in neurofibromas. Both may show homogeneous or inhomogeneous gadolinium enhancement, but schwannomas may have the typical ring or target type of enhancement in which the central portion of the mass remains relatively hypointense after contrast administration (Fig. 16.13). Chronic compression of the spinal cord may result in formation of syringomyelia.

MENINGIOMA

Intraspinal meningioma is the second most common (25%) primary tumor of the spine after nerve sheath tumors (7). Most meningiomas are benign and of "classic" histology (fibroblastic, meningothelial, and transitional). Aggressive meningiomas are very rare in the spine. Over two-thirds of spinal meningiomas are found in middle-aged women (9).

A

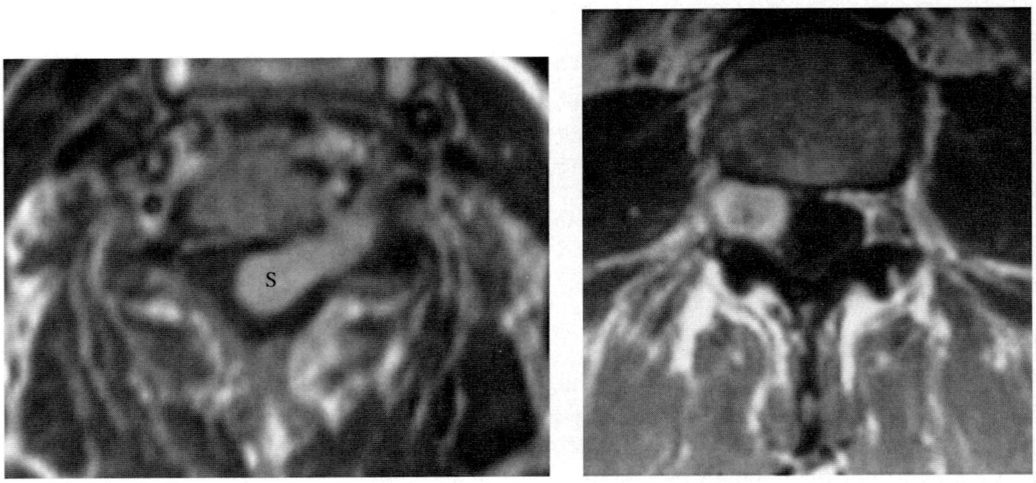

B

Figure 16.13 *Schwannoma. A.* Axial postcontrast T1-weighted image shows an enhancing dumb-bell–shaped mass *(S)* in the left C5 to C6 neural foramen. The foramen is expanded and the tumor compresses the spinal cord. *B.* In a different patient, a postcontrast T1-weighted image shows a rounded and enhancing schwannoma slightly expanding the neural foramen. The tumor shows some degree of target-type enhancement, with less enhancement centrally.

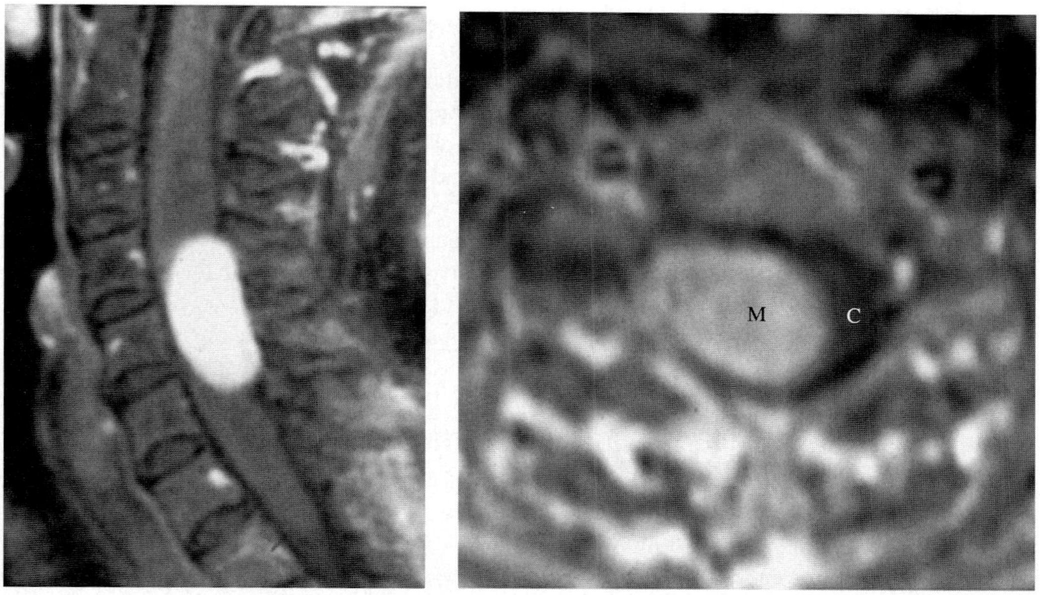

A B

Figure 16.14 *Meningioma. A.* Sagittal postcontrast fat-suppressed T1-weighted image shows a homogeneously enhancing mass in the mid-cervical region. The lesion compresses the spinal cord, which also appears edematous. Based on this image, it is difficult to establish the compartment from which this mass arose. *B.* Axial postcontrast image shows that the mass *(M)* is extramedullary *(C,* spinal cord). Note compressed spinal cord.

Most spinal meningiomas are found the thoracic spine, followed by the craniocervical junction and the lumbar region. Multiple spinal meningiomas may be seen in patients with NF-2 (Chapter 2). The most common symptoms are pain and neurologic abnormalities (radiculopathy, sensory deficits, myelopathy). Although most thoracic and lumbar meningiomas are based on the posterior dura, craniocervical ones may be anterior or posterior in location. Meningiomas are smooth, well marginated masses attached to the dura by a broad base. They are nearly isointense to the spinal cord on both T1 and T2 images. Attempting to differentiate between the different histologic grades of meningioma by MRI is not practical and not clinically relevant. Similar to intracranial meningiomas, spinal ones may show a tail of dural enhancement. Most meningiomas show robust gadolinium enhancement (Fig. 16.14). CT may show intratumoral calcifications, and this finding may aid in distinguishing between meningioma and nerve sheath tumors, which do not contain calcifications. Occasionally, spinal meningiomas have a plaquelike configuration. Chronic compression of the spinal cord by a meningioma may result in the formation of a syrinx.

Most spinal meningiomas are found the thoracic spine, followed by the craniocervical junction and, last, the lumbar region.

Cerebrospinal Fluid–Filled Cysts

CSF-filled cysts in the spinal canal usually are classified as follows (7):

1. Cysts containing no neural elements (type 1)
   i. Type 1A: extradural, either projecting into the neural foramina or into the epidural spaces
   ii. Type 1B: intrasacral "meningoceles"
2. Cysts containing neural elements (type 2), these typically are perineurial (Tarlov cysts).
3. Intradural meningeal cysts (type 3).

Most of these cysts are congenital, although some may appear after trauma. Midline cysts are due to a congenital defect in the dura (26) (Fig. 16.15A). CSF is then hydrostatically forced into the defect, expanding it. A valve–ball mechanism results in trapping of CSF inside the cyst. The wall of these cysts may contain arachnoid and fibroid tissues. Rarely, the spinal cord herniates into one of the cysts (27). Most of these cysts are found in the thoracic spine, followed by the thoracolumbar, lumbosacral, and cervical regions (28) (Fig. 16.15B). Nearly all cysts are posterior, but they may have lateral extension (Fig. 16.15A). They are more common in boys and usually are large (>5 cm in diameter) at presentation. Their early presentation probably reflects the fact that these cysts may compress the spinal cord and nerve roots and produce symptoms. Before surgical resection, it is imperative to try to find their ostium. This usually necessitates myelography, and in most of these cysts the opening is located in the cephalad aspect. These lesions are equivalent to CSF in signal intensity in all MRI sequences (29). They tend to be surrounded by epidural fat and show no gadolinium enhancement. Other causes of intraspinal CSF-filled cysts are NF-1 (dural ectasia), Marfan's syndrome (dural ectasia), postoperative pseudomeningoceles, and posttraumatic pseudomeningoceles.

A

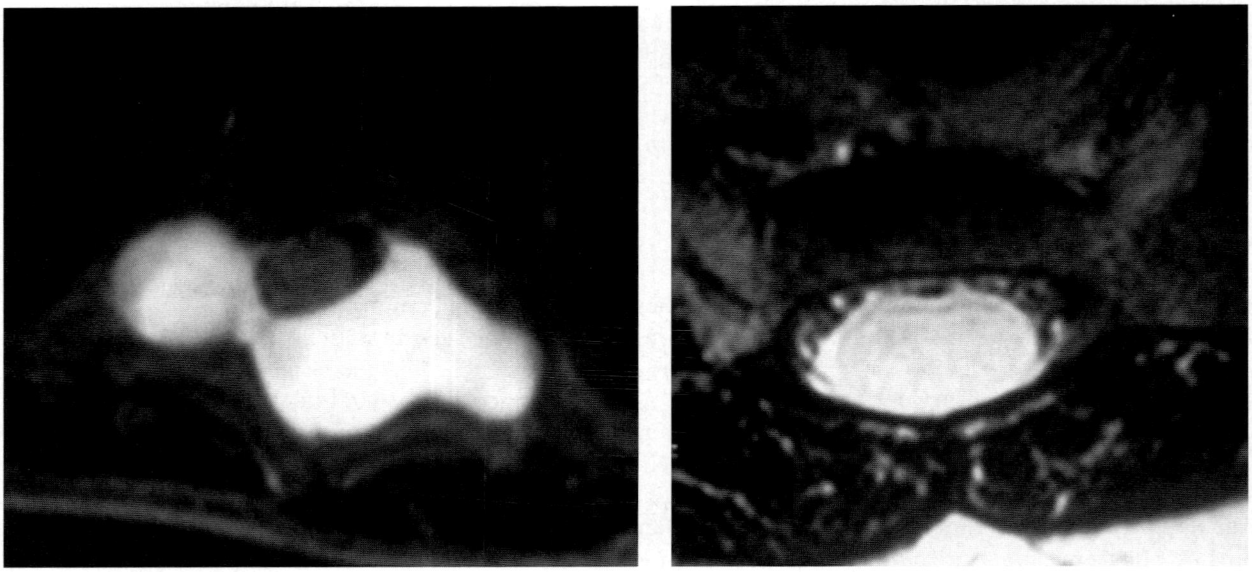

C

B

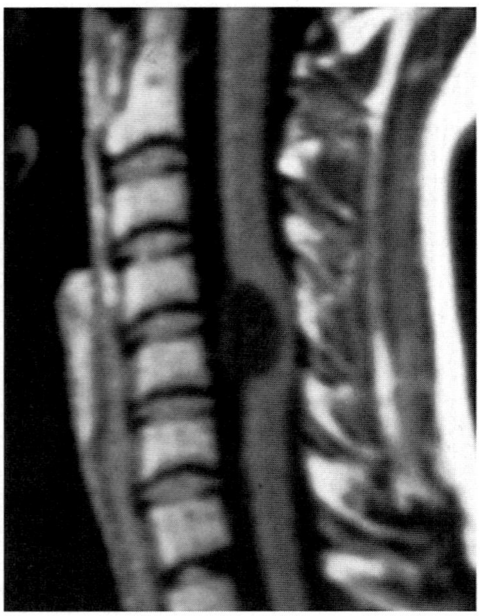

Figure 16.15 *Intraspinal Cysts. A.* Axial T2-weighted image shows a large extradural cerebrospinal fluid–containing cyst in the mid-thoracic region extending laterally through the neural foramina, which are expanded. This is a surgically proven arachnoid cyst. *B.* In a different patient, sagittal T1-weighted image shows a ventrally located arachnoid cyst at the C5 level insinuating itself into the spinal cord. The differential diagnosis was that of a duplication cyst, which is unlikely in the presence of normally developed vertebrae. (Case courtesy of R. M. Quencer, Miami, FL.) *C.* Axial T2-weighted image shows an intrasacral cyst compressing the nerve roots and displacing them laterally. This represents the so-called intrasacral meningocele.

In addition, intradural arachnoid cysts may be acquired. These also may be secondary to prior infection or inflammation, as well as inflammation induced by older myelographic contrast media and epidural anesthesia. Like any other lesion compressing the spinal cord, any of these cysts may result in the formation of syringomyelia.

Cysts involving the nerve roots are much more common than midline cysts and tend to be found mostly incidentally in older adults. However, these cysts also may cause symptoms by virtue of compression of nerve roots between the wall of the cyst and adjacent bone. The slow growth of the cysts and constant internal pulsations may lead to radiculopathies. A focal dilatation of the dura and arachnoid filled with CSF and located proximal to the dorsal root ganglion is called a *meningeal diverticulum* (type 1) and usually does not contain the nerve root in it (30). These cysts may or may not communicate freely with the rest of the subarachnoid space. A CSF-filled cyst arising distal to the dorsal root ganglion in which its outer layer is formed by dura and the arachnoid (perineurium) and its basal layer is formed by the endoneurium is called a *Tarlov cyst* (type 2) (30). From a practical standpoint, a Tarlov cyst is diagnosed if a cyst arises distal to the dorsal root ganglion. Its importance lies in the fact that Tarlov cysts have poor communication with rest of the CSF, and if they grow (presumably by a valve–ball-like mechanism that allows CSF to enter but not to exit) and produce symptoms, surgery may be indicated. To assess the success of surgery on a preoperative basis, some authors recommend puncturing the cyst, evacuating its fluid, and observing a positive response with diminution of symptoms (31). The etiology of Tarlov cysts is uncertain. Most are 3 cm or more in diameter when they are found. Their most common location is the sacrum. Tarlov cysts may protrude into the presacral space. Conversely, focal dilatations of the arachnoid and dura mater in the sacrum may form intrasacral cysts (Fig. 16.1C). These also may compress nerve roots and produce symptoms. Both types of cysts result in smooth, benign-appearing bone expansion. They are of similar signal intensity to CSF in all MRI sequences. Occasionally, the cysts may contain increased levels of proteins (particularly if they do not communicate with the rest of the subarachnoid space) or pulsations that may alter their MRI signal intensity.

A Tarlov cyst occurs distal to the level of the dorsal root ganglion. I suggest reading the following article: Khosla A, Wippold FJ. CT myelography and MR imaging of extramedullary cysts of the spinal canal in adult and pediatric patients. AJR Am J Roentgenol 2002;178:201–207.

Intramedullary Lesions

Ependymoma

Ependymomas and astrocytomas are the most common primary tumors of the spinal cord (32). Overall, their incidence is roughly equal, but ependymomas are more common in adults than children. Spinal cord ependymomas may be divided as follows:

Distal: Approximately 50% of all cord ependymomas occur in the filum terminale and conus medullaris region; these can be "classic" ependymomas or of the myxopapillary type (which occur nearly exclusively in this region).

Others: These involve the cervical and thoracic cord and account for the other 50% of spinal ependymomas.

Ependymomas are slightly more common in women 40 to 50 years of age (32). There is an increased incidence of these tumors in patients with NF-2 (33). The symptoms are chronic and consist mainly of pain, myelopathy, and radiculopathies. Occasionally, these ependymomas may bleed and produce subarachnoid hemorrhage or hematomyelia and acute symptoms (34). In addition, spinal cord ependymomas may undergo repeated and subclinical bleeds, leading to chronic deposition of blood products on the surface of the brain and cord (superficial siderosis). Ependymomas grow very slowly and may reach a very large size, particularly in the lumbar region. The MRI appearance of spinal cord ependymoma varies (Fig. 16.16A and B). The solid portions of the tumors are of low T1 and high T2 signal and enhance after contrast is given (35). These tumors tend to harbor cysts. The signal intensity of these cysts is variable

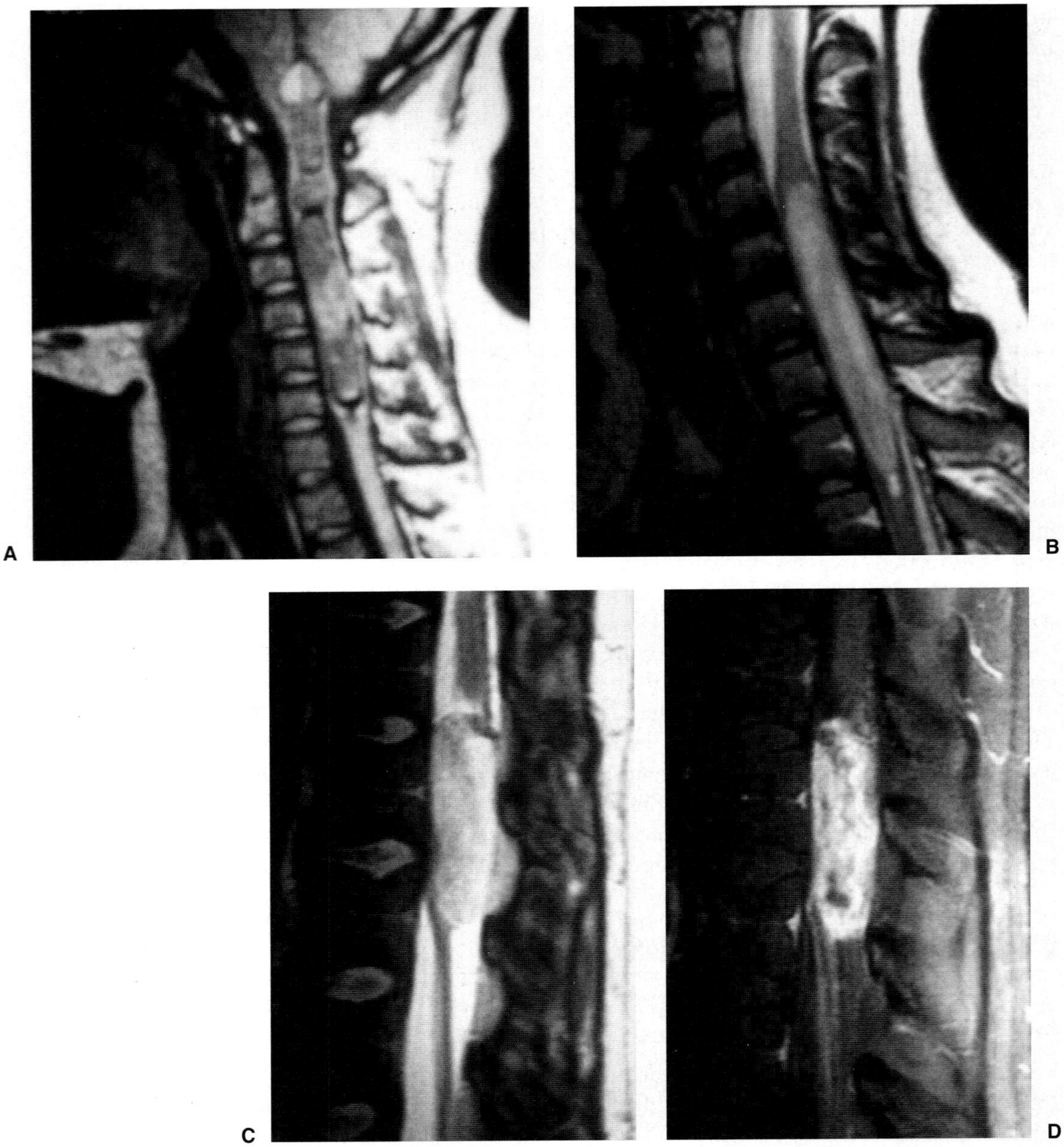

Figure 16.16 *Ependymoma. A.* Sagittal T1-weighted image shows a complex-appearing intramedullary spinal cord tumor in the cervical region. Note that the tumor contains multiple areas of hemorrhage that are suggestive of ependymoma. (Case courtesy of M. Smith, Milwaukee, WI.) *B.* In a different patient, a sagittal T2-weighted image shows a nonspecific–appearing ependymoma involving the middle to low cervical spinal cord. *C.* Sagittal T2-weighted image shows a mostly bright intradural mass in the region of the cauda equina. *D.* Corresponding postcontrast fat-suppressed T1-weighted image shows significant enhancement of this sausage-shaped myxopapillary ependymoma. Note enhancement of the distal conus medullaris and some nerve roots, suggesting tumor extension.

because some contain clear fluid, whereas in others the fluid is xanthochromic (36). Although the walls of the cysts usually are made up of gliotic tissue, enhancing tumor may surround the cysts. Chronic blood products may be deposited along the margins of the tumors (37). This feature is well seen on gradient-echo T2-weighted images and is typical of ependymomas. Syrinxes may form above or below the tumor. Expansion of the bony spinal canal and scoliosis may occur. Ependymomas arising distally also have a somewhat typical appearance. They tend to be sausage shaped and are centered in the region of the proximal filum terminale (38). These solid tumors are of low T1 and high T2 signal intensity and tend to enhance mostly in a homogeneous fashion after gadolinium administration (Fig. 16.16C and D). They may invade the distal conus medullaris and also extend along the length of the filum terminale. Both distal and spinal cord ependymomas may result in metastases in the subarachnoid space. Although these tumors are histologically benign, they are difficult to resect and multiple recurrences are common. The differential diagnosis of a mass arising in the filum terminale is as follows:

- Ependymoma
- Astrocytoma
- Nerve sheath tumor
- Metastases
- Paraganglioma
- Hemangioblastoma

Astrocytoma

Overall, astrocytomas in the spinal cord are as common as ependymomas, but astrocytomas are more common in children and in young adults (32). Astrocytomas also are more common in the cervical and thoracic regions and relatively unusual in the conus medullaris and filum terminale (unlike ependymomas). Most spinal cord astrocytomas are histologically benign, and only approximately 10% show malignant features (32). Astrocytomas are slow growing and may attain very large size by the time of diagnosis. Indeed, many of them involve most of the spinal cord (holocord type) at presentation. The symptoms are chronic and depend on the location of the tumor. Spinal cord astrocytomas may produce proteins that are excreted into the CSF and that may result in communicating hydrocephalus. Spinal cord astrocytomas also are seen in patients with NF-1 (33). The MRI appearance of spinal cord astrocytomas is nonspecific (39). The cord is expanded and the solid portions of the mass show low T1 and high T2 signal, and enhance after gadolinium is given (Fig. 16.17). Cysts are common (although less common than in ependymomas) and are of low T1 and high T2 signal intensity, with a rim that may or may not enhance (40). Blood products usually are not seen in astrocytomas, and this feature may be used to differentiate them from ependymomas. Syringomyelia may develop above or below the tumor. Spread of tumor through the CSF is less common than with ependymomas. Scoliosis may be present.

Although the overall incidence of cord astrocytomas and ependymomas is roughly equal, astrocytomas are more common in children and ependymomas are more common in adults.

Hemangioblastoma

Hemangioblastoma (HB) is the third most common primary tumor arising in the spinal cord (41). Approximately 10% of all HBs arise in the cord. Most are purely intramedullary, but approximately 20% of them have an exophytic component. HBs are associated with von Hippel-Lindau disease (VHL; Chapter 2). Up to one-third of spinal cord HBs occur in the presence of VHL, and spinal cord HB eventually develops in approximately 15% of patients with this disease (42). These tumors are more common in adult men 30 to 40 years of age. When they are found in children, it is almost exclusively in the context of VHL. The symptoms related to HB are of shorter duration than those seen with spinal cord ependymomas and astrocytomas. Symptoms depend on the site at which the tumor arises. Although polycythemia (due to production of erythropoietin) occurs with cerebral and cerebellar HBs, it does not occur when the tumor originates in the cord. Occasionally, HBs bleed and tend to present with acute subarachnoid hemorrhage or hematomyelia. HBs in the absence of VHL have cysts up to 70% of the time. HBs associated with VHL usually are multiple and tend to be solid. As in any other

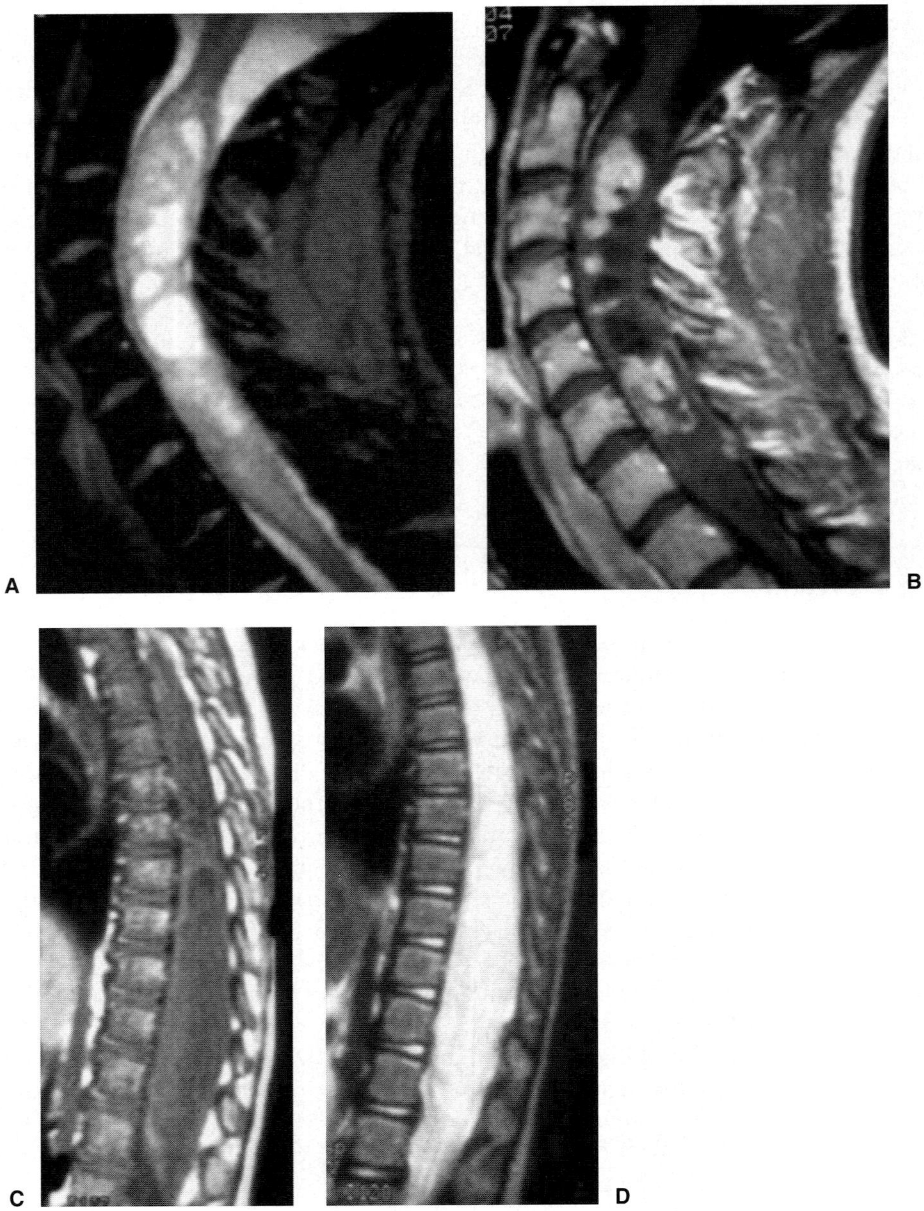

Figure 16.17 *Astrocytoma. A.* Sagittal T2-weighted image shows a large, expansile, and heterogeneously appearing intramedullary cervical spinal cord tumor containing solid and cystic regions. *B.* Corresponding postcontrast T1-weighted image shows enhancement of solid tumor and nonenhancing cysts. *C.* In a different patient, sagittal noncontrast T1-weighted image shows hypointense holocord astrocytoma with expansion of the spinal canal. *D.* On a corresponding T2-weighted image, the tumor is bright.

intramedullary tumor, MRI is the imaging method of choice. The solid tumor nodule usually is pial based and of low T1 and high T2 signal (43) (Fig. 16.18). Serpiginous areas of flow void may be associated with the tumor and are highly suggestive of HB, but in my experience it is rare to visualize them (44). Cysts, which may be unilocular or septated, may arise distal or proximal to the tumor. The cysts usually are of low T1 and high T2 signal but their features may be variable, particularly if intracyst bleeding has occurred. The wall of the cysts does not enhance.

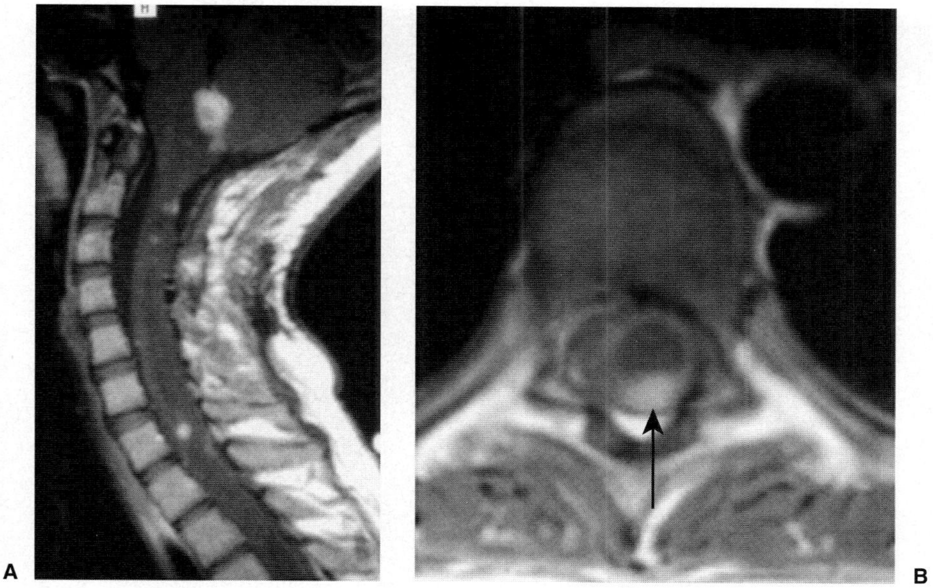

Figure 16.18 *Hemangioblastoma. A.* Sagittal postcontrast T1-weighted image in a patient with von Hippel-Lindau disease shows multiple enhancing hemangioblastomas in the cerebellum and cervical spinal cord. There also is a cyst in the cervical cord. *B.* Axial postcontrast T1-weighted image at mid-thoracic level in the same patient shows an enhancing lesion *(arrow)* that is pial based and has a cyst anteriorly.

Paragangliomas

Although spinal paragangliomas are rare, they are the third most common primary tumor to arise in the filum terminale (after ependymoma and astrocytoma) (45). Although most spinal paragangliomas arise in the filum terminale, occasionally they are found in the nerves of the cauda equina and in the spinal cord (46). Paragangliomas are the third most common primary spinal cord tumor to bleed, after ependymoma and HB. Unlike paragangliomas elsewhere, those arising in the filum terminale do not produce catecholamines. The MRI appearance of the lesions is nonspecific and they are indistinguishable from myxopapillary ependymomas (47) (Fig. 16.19). However, filar paragangliomas are hypervascular and occasionally contain punctate areas of flow void or enhancing blood vessels.

Paragangliomas are the third most common primary spinal cord tumor to bleed, after ependymoma and hemangioblastoma.

Ganglioglioma

Gangliogliomas are rare tumors accounting for 1% to 3 % of central nervous system tumors (Chapter 6). Less than 1% of spinal tumors are gangliogliomas (48). Spinal cord gangliogliomas are found more often in the cervical spine, followed by the thoracic region, but also may occur in the filum terminale. Gangliogliomas grow slowly and achieve a large size by the time of diagnosis (they are perhaps the second most common tumor after astrocytomas to have a holocord distribution) (48). By diagnosis, most cord gangliogliomas are approximately eight vertebral segments in length. Scoliosis and bone erosion are seen in approximately 50% of patients. Cysts are said to be more common than in astrocytomas and ependymomas. The cysts are of low T1 and high T2 signal intensity, and hemorrhage does not occur in them (48) (Fig. 16.20). The solid portions of the mass are of low T1 and high T2 signal intensity, and enhance after gadolinium. The solid portions of the tumor usually are eccentrically located in the cord and may be exophytic. Enhancement along the surface of the spinal cord is not unusual. Ganglioglioma is the only spinal cord tumor where contrast enhancement occasionally is absent.

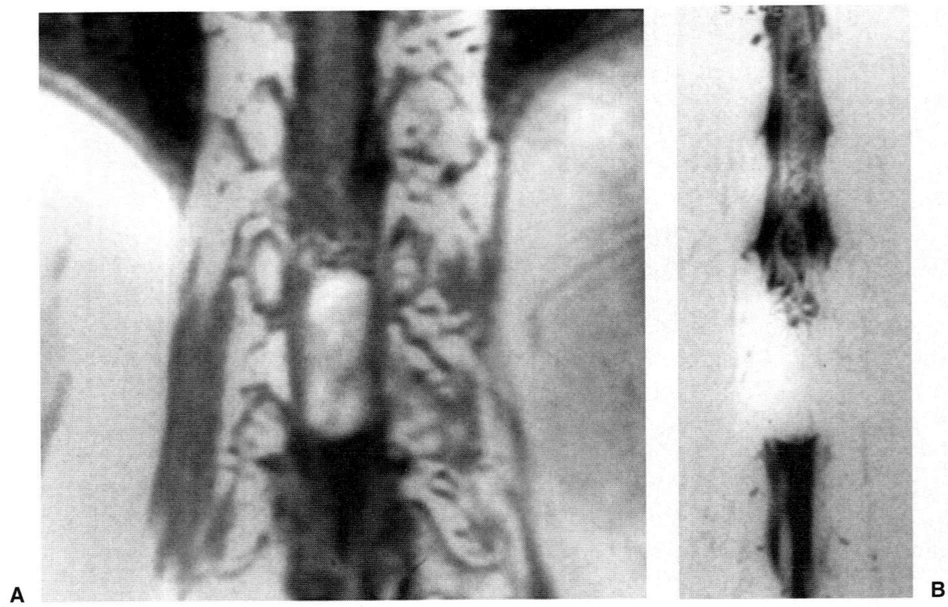

Figure 16.19 *Paraganglioma. A.* Coronal postcontrast T1-weighted image shows an enhancing tumor in the region of the cauda equina. There are serpiginous enhancing structures superior to the mass that likely are blood vessels. The tumor is indistinguishable from a myxopapillary ependymoma. *B.* In the same patient, a coronal view from a magnetic resonance myelogram shows that the lesion "blocks" the cerebrospinal fluid and demonstrates the large blood vessels well.

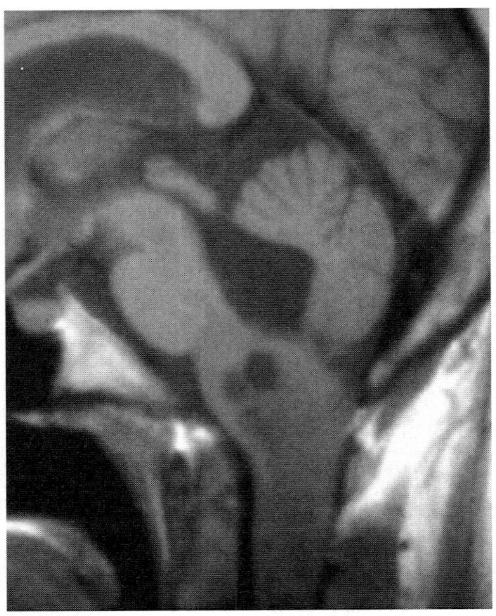

Figure 16.20 *Ganglioglioma. A.* Sagittal noncontrast T1-weighted image shows a complex-appearing tumor with cystic and solid regions involving the upper cervical cord and medulla. The outlet foramina of the fourth ventricle are obstructed, resulting in hydrocephalus.

Spinal Cord Cysts

Although many of these cysts occur without associated tumors, they behave like true masses, produce symptoms as such, and may need surgical intervention, and therefore are addressed here. Histologically, these cysts may represent expansion of the central cord canal and be lined by ependyma (hydromyelia), or they may be eccentric from the central canal and lined by gliotic tissues (syringomyelia). From a clinical standpoint, it makes little sense to attempt this classification because both have identical appearances (clinical and by imaging studies) and need to be treated similarly. Thus, I refer to both types simply as *spinal cord cysts*. The mechanism by which these cysts form has been a matter of considerable debate (49–51). In most patients, there is a history of abnormal CSF flow (Chiari malformations, arachnoiditis), injury to the cord (trauma), chronic compression of the cord by extramedullary masses, or intramedullary tumors. However, in some patients no predisposing factors are found. A current (and favorite) hypothesis states that abnormal CSF flow around the cord forces the fluid into the cord through abnormal perivascular and extracellular spaces (52). Once intramedullary microcysts have formed, the normal pulsations related to blood flow cause "sloshing" and fluid turbulence, resulting in expansion of these cystic cavities. This observation is supported by the fact that in many patients, areas of high T2 signal intensity in the cord (caused by increased fluid) develop just before a cyst becomes obvious (this has been called a *presyrinx state*) (53). The cysts expand the cord and may be focal, multiple, unilocular, or multiseptated. When they are seen in association with a Chiari 1 malformation (Chapter 1) or there is clear antecedent trauma, administration of contrast is not necessary (Fig. 16.21). Otherwise, contrast needs to be given to rule out an underlying tumor as the cause of the cyst. Cysticercosis (Chapter 15) is perhaps the only infectious process in the cord to produce cysts. In children, a cyst in the conus medullaris may be related to a persistent ventriculus terminalis (Chapter 13).

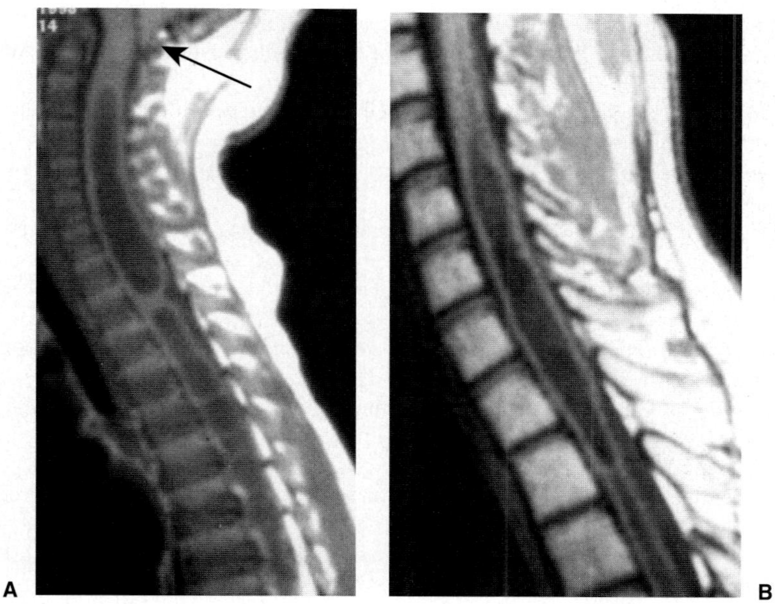

Figure 16.21 *Spinal Cord Cyst. A.* Sagittal T1-weighted image shows a Chiari type 1 malformation *(arrow)* and a multiseptated cervical and thoracic spinal cord cyst that expands the cord and the spinal canal. *B.* In a different patient, a sagittal T1-weighted image shows an idiopathic septated cyst involving the lower cervical and upper thoracic spinal cord.

References

1. Laredo JD, Lakhdari K, Bellaïche L, et al. Acute vertebral collapse: CT findings in benign and malignant nontraumatic cases. Radiology 1995;194:41–48.
2. Cuénod CA, Laredo JD, Chevret S, et al. Acute vertebral collapse due to osteoporosis or malignancy: appearance on unenhanced and gadolinium-enhanced MR images. Radiology 1996;199: 541–549.
3. Castillo M, Malko JA, Hoffman JC. The bright intervertebral disk: an indirect sign of abnormal spinal bone marrow on T1-weighted MR images. AJNR Am J Neuroradiol 1990;11:23–26.
4. Schellinger D. Patterns of anterior spinal canal involvement by neoplasms and infections. AJNR Am J Neuroradiol 1996;17:953–959.
5. Baur A, Huber A, Ertl-Wagner B, et al. Diagnostic value of increased diffusion weighting of a steady-state free precession sequence for differentiating acute benign osteoporotic fractures from pathologic vertebral compression fractures. AJNR Am J Neuroradiol 2001;22:366–372.
6. Rahmouni A, Divine M, Mathieu D, et al. Detection of multiple myeloma involving the spine: efficacy of fat-suppression and contrast-enhanced MR imaging. AJR Am J Roentgenol 1993;160: 1049–1052.
7. St. Amour TE, Hodges SC, Laakman RW, et al. MRI of the spine. New York: Raven Press, 1994.
8. Rahmouni A, Divine M, Mathieu D, et al. MR appearance of multiple myeloma of the spine before and after treatment. AJR Am J Roentgenol 1993;160:1053–1057.
9. Ortiz O, Lefkowitz D. Imaging spinal tumors. In: Castillo M, ed. Spinal imaging. Philadelphia: Hanley & Belfus, 2001:145–168.
10. Friedman DP. Symptomatic vertebral hemangiomas: MR findings. AJR Am J Roentgenol 1996; 167:359–364.
11. Murphey MD, Andrews CL, Flemming DJ, et al. Primary tumors of the spine: radiologic-pathologic correlation. Radiographics 1996;16:1131–1158.
12. Vergel De Dios AM, Bond JR, Shives TC, et al. Aneurysmal bone cyst: a clinicopathologic study of 238 cases. Cancer 1992;69:2921–2931.
13. Meyers SP, Yaw K, Devaney K. Giant cell tumor of the thoracic spine: MR appearance. AJNR Am J Neuroradiol 1994;15:962–964.
14. Assoun J, Richardi G, Raihac JJ, et al. Osteoid osteoma: MR imaging versus CT. Radiology 1994; 191:217–223.
15. Omojola MF, Fox AJ, Vinuela FV. Computed tomographic metrizamide myelography in the evaluation of thoracic spinal osteoblastoma. AJNR Am J Neuroradiol 1982;3:670–673.
16. Llauger J, Palmer J, Amores S, et al. Primary tumors of the sacrum: diagnostic imaging. AJR Am J Roentgenol 2000;174:417–424.
17. Meyer JE, Lepke RA, Lindfors KK, et al. Chordomas: their CT appearance in the cervical, thoracic and lumbar spine. Radiology 1984;153:693–696.
18. Wippold FJ, Koeller KK, Smirniotopoulos JG. Clinical and imaging features of the cervical chordoma. AJR Am J Roentgenol 1999;172:1423–1426.
19. Sze G, Uichanco LS, Brant-Zawadzki MN, et al. Chordomas: MR imaging. Radiology 1988;166: 187–191.
20. Provenzale JM, McLendon RE. Spinal angiolipomas: MR features. AJNR Am J Neuroradiol 1996; 17:713–719.
21. Sakaida H, Waga S, Kojima T, et al. Thoracic spinal angiomyolipoma with extracanal extension to the thoracic cavity. Spine 1998;23:391–394.
22. Bouramas D, Korres DS, Roussos L, et al. Spinal extradural angiolipoma. J Spinal Disord 1995; 8:324–327.
23. Quint DJ, Boulos RS, Sanders WP, et al. Epidural lipomatosis. Radiology 1988;169:485–490.
24. Schild SE, Wharen RE, Menke DM, et al. Primary lymphoma of the spinal cord. Mayo Clin Proc 1995;70:256–260.
25. Burk DL, Brunberg JA, Kanal E, et al. Spinal and paraspinal neurofibromatosis: surface coil MR imaging at 1.5 T. Radiology 1987;162:797–801.
26. Congia S, Coraddu M, Tronci S, et al. Myelographic and MRI appearances of a thoracic spinal extradural arachnoid cyst of the spine with extra- and intraspinal extension. Neuroradiology 1992;34:444–446.
27. Watters MR, Stears JC, Osborn AG, et al. Transdural spinal cord herniation: imaging and clinical spectra. AJNR Am J Neuroradiol 1998;19:1337–1344.
28. Rimmelin A, Clouet PL, Salatino S, et al. Imaging of thoracic and lumbar spinal extradural arachnoid cysts: report of two cases. Neuroradiology 1997;39:203–206.

29. Gindre-Barrucand T, Charleux F, Turjman F, et al. Magnetic resonance imaging contribution to the diagnosis of spinal cord compression by a subdural arachnoid cyst. Neuroradiology 1991; 33:87–89.
30. Wilkins RH. Prevalence and percutaneous drainage of cysts of the sacral nerve root sheath (Tarlov cysts). AJNR Am J Neuroradiol 1994;15:298–299.
31. Paulsen RD, Call GA, Murtagh FR. Prevalence and percutaneous drainage of cysts of the sacral nerve root sheath (Tarlov cysts). AJNR Am J Neuroradiol 1994;15:293-297.
32. Koeller KK, Rosenblum RS, Morrison AL. Neoplasms of the spinal cord and filum terminale: radiologic-pathologic correlation. Radiographics 2000;20:1721–1749.
33. Egelhoff JC, Bates DJ, Ross JS, et al. Spinal MR findings in neurofibromatosis types 1 and 2. AJNR Am J Neuroradiol 1992;13:1071–1077.
34. Shen WC, Ho YJ, Lee SK, et al. Ependymoma of the cauda equina presenting with subarachnoid hemorrhage. AJNR Am J Neuroradiol 1993;14:399–400.
35. Kahan H, Sklar EM, Post MJ, et al. MR characteristics of histopathologic subtypes of spinal ependymoma. AJNR Am J Neuroradiol 1996;17:143–150.
36. Fine MJ, Kricheff II, Freed D, et al. Spinal cord ependymomas: MR imaging features. Radiology 1995;197:655–658.
37. Nemoto Y, Inoue Y, Tashiro T, et al. Intramedullary spinal cord tumors: significance of associated hemorrhage at MR imaging. Radiology 1992;182:793–796.
38. Wippold FJ, Smirniotopoulos JG, Moran CJ, et al. MR imaging of myxopapillary ependymoma: findings and value to determine extent of tumor and its relation to intraspinal structures. AJR Am J Roentgenol 1995;165:1263–1267.
39. Bourgouin PM, Lesage J, Fontaine S, et al. A pattern approach to the differential diagnosis of intramedullary spinal cord lesions on MR imaging. AJR Am J Roentgenol 1998;170:1645–1652.
40. Goy AMC, Pinto RS, Raghavendra BN, et al. Intramedullary spinal cord tumors: MR imaging, with emphasis on associated cysts. Radiology 1986;161:381–386.
41. Baker KB, Moran CJ, Wippold FJ, et al. MR imaging of spinal hemangioblastoma. AJR Am J Roentgenol 2000;174:377–382.
42. Ho VB, Smirniotopoulos JG, Murphey FM, et al. Radiologic-pathologic correlation: hemangioblastoma. AJNR Am J Neuroradiol 1992;13:1343–1352.
43. Rebner M, Gebarski SS. Magnetic resonance imaging of spinal-cord hemangioblastoma. AJNR Am J Neuroradiol 1985;6:287–289.
44. Chu BC, Terae S, Hida K, et al. MR findings in spinal hemangioblastoma: correlation with symptoms and with angiographic and surgical findings. AJNR Am J Neuroradiol 2001;22:206–217.
45. Levy RA. Paraganglioma of the filum terminale: MR findings. AJR Am J Roentgenol 1993;160: 851–852.
46. Aggarwal S, Deck JH, Kucharczyk W. Neuroendocrine tumor (paraganglioma) of the cauda equina: MR and pathologic findings. AJNR Am J Neuroradiol 1993;14:1003–1007.
47. Silverstein AM, Quint DJ, McKeever PE. Intradural paraganglioma of the thoracic spine. AJNR Am J Neuroradiol 1990;11:614–616.
48. Patel U, Pinto RS, Miller DC, et al. MR of spinal cord ganglioglioma. AJNR Am J Neuroradiol 1998;19:879–887.
49. Castillo M, Quencer RM, Green BA, et al. Syringomyelia as a consequence of compressive extramedullary lesions: postoperative clinical and radiologic manifestations. AJNR Am J Neuroradiol 1987;8:973–978.
50. Schwartz ED, Falcone SF, Quencer RM, et al. Posttraumatic syringomyelia: pathogenesis, imaging, and treatment. AJR Am J Roentgenol 1999;173:487–492.
51. Quencer RM, el Gammal T, Cohen G. Syringomyelia associated with intradural extramedullary masses of the spinal canal. AJNR Am J Neuroradiol 1986;7:143–148.
52. Brugières P, Idy-Peretti I, Iffenecker C, et al. CSF flow measurement in syringomyelia. AJNR Am J Neuroradiol 2000;21:1785–1792.
53. Fischbein NJ, Dillon WP, Cobbs C, et al. The "presyrinx" state: a reversible myelopathic condition that may precede syringomyelia. AJNR Am J Neuroradiol 1999;20:7–20.

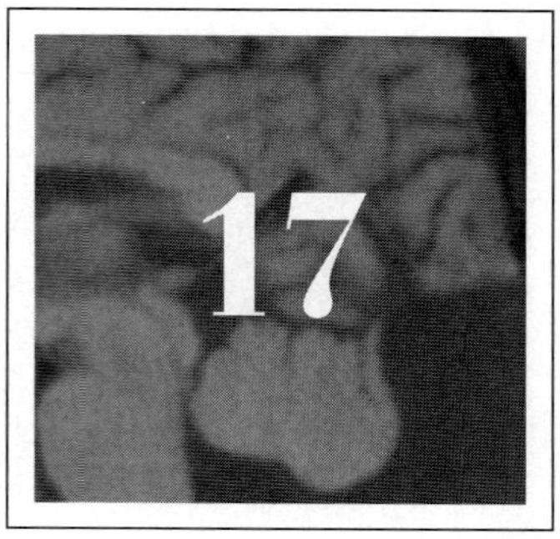

DEGENERATIVE DISORDERS

- The Intervertebral Disk Unit
- Bulging Annulus
- Disk Herniations
- Endplate Changes
- Facet and Ligament Changes
- Neural Foramina
- Conjoined Nerve Roots
- Synovial Cysts
- Spondylolisthesis and Spondylolysis
- Ossification of the Posterior Longitudinal Ligament
- Scheuermann's Disease
- Paget's Disease

THE INTERVERTEBRAL DISK UNIT

The intervertebral disk is composed of the central nucleus pulposus and the peripheral annulus fibrosis. The nucleus contains collagen and proteoglycans that bind to water and give it a gel-like consistency (1). The peripheral aspect of the nucleus merges imperceptibly with the annulus, which is composed of collagen arranged in concentric lamellae. Sharpey's fibers attach the periphery of the annulus to the vertebral body endplates and to the posterior and anterior longitudinal ligaments. The endplates are composed of hyaline cartilage. Early in life, water comprises over 90% of the weight of the disk (1). With progressing age, the amount of proteoglycans diminishes and water is lost. By 75 years of age, approximately 75% to 80% of disk has been replaced by collagen (1). Normally, fissures in the annulus appear by 30 years and degeneration of the disk by 40 years of age; desiccation and loss of height of the disk is nearly universal by 60 years of age. The term *degenerative disk disease* is inappropriate because the entire intervertebral unit (disk, endplates, facets, and ligaments) degenerates synchronously, not just the disk. More than anywhere else in neuroimaging, spine imaging does not rely only on scientific knowledge but on the philosophy of the physicians and institution caring for the patient. The significance attached to abnormalities varies among radiologists and other clinicians. This review represents my point of view with regard to imaging degenerative spine disorders.

BULGING ANNULUS

Relaxation of the fibers of the annulus leads to bulging (2) of the disk. This bulging usually is due to tears in the annulus that may be crescent, radial, or located at the insertions of Sharpey's fibers (3). All types of tears result in a bulging annulus, but usually only radial ones allow for extrusion of the nucleus and development of "herniated disks." All types of annular tears may produce symptoms. These tears may irritate numerous somatic and autonomic nerve endings located at the edge of the annulus (4). This probably is the reason why anterior bulges sometimes are symptomatic. As the annulus bulges, it may result in spinal canal stenosis (I like the analogy of a bulging disk appearing like a hamburger patty protruding from all of the edges of the bun). Isolated bulging annuli are not surgical

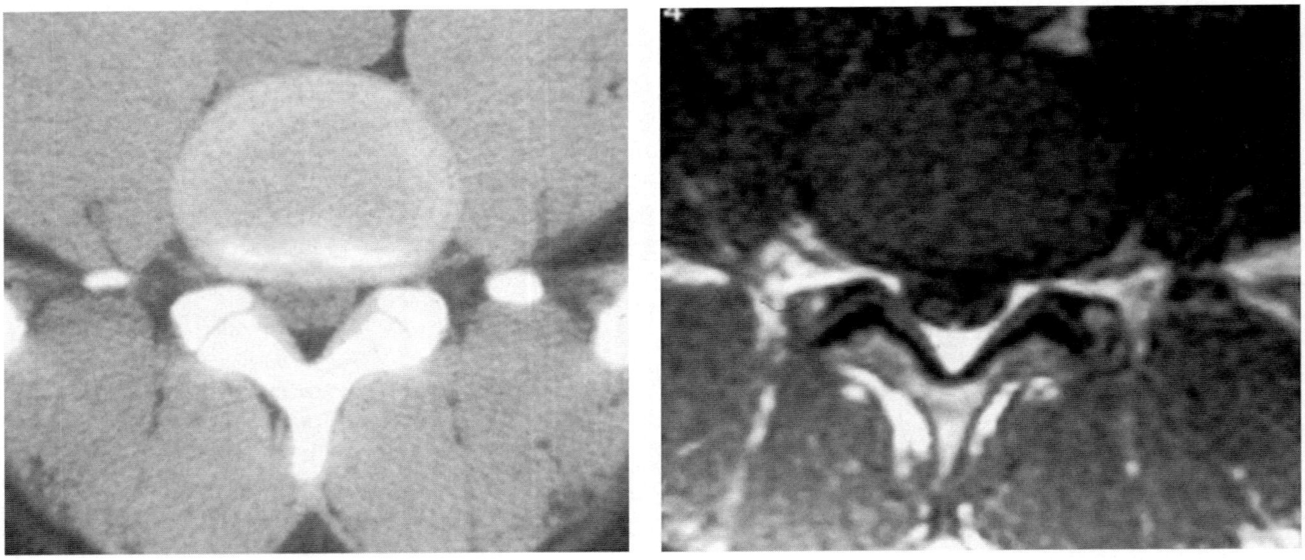

A B

Figure 17.1 *Bulging Disk. A.* Axial computed tomography shows a diffuse bulging disk at L4 to L5 (note loss of central posterior concavity) that, in combination with mild degenerative changes in the facets, narrows the circumference of the spinal canal. *B.* Axial T1-weighted image in a different patient shows diffuse disk bulge.

conditions. However, when this bulging is associated with thick ligamentum flavum and degenerated facet joints, it may lead to central spinal canal stenosis and surgery (unroofing) may be indicated in symptomatic patients (Fig. 17.1). Bulging annuli are common in the lumbar region, particularly at the L4 to L5, L5 to S1, and L3 to L4 levels, in which the change in curvature of the spine results in redistribution of the mechanical forces and increased stress. Many authors do not believe that bulging annuli occur in the thoracic and cervical regions. I do, however, believe cervical disk bulging occurs, and that it usually is accompanied by osteophytes. Again, in the cervical spine the most commonly affected sites are where the curvature changes (C4 to C5, C5 to C6, C6 to C7, C7 to T1, and, less commonly, C3 to C4). Cervical bulging disks/osteophyte complexes may narrow the canal

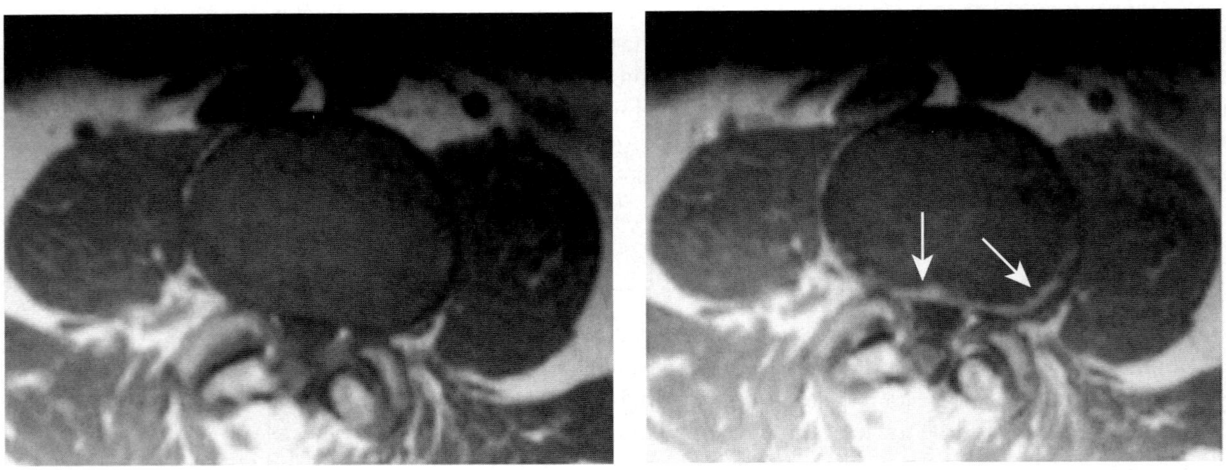

A B

Figure 17.2 *Annular Tears. A.* Axial noncontrast T1-weighted image shows diffuse disk bulge at the L4 to L5 level. In combination with degeneration of the facets, this results in spinal canal narrowing. *B.* Corresponding postcontrast T1-weighted image shows linear enhancement in annular tears *(arrows).* This enhancement presumably is caused by ingrowth of granulation and vascular tissues into the tear.

with or without associated degeneration of the facet joints and thickening of the ligamentum flavum.

On both T1 and T2 images, the normal annulus is slightly darker than the nucleus. The annulus also is thicker anteriorly than posteriorly. Annular tears appear as small focal areas of increased T2 signal usually in the posterior aspect and are easier to see on sagittal images. After gadolinium administration, annular tears may enhance, and this is thought to be secondary to ingrowth of granulation tissues (3) (Fig. 17.2).

DISK HERNIATIONS

Because it contains mostly water, the normal nucleus pulposus is of intermediate T1 signal and bright on T2-weighted images (1). There is a line of low T2 signal intensity through the mid-portion of the nucleus pulposus. This is called the *internuclear cleft* and represents an accumulation of collagen fibers rather than a true anatomic structure. In the young spine, the cleft is seen clearly, and it disappears with age as the rest of the nucleus becomes collagenized and darker on T2 images. The most common way nuclear material herniates is through a radial tear in the annulus and into the epidural space. What distinguishes a disk herniation from a disk bulge is the focal nature of the former. Although there are many terms such as *protrusion* and *extrusion*, I personally find these terms very confusing despite many recent attempts by investigators to create a uniform lexicon. Thus, I use only *bulging* and *herniation* to describe disk pathology. Herniations are focal extrusions of the nucleus pulposus into the epidural space. If they remain contained under the posterior longitudinal ligament, they are called *subligamentous* herniations. Because the ligament is attached to the mid-portion of the vertebral body by the median raphe, most herniations are slightly off midline (Fig. 17.3). A herniated fragment also may erode the posterior longitudinal ligament. The diagnosis of a ruptured posterior longitudinal ligament is difficult to make, and is possible only in approximately 50% of imaging studies. The disk fragment may detach from the parent disk, in which case it is called a *free fragment* (it also is called a *sequestered* fragment because it lies in the epidural space and away from its parent disk; Fig. 17.4). These free fragments may migrate inferiorly or superiorly with equal frequency (in the past it was thought that inferior migration was more common owing to the influence of gravity) (5). A free disk (nuclear) fragment may migrate inferiorly or laterally into a lateral recess (6). A herniated disk may be paracentral, foraminal, and even extraforaminal (and large ones may be in all three locations simultaneously). Foraminal disks may remodel and expand a neural foramen if they are of long standing. Rarely, a herniated disk erodes through the dura and becomes intradural in location (7).

The most common cause for herniated disks is undue force exerted on them. As such, herniated disks are rare in children and older patients and are more common during the most active part of life (20 to 50 years of age). They also are more common in men. Most disk herniations affect the lumbar region (Table 17.1).

The symptoms produced by disk herniations often are baffling, and sometimes the location of the diseased disk does not correlate with the symptoms. Radiculopathies are common, as is low back pain (8). Most patients with symptoms return to normal after 8 to 10 weeks of conservative therapy (9). This is thought to be due to a reduction in the size of the herniated disk, resolution of the hematoma associated with the herniated disk, and resolution of an accompanying inflammatory process (10). Often it is believed that foraminal or extraforaminal disk herniations can cause pain only when they migrate superiorly and laterally to compress exiting nerve roots. In reality, a foraminal disk herniation compresses the normal fat in this location, which in turn may compress the nerve root and produce symptoms (i.e., a lateral disk does not need to compress the nerve root itself to produce symptoms).

In the cervical region, the most common sites for disk herniations are the C5 to C6, C7 to C6, C7 to T1, C4 to C5, and C3 to C4 levels (11). Remember that (unlike the lumbar spine) there are eight pairs of cervical nerve roots and only seven pairs of neural

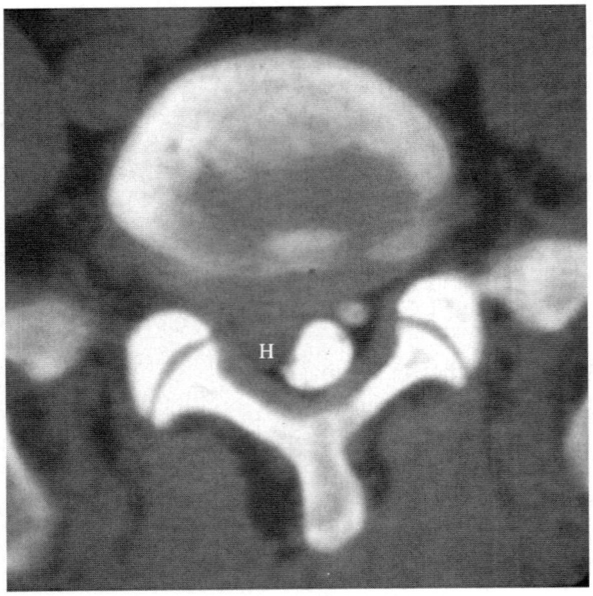

A

Figure 17.3 *Disk Herniation. A.* Postmyelogram axial computed tomography shows a right paramedian L5 to S1 disk herniation *(H)* with compression of the corresponding S1 nerve root. *B.* Axial T1-weighted image shows similar findings (*H*, disk herniation). *C.* Corresponding T2-weighted image shows the disk herniation to be isointense to the parent disk. The facet joints are degenerated and contain bright fluid. *D.* In a different patient, a sagittal T1-weighted image shows a subligamentous, nearly central disk herniation *(H)* at the L5 to S1 level. The disk extends caudally in the ventral epidural space. *E.* Corresponding T2-weighted image shows the herniated disk to be slightly bright.

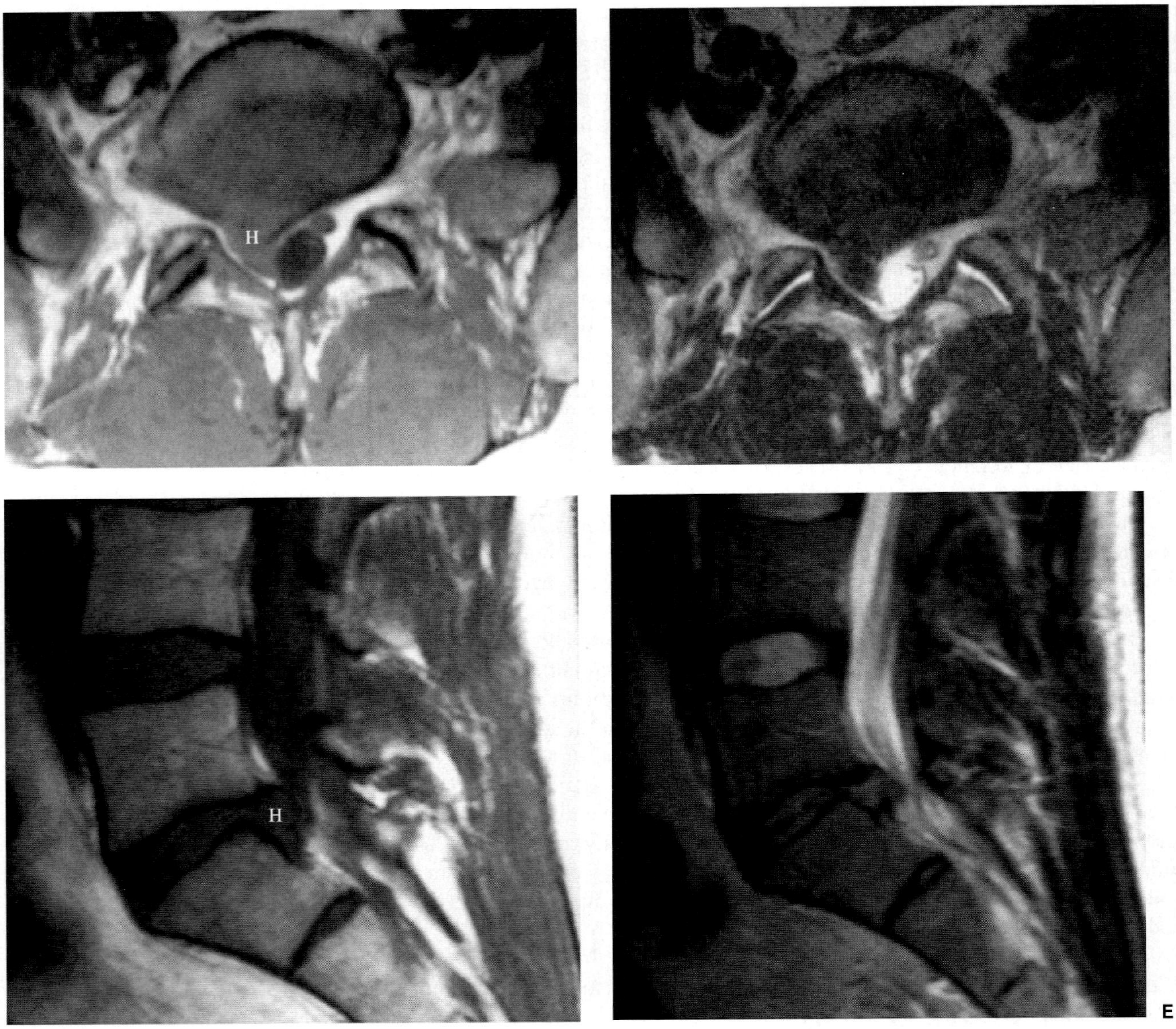

B C D E

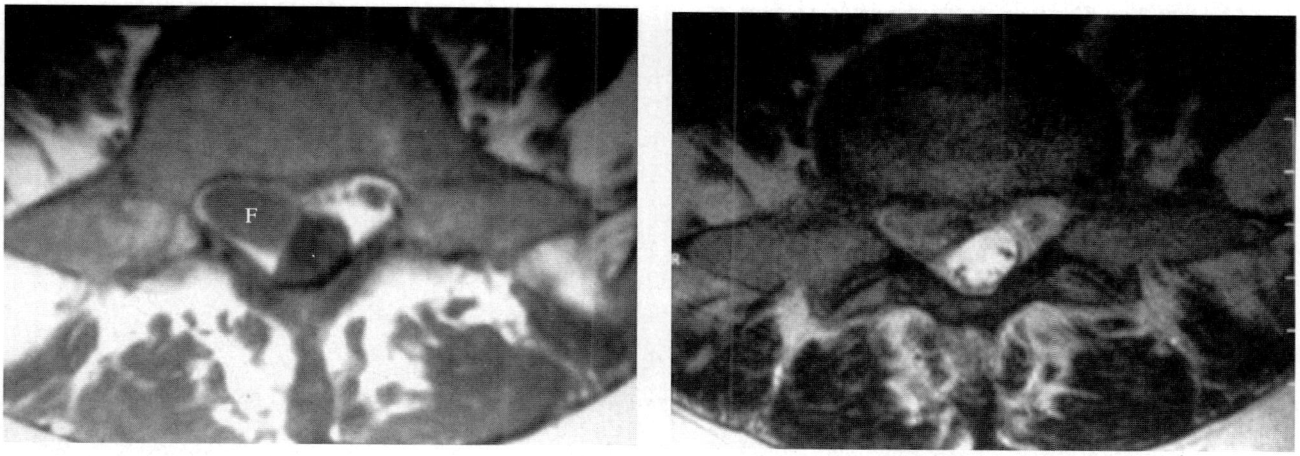

A B

Figure 17.4 *Sequestered Disk Fragment. A.* Axial T1-weighted image shows large hypointense disk fragment *(F)* in the right lateral recess of S1. The adjacent nerve is compressed and not seen. *B.* Corresponding T2-weighted image shows that the sequestered disk fragment is slightly bright.

foramina (12). So, in the cervical region, the nerve exiting at the C5 to C6 level is C6; at the C6 to C7 level, C7; and at the C7 to T1 level, C8. Another difference between the lumbar and cervical regions is that the median raphe attaching the posterior longitudinal ligament to the dorsal aspect of the vertebral bodies and annuli is ill defined in the cervical spine. This is the reason why central herniated disks are not uncommon in the cervical spine (Fig. 17.5). Another difference between the cervical spine and the lumbar spine lies in the fact that the former contains the spinal cord and thus the symptoms from spondylolysis may include not only radiculopathies but myelopathies (including progressive painless paraparesis, gait abnormalities, pain, hyperreflexia). A myelopathy usually occurs when the cervical anteroposterior diameter is reduced to less than 8 mm regardless of the underlying cause (13). Normal dimensions in the spine are listed in Table 17.2. As in the lumbar region, cervical disk herniations also may be paracentral, foraminal, or extraforaminal (Fig. 17.6B). Free fragments are less common in the cervical spine.

The magnetic resonance imaging (MRI) evaluation of disk herniations usually is straightforward. In the lumbar and thoracic regions, they are readily seen on sagittal T1 and T2 sequences (14,15). On axial T1 images, the normal bright epidural fat serves as contrast and outlines these herniations. The presence of fat is particularly helpful in the lumbar region. Because of the presence of epidural fat providing good contrast between the thecal sac and its adjacent structures, T1-weighted images traditionally have been considered sufficient. In the past, conventional T2-weighted images were not used because the fat lost signal and because of artifacts from cerebrospinal fluid (CSF) movement. Today, fast spin-echo T2 images of the lumbar spine are very helpful. They benefit from bright fat (thus creating a good contrast with the adjacent bones and ligaments) and from homogeneous signal intensity from the CSF owing to the inherent rephrasing of the long echo train. I used both T1 and fast spin-echo T2 images in axial projection when examining the lumbar spine.

Table 17.1: Location and Incidence of Lumbar Herniated Disks

Level	*Incidence*
L4–L5 and L5–S1	85%–90%
L3–L4	5%–10%
L2–L3 and L1–L2	<5%

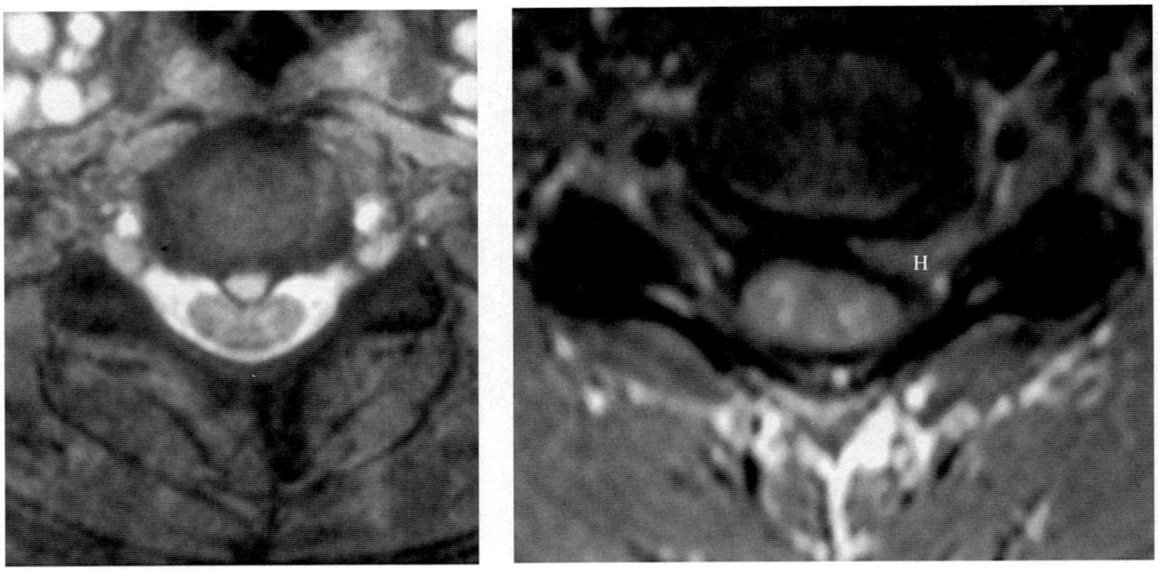

A B

Figure 17.5 *Cervical Disk Herniations. A.* Axial T2-weighted image shows a bright and central disk herniation at the C4 to C5 level. The herniation indents the ventral surface of the spinal cord. *B.* In a different patient, an axial T1-weighted image shows a left lateral and foraminal disk herniation *(H)* at the C5 to C6 level.

Table 17.2: Normal Dimensions of the Bony Spinal Canal (Anteroposterior)

Level	*Size*
Cervical	>10 mm
Thoracic	>8 mm
Lumbar	>12 mm

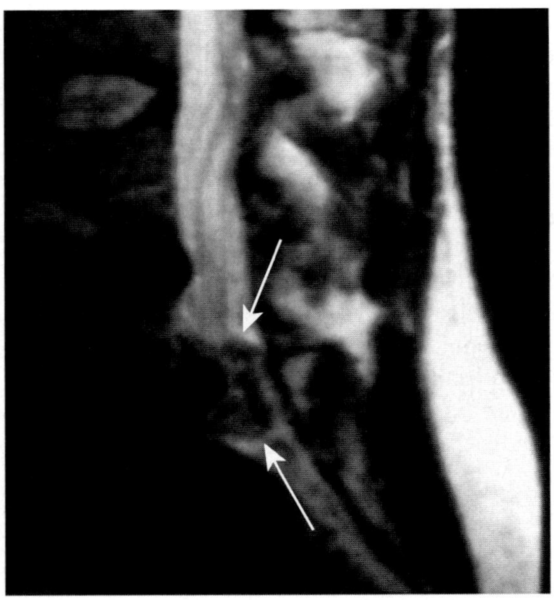

Figure 17.6 *Giant Disk Herniation.* Sagittal T2-weighted image shows a very large disk herniation at the L5 to S1 level. On close inspection, the disk herniation has a component of slightly higher signal intensity *(arrows)* projecting into the spinal canal. This component disappeared 2 weeks later and is believed to be due to hematoma. The patient's symptoms improved after resolution of the hematoma.

Most lumbar herniated fragments are isointense on T1 and may be dark, intermediate, or bright on T2. Bright T2 disk herniations are thought to be related to the presence of edema and thus are common in the acute period. The herniated disk compresses the ventral aspect of the thecal sac or adjacent nerve roots. On sagittal images, a linear area of low signal intensity outlining the herniated disk usually is related to an intact posterior longitudinal ligament. Many disks show peripheral contrast enhancement, which is thought to be related to the presence of granulation tissues. This finding is more common in long-standing rather than acute disks and also more common in the lumbar spine. A significant amount of enhancement may be seen in so-called inflammatory disk herniations, and this finding correlates with acute symptoms (16). A specific type of herniation, called a *giant disk herniation*, deserves special mention. In this situation, there is a large disk herniation often in combination with an epidural hematoma (Fig. 17.6). This may be suspected because hematoma is of low T2 signal, particularly on gradient-echo images. In these patients, the hematoma resolves with time and thus the size of the herniation improves. It is believed that epidural hematomas may accompany many disk herniations that improve spontaneously. I usually do not use gadolinium for the evaluation of lumbar herniated disks. Contrast administration is helpful when the presence of a herniation is in doubt. In this situation, the enhancing epidural space outlines the disk. Similarly, contrast administration may improve visualization of foraminal and extraforaminal disk herniations.

In the cervical spine, herniated disks appear similar to those found in the lumbar region. Cervical herniated disks (unless hyperacute and posttraumatic) have associated osteophytes (17). Because there is little or no epidural fat in the cervical region, an MRI sequence that maximizes the contrast between CSF and adjacent bone/ligaments is desirable. This is performed by using low–flip-angle T2-weighed imaging that results in a "myelographic" effect with minimal degradation by the motion of CSF. Unfortunately, these sequences are sensitive to magnetic susceptibility and result in artifactual narrowing of the diseased spinal canal and the neural foramina. Occasionally, cervical herniated disks are bright on T1 images (18,19) (Fig. 17.7). This is believed to be due to the presence of hydrated calcium or subacute hemorrhage in the herniated fragments. In the presence of herniated disks it is important to evaluate the spinal cord. Intramedullary areas of T2 signal intensity may be related to long-standing myelomalacia or to acute edema, and in patients with multilevel disease may serve as an indication that the site needs prompt decompression (20–23). Because of poor intrinsic contrast owing to the lack of epidural fat in the cervical spine, contrast enhancement is helpful in assessing some cervical herniated disks. Enhancement of the epidural plexus makes them more obvious visually.

Disc herniations that are bright on T1 weighted images are more common in the cervical spine, and are thought to be due to the presence of hydrated calcium and less commonly subacute blood products.

Thoracic disk herniations are thought to be rare (<1% of all disk herniations), but I think that this reflects data that were acquired before MRI. In reality, the incidence of tho-

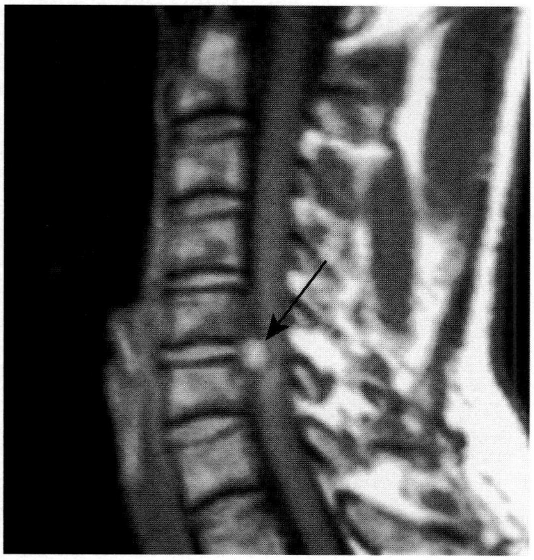

Figure 17.7 *"Bright" Cervical Disk Herniation.* Sagittal T1-weighted image shows a bright central disk herniation *(arrow)* at the C5 to C6 level. This degree of brightness probably is due to the presence of hydrated calcium and not subacute hemorrhage.

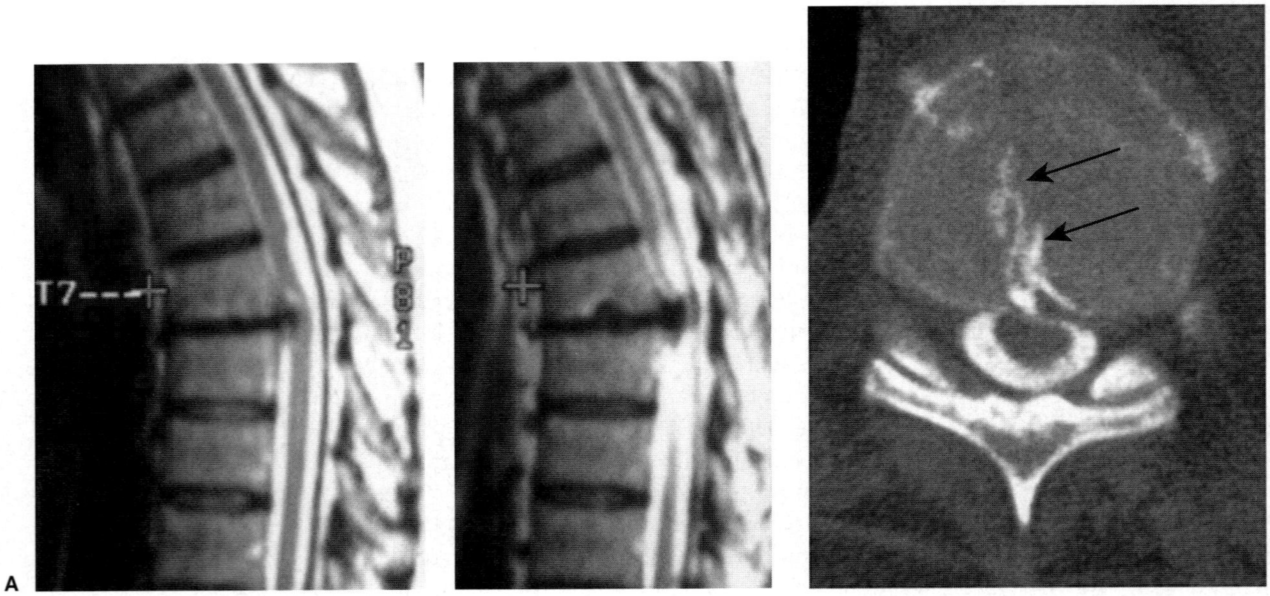

Figure 17.8 *Thoracic Disk Herniation. A.* Two consecutive sagittal T2-weighted images show a disk herniation at the T7 to T8 level. *B.* In a different patient, axial postmyelogram image shows a sclerotic "nuclear trail" *(arrows)* terminating in a small left paracentral disk herniation that indents the ventral surface of the spinal cord.

racic disk herniations probably is approximately 7% to 10% (14). The most common symptoms due to thoracic disk herniation are pain (local or in the chest), lower extremity weakness, gait disturbance, bowel/bladder dysfunction, and sensory loss. Because of the smaller size of the spinal canal in this region and the limited epidural space, intradural disk herniations are more common in the thoracic region than elsewhere. Over 75% of thoracic disk herniations occur between T8 and L1, but other levels also may be affected (Fig. 17.8A). Many lower thoracic disk herniations are found incidentally when examining the lumbar spine. Thoracic disk herniations usually are smaller than cervical and lumbar ones but produce symptoms early because of the reduced diameter of the spinal canal in this region (14). These herniations are isointense or of low signal on T1 images and may be difficult to visualize. They nearly always are hypointense on T2 images because over 55% of them contain calcium on radiographs (16). An interesting finding seen with thoracic disk herniations is that of a "nuclear tail" or "trail" (14) (Fig. 17.8B). These terms reflect the presence of abnormal linear areas extending from the nucleus pulposus to the herniated fragment. It is thought that this tail represents a scar left by the nucleus along its path of herniation (like the tail of a comet). Often, this tail is more obvious than the herniated disk fragment. In the presence of a nuclear tail, the radiologist always should follow it to where it ends in the region of the epidural space to exclude a disk herniation. Remember that the ventral epidural space in the thoracic region also contains little fat, and that contrast enhancement is helpful in many instances to document the presence of herniated disks. Axial T2 images also are very helpful, but tend to be degraded by artifacts from pulsations in the aorta and heart.

I do not address myelography here because MRI is the imaging method of choice except when the patient cannot be placed in the unit. I still believe that the fourth edition of *Myelography* by Robert Shapiro is the best book to read on this topic.

ENDPLATE CHANGES

As the disk degenerates, changes in the vertebral body endplates occur. Radiographs and computed tomography (CT) reveal only the end-stage changes as sclerosis. On MRI, these changes were classified by Modic et al. (24) (Table 17.3) (Figs. 17.9 and 17.10).

Table 17.3: Modic Changes in the Vertebral Endplates

Type/Cause	*T1 Images*	*T2 Images*
I/edema and vascularized bone marrow (Fig. 17.9)	Low signal	High signal
II/fatty infiltration (Fig. 17.10)	High signal	Moderately high signal
III/fibrous and osseous changes	Low signal	Low signal

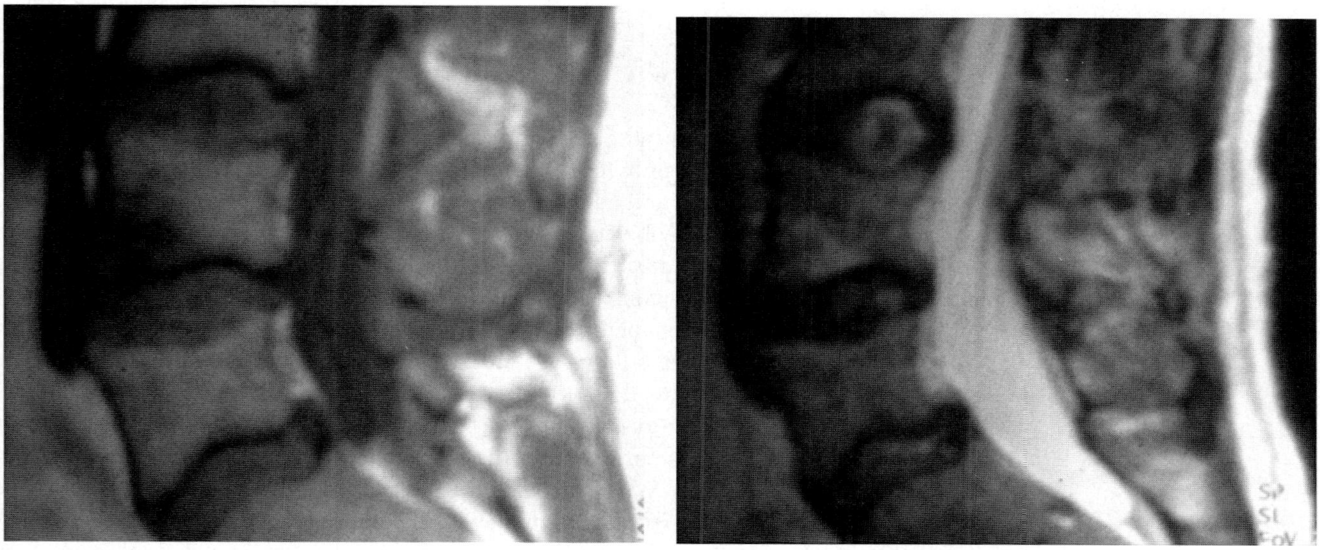

A B

Figure 17.9 *Early Degenerative Changes of the Vertebral Endplates (Modic Type 1). A.* Sagittal T1-weighted image shows low signal intensity from the inferior and anterior aspect of L4. *B.* Corresponding T2-weighted image shows that the abnormal area is bright. The L4 to L5 disk is dark, probably related to loss of proteoglycans and desiccation.

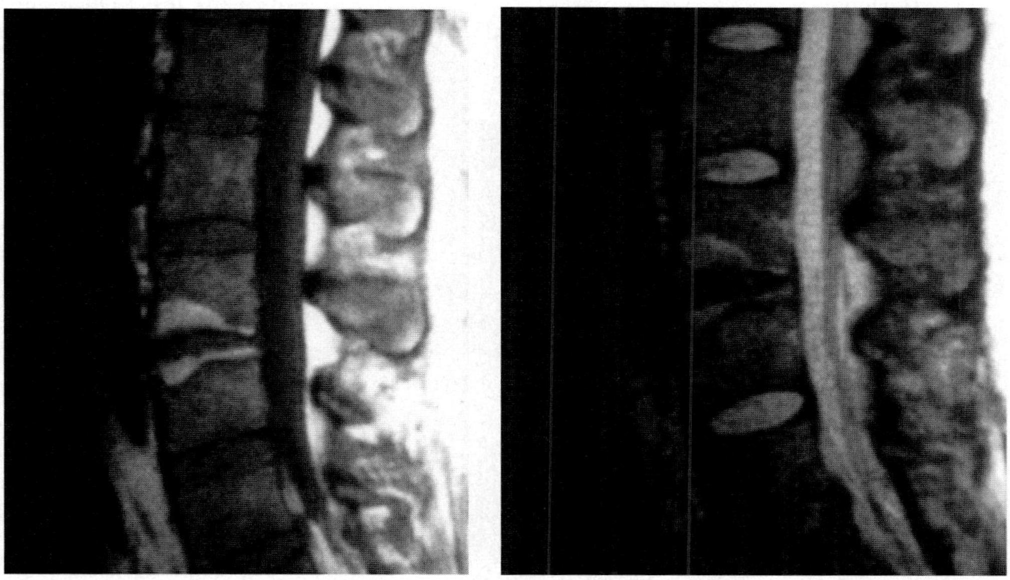

A B

Figure 17.10 *Intermediate Degenerative Changes of the Vertebral Endplates (Modic Type 2). A.* Sagittal T1-weighted image shows high signal intensity from the superior endplate of L4 and inferior endplate of L3. *B.* On a corresponding T2 (fast spin-echo) image, the endplate changes remain bright. The intervening disk has lost height and is dark. The findings probably are due to fibrofatty changes in the endplate and adjacent bone marrow.

Important aspects of these observations include:

1. Vertebral endplate changes begin before they are seen on radiographs and CT.
2. Type I and II changes may be reversible.
3. Type I changes should not be confused with edema due to early infection (in cases of infection, the disk is T2 bright, whereas in most diskogenic changes, the disk is of low T2 signal; in both instances the disk space may be narrowed).
4. Occasionally, the endplates may enhance, and this normally is due to the presence of vascularized tissues (type I).

Facet and Ligament Changes

A ligamentum flavum measuring between 3 and 5 mm is somewhat large, and one above 5 mm is definitely abnormal.

Like any other synovial joint, the facet joint may suffer the formation of subchondral cysts, sclerosis, formation of osteophytes (particularly at the level of attachment of the ligamentum flavum), hypertrophy, and narrowing. Vacuum phenomenon (due to accumulation of nitrogen) is common in the lower lumbar region and less common elsewhere. As the facet joints (especially in the lumbar region) settle on each other, the superior one slides rostrally and slightly anterior while the posterior one slides down and backward (12). When this happens, the normal ligamentum flavum becomes too long and buckles over the facet, appearing thick on imaging studies. The term *hypertrophied ligamentum flavum* is a misnomer because the ligaments do not hypertrophy. Thus, changes in the facets and the ligamentum flavum nearly always occur at the same time. The hypertrophy of the facets and ligament buckling result in narrowing of the spinal canal (in addition to narrowing of the neural foramina; see later). When these findings are accompanied by a disk bulge or herniation, the spinal canal is reduced in diameter from all sides. On axial images this is seen as a triangular-shaped thecal sac and receives the name of *central spinal canal stenosis* (Fig. 17.11). There are many variations of spinal stenosis. In most instances it is the central type, but may be lateral or just anteroposterior depending on its underlying cause. Degeneration of the facet joints and buckling of the ligamentum flavum also occur in the cervical region, but are uncommon in the thoracic spine. The anatomy of the cervical spine is further complicated by the presence of the uncovertebral joints of Luschka, which also may degenerate. I consider a normal ligamentum flavum to measure less than 3 mm on

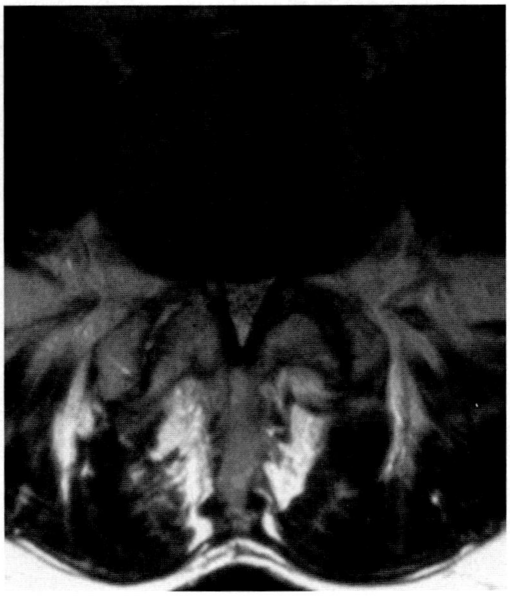

Figure 17.11 *Central Spinal Canal Stenosis.* Axial T2-weighted image shows a diffuse L5 to S1 disk bulge, degenerated facet joints (the right one contains bright fluid), and mild thickening of the ligamentum flavum, all of which result in the central type of spinal canal narrowing.

axial images. A ligamentum flavum measuring between 3 and 5 mm is somewhat large, and one above 5 mm is definitely abnormal.

NEURAL FORAMINA

The cervical neural foramina are difficult to examine. Axial images show them to be oriented at approximately 45 degrees off midline (12). Thus, they are incompletely visualized on sagittal images. The posterior wall of a cervical neural foramen is formed by the superior articular facet (from the underlying vertebra), the inferior wall by the pedicle of the vertebra below, the anterior superior wall by the pedicle of the vertebra above, and the superiormost aspect of its posterior wall by the inferior articular facet of the vertebra above. The nerve roots lie in the middle to inferior aspect of the foramen. In the thoracic spine the foramina assume a more vertical position, and on axial images are oriented nearly 90 degrees from the midline. The nerve roots are contained in their middle to superior portion. In the lumbar region, the inferior and posterior wall of a foramen is formed by the superior articular facet of the vertebra below, the posterior and superior wall by the inferior articular facet of the vertebra above, the superior margin by the pedicle of the vertebra above, the anterior and superior wall by the body of the vertebra above and disk, and the inferior and anterior wall by the body of the vertebra below (25). Note that the ligamentum flavum forms part of the posterior wall of the neural foramina at all levels. On axial images, the lumbar foramina are oriented 90 degrees from the midline. They are seen clearly on sagittal images and have an inverted teardrop shape (bulbous superiorly and narrow inferiorly). The nerve roots (and corresponding blood vessels) are located in their superior aspect. All neural foramina are filled with fat and contain the radicular artery and vein, exiting epidural veins, the nerve roots, and, laterally, the dorsal root ganglia.

All neural foramina may be considered narrowed if they measure less than 5 mm in diameter on axial images. In the cervical region, the major cause of narrowing is hypertrophy and degeneration of the uncovertebral joint, which nearly always is accompanied by degeneration of the facet joints and buckling of the ligamentum flavum. In the thoracic and particularly the lumbar spine, narrowing of the neural foramina is due to degeneration of the facet joints and buckling of the ligamentum flavum. Laterally herniated disks may compress the exiting nerve roots and dorsal root ganglia at every level. Often, narrowing of the neural foramina is asymptomatic or does not correspond with the patient's symptoms. Axial MRI using low–flip-angle techniques tends to overestimate the degree of narrowing always (one of the benefits of CT is that this does not occur).

CONJOINED NERVE ROOTS

It is important not to confuse conjoined nerve roots with herniated disk or with masses (such as nerve sheath tumors) (16). These normal variations occur exclusively in the lower lumbar spine and may result in conflicting clinical findings. They are seen in approximately 1% of lumbar spine MRI studies (25). Nearly always, conjoined nerve roots are unilateral. In these anomalies, two nerve roots travel in the same meningeal sleeve and more commonly leave the spine through their separate and distinct neural foramina. Occasionally, both nerve roots exit through one neural foramen. On axial images, the nerve root sleeve is large (resulting in enlargement of the corresponding lateral recess) and the nerves in the neuroforamen appear large, as does the dorsal root ganglion (Fig. 17.12). Most conjoined nerve roots are found at L4 to L5, L5 to S1, and rarely at L3 to L4. They are important to the neurosurgeon operating for herniated disks. If a conjoined nerve is present at the level of a laterally herniated disk, it is possible for the surgeon to be unable to distinguish between them and potentially injure the conjoined nerve roots. Because of this, they should always be reported.

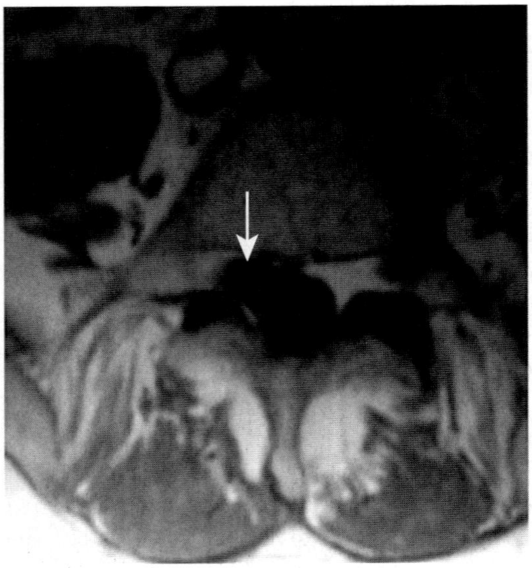

Figure 17.12 *Conjoined Nerve Root.* Axial T1-weighted image shows large right S1 nerve root sleeve *(arrow)*. This widening of the sleeve is due to the fact that it contains both the L5 and S1 nerve roots. Note that the corresponding lateral recess also is widened.

Synovial Cysts

Although histologically, cysts arising from a facet joint may be true synovial, pseudosynovial or ganglion cysts, this classification has little practical importance and by imaging, they are all nearly identical in appearance.

Facet joint synovial cysts may be of the following types (16):

1. True synovial cysts contain fluid, communicate with the joint space, and are lined by synovium.
2. Pseudosynovial cysts contain fluid, communicate with the joint space, and are lined by a fibrous capsule.
3. Ganglion cysts contain fluid, do not communicate with joint space, and are lined by a fibrous capsule.

For practical purposes, all have a similar imaging appearance and are treated in the same fashion, and hence I call all of them synovial cysts. Their origin probably is an inflammatory process in the joint leading to weakening and erosion of the synovial lining. This same inflammatory activity later may obliterate the communication between cyst and joint space. This inflammation in the wall of the cyst may lead to calcification or hemorrhage and may change the characteristics of the fluid in the cyst. If the joint space contains gas, it also may extend into the cyst. These cysts may be contained by the ligamentum flavum or erode through it. They are located in the dorsolateral aspect of the spinal canal. The joint adjacent to a synovial cyst always is degenerated. This change results in nonspecific back pain and at times radiculopathy. Nearly three-fourths of synovial cysts occur at the L4 to L5 level, but they are also found at L5 to S1 and L3 to L4. The appearance of synovial cysts by MRI is variable (26) (Fig. 17.13A). They may have low or high T1 signal intensity (depending on the protein concentration of their fluid and presence or absence of hemorrhage). On T2 images, their signal nearly always is high. Occasionally, they may be of very low signal on T1 and T2 images, and this is related to the presence of gas or calcifications. After contrast administration, their periphery often enhances, reflecting adjacent inflammation. The differential diagnosis of a synovial cyst is as follows:

- Herniated free disk fragment
- Cystic nerve sheath tumor
- Meningeal CSF-filled cyst

Often, the diagnosis of synovial cyst is made on images and the surgeon is unable to find it. This usually results from the fact that the surgeon opens the lining of the facet and fluid filling the cyst extravasates and the cyst collapses. On CT, synovial cysts may contain gas and show a calcified or partially calcified wall (Fig. 17.13B). Last, synovial cysts also

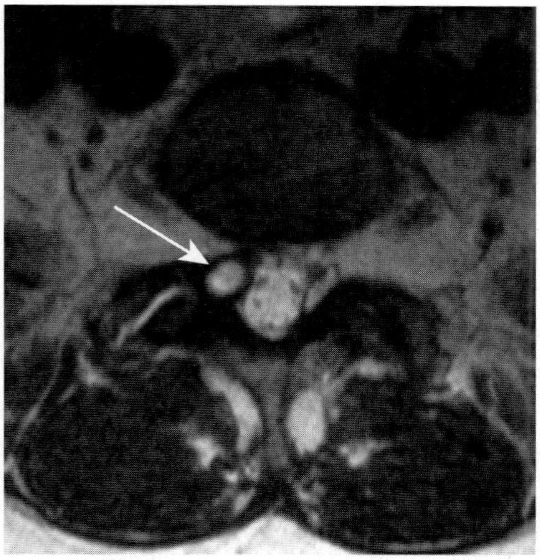

A

Figure 17.13 *Synovial Cyst. A.* Axial T2-weighted image shows a right bright synovial cyst *(arrow)* arising from the ipsilateral L5 to S1 facet joint that is degenerated and also contains fluid of high signal intensity. *B.* Axial computed tomography shows left-sided synovial cyst *(small arrows)* that contains gas. Gas also is seen in the corresponding degenerated facet joint *(large arrow)*. The walls of the cyst are hyperdense, probably because of calcification. *C.* Axial T2-weighted image shows an incidental left-sided posterior synovial cyst *(arrow)*.

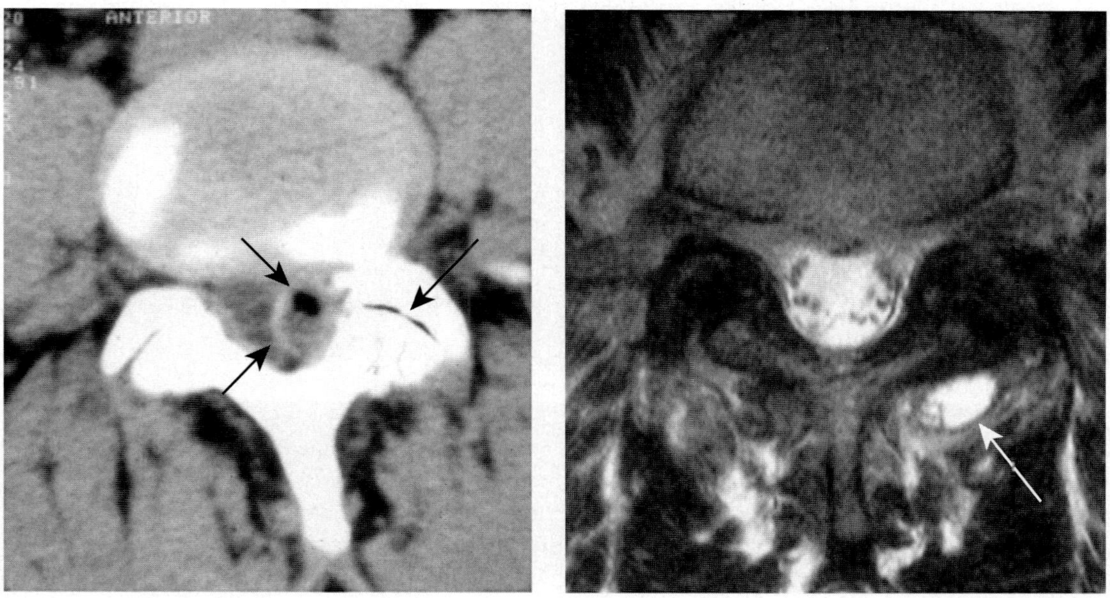

B C

may arise from the posterior aspect of the facet joints and project into the posterior paraspinal fat and musculature (Fig. 17.13C). These patients often have pain associated with the degenerative changes of the facet joint from which the cyst arises. They commonly are seen on MRI studies of the lumbar spine.

Spondylolisthesis and Spondylolysis

Spondylolisthesis is a nonspecific term describing the slippage of one vertebra with respect to the one below (16). It may be caused by spondylolysis, degenerative facet disease, trauma, and postsurgical instability. Most spondylolistheses occur at the L5 and L4 levels, regardless of their underlying etiology. By convention, the slippage is graded on lateral radiographs or sagittal CT reformations (27). The slipped vertebral body is divided into three equal parts. If the slippage is no greater than the posterior one-third of the caudal vertebral body, it is grade I. If the slippage places the posterior edge of the slipped vertebral body in the middle one-third of the caudal vertebral body, it is called grade II, and if it lies in the anterior one-third, it is grade III. Some refer to grade IV slips when the dis-

In degenertive spondylolisthesis, the width of the spinal canal is generally decreased, while in spondylolisthesis due to spondylolysis, the width of the canal is generally increased.

placed vertebral body is located completely ventral to the underlying vertebra. On sagittal images (either reformatted CT or MRI), the anteroposterior diameter of the spinal canal at the level of the spondylolisthesis provides a clue as to its underlying etiology. If the canal is wide and the patient has not received surgery, the cause nearly always is spondylolysis. Conversely, if the spinal canal is narrowed, the underlying cause nearly always is degeneration and laxity of the facet joints. Multilevel spondylolisthesis nearly always is degenerative in nature.

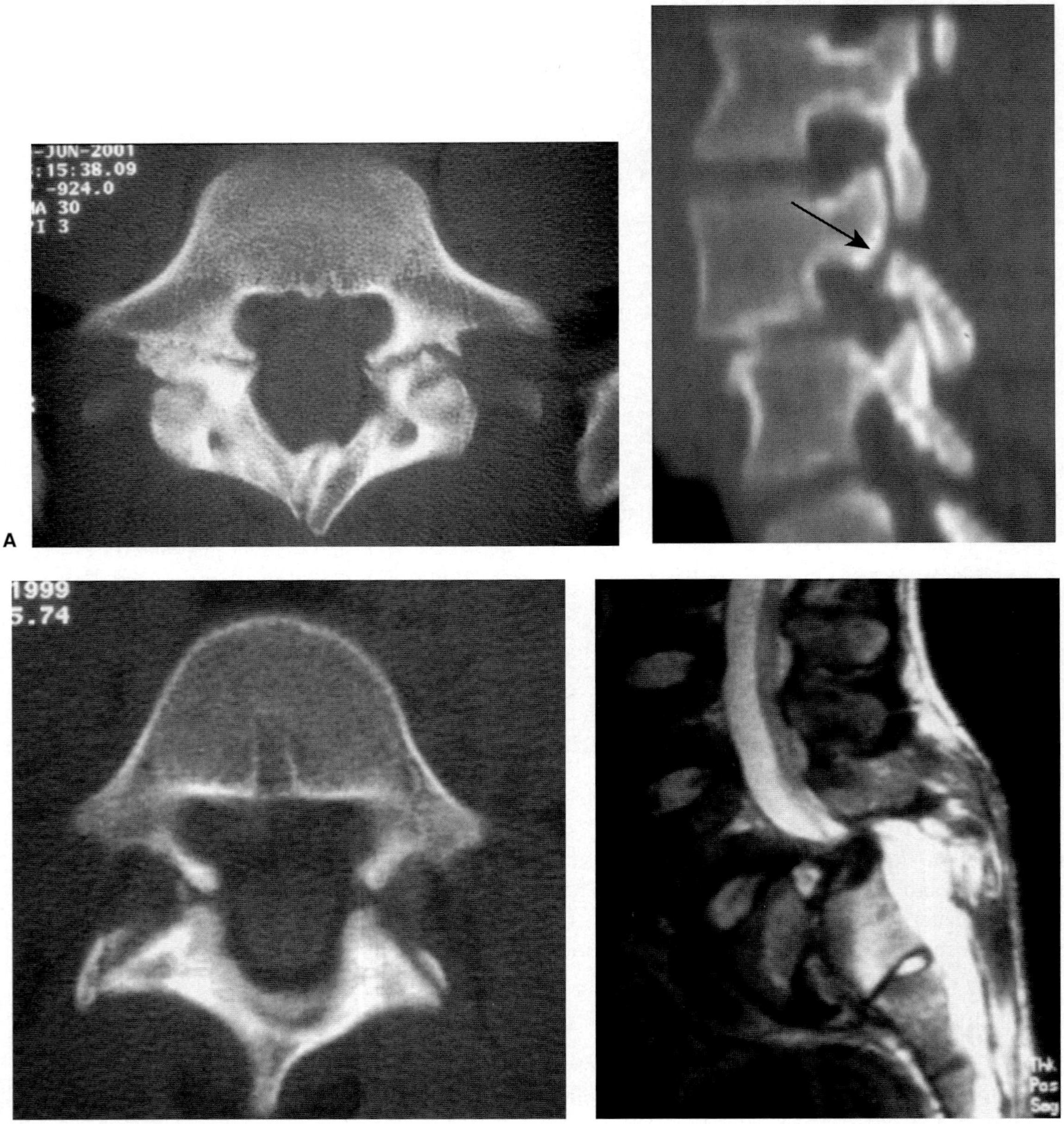
A B C D

Figure 17.14 *Spondylolysis and Spondylolisthesis. A.* Axial computed tomography (CT) shows sclerotic clefts in both pars interarticularis. These clefts are not the facet joints. They are located anterior to the facet joints, are nearly horizontal in orientation, and are markedly irregular. *B.* Parasagittal CT reformation in a different patient shows a pars defect *(arrow)* at the L4 to L5 level and a mild (grade I) anterior displacement of L4 on L5. C. In a different patient, axial CT shows bilateral spondylolysis and severe spondylolisthesis. *D.* In the same patient, a sagittal T2-weighted image shows complete anterior dislocation of L5 on S1, edema of the endplates, and significant narrowing of the spinal canal at that level.

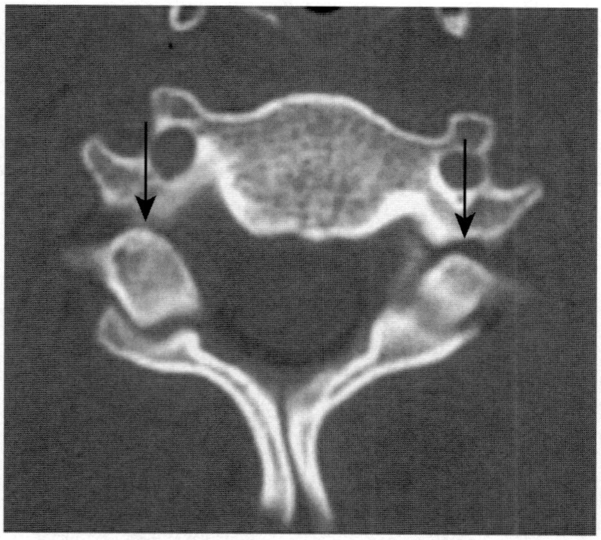

Figure 17.15 *Cervical Spondylolysis.* Axial computed tomography shows bilateral clefts *(arrows)* anterior to the facet joints at the C4 to C5 level. Associated bifid spinous process is present.

Spondylolysis was thought to be congenital, but because it is extremely rare in young children (<6 years of age), a traumatic etiology is now favored (28). It is a common anomaly seen in up to 5% of the general population. It appears that commencing sports at school results in undue stress on the thin pars interarticularis, causing multiple microstress fractures. Once the pars defect is established, further stress by exercising (particularly during the high school years) results in anterior slippage of the affected vertebra (Fig. 17.14). The presence of minor underlying congenital defects (e.g., spina bifida occulta) appears to increase the risk for development of spondylolysis. Most patients with spondylolysis have only nonspecific low back pain, but as the slippage increases, compression of the nerve roots ensues. Because the disk remains in its normal position, the thecal sac drapes over the disk at the level of the slippage, and on axial images gives the appearance of a "pseudodisk herniation." The clefts may be difficult to identify on axial images, and in my opinion one of the best clues to the presence of underlying spondylolysis is seeing "too many facets." The clefts in the pars interarticularis nearly always are irregular and sclerotic. If a unilateral defect is present, the contralateral facet degenerates (because it sustains the normal alignment and motion of the spine) and the contralateral pedicle hypertrophies. The clefts may be difficult to visualize on MRI, and in these cases spondylolisthesis on the sagittal images provides an important clue. Pain at the level of a spondylolysis usually is due to instability. Motion and slippage are best assessed with flexion and extension lateral radiographs. Most spondylolyses are found at the L5 level. Cervical spondylolysis is known to occur, but is rare (Fig. 17.15).

Ossification of the Posterior Longitudinal Ligament

This disorder is being recognized with increasing frequency in the United States. It was first described in Japan where it is considered to be endemic and affects approximately 5% of the population, particularly men 60 to 70 years of age (16). In the United States, there is a strong association between ossification of the posterior longitudinal ligament (OPLL) and diffuse idiopathic skeletal hyperostosis (DISH). Most patients present with symptoms of a myelopathy (secondary to narrowing of the spinal canal), although radiculopathies also occasionally may be encountered. The etiology of the disease is unknown, but it is believed that underlying disk herniations and repetitive stress on the ligaments induce calcification and later ossification. The three types of OPLL are segmental, continuous, and

Patients with ossification of the cervical posterior longitudinal ligament and a spinal canal width of <8mm will generally present with a myelopathy.

mixed, and these findings easily are seen on radiographs (28) (Fig. 17.16A). The incidence of the three types is roughly equal. OPLL usually begins at the C3 to C5 levels and then extends inferiorly and superiorly. One of the easiest ways to visualize OPLL is with radiographs. CT with intrathecal contrast also is helpful in the diagnosis (Fig. 17.16B). Some authors advise caution because they believe that the high density of the myelographic contrast may be confused with the ossified ligament. This, however, is extremely rare because the ossified ligament usually is much denser than the contrast material. By MRI, the

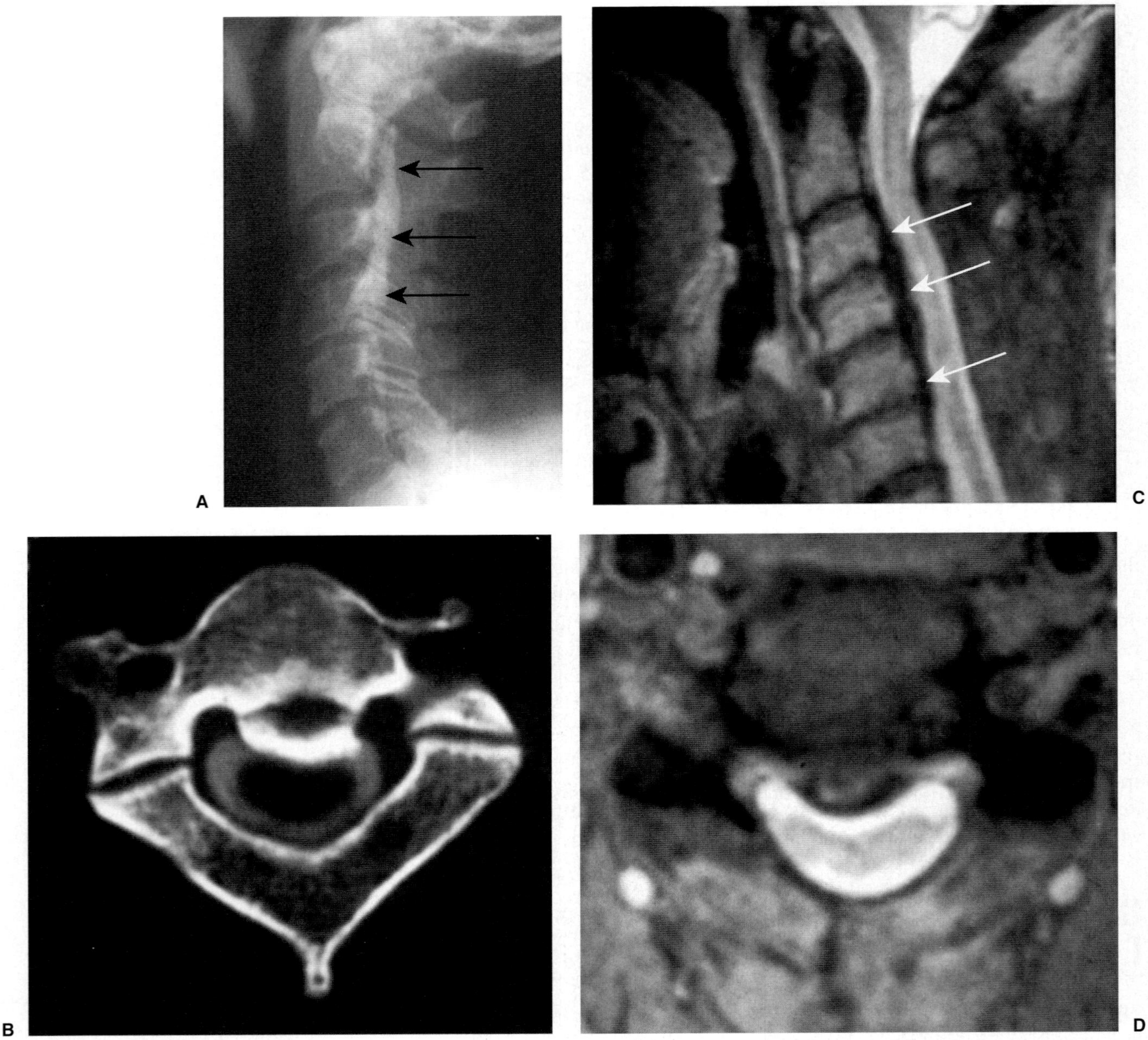

Figure 17.16 *Ossification of the Posterior Longitudinal Ligament (OPLL). A.* Lateral radiograph shows OPLL *(arrows)* extending from C2 to C4. *B.* In the same patient, axial postmyelogram computed tomography shows that the ossified ligament narrows the spinal canal and deforms the ventral surface of the spinal cord. *C.* In a different patient, a sagittal T2-weighted image shows OPLL *(arrows)* extending from C3 to C6 and narrowing the spinal canal. There are focal hyperintense areas in the compressed spinal cord. *D.* Axial T2-weighted image in the same patient shows the OPLL and the deformed spinal cord and narrowed spinal canal.

abnormal ligament is T1 dark and may be difficult to distinguish from the CSF. The ossified ligament always is seen clearly on T2 images and becomes quite obvious on axial gradient recalled echo images owing to magnetic susceptibility effects and an artifactual "blooming" of the abnormality (Fig. 17.16C and D). The abnormal ligament may contain areas of high T1 signal because of the presence of fatty bone marrow in it. T2 images help in assessing the degree of compression, edema, and malacia. In combination with DISH, the anterior longitudinal ligament commonly is ossified. Ossification of the ligamentum flavum also occurs with OPPL, particularly in the thoracic region. Isolated ossification of the ligamentum flavum is more common in Southeast Asia. Ossification of the cephalic portion of the ligamentum flavum almost always is a normal variant and usually does not result in symptoms (29).

Scheuermann's Disease

Scheuermann's disease is a disorder of boys affecting approximately 0.5% of the population (30). It eventually leads to the so-called juvenile kyphotic disorder. Its etiology is not clear, but aseptic necrosis of the vertebral body endplates with herniation of the nucleus pulposus (Schmorl's nodes) is favored. Progressive compression of the endplates leads to kyphosis. The disease usually commences at approximately 10 years of age. Pain and myelopathy are common symptoms. The diagnosis of Scheuermann's disease may be confirmed on lateral spinal radiographs when the following are present: irregular vertebral endplates, loss of disk space height, vertebral body wedging of more than 5 degrees, and kyphosis greater than 40 degrees measured by the Cobb method. Schmorl's nodes are common, and more than three consecutive vertebral bodies usually are affected (Fig. 17.17). Schmorl's nodes occasionally may enhance, particularly when they are acute (31). Some vertebral endplate fractures develop into a Schmorl's node as they heal.

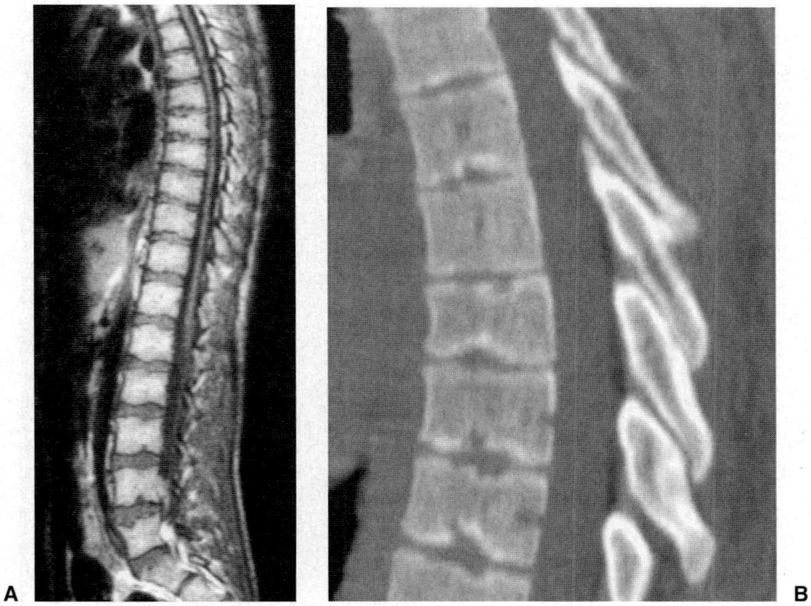

Figure 17.17 *Multiple Schmorl's Nodes. A.* Sagittal T1-weighted image shows multiple Schmorl's nodes in the vertebral endplates and minimal thoracic kyphosis, in this case presumed to represent early Scheuermann's disease. *B.* Sagittal computed tomography reformation in a different patient shows multiple central endplate depressions and slight kyphosis, suggesting Scheuermann's disease.

Paget's Disease

Paget's disease is initially characterized by acute bone resorption, which may be focal, diffuse, or in multiple sites in one bone (31). It affects approximately 3% of the general population and usually becomes clinically evident after 40 years of age. Men are affected more than women. In 70% of cases, the disease is polyostotic, and it is monostotic in 30% of individuals. When multiple bones are involved, the most common sites are the spine, skull, and pelvis (Table 17.4). The most common symptoms are back pain (in up to 50% of patients) and those related to spinal canal stenosis (occurring in nearly all patients). Other symptoms are those related to spinal cord compression, microfractures or macrofractures of the vertebral bodies, basilar invagination, laxity of the transverse ligament with atlantoaxial subluxation, spinal cord ischemia, motor weakness, and sarcomatous degeneration. New onset of pain and a change in the quality and severity of pain in a bone affected by Paget's disease always is suspect for sarcomatous degeneration. Thickening of the bone cortex and the vertebral body trabeculae is the hallmark of the disease on radiographs and CT (Fig. 17.18A). The affected vertebral body may appear to be expanded. By MRI, three phases of the disease are known to occur (32) (Table 17.5). In reality, on MRI the signal intensity of Paget's disease tends to be mixed in most patients (Fig. 17.18B). Bone expansion in the later phases of the disease affects the vertebral body

Table 17.4: Common Sites of Involvement in Paget's Disease

Site	*Incidence*
Spine	30%–75%
Skull	65%
Pelvis	40%

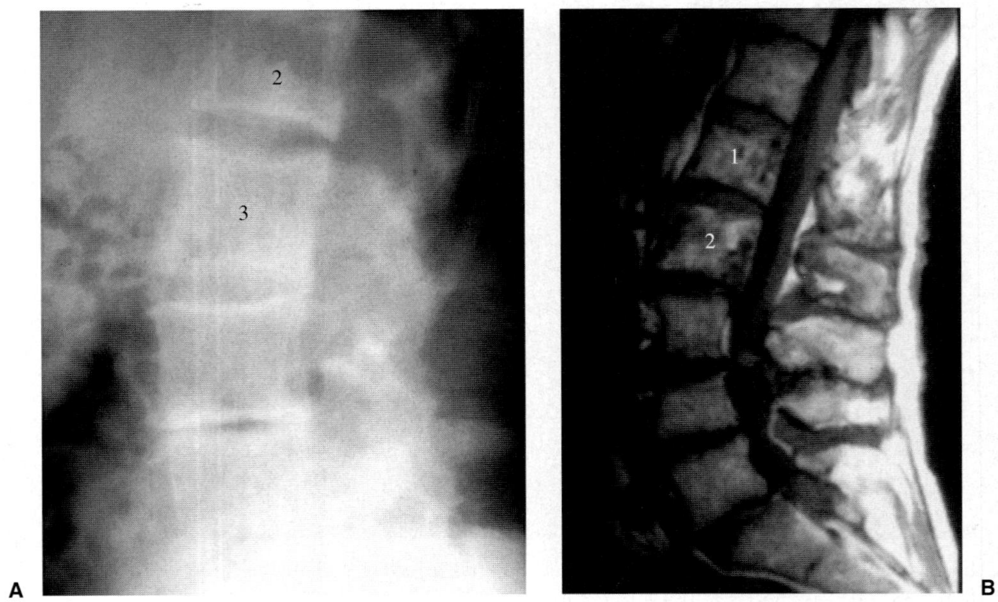

Figure 17.18 *Paget's Disease. A.* Lateral radiograph shows that the L3 and L2 vertebral bodies are sclerotic, contain thick trabeculae, and are slightly enlarged. *B.* In a different patient, a sagittal T1-weighted image shows patchy signal intensity and slight enlargement of the L2 and L1 vertebral bodies.

Table 17.5: Magnetic Resonance Imaging Phases of Paget's Disease

Phase	*Etiology*	*T1 Images*	*T2 Images*	*Contrast Enhancement*
Lytic	Fibrous conversion of the marrow and presence of multiple large blood vessels	Mixed patchy areas of low and high signal	Same as T1	Yes
Mixed	Slow disappearance of changes seen during the lytic phase	Mixed patchy areas of low and high signal	Same as T1	Yes
Sclerotic	Bone marrow returns to near normal, cortex and trabeculae become thick, bone may be expanded	Near-normal signal from bone marrow framed by a thick and low-intensity cortex	Same as T1	Variable

and the neural arch. This may lead to stenoses of the neural foramina and radiculopathies. Compression of the spinal cord may be due to bone expansion and associated soft tissue masses. The complications arising from Paget's disease are spinal cord compression, pathologic fractures, osteomyelitis (due to increased circulation?), and development of tumors (osteosarcoma, chondrosarcoma, and fibrosarcoma) (33).

References

1. Modic MT, Masaryk TJ, Ross JS, et al. Imaging of degenerative disk disease. Radiology 1988;168: 177–186.
2. Yu S, Haughton VM, Sether LA, et al. Anulus fibrosus in bulging intervertebral disks. Radiology 1988;169:761–763.
3. Stadnik TW, Lee RR, Coen HL, et al. Annular tears and disk herniation: prevalence and contrast enhancement on MR images in the absence of low back pain or sciatica. Radiology 1998;206:49–55.
4. Jinkins JR. The pathoanatomic basis of somatic and autonomic syndromes originating in the lumbosacral spine. Neuroimaging Clin North Am 1993;3:443–464.
5. Schellinger D, Manz HJ, Vidic B, et al. Disk fragment migration. Radiology 1990;171:831–836.
6. Masaryk TJ, Ross JS, Modic MT, et al. High-resolution MR imaging of sequestered lumbar intervertebral disks. AJNR Am J Neuroradiol 1988;9:351–358.
7. Castillo M. Neural foramen remodeling caused by a sequestered disk fragment: case report. AJNR AM J Neuroradiol 1991;12:566.
8. Czervionke LF. Lumbar intervertebral disc disease. Neuroimaging Clin North Am 1993;3: 465–486.
9. Bush K, Cowan N, Katz DE, et al. The natural history of sciatica associated with disc pathology: a prospective study with clinical and independent radiologic follow-up. Spine 1992;17: 1205–1212.
10. Bozzao A, Galluci M, Masciocchi C, et al. Lumbar disk herniation: MR imaging assessment of natural history in patients treated surgery. Radiology 1992;185:135–141.
11. Russell EJ. Computed tomography and myelopathy in the evaluation of cervical degenerative disease. Neuroimaging Clin North Am 1995;5:329–348.
12. Haughton VM. Anatomy of cervical spine. Neuroimaging Clin North Am 1995;5:309–320.
13. Sweeney PJ. Clinical evaluation of cervical radiculopathy and myelopathy. Neuroimaging Clin North Am 1995;5:321–328.
14. Ross JS, Perez-Reyes N, Masaryk TJ, et al. Thoracic disk herniation: MR imaging. Radiology 1987;165:511–515.
15. Takahashi M, Shimomura O, Sakae T. Comparison of magnetic resonance imaging with myelography and computed tomography–myelography in the diagnosis of lumbar disc herniation. Neuroimaging Clin North Am 1993;3:487–498.
16. St. Amour TE, Hodges SC, Laakman RW, et al. MRI of the spine. New York: Raven Press, 1994.
17. Teresi LM, Lufkin RB, Reicher MA, et al. Asymptomatic degenerative disk disease and spondylosis of the cervical spine: MR imaging. Radiology 1987;164:83–88.
18. Bangert BA, Modic MT, Ross JS, et al. Hyperintense disks on T1-weighted MR images: correlation with calcification. Radiology 1995;195:437–443.

19. Major NM, Helms CA, Genant HK. Calcification demonstrated as high signal intensity on T1-weighted MR images of the disks of the lumbar spine. Radiology 1993;189:494–496.
20. Nagata K, Kiyonaga K, Ohashi T, et al. Clinical value of magnetic resonance imaging for cervical myelopathy. Spine 1990;15:1088–1096.
21. Kameyama T, Yanagi T, Yasuda T, et al. Intramedullary high intensity lesion on T2-weighted MR images in compressive cervical myelopathy. Rinsho Shinkeigaku 1991;31:1177–1181.
22. Statham PF, Hadley DM, Macpherson P, et al. MRI in the management of suspected cervical spondylotic myelopathy. J Neurol Neurosurg Psychiatry 1991;54:484–489.
23. Al-Mefty O, Harkey LH, Middleton TH, et al. Myelopathic cervical spondylotic lesions demonstrated by magnetic resonance imaging. J Neurosurg 1988;68:217–222.
24. Modic MT, Steinberg PM, Ross JS, et al. Degenerative disk disease: assessment of changes in vertebral body marrow with MR imaging. Radiology 1988;166:193–199.
25. Firooznia H, Rauschning W, Rafii M, et al. Normal correlative anatomy of the lumbosacral spine and its contents. Neuroimaging Clin North Am 1993;3:411–424.
26. Jackson DE, Atlas SW, Mani JR, et al. Intraspinal synovial cysts: MR imaging. Radiology 1989;170:527–530.
27. Ulmer JL, Elster AD, Mathews VP, et al. Distinction between degenerative and isthmic spondylolisthesis on sagittal MR images: importance of increased anteroposterior diameter of the spinal canal ("wide canal sign"). AJR Am J Roentgenol 1994;163:411–416.
28. Yamashita Y, Takahashi M, Matsuno Y, et al. Spinal cord compression due to ossification of ligaments: MR imaging. Radiology 1990;175:843–848.
29. Williams DM, Gabrielsen TO, Latack JT, et al. Ossification in the cephalic attachment of the ligamentum flavum. Radiology 1984;150:423–426.
30. Ascani E, La Rosa G. Scheuermann's kyphosis. In: Weinstein SL, ed. The pediatric spine: principles and practice. New York: Raven Press, 1994:557.
31. Stabler A, Bellan M, Weiss M, et al. MR imaging of enhancing intraosseous disk herniation (Schmorl's nodes). AJR Am J Roentgenol 1997;168:933–938.
32. Roberts MC, Kressel HY, Fallon MD, et al. Paget disease: MR imaging findings. Radiology 1989;173:341–345.
33. Boutin RD, Spitz DJ, Newman JS, et al. Complications in Paget disease at MR imaging. Radiology 1998;209:641–651.

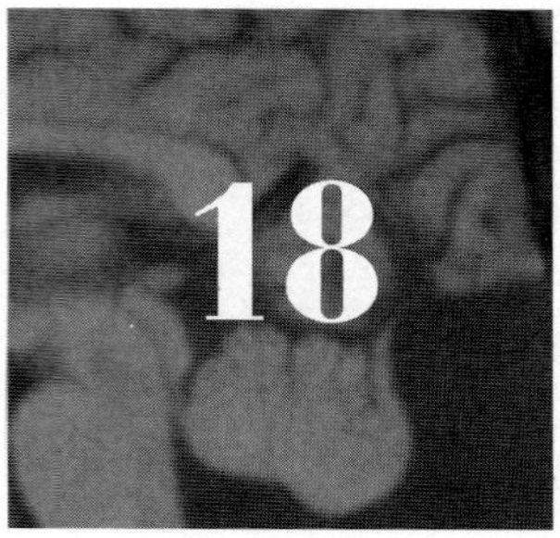

Vascular Diseases of the Spinal Cord

- Vascular Anatomy
- Arteriovenous Malformations
- Spinal Arteriovenous Fistula
- Complex Vascular Malformations
- Cavernous Angioma
- Spinal Cord Infarction
- Vasculitis

Vascular Anatomy

The major blood supply to the spinal cord is through the longitudinal anterior spinal artery (which courses in the anterior median sulcus) and the paired longitudinal posterior spinal arteries (which course in the posterior paramedian sulci) (1). These three arteries receive their blood supply from the radiculomedullary arteries, which in turn are fed as follows (2):

- Cervical radiculomedullary arteries: fed by branches from the vertebral and deep cervical arteries
- Thoracic radiculomedullary arteries: fed by intercostal arteries
- Lumbar radiculomedullary arteries: fed by lumbar arteries

Both the intercostal and lumbar arteries are branches of the aorta. In the superiormost aspect of the spine, the upper cervical spinal cord and cervicomedullary junction receive their blood supply from the anterior spinal branch arising from the distal intradural vertebral arteries. Not all radiculomedullary arteries supply the spinal cord, but most do. The largest of the radiculomedullary arteries is the artery of Adamkiewicz. This artery provides the major blood supply to the distal thoracic spinal cord and the conus medullaris. In approximately 80% of individuals, the artery of Adamkiewicz arises in the left side between T7 and L3 (2). In approximately 15% of individuals, it arises at similar levels, but from the right side, and in the remaining 5% it may arise from other branches. Anastomoses between the anterior and posterior spinal arteries are common in the region of the conus medullaris.

The anterior spinal artery has many radial branches wrapping around the spinal cord (1). From these branches, many tiny perforation arteries supply the cord. On an axial section, the anterior spinal artery supplies the anterior two-thirds of the transverse diameter of the cord and most of its periphery and gray matter. The territory supplied by the posterior spinal arteries is mostly the central posterior one-third of the cord. Because of this, occlusion of the anterior spinal arteries is catastrophic, whereas occlusion of the posterior spinal arteries is tolerated (despite the development of a "posterior spinal cord syndrome"). Traditionally, lesions supplied by the anterior spinal arteries are difficult to treat and require a combination of embolization and surgery, and lesions supplied by the posterior spinal arteries usually are surgically treated.

The cervical venous epidural plexus may become enlarged in cases of obstruction of the jugular veins, in intracranial hypotension and in patients with Marfan syndrome.

Longitudinal spinal veins accompany the arteries (2). These longitudinal veins drain through the emissary veins that in turn drain into the venous epidural plexus. The venous epidural plexus drains through the veins of the neural foramina into the paraspinal venous plexus. Any lesion that increases the venous pressure by overloading the veins [e.g., an arteriovenous malformation (AVM) or fistula] delays the venous filling on angiography. Thus, it is very rare to have a spinal AVM or fistula when the venous drainage follows a normal time sequence. In the caudal spine, the normal radicular veins enhance, and this should not be misconstrued as being abnormal or representing enhancing abnormal nerve roots. Below L2, the radicular veins course downward to join (and drain into) the iliolumbar veins.

Arteriovenous Malformations

Spinal AVMs are complex lesions that may be purely intramedullary, pial, or mixed (2). They usually are supplied by multiple arterial pedicles. When the AVM is intramedullary, most of its supply is through feeders arising from the anterior spinal artery. When the AVM is pial, most of its supply is through feeders arising from the posterior radiculomedullary arteries. Spinal AVMs also may be divided according to their appearance (Table 18.1).

Although spinal AVMs are thought to be congenital, they are very rare in childhood and most are found in men age 20 to 30 years of age (3). Most patients present with a slowly progressive myelopathy called the *Foix-Alajouanine syndrome* (subacute progressive necrotizing myelitis) due to venous hypertension (2). Other symptoms are progressive paraparesis, sensory disturbances, autonomic dysfunction, and impotence. Some present with acute subarachnoid or intramedullary hemorrhage (hematomyelia) or a combination of both. Lesions that bleed have an increased incidence of associated aneurysms. These AVMs need to be treated because hemorrhage (hematomyelia) usually has dire consequences. They may be treated with a combination of endovascular techniques and surgery, but embolization by itself seldom results in a complete cure (2,4). Rarely, a spinal AVM is found in combination with a spinal arteriovenous fistula (AVF).

Considerable improvements in magnetic resonance imaging (MRI) and MR angiography (MRA) have led some authors to recommend these methods as the best ones to screen patients suspected of harboring a spinal AVM (5–7). In addition, MRA may be useful in the evaluation of treated spinal AVMs. The role of MRI in this malformation is, in my opinion, limited to screening and perhaps posttreatment follow-up. MRI identifies the location of the abnormal vessels guiding the catheter angiogram (Fig. 18.1). MRI also identifies the presence of cord edema (which should improve after adequate treatment) and of hematomyelia. MRI also may identify residual patent blood vessels, indicating the need for further treatment.

Table 18.1: Classification of Spinal Arteriovenous Malformations

Type	*Characteristics*
Type 1 (glomus-like)	Small, compact nidus with multiple feeders from the anterior and posterior spinal arteries
Type 2 (juvenile)	Large nidus with multiple feeders from the anterior and posterior spinal arteries, may extend outside of the spinal cord
Type 3 (metameric)	Large lesion involving cord, meninges, epidural space, and vertebrae

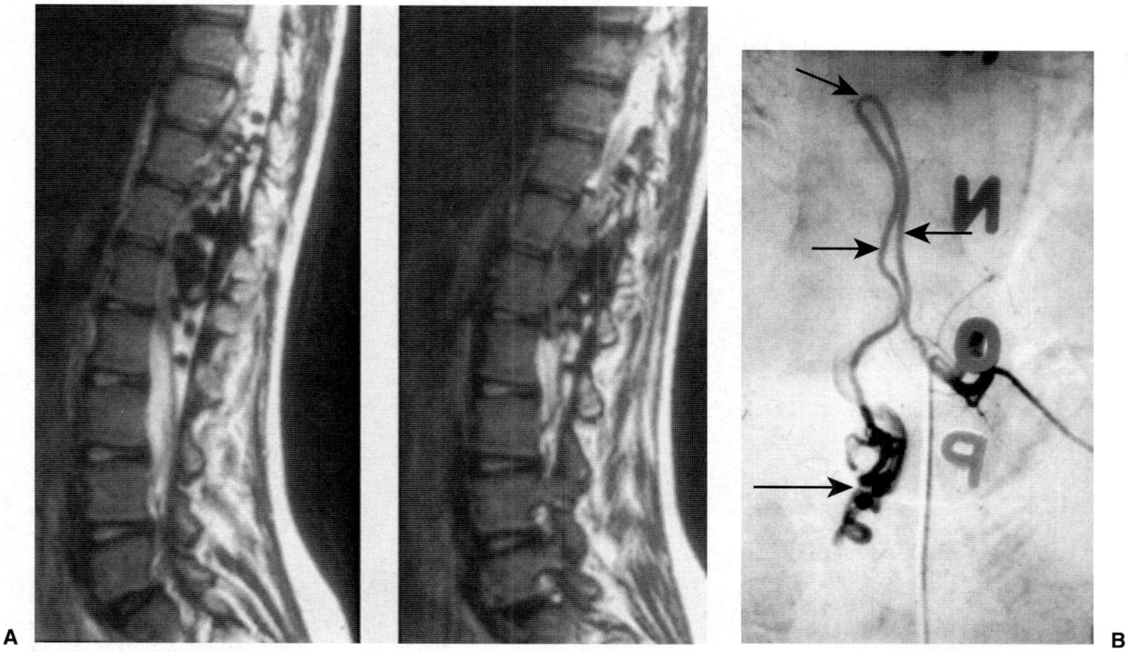

Figure 18.1 *Spinal Cord Arteriovenous Malformation (AVM). A.* Consecutive sagittal T2-weighted images show a large AVM located in the conus medullaris and cauda equina regions. There are multiple large draining veins and aneurysms. *B.* In a different patient, a frontal projection from a conventional catheter angiogram during early injection of the left T11 intercostal artery shows filling of an enlarged artery of Adamkiewicz *(small arrows)* filling the nidus *(large arrow)* of a distal spinal cord AVM. The draining veins are not visualized in this early view.

Spinal Arteriovenous Fistula

Spinal AVFs probably are more common than spinal AVMs. They are found in men, usually older than 50 years of age. Histologically, they represent communications between the radiculomedullary arteries and the adjacent veins (8). AVFs have no nidus. The high-pressure blood from the arteries then backs up into the low-pressure venous system and the radiculomedullary veins and perimedullary (around the cord) veins become dilated. This results in venous hypertension that is responsible for the symptoms, which usually are slowly progressive in the form of the Foix-Alajouanine syndrome. However, spinal subarachnoid hemorrhage may occur. They may be classified according to their size (2) (Table 18.2).

If the AVF is located posteriorly, surgery is the treatment of choice, but if it is located anteriorly, embolization is best. By MRI, these fistulas appear as dilated vessels of the surface of the spinal cord, particularly its dorsal aspect (8) (Fig. 18.2A). These vessels are not the fistula itself (which requires catheter angiography to be identified), but represent its venous drainage. If the patient is symptomatic, the spinal cord always shows high T2 sig-

All symptomatic spinal arteriovenous fistulas show high T2 signal in the spinal cord, and many of them result in intramedullary spinal cord contrast enhancement.

Table 18.2: Classification of Spinal Arteriovenous Fistulas

Type	*Size*
Type I	Small
Type II	Voluminous (most frequent type)
Type III	Giant

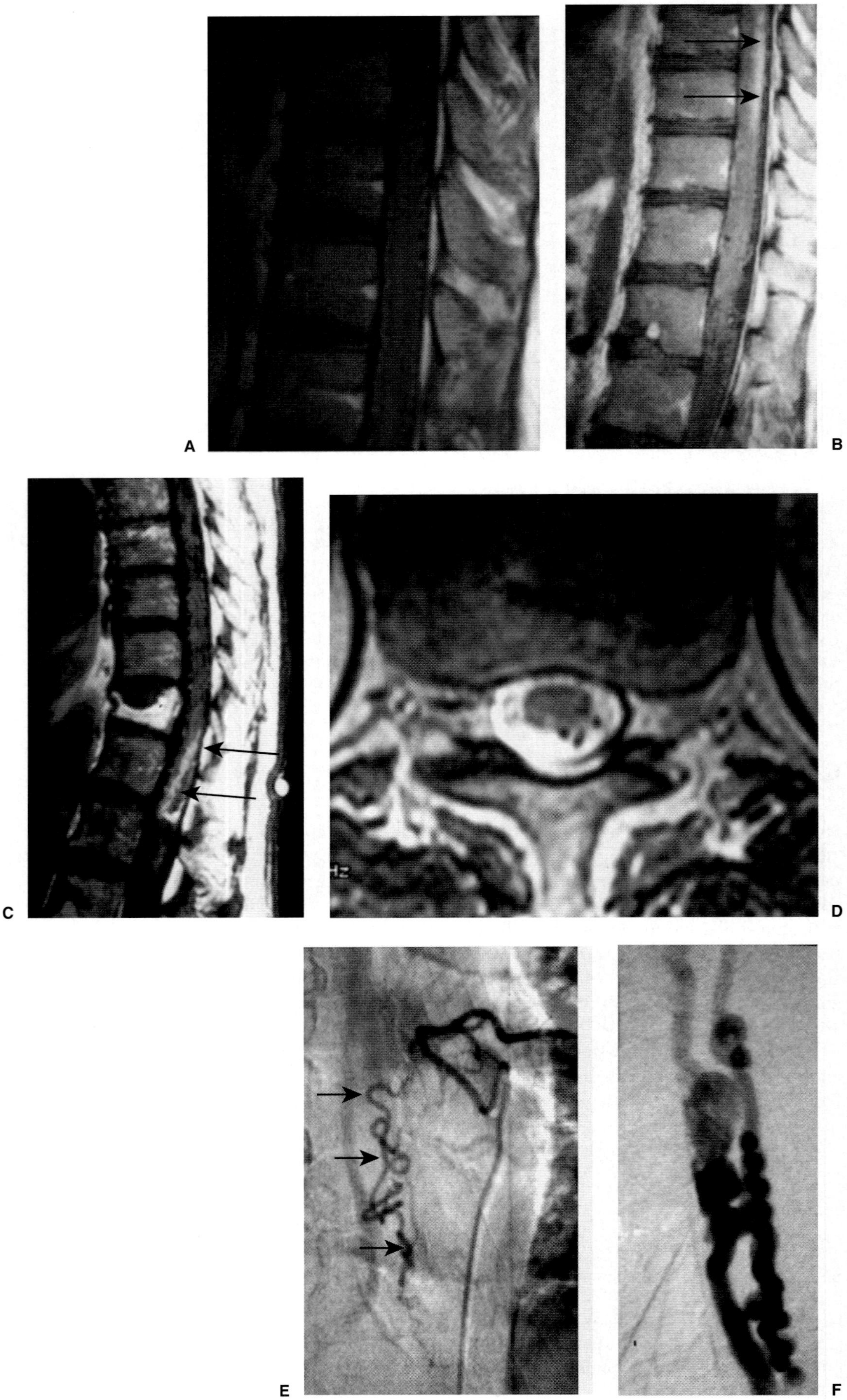
A
B
C
D
E
F

nal. This area of presumed myelomalacia and ischemia also may enhance after gadolinium is given (Fig. 18.2B–D). Although the etiology of spinal AVFs is uncertain, trauma may play a role. As such, it is not unusual to find the fistula at the same level as a compression fracture involving a vertebra. Dural fistulas located in the posterior fossa may recruit spinal venous drainage and present in an identical fashion to pure spinal AVFs. Catheter angiography is the definitive diagnostic study and shows the site of the fistula and the anatomy of the draining veins. The fistula usually is from the intradural portion of a radicular artery and fills the intradural veins rapidly (Fig. 18.2E). These veins may be very prominent and compress the spinal cord (Fig. 18.2F). The fistula may be occluded surgically or by endovascular techniques.

Complex Vascular Malformations

The syndromes associated with complex spinal vascular malformations are very rare (2) (Table 18.3; Fig. 18.3).

Cavernous Angioma

A discussion of cavernous angiomas is found in Chapter 9. Spinal cord cavernous angiomas usually become manifest between 15 and 60 years of age (9). The symptoms usually are chronic and there may be periods of improvement followed by periods of deterioration. Abrupt and catastrophic symptoms of a myelopathy may occur after the lesion bleeds spontaneously. Most of the hemorrhage occurs in the cord (hematomyelia), but subarachnoid hemorrhage also occasionally may be found. Spinal cord cavernous angiomas usually are small, 0.5 to 1.5 cm in length, but occasionally they may be larger (up to 3 cm in length). The lesions result in only mild expansion of the cord. Their MRI features are identical to those previously described (Chapter 9) for intracerebral cavernous angiomas (Fig. 18.4).

Spinal Cord Infarction

Spinal cord infarctions are rare and mostly occur in patients with hypertension, diabetes, trauma, sickle cell disease, Caisson disease, and atherosclerosis (10,11). They also may follow surgery for treatment of aortic aneurysm and hypotensive events. Most patients are older than 60 years of age, and there is no gender predilection. The patients usually present with acute onset of paraplegia and bowel and bladder dysfunction. Most spinal cord infarctions are secondary to occlusion of the largest anterior spinal artery (artery of Adamkiewicz; see earlier). Dissecting aortic aneurysms with a left-sided lumen may lead to occlusion of this artery. Venous infarctions also may occur, and their onset is insidious

In spinal cord ischemia, the "owl-eye" appearance on axial T2 images is due to swelling of the ventral and dorsal gray matter horns and is probably related to cytotoxic edema.

Figure 18.2 *Dural Arteriovenous Fistula (AVF). A.* Sagittal postcontrast T1-weighted image shows fine and enhancing veins on the surface of the spinal cord due to an AVF. There is no enhancement of the cord. *B.* In a different patient, sagittal postcontrast T1-weighted image shows enlarged draining veins in the region of the conus medullaris and cauda equina, and dorsal enhancement *(arrows)* of the lower thoracic spinal cord. *C.* In another patient, postcontrast sagittal T1-weighted image shows enhancement *(arrows)* of the conus medullaris due to an AVF, presumably a sequela of trauma (note enhancing compression fracture). *D.* Axial T2-weighted image shows enlarged veins with flow void in the subarachnoid space and some high signal in the spinal cord. *E.* Frontal projection from a catheter angiogram after injection of the left T9 intercostal artery shows a fistula with immediate filling of intradural veins *(arrows)*. *F.* In a different patient with a vertebral artery fistula, a lateral projection from the angiogram shows filling of markedly enlarged intradural cervical veins.

Table 18.3: Syndromes Associated with Complex Spinal Vascular Malformations

Syndrome	*Characteristics*
Cobb's syndrome	Metameric AVM with cutaneous capillary angiomas
Osler-Weber-Rendu syndrome	Multifocal telangiectasias of the mucosa, meninges, and central nervous system with multiple AVMs of the brain and spinal cord
Klippel-Trenaunay syndrome	AVMs, arteriovenous shunts, and lymphatic malformations of the extremities, segmental gigantism and metameric spinal AVMs

AVM, arteriovenous malformation.

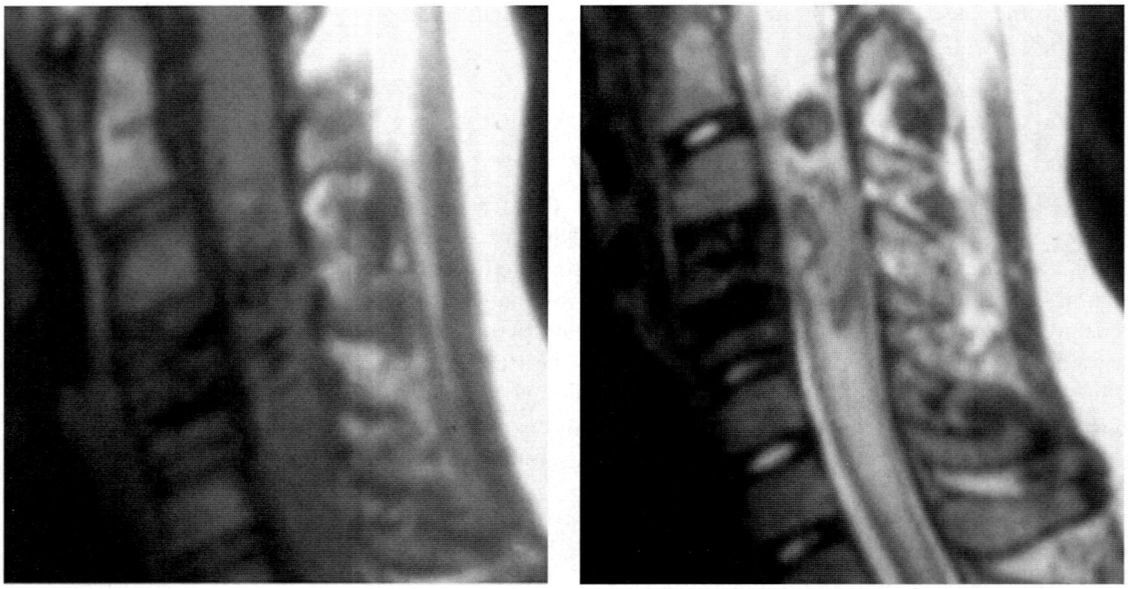

A B

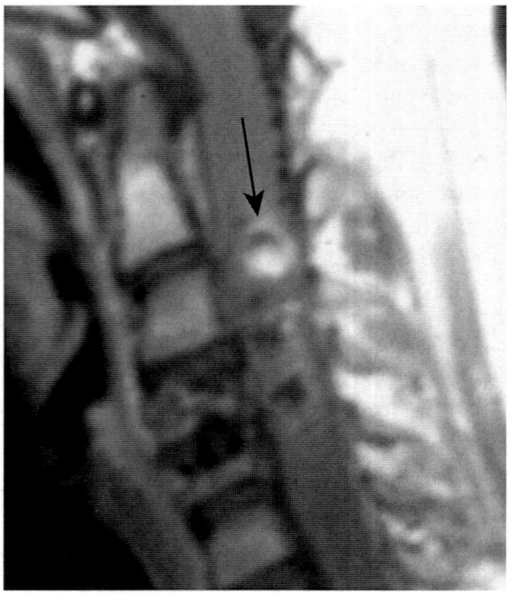

C

Figure 18.3 *Complex Spinal Arteriovenous Malformation (AVM) in Cobb's Syndrome. A.* Noncontrast sagittal T1-weighted image shows complex flow voids inside the spinal cord at the C3 to C4 levels and extension of the vascular malformation into the C4 vertebral body. *B.* Corresponding T2-weighted image shows the metameric AVM and high signal intensity diffusely involving the cervical spinal cord. *C.* Corresponding postcontrast T1-weighted image shows enhancement of some vessels and an intranidal aneurysm *(arrow)* inside the spinal cord.

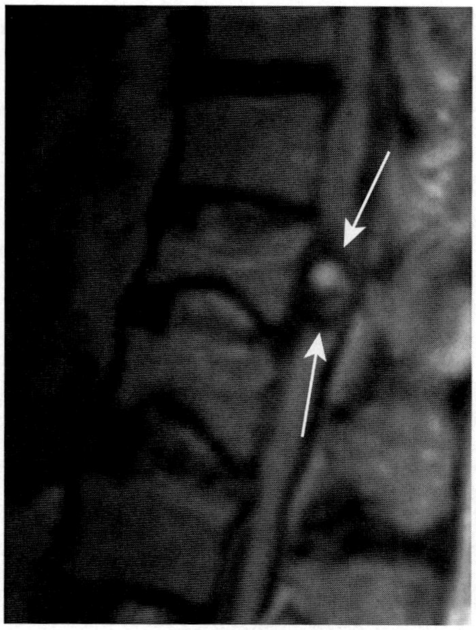

Figure 18.4 *Cavernous Angioma.* Sagittal T2-weighted image shows the typical appearance (central high signal surrounded by a hypointense rim) of an intramedullary cavernous angioma *(arrows)* in the distal thoracic spinal cord.

(10). Venous infarctions are associated with AVFs, hypercoagulable states, and fibrocartilaginous emboli. These infarctions present with symptoms identical to those found in patients with subacute necrotizing myelopathy (Foix-Alajouanine syndrome). Occlusion of the anterior spinal artery produces abnormalities that are more prominent at the level of the distal portions of the deep perforating branches. Therefore, the gray matter is affected first. In addition, the gray matter is more vulnerable to ischemia because it is relatively hypermetabolic compared with the spinal cord white matter. MRI is the imaging method of choice (12). On T1-weighted images, the involved portion of the spinal cord may be expanded and show subtle hyperintense or hypointense regions. The anterior two-thirds of the spinal cord may be bright on T2-weighted images. Acutely, the central gray matter appears swollen and bright on T2 images (Fig. 18.5A–D). The central gray matter also may enhance after contrast administration. Enhancement may be more prominent in the swollen gray matter, resulting in the so-called owl eyes appearance on axial postcontrast T1-weighted images (Fig. 18.5E). The imaging features of spinal cord infarction are quite typical, excluding other etiologies for the patient's symptoms. The chronic sequela of spinal cord infarction is severe atrophy of the spinal cord. In children, the cervicothoracic area is a watershed region and is especially vulnerable to ischemia (13). This ischemia may follow traumatic breech delivery (14).

VASCULITIS

Vasculitis involving the spinal cord is rare and usually occurs in the presence of vasculitis involving the brain. Isolated vasculitis of the spinal cord is very rare. Vasculitides that can involve the spinal cord include granulomatous angiitis, antiphospholipid syndrome, scleroderma, Sjögren's syndrome, polyarteritis nodosa, and rheumatoid arthritis (15). Infectious causes such as the human immunodeficiency virus (HIV), tuberculosis, cytomegalovirus, and Chagas disease also may result in a vasculitis involving the spinal cord. Sarcoidosis may result in direct infiltration of the spinal cord or in a vasculitis. Rhabdomyolysis and paraneoplastic syndromes may affect the spinal cord in an identical fashion to a vasculitis. Granulomatous angiitis is a rare disorder that may be primary or occur in association with lymphoma, sarcoidosis, herpes virus infections, and HIV infection (15). Patients with spinal cord involvement by granulomatous angiitis present with back

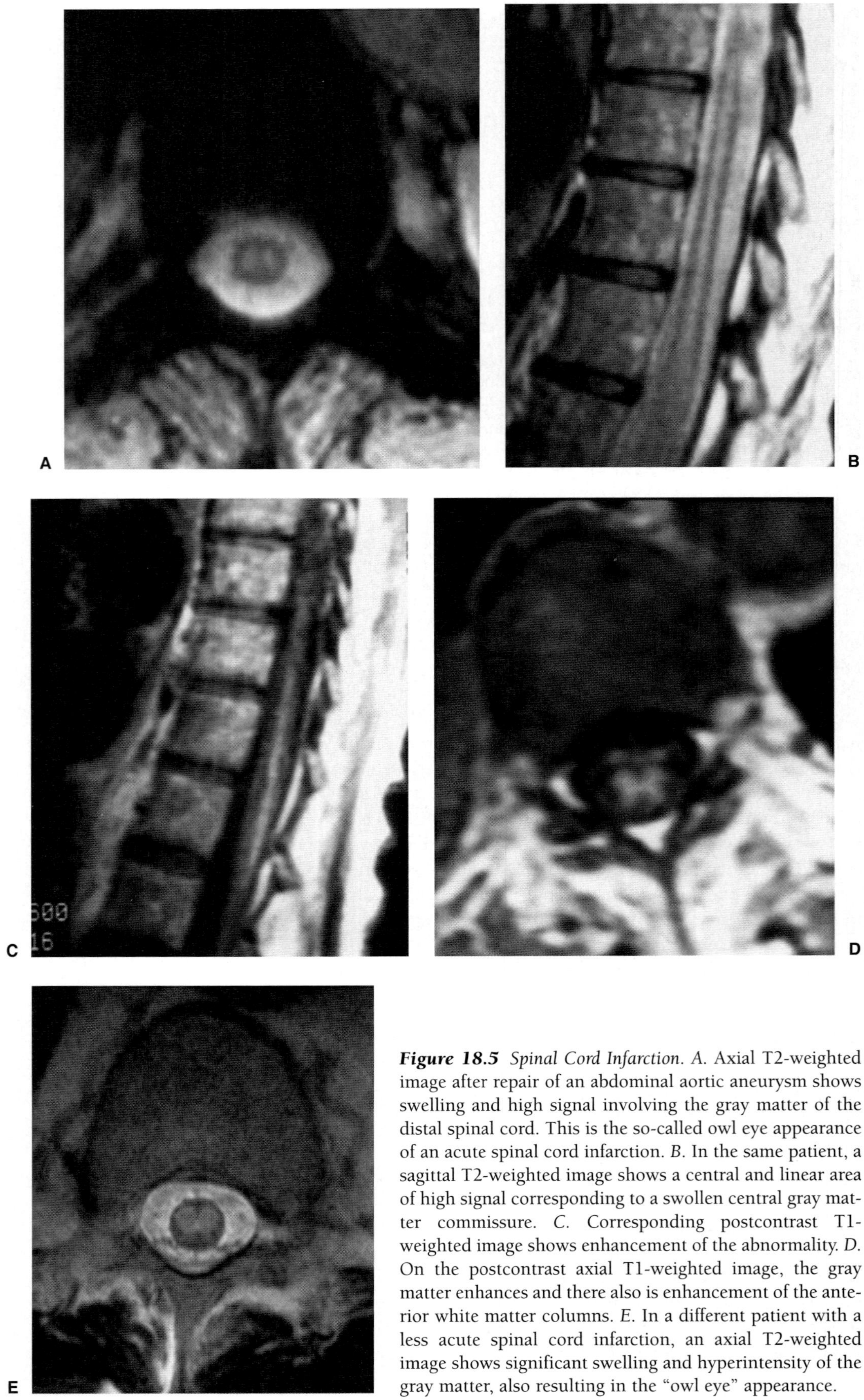

Figure 18.5 *Spinal Cord Infarction. A.* Axial T2-weighted image after repair of an abdominal aortic aneurysm shows swelling and high signal involving the gray matter of the distal spinal cord. This is the so-called owl eye appearance of an acute spinal cord infarction. *B.* In the same patient, a sagittal T2-weighted image shows a central and linear area of high signal corresponding to a swollen central gray matter commissure. *C.* Corresponding postcontrast T1-weighted image shows enhancement of the abnormality. *D.* On the postcontrast axial T1-weighted image, the gray matter enhances and there also is enhancement of the anterior white matter columns. *E.* In a different patient with a less acute spinal cord infarction, an axial T2-weighted image shows significant swelling and hyperintensity of the gray matter, also resulting in the "owl eye" appearance.

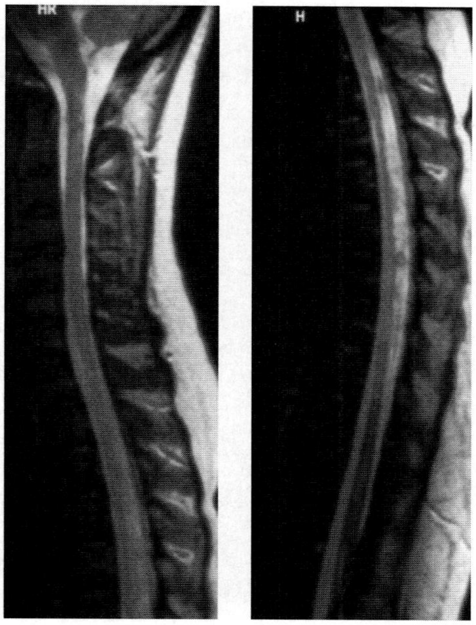

A B

Figure 18.6 *Spinal Cord Vasculitis. A, B.* Sagittal T2-weighted images shows diffuse and patchy increased signal intensity throughout the spinal cord in this patient with granulomatous angiitis.

pain, a progressive myelopathy, elevated cerebrospinal fluid proteins, and a normal erythrocyte sedimentation rate. MRI is the imaging method of choice for the evaluation of these patients. The findings are nonspecific and include increased T2 signal intensity and widening of the spinal cord (Fig. 18.6). Usually, there is no enhancement after contrast administration. The correct diagnosis requires biopsy. Treatment with steroid or cytotoxic drugs may lead to rapid stabilization or disappearance of the symptoms.

References

1. McCulloch JA, Young PH. Surgical anatomy of the cervical spine, spinal cord, and surrounding structures. In: McCulloch JA, Young PH, eds. Essentials of spinal microsurgery. Philadelphia: Lippincott–Raven, 1998:121–150.
2. Guimaraens L, Arbelaez A, Sola-Martinez T, et al. Image-guided interventions in the spine and spinal cord. In: Castillo M, ed. Spinal imaging. Philadelphia: Hanley & Belfus, 2001:169–186.
3. Minami S, Sagoh T, Nishimura K, et al. Spinal arteriovenous malformation: MR imaging. Radiology 1988;169:109–115.
4. Biondi A, Merland JJ, Reizine D, et al. Embolization with particles in thoracic intramedullary arteriovenous malformations: long-term angiographic and clinical results. Radiology 1990; 177:651–658.
5. Mascalchi M, Ferrito G, Quilici N, et al. Spinal vascular malformations: MR angiography after treatment. Radiology 2001;219:346–353.
6. Bowen BC, DePrima S, Pattany PM, et al. MR angiography of normal intradural vessels of the thoracolumbar spine. AJNR Am J Neuroradiol 1996;17:483–494.
7. Bowen BC, Fraser K, Kochan JP, et al. Spinal dural arteriovenous fistulas: evaluation with MR angiography. AJNR Am J Neuroradiol 1995;16:2029–2043.
8. Masaryk TJ, Ross JS, Modic MT, et al. Radiculomeningeal vascular malformations of the spine: MR imaging. Radiology 1987;164:845–849.
9. Fontaine S, Melanson D, Cosgrove R, et al. Cavernous hemangiomas of the spinal cord: MR imaging. Radiology 1988;166:839–841.
10. Manabe Y, Sakai K, Kashihara K, et al. Presumed venous infarction in spinal decompression sickness. AJNR Am J Neuroradiol 1998;19:1578–1580.
11. Mawad ME, Rivera V, Crawford S, et al. Spinal cord ischemia after resection of thoracoabdominal aortic aneurysms: MR findings in 24 patients. AJNR Am J Neuroradiol 1990;11:987–991.
12. Yuh WT, Marsh EE 3rd, Wang AK, et al. MR imaging of spinal cord and vertebral body infarction. AJNR Am J Neuroradiol 1992;13:145–154.

13. Davis PC, Reisner A, Hudgins PA, et al. Spinal injuries in children: role of MR. AJNR Am J Neuroradiol 1993;14:607–617.
14. Castillo M, Quencer RM, Green BA. Cervical spinal cord injury after traumatic breech delivery. AJNR Am J Neuroradiol 1989;10[Suppl]:99.
15. Giovanini MA, Eskin TA, Mukherji SK, et al. Granulomatous angiitis of the spinal cord: a case report. Neurosurgery 1994;34:540–543.

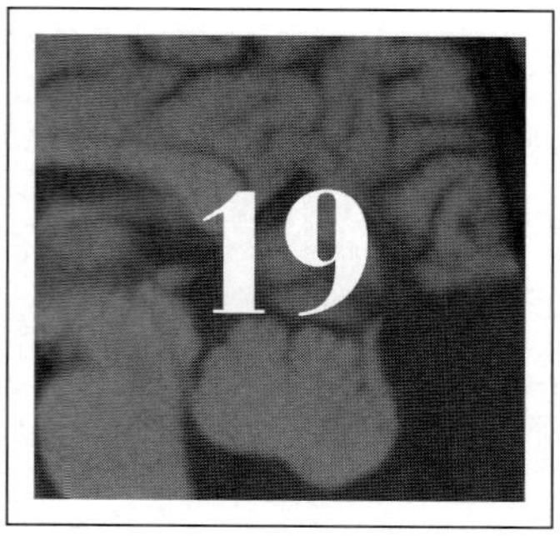

THE POST-SURGICAL SPINE

- Lumbar Spine
- Complications of Lumbar Spine Surgery
- Cervical Spine
- Thoracic Spine
- Complications of Cervical and Thoracic Spine Surgery
- Imaging Sequences

LUMBAR SPINE

I begin this chapter by briefly addressing some important aspects of surgery and its complications, first in the lumbar region (because this is where most spine surgery is done) and then in the cervical and thoracic regions. Most lumbar spine surgery is done for degenerative disk disease, trauma, tumors, and infection (1). Nearly all surgery (for degenerative disease) in the lumbar region is done through a posterior approach. After localization of the level with intraoperative fluoroscopy or computer-guided navigation systems, a midline incision is done, followed by subperiosteal muscle dissection to approach the interlaminar space. According to the level of exposure desired, a partial hemilaminectomy to full laminectomies and facetectomies may be used. Despite adequate surgical technique, it is estimated that 10% to 40% of operated patients have recurrent or residual symptoms ("failed back surgery syndrome") (2). The main features of this syndrome are low back pain, lower extremity pain, and varying degrees of muscle dysfunction in the lower extremities. The causes of the failed back surgery syndrome are listed in Box 19.1 (2).

Intervertebral body fusion cages are being used with increasing frequency. These devices presumably increase the intervertebral space and thus relieve compression on the nerve roots (by virtue of expanding the neural foramina). They also promote fusion and increase stability at the level fused. Most are used in the lumbar spine, but they also may be used in the cervical region. The devices are place through open or minimally invasive endoscopic surgery. The major indications for these devices are segmental disk degeneration, foraminal stenosis, mild spondylolisthesis, and acquired or iatrogenic instability. The most commonly used devices are made of stainless steel or titanium (newer materials include carbon fiber) and have varying shapes (e.g., cylindrical, square, rectangular). Many of them are threaded on the outside, and many are filled with bone chip grafts before insertion. One or more devices may be used per level, and one or more levels fused. They may be successfully imaged with radiographs, computed tomography (CT; with sagittal reformations), and magnetic resonance imaging (MRI; Fig. 19.1). The devices should not protrude into the spinal canal, nor should they protrude excessively from the anterior and lateral margins of the vertebral bodies.

The types of postoperative complications in the lumbar region differ from those seen in the cervical and thoracic regions because of the absence of spinal cord and because the

In order to differentiate a recurrent/residual herniated disc from epidural scar, postcontrast T1 images need to be obtained immediately after the administration of gadolinium.

Box 19.1: Etiologies for the Failed Back Surgery Syndrome

Recurrent or residual disk hernation
Epidural fibrosis (scar)
Arachnoiditis
Pseudomeningocele formation
Unrecognized lateral recess stenoses
Unrecognized stenoses of neuroforamina
Limited unroofing of central spinal canal stenosis

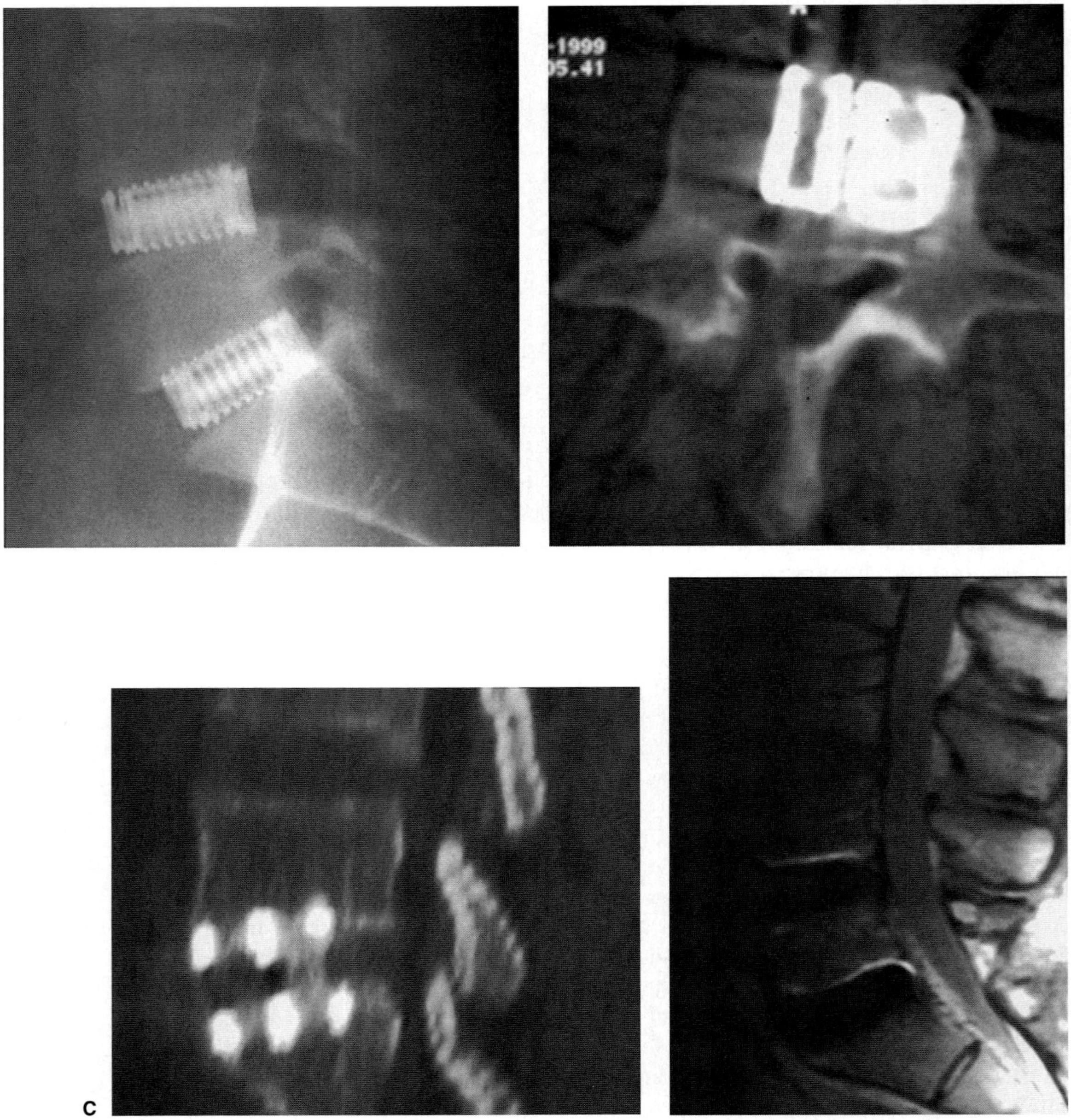

Figure 19.1 *Intervertebral Fusion Cages. A.* Lateral radiograph shows threaded cages at the L5 to S1 and L5 to L4 spaces. These spaces are expanded (compared with height of the L3 to L4 space). The cages do not protrude anteriorly or posteriorly and do not "settle" into the vertebral bodies. *B.* Axial computed tomography in a different patient shows paired cages in good position at the L5 to S1 space. *C.* Sagittal reformation in the same patient through the middle aspect of a cage shows it to be in adequate position. *D.* Sagittal T1-weighted image in the same patient as *A* shows minimal artifact from the cages and normal-appearing spinal canal at those levels.

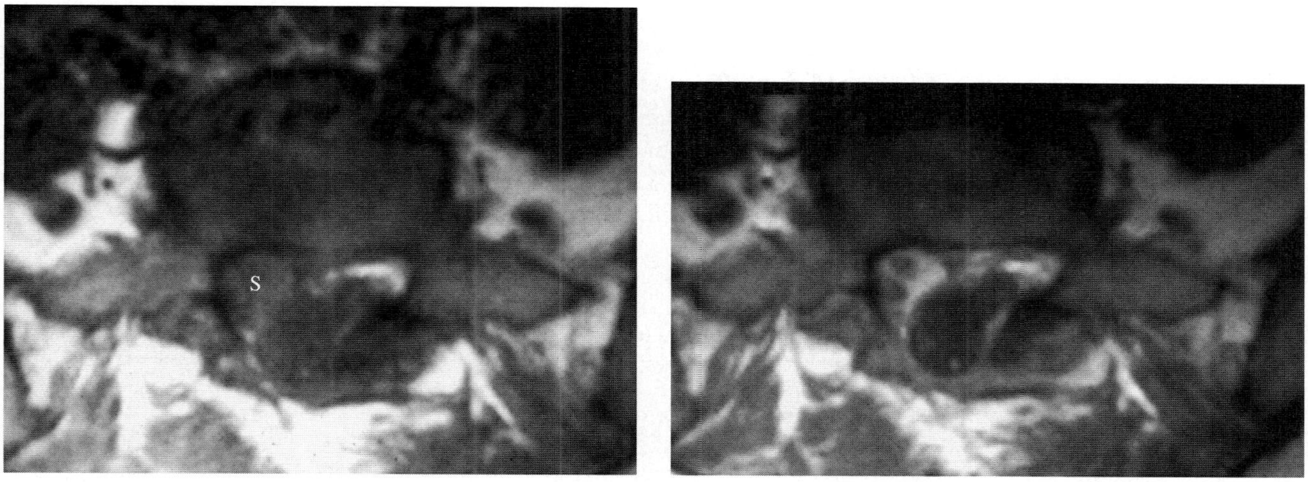

A B

Figure 19.2 *Epidural Fibrosis (Scar). A.* Precontrast axial T1-weighted image months after an L5 laminectomy shows abnormal soft tissue *(S)* of intermediate signal intensity in the right lateral recess. *B.* Corresponding postcontrast image shows enhancement of most of that soft tissue compatible with scar. Note that nerve roots coursing amid the scar now can be visualized.

lumbar epidural space responds to inflammation in a peculiar fashion (note that there is no formation of symptomatic postsurgical scar in the cervical and thoracic epidural space). The best way to evaluate for scar/disk is with the use of contrast-enhanced MRI. It is generally accepted that scar enhances, whereas disk material does not (Figs. 19.2 and 19.3). The images need to be obtained within 2 minutes of the injection of contrast because some disks are highly vascularized and will enhance, making them indistinguishable from scar (3). Contrast enhancement about the margins of a recurrent/residual herniated disk is not uncommon. Thus, delayed postcontrast imaging of the postsurgical spine is not useful. Although we usually also give contrast for the evaluation of the postsurgical cervical spine,

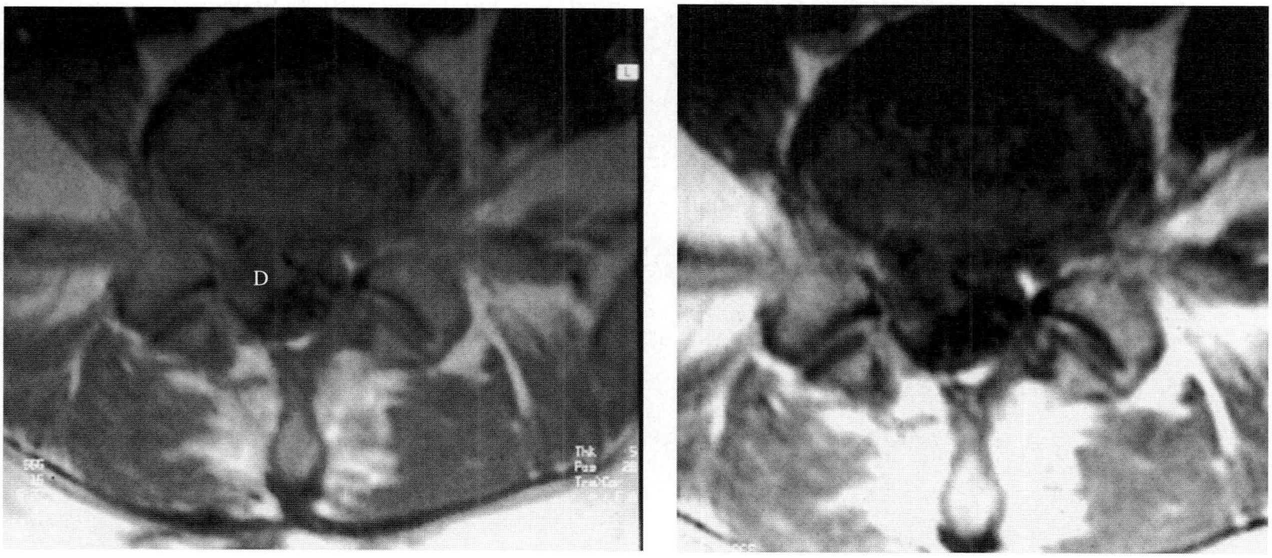

A B

Figure 19.3 *RecurrentResidual Disk Herniation. A.* Precontrast axial T1-weighted image shows abnormal soft tissue *(D)* of intermediate signal intensity in the right lateral recess in a patient after ipsilateral hemilaminectomy. *B.* Corresponding postcontrast image shows that there is no significant enhancement of the abnormal soft tissue that is compatible with herniated disk material.

I am not sure that it really is needed. An important aspect to remember is that imaging the postsurgical back during the initial 6 to 8 weeks may be tricky (4,5). There usually is considerable edema and mass effect and significant contrast enhancement, and the resected herniated disk tends to appear very similar in size and configuration compared with the preoperative images. The surgical tract also shows contrast enhancement. All of these findings slowly resolve, and by 3 months, most have disappeared. However, if neurologic damage or infection is suspected, immediate imaging is indicated.

Complications of Lumbar Spine Surgery

Epidural Scar

Epidural scar formation begins at about the fifth postoperative week and continues until the scar matures (4 to 5 months) (2). Scar tends to vascularize, and the tight junctions of these neocapillaries are loose, allowing for the leakage of gadolinium. Because of this, epidural scar enhances significantly during the first minute after contrast is administered (Fig. 19.2). Scar may continued to enhance for years (even throughout the life of the patient). CT with contrast demonstrates enhancing scar in 50% to 80% of patients who harbor it (6). MRI shows scar to be mostly hypointense (with respect to the epidural space), but occasionally it is hyperintense on T2 images. MRI with contrast differentiates between scar and herniated disk in 96% to 100% of patients (7–9). Scar, particularly that located in the ventral epidural space, enhances considerably on immediate postcontrast MRI. It is said that all scar enhances by 5 minutes after contrast administration.

Residual or Recurrent Disk Herniations

Residual or recurrent disk herniations do not enhance homogeneously on immediate postcontrast MRI (Fig. 19.3). As mentioned earlier, care is needed because many disks enhance homogeneously at 10 to 15 minutes after administration of contrast and become indistinguishable from scar (1). Most residual/recurrent disk herniations show peripheral contrast enhancement that correlates with infiltration by granulation tissues.

Arachnoiditis

Sterile arachnoiditis occurs in up to 15% of patients after lumbar spine surgery (10). This process involves not only the arachnoid membranes but the dura and pia mater. The causes for arachnoiditis are listed in Box 19.2 (10).

The severity of the imaging findings is only loosely correlated with the patient's symptoms (Table 19.1).

The overall sensitivity of MRI for the detection of arachnoiditis varies from 90% to 100% (10).

Box 19.2: Relatively Common Causes of Spinal Arachnoiditis

Surgery or trauma
Intradural blood or anesthetics and antiinflammatory medications
Infection
Previous use of oil-based myelographic contrast (uncommon today)

Table 19.1: Imaging Features of Arachnoiditis

Type	*Myelography*	*Magnetic Resonance Imaging*
I (mild to moderate)	Blunting of the distal end of the thecal sac and nerve root sleeves (Fig. 19.4A)	Probably none
II (moderate to severe)	The above, plus clumping of the nerve roots; the nerve roots may be adherent to the walls of the thecal sac, creating an "empty sac" sign (Fig. 19.4B)	Clumping and thickening of nerves roots (particularly on T2 images), "empty sac" sign, contrast enhancement of nerve roots
III (fibrosing or ossifying)	The above, plus a mass (soft tissue density or calcified) blocking the flow of myelographic contrast (Fig. 19.4C)	Mass of low T2 signal compressing the sac; this mass enhances after contrast administration

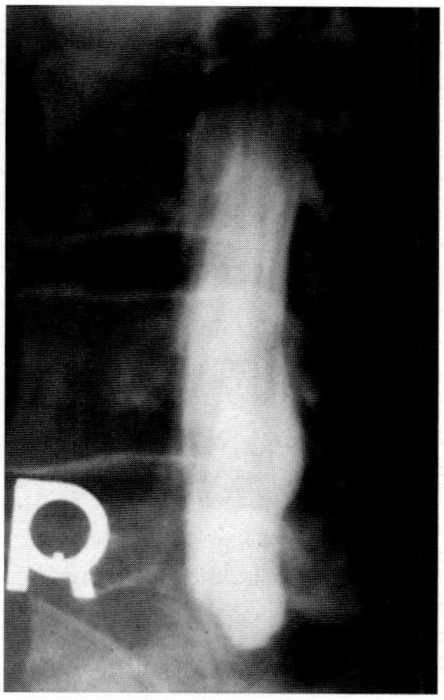

A

Figure 19.4 *Arachnoiditis. A.* Oblique view from a conventional myelogram shows blunting and nonvisualization of the nerve root sleeves and the distal thecal sac (so-called featureless thecal sac). *B* Axial T2-weighted image in a different patient shows that all nerve roots are adhered to the walls of the thecal sac (so-called empty sac sign). There is a left-sided laminectomy. *C.* In a different patient, axial computed tomography after myelography shows conglomeration of nerve roots (fibrosing arachnoiditis) in the center of the thecal sac. Note contrast/cerebrospinal fluid level due to inadequate mixing.

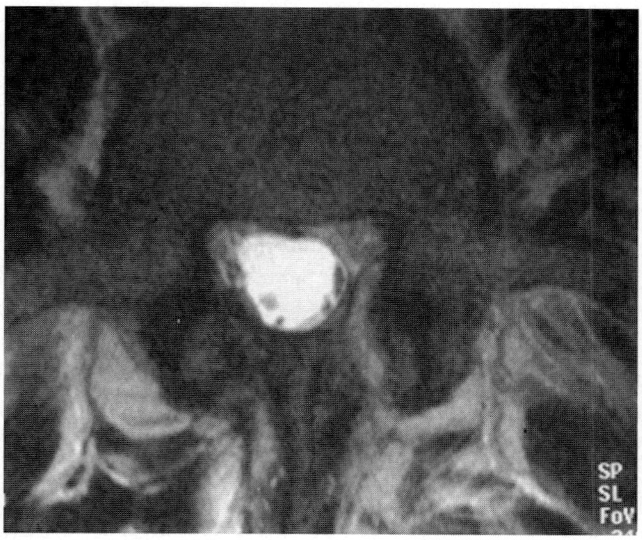

B

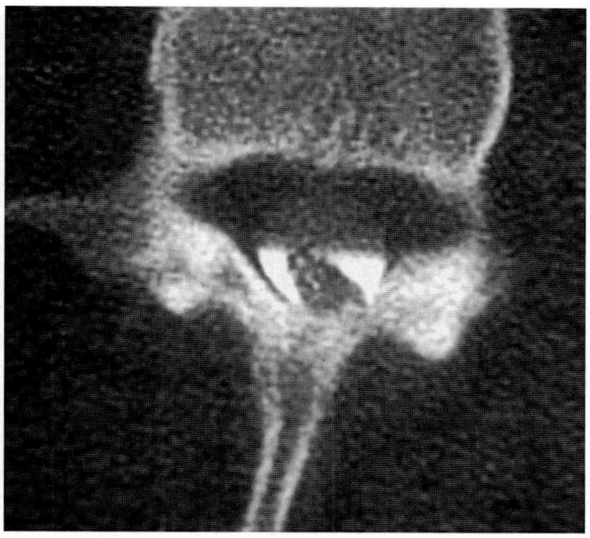

C

Cervical Spine

Most cervical spine surgery for radiculopathies and diskectomies is done with microsurgical techniques (11). The traditional laminectomy–diskectomy is supplanted by a microdiskectomy, and facetectomies and laminotomies are supplanted by facetoplasties and laminoplasties. Limited microscopic exposure reduces morbidity, shortens hospital stay, and results in fewer complications. In the cervical region, surgical approaches may be posterior or anterior. The advantages of the anterior approach over the posterior one are (11,12):

- Allows for exposure of C2 to C7 with minimal blood loss
- Offers a direct route to anterior disk herniations or osteophytes
- Allows for fusion
- Allows for subsequent posterior fusion

The disadvantages of the anterior approach are (11,12):

- Limited exposure to posteriorly localized disease
- May result in significant loss of motion if multiple levels are treated
- Fusion may lead to development of degenerative changes at other levels (particularly worrisome in younger patients)

The advantages of the posterior approach are (11,13):

- Provides direct visualization of pathology occurring posteriorly
- Permits multilevel exposure with preservation of stability
- Permits access to neural foramina without diskectomies
- A fusion may not be needed

The disadvantages of the posterior approach are (11,13):

- Patient position during surgery is difficult and dangerous
- Does not allow visualization of pathologic processes occurring anteriorly and is incapable of decompression of anterior lesions
- It has more complications, longer hospital stay, and increased incidence of long-term neck deformities

From the foregoing, it stems that older patients with single-level disease caused by anterior lesions ideally are approached anteriorly. Radiculopathies may be approached anteriorly or posteriorly, whereas patients with a myelopathy benefit from wide posterior decompressions. However, patients with single-level myelopathy benefit from a single-level anterior approach. Ultimately, the type of approach is surgeon dependent and varies at different institutions.

Anterior Approach for Disk Herniations

This type of surgery is indicated in patients with a myelopathy due to anterior central or paracentral disk herniations and radiculopathies caused by paracentral or foraminal disk herniations (11,12). After exposure of the disk, it is removed by curettage and, if necessary, the posterior longitudinal ligament also is removed. Lateral exploration permits visualization of the first 5 mm of the nerve root sleeve and allows for removal of foraminal disk herniations. Most surgeons perform a fusion after the diskectomy. Fusion reduces postoperative pain, increases stabilization, and reestablishes the disk space, opening the neural foramina (14).

Regardless of their level, anterior intervertebral bone grafts should not protrude posteriorily into the canal but may protrude slightly anteriorly.

Grafts should restore the intervertebral space to a normal dimension (15,16). They normally should lie 1 to 2 mm deep to the anterior cortex of the vertebral bodies and should not protrude posteriorly (Fig. 19.5). The residual spaces surrounding a graft are filled with cancellous bone chips. Bone grafts have the following shapes:

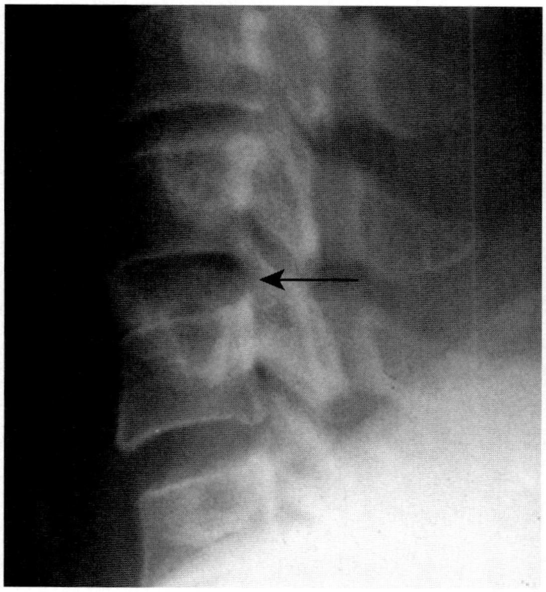

A

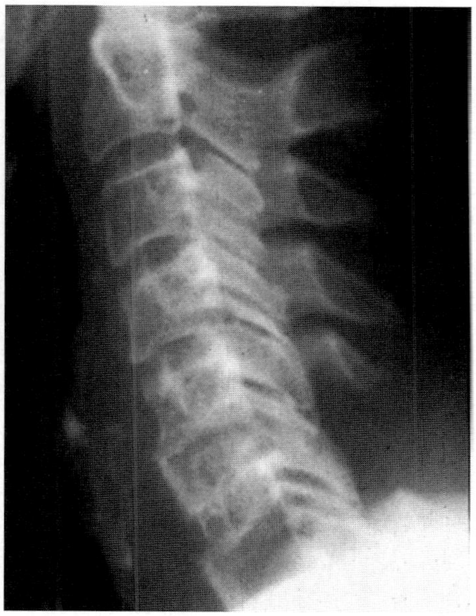

B

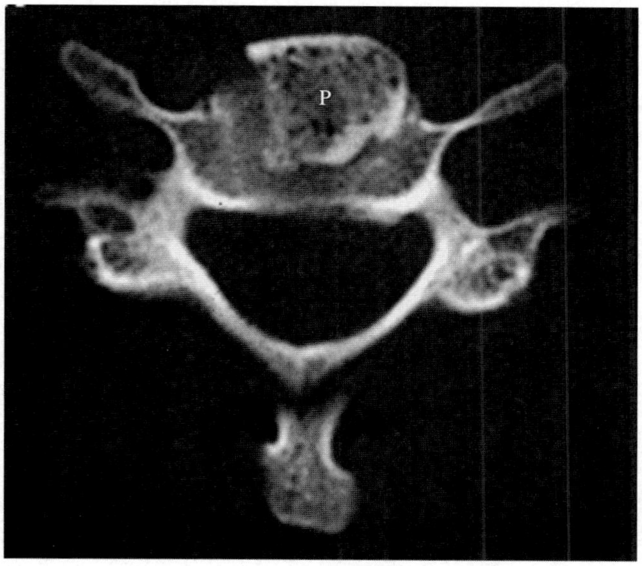

C

Figure 19.5 *Anterior Diskectomy and Fusion. A.* Lateral radiograph shows bone plug *(arrow)* at the C4 to C5 level. The plug does not protrude anteriorly or dorsally. *B.* In a patient who has undergone multi-level fusions, a lateral radiograph shows C4 to C5, C5 to C6, and C6 to C7 bone plugs that are in good position and well incorporated. *C.* Axial computed tomography in a different patient shows a bone plug (P). Although the graft protrudes slightly anteriorly, this is less than 3 mm and it was considered to be in good position.

- Plug (Smith-Robinson procedure)
- Rectangle (Bailey-Badgley procedure)
- Dowel (Cloward fusion)

Partial or complete corpectomies necessitate larger grafts usually obtained from iliac crests. After this type of surgery, most patients are discharged in their second postoperative day. More than 80% of them resume home activities at 2 weeks and return to work at 2 months.

ANTERIOR APPROACH FOR OSTEOPHYTOSIS

Usually, these patients have anterior spurs that need to be drilled out before encountering the disk space (11). The vertebral bodies are distracted to open up the space. In cases of advanced degenerative disease, no disk may be present. The residual disk is curetted and the endplates are drilled in an attempt to recreate the space. The posterior longitudinal ligament (which, in these patients, tends to be very thin) is preserved and the canal is resculpted with the drill. The dissection may be extended laterally to decompress the neural foramina. Anterior graft placement is then done.

Posterior Approach for Herniated Disks and Osteophytes

A paraspinal dissection under the periosteum of a spinous process is done until the desired lamina is exposed (13). Using the drill, mostly the upper lamina is resected. The resection may be extended to involve part of the facet joint. Progressive lateral exploration is done until a nerve root is seen. Removal of the facets allows for exposure of the neural foramen. Retraction of the nerve root allows for removal of disk material and osteophytes.

Laminoplasties are being done with increasing frequency for spinal canal stenosis. The advantages of this procedure are:

- Greater safety because the bone incision is lateral and distal from the compressed spinal cord
- Increased postsurgical stability
- Reduced hospitalization and recovery period
- Decreased incidence of postoperative deformities

One of the most common techniques is the "open-door" laminoplasty. The "door side" may be held open by insertion of bone grafts, methylmethacrylate, or metal plates (Fig. 19.6). This may be done at every other level. The "hinge" side may or may not be held in place by wires. In the bifid type of laminoplasty, the spinous process is opened in the midline, and after bilateral laminotomies the posterior elements are opened in a "French door" type of configuration. Again, the door may be kept open by bone or synthetic materials. In the Z-type laminoplasty, the laminae are cut, elevated, split laterally, and then sutured to the higher arch.

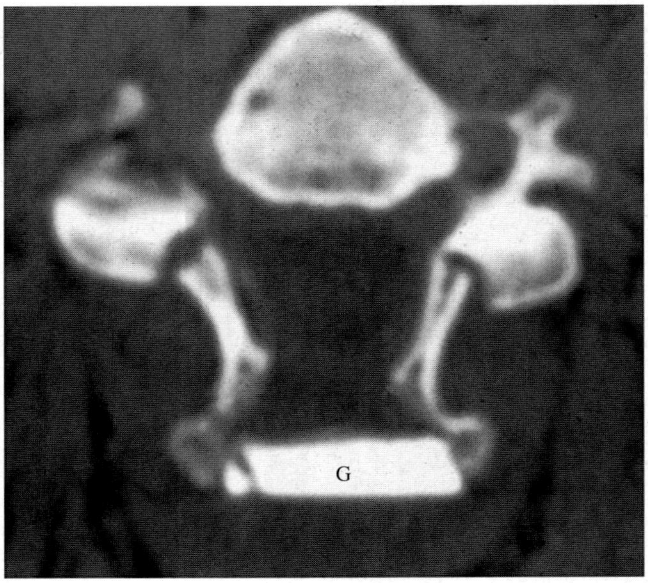

Figure 19.6 *Laminoplasty*. Axial computed tomography shows laminoplasty of the "French door" type. The "open door" aspect of the laminoplasty is reinforced with a methylmethacrylate graft (*G*). (Case courtesy of J. Cinnamon, Atlanta, GA.)

THORACIC SPINE

Anterior and posterior approaches also are used in the thoracic region (17) (Fig. 19.7). Devices usually are placed to provide initial stabilization, but most eventually fail and an underlying bone fusion is done in nearly all patients. This bone fusion maintains the long-term stability of the spine. The most common indications for thoracic surgery are correction of scoliosis, trauma, and degenerative disk disease (18). MRI always should be obtained before the correction of kyphosis or scoliosis to exclude tethering of the spinal cord and the presence of spinal cord cysts. Spinal cord cysts are present in up to 20% of patients with scoliosis. In patients with thoracic scoliosis, surgery is indicated when the curvature is greater than 45 degrees as measured by the Cobb method.

Before the surgical stabilization of scoliosis, MR imaging of the spine is done to exclude tethering of the cord tumor or a syrinx.

ANTERIOR APPROACH

The anterior thoracic approach is indicated in the patients with a failed posterior fusion, degenerative disk disease, high-grade spondylolisthesis, trauma, infection (particularly tuberculosis), and some tumors (11). Plates and screws usually are attached to the lateral aspect of the vertebrae for immediate stabilization, allowing the time needed for a bone graft to become incorporated (Fig. 19.7). Anterior plating aids in maintaining a normal position. Plating reduces the risk of pseudoarthrosis formation.

POSTERIOR APPROACH

This is the most common approach used for stabilization of the thoracic spine. After a midline incision, laminectomies or laminotomies are used to decompress the spinal canal (11). The most commonly used stabilization devices are rods (Harrington and Luque

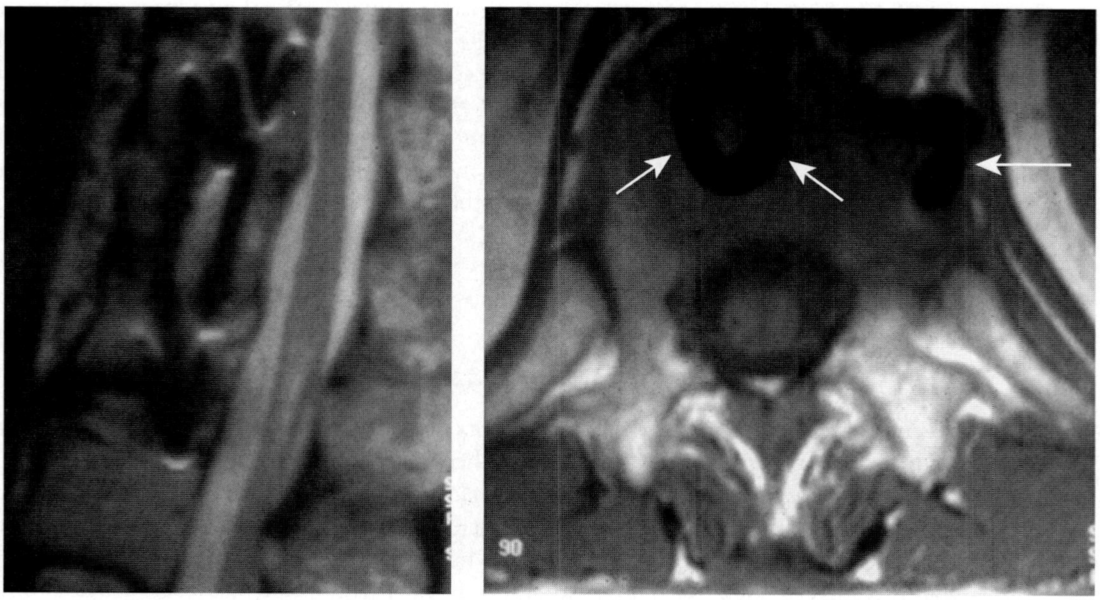

A B

Figure 19.7 *Anterior Thoracic Fusion. A.* Sagittal T2-weighted image shows anterior corpectomy and graft fusion at the T12 to L1 level. The fibular graft is well seen and the artifacts superior and inferior to it are due to screws holding a lateral plate in place. The spinal canal is well visualized and its diameter is not compromised. *B.* Axial T1-weighted image in the same patient clearly shows the fibular graft *(small arrows)* and the lateral plate *(large arrow)*. The spinal canal size is well preserved.

types). These rods are capable of spanning long segments. These rods usually are attached with the use of sublaminar wires or braided steel cables, hooks, or screws. These devices correct deformities by means of compression or distraction.

Complications of Cervical and Thoracic Spine Surgery

Several complications do not require imaging, and these include incorrect initial clinical diagnosis, choice of poor therapy, wrong operative approach, and lack of patient motivation (19).

In the postoperative patient, MRI may be helpful in the evaluation of the following (17):

Status of the spinal cord and meninges
Epidural/subdural hematomas
Infections
Instability and incorporation of bone grafts
Unusual complications

Spinal Cord, Meninges, and Nerve Roots

Spinal cord infarction occurs in approximately 0.2% of patients who receive surgery in the cervical region (17). Spinal cord infarctions are more common after anterior surgical approaches, but also may occur after posterior approach surgery. In these patients, T2 images show increased signal intensity and expansion of the cord at the level of the surgery (Fig. 19.8). When the infarction involves the lower spinal cord, edema of the gray matter may be seen acutely on T2 images (Chapter 18). Postsurgical myelomalacia may be static or progressive. Progressive posttraumatic myelomalacia is a recently recognized condition usually seen in patients with prior spinal cord injuries (20). Most patients have progressive loss of motor function, sensory level changes, increasing spasticity, radicular pain, autonomic dysreflexia, and loss of bowel/bladder control. MRI shows increased T2 signal intensity and tethering and expansion of the spinal cord by adhesions (Fig. 19.9). This condition should be recognized because these patients benefit from timely surgical intervention. Vascular injury to the spinal cord also may be indirect. Injury to the vertebral arteries may result in formation of arteriovenous fistulas, which then may result in spinal cord edema or infarction (17). Injury to the meninges may result in the formation of postoperative pseudomeningoceles, which may be identified with MRI or after myelography (Fig. 19.10). The syndrome of intracranial and intraspinal hypotension may accompany the pseudomeningoceles, and these patients may show thick and enhancing dura in the spinal canal. Damage to nerve roots also may result in worsening of a radiculopathy.

Epidural/Subdural Hematoma

Most epidural hematomas are spontaneous in nature but about 14% of them are related to trauma.

In one large series, only 0.17% of patients were found to have postoperative spinal epidural hematomas (21). Most patients had a 5-hour symptom-free period between surgery and the discovery of the hematoma. The most common symptoms were pain, paresthesia, radiculopathies, and neurologic palsies. Because of cord compression, the diagnosis is established earlier when the hematoma is located in the cervicothoracic regions. Early reoperation allows for full recovery. The exact incidence of postsurgical subdural hematomas is not known. For a description of the appearance of spinal epidural and subdural hematomas, see Chapter 14.

Infections

The overall risk of infection after spinal surgery is approximately 1% to 2% (2). This risk increases with the duration of the procedure and use of grafts and instrumentation. In trau-

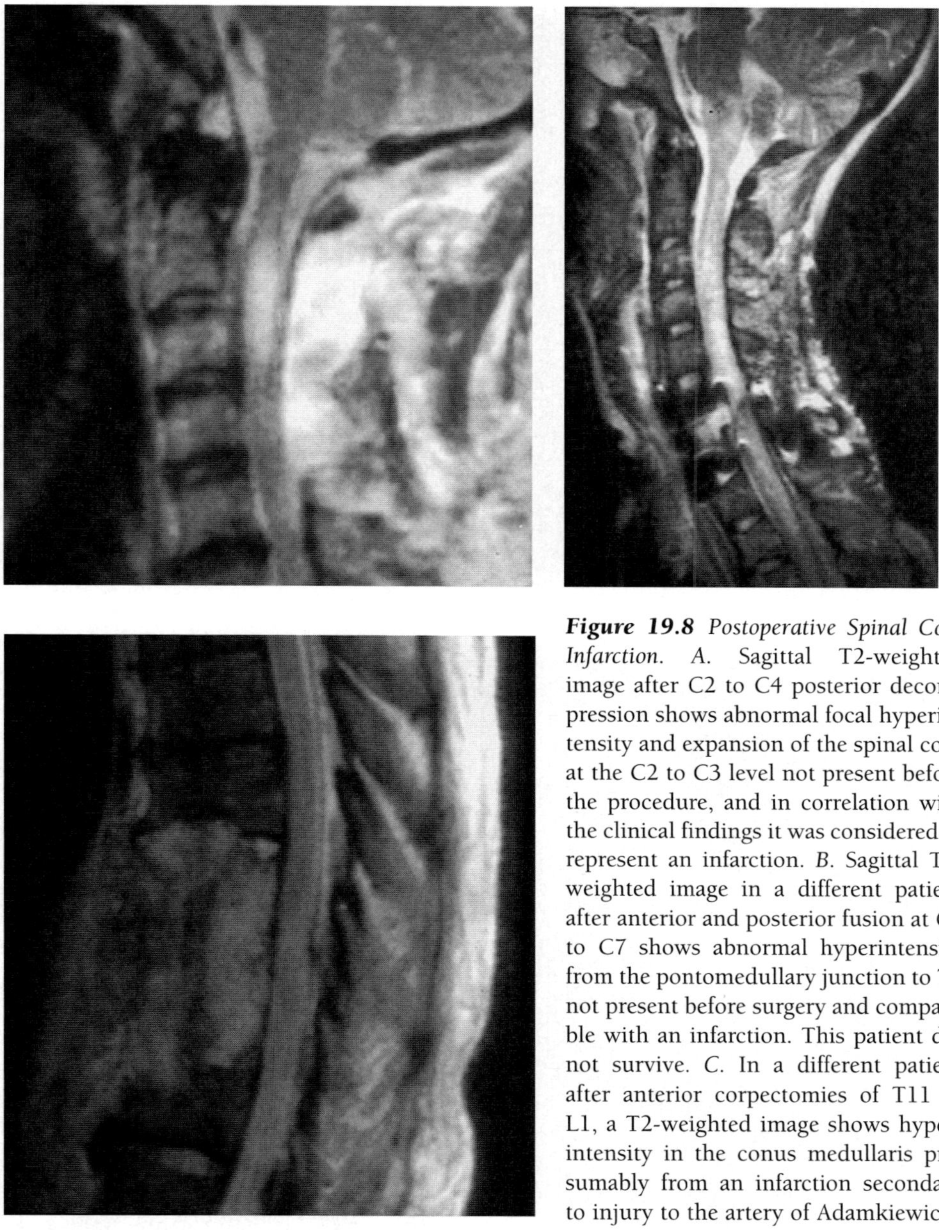

A B C

Figure 19.8 *Postoperative Spinal Cord Infarction. A.* Sagittal T2-weighted image after C2 to C4 posterior decompression shows abnormal focal hyperintensity and expansion of the spinal cord at the C2 to C3 level not present before the procedure, and in correlation with the clinical findings it was considered to represent an infarction. *B.* Sagittal T2-weighted image in a different patient after anterior and posterior fusion at C6 to C7 shows abnormal hyperintensity from the pontomedullary junction to T2 not present before surgery and compatible with an infarction. This patient did not survive. *C.* In a different patient after anterior corpectomies of T11 to L1, a T2-weighted image shows hyperintensity in the conus medullaris presumably from an infarction secondary to injury to the artery of Adamkiewicz.

matized patients who require a tracheostomy and thereafter undergo cervical spine surgery, the risk of infection also may be increased. Other predisposing factors for infection in spine surgery are diabetes, corticosteroid therapy, prior spinal surgery, obesity, chronic infection, smoking, extended hospitalization, and high blood loss. The benefit of prophylactic antibiotic therapy after spinal surgery is debatable. After diskectomies, suspected infection is uncommon and is an indication for immediate MRI. If infection is suspected, gadolinium administration is warranted. See Chapter 15 for a complete discussion of spinal infections.

Incorporation of Bone Grafts

MRI has been used to follow the incorporation (or lack thereof) of bone grafts. Within the first month after surgery, bone grafts are of high signal intensity in T1- and T2-weighted sequences, probably reflecting the presence of hematoma (22). The same signal characteristics persist until 3 months, but the signal intensity becomes progressively less homogeneous. Six months after surgery, nearly all of the hyperintensity in the graft disappears (Fig. 19.11). The adjacent endplates and vertebral body bone marrow become infiltrated

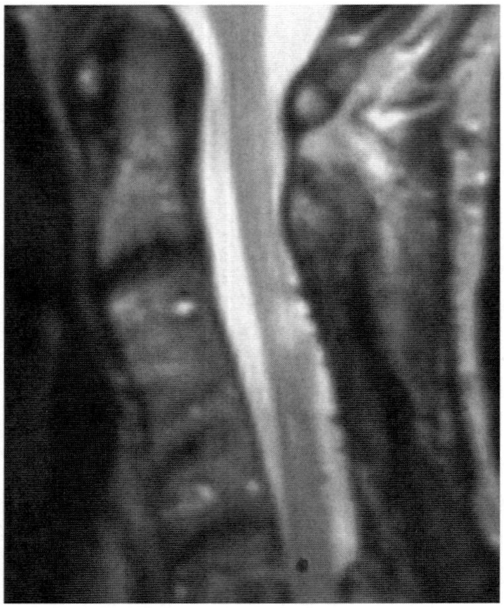

Figure 19.9 *Postsurgical Progressive Myelomalacia.* Sagittal T2-weighted image shows an area of increased signal intensity in the spinal cord at the C3 level, where it is tethered posteriorly by scar.

A

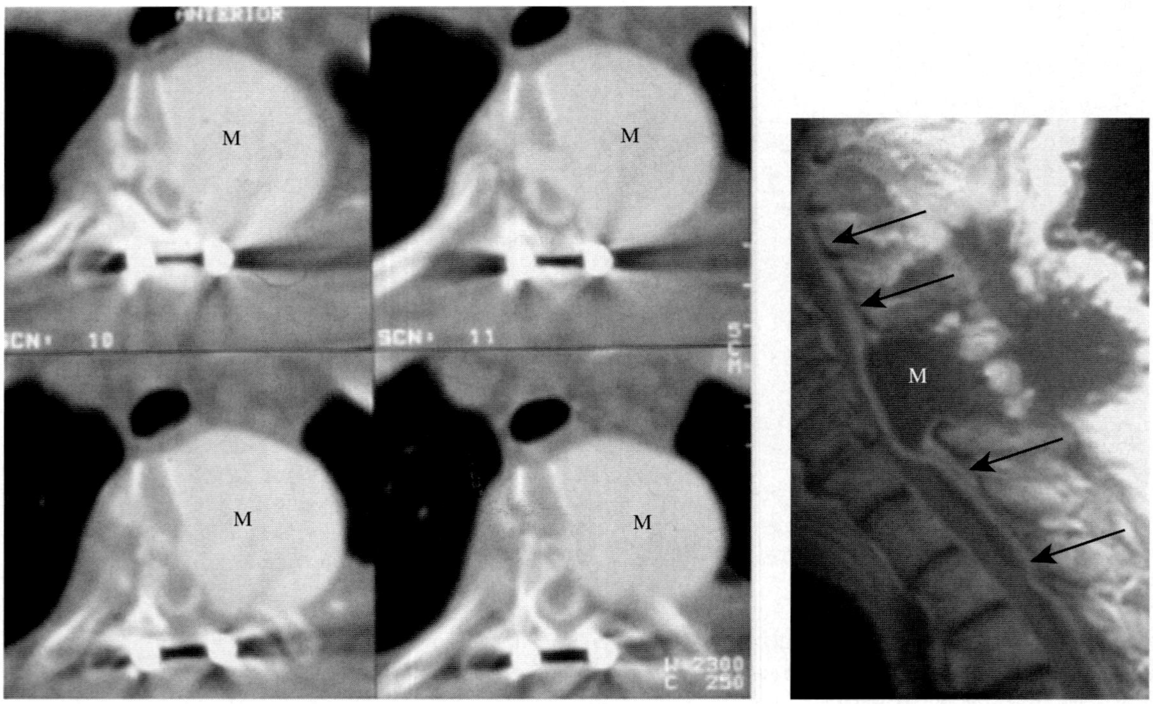

B

Figure 19.10 *Postoperative Pseudomeningocele. A.* Axial views from postmyelogram computed tomography show a large, contrast-filled pseudomeningocele *(M)* on the left in this patient after an anterior corpectomy. Note that the spinal cord is compressed by the pseudomeningocele, which communicates freely with the subarachnoid space. *B.* In a different patient after posterior cervical decompression, sagittal postcontrast T1-weighted image shows a dorsal pseudomeningocele *(M)* at C6 to C7 that compresses the spinal cord. Note thick dural enhancement *(arrows)* secondary to intracranial and intraspinal hypotension.

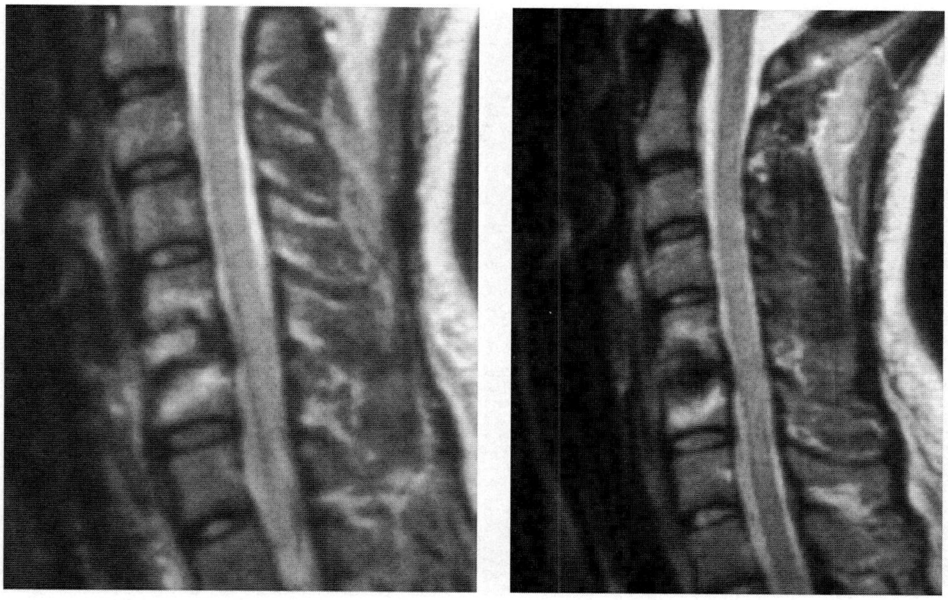

Figure 19.11 *Bone Graft Incorporation. A.* Sagittal T2-weighted image 10 days after surgery shows a bright bone plug at the C5 to C6 level. Note that adjacent endplates also are bright. *B.* Corresponding T2-weighted image 3 months after surgery shows that the bone plug and adjacent endplates are dark, indicating incorporation of the graft and lack of motion at this level. There is residual high signal in the adjacent vertebral bodies owing to the presence of prior degenerative changes (so-called Modic type 2 changes).

by fat, simulating the so-called type 2 Modic changes. After 6 months, the normally incorporated bone graft should be difficult to distinguish from the adjacent vertebrae, and the parent disk space should not be visible (23). Lack of fusion and instability leads to edema and prevents fatty infiltration of the endplates and vertebrae. The most common abnormalities in patients with postcervical spine fusion include disk herniations below or above the level of the fusion (occurring with equal frequency) and spinal canal stenosis at the level of the fusion (Fig. 19.12). Acute expulsion of grafts may lead to damage of the spinal cord or the esophagus (Fig. 19.13). Kyphosis at the site of fusion also may occur.

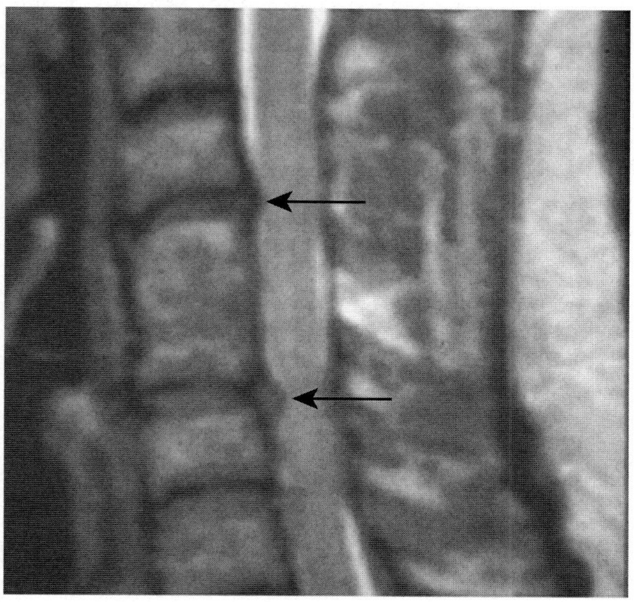

Figure 19.12 *Postfusion Degenerative Changes.* Sagittal T2-weighted image years after a C4 to C5 anterior fusion shows disk herniations *(arrows)* above and below the levels of the fusion.

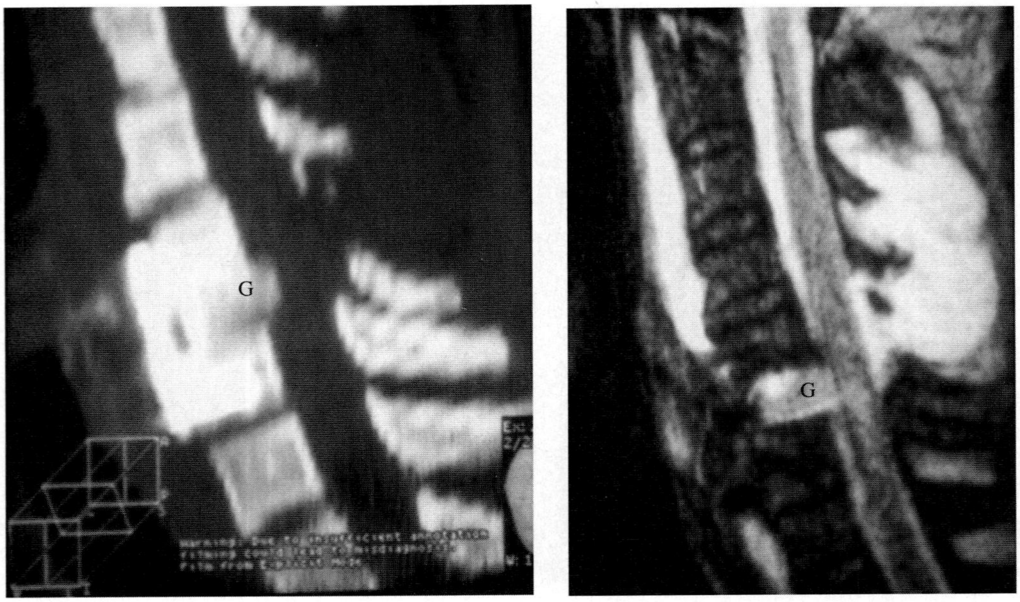

A B

Figure 19.13 *Extruded Bone Graft. A.* Sagittal computed tomography reformation after a C5 to C6 anterior diskectomy and bone plug insertion shows that the graft *(G)* is posteriorly displaced. *B.* Corresponding T2-weighted image shows the bright plug *(G)* posteriorly displaced and touching the spinal cord, which harbors high signal at that level as well. The patient also had undergone a C5 posterior decompression. (Case courtesy of T. P. Naidich, New York, NY.)

Complications Related to Hardware

An underlying pseudoarthrosis is perhaps the most important cause for plate/screw failure.

Hardware complications are less common in the cervical spine and increase in the thoracic and lumbar because of the increased weight load in those regions. Since the routine introduction of intraoperative fluoroscopy, misplaced instrumentation is an uncommon event. With the use of computer-guided intraoperative navigation aids, this complication is even rarer. Plain radiographs usually suffice in identifying the misplaced instrument. Misplaced screws may be identified by radiographs and CT, but when isolated they seldom are the cause of underlying neurologic symptoms (Fig. 19.14). These patients should be imaged with MRI to identify other potential causes for the symptoms. Screws may be considered misplaced when located in a disk or within 2 mm of an endplate. Some plates require the placement of bicortical screws. Inadequate calculation as to length of the screws may result in a breaching of the posterior cortical margin and damage to the epidural space, meninges, and spinal cord. Plates of the Morscher, H-shape, and Orozco types usually require only unicortical screws. Loosening of a screw may lead to screw–plate separation. When lateral mass plates are used, long screws may result in damage to the nerve roots, epidural hematoma, and injury to the vertebral arteries. Progressive extrusion of screws is uncommon and may be identified by serial radiographs. The importance of comparison with prior studies in these patients needs to be stressed. The metal plates may fracture as the sequela of an underlying pseudoarthrosis (due to lack of bone fusion at the level of a graft placement; Fig. 19.15A). Fracture of the hardware is perhaps more common in the lumbar region, where it is submitted to greater stresses (Fig. 19.15B). If the initial curvature of a plate is miscalculated, it may not conform to the shape of the spine, and there is an increased incidence of plate dislodgement (Fig. 19.16).

Fractures of wires are not uncommon (7). This usually is seen after posterior fixation and fusion. Songer-type braided steel or titanium cables tend to fracture much less often than monofilament wires. Fatigue and fracture of most metal instrumentation usually is

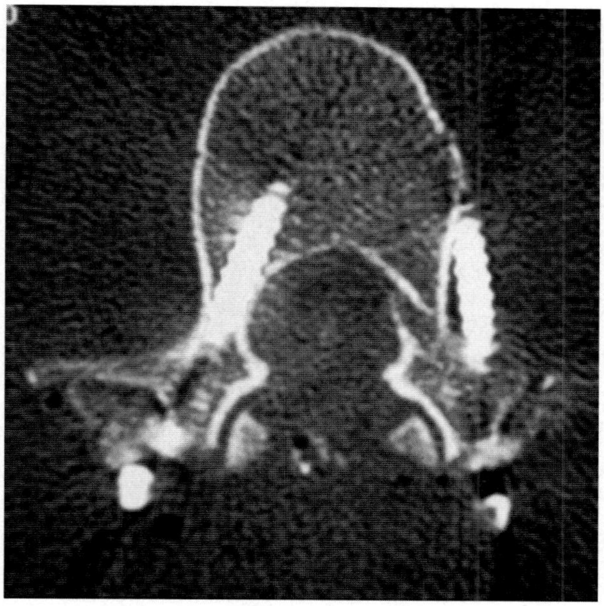

A

Figure 19.14 *Misplaced Screws. A.* Axial computed tomography (CT) shows left-side screw to be outside of the corresponding pedicle and vertebral body. The right-side screw is in good position. *B.* Lateral radiograph after anterior corpectomies and fibular graft placement shows that the superior unicortical screw is in a disk space and not in the vertebral body. *C.* Axial CT in a different patient shows that plate is not centered correctly and that the left-side bicortical screw *(arrow)* has breached the posterior margin and its tip is in the ventral epidural space.

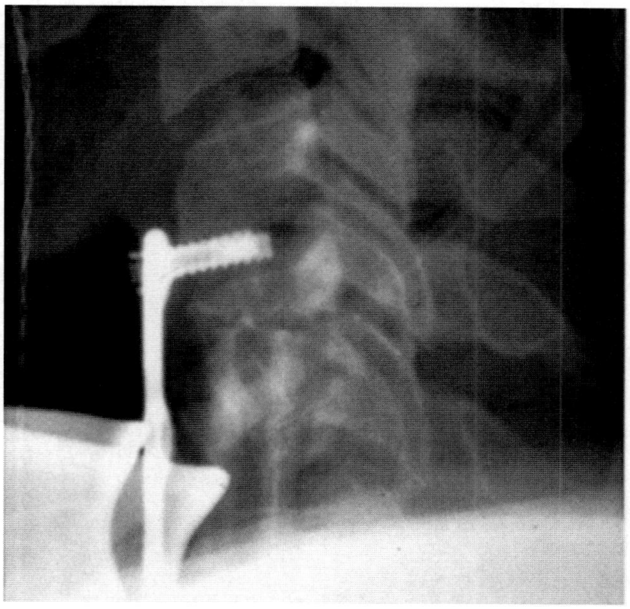

B

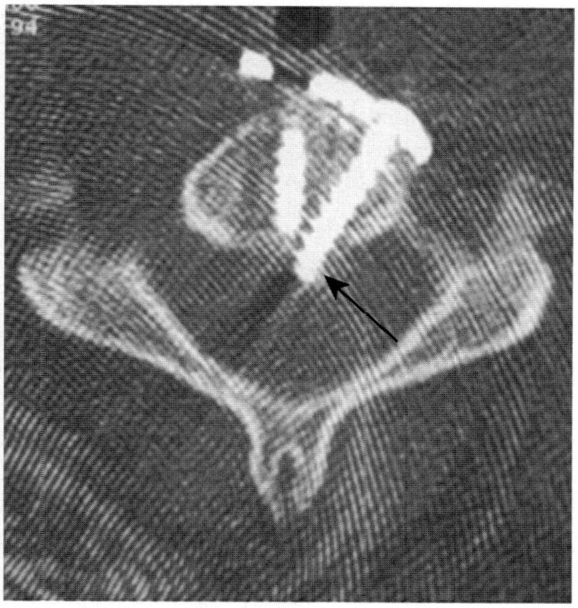

C

accompanied by an underlying pseudoarthrosis. Wires and cables may result in the formation of extradural hematomas. The combination of hematoma and wires may encroach on the spinal canal. Monofilament wires may cut into the underlying bone. This complication is less common when braided cables are used. Plastic ties, which rarely are used, may not be evaluated by imaging. Arachnoiditis is uncommon in the cervical region. The reason for this is not known.

Unusual Complications

Perforation of the pharynx, trachea, larynx, and esophagus is rare and may result in infections (24) (Fig. 19.17). These abscesses are seen as areas of low density on CT that may

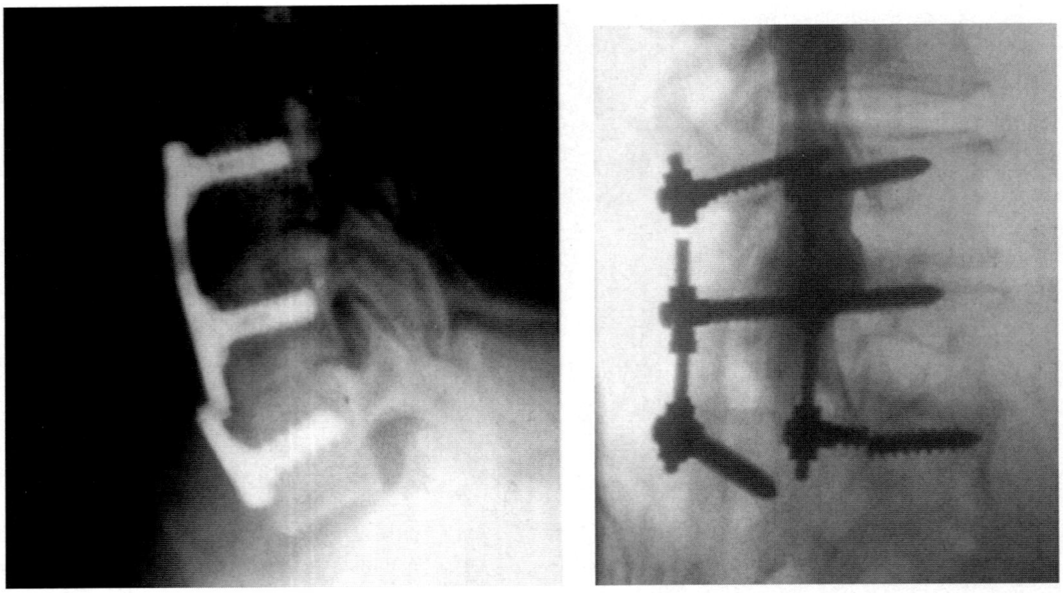

A B

Figure 19.15 *Hardware Fracture. A.* Lateral radiograph shows fracture in the lower aspect of a plate secondary to fatigue induced by the pseudoarthrosis that has developed at C6 to C7. (Case courtesy of D. Karasick, Philadelphia, PA.) *B.* Oblique view from a myelogram shows a fractured right-side laminar plate and a fractured left-side screw.

or may not have peripheral enhancement. Inflammatory changes in the adjacent tissues help in confirming the diagnosis. Cerebral infarction due to injury to the carotid or vertebral arteries may be the result of direct damage to a vessel or a complication of previously unrecognized atherosclerosis. Other very uncommon complications are ligation of the thoracic duct and blindness due to direct injury to a globe from the hand of the surgeon resting on it. Cerebral edema due to a malpositioned endotracheal tube during posterior approaches has been reported. During a posterior approach, the eyes also may be damaged.

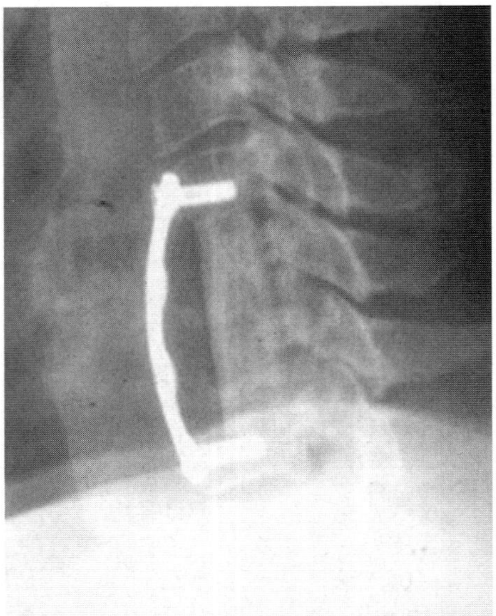

Figure 19.16 *Exaggerated Bending of Plate.* Lateral radiograph shows that the anterior cervical plate has been given too much curvature and is separated from the graft by a wide space.

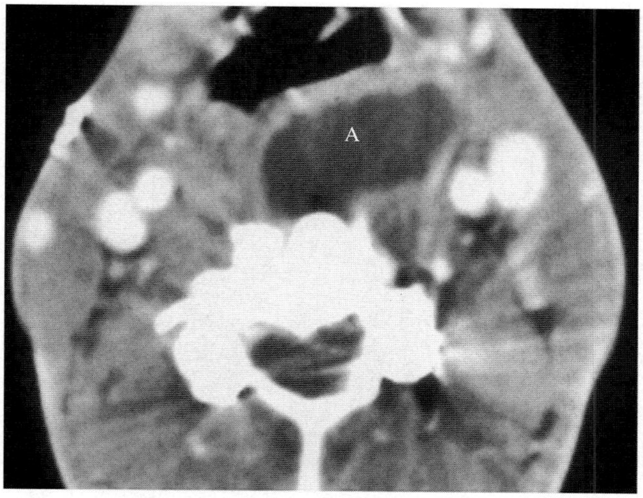

Figure 19.17 *Postgrafting Abscess.* Axial postcontrast computed tomography shows a precervical low-density fluid collection *(A)* in a patient 6 days after an anterior cervical corpectomy and fusion. This abscess was secondary to an esophageal perforation during surgery.

IMAGING SEQUENCES

MRI of the postsurgical spine may be challenging because of the artifacts introduced by metallic hardware. Today, most of these instruments are said to the "MRI compatible." This means that no harm to the patient will occur when he or she is placed in the magnet, but does not guarantee that artifacts will not obscure and degrade the images. Metallic artifacts are worse on gradient-recalled echo sequences, and hence these should not be used in patients with hardware. T1-weighted sequences also are somewhat degraded by metal, but to a lesser degree than gradient-recalled echo imaging (Fig. 19.18). T2 fast

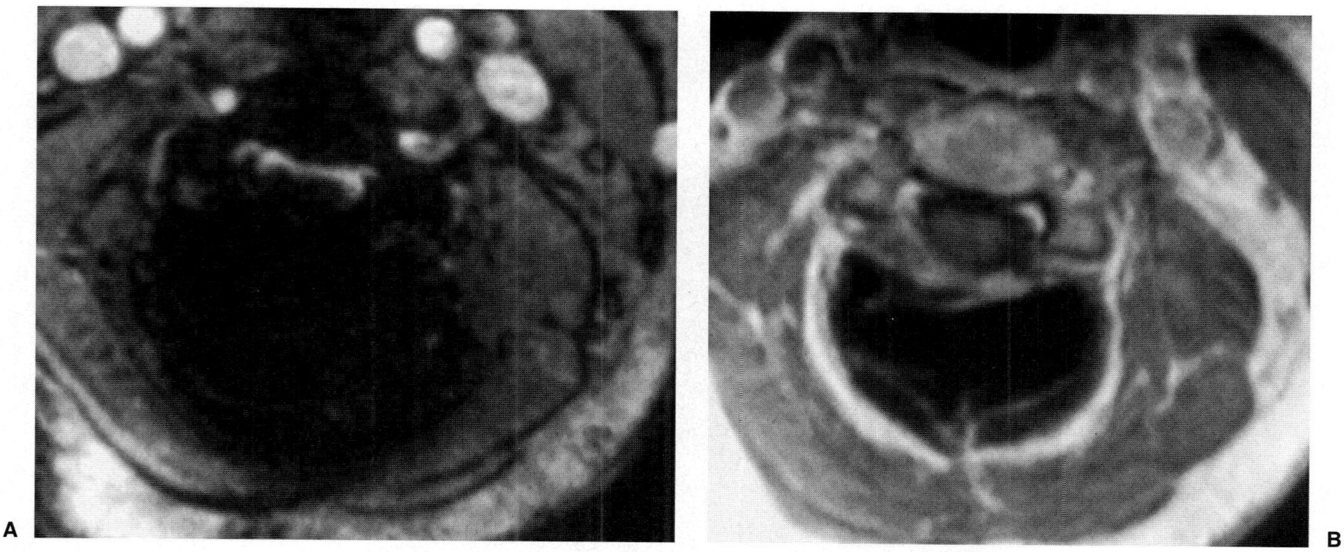

Figure 19.18 *Artifact from Wires. A.* Axial gradient echo T2-weighted image (T2*) shows large blooming artifact obscuring the spinal canal. This artifact is due to magnetic susceptibility effects accentuated by the type of imaging sequence used. *B.* Corresponding T1-weighted image shows much less artifact and now permits visualization of the spinal canal.

A,B 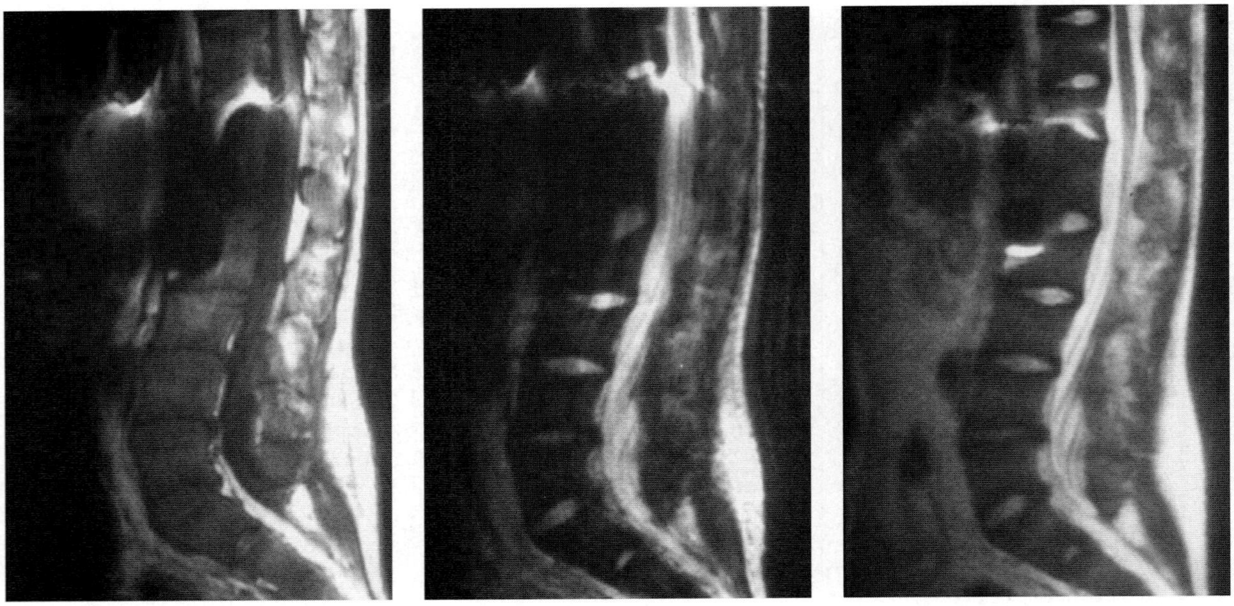 C

Figure 19.19 *Metal Artifact on Different Magnetic Resonance Imaging Sequences. A.* Sagittal T1-weighted image in a patient after anterior corpectomies and graft and metal hardware placement. The artifact partially obscures the spinal canal and results in brightness in the region of the conus medullaris. *B.* Corresponding T2-weighted image shows less artifact but still some interference with visualization of the spinal canal. *C.* Corresponding HASTE (half-Fourier acquisition single-shot turbo spin-echo) image reduces the artifact considerably and allows for visualization of the spinal canal.

spin-echo images are less sensitive to magnetic susceptibility artifacts and often provide adequate images (25). Half-Fourier acquisition single-shot turbo spin-echo (HASTE) images decrease the amount of artifact considerably but offer limited contrast resolution, and I use them as a last resort (Fig. 19.19). Using a frequency encoding direction that is parallel to the long axis of screws and other hardware also improves the image quality (26) (Fig. 19.20).

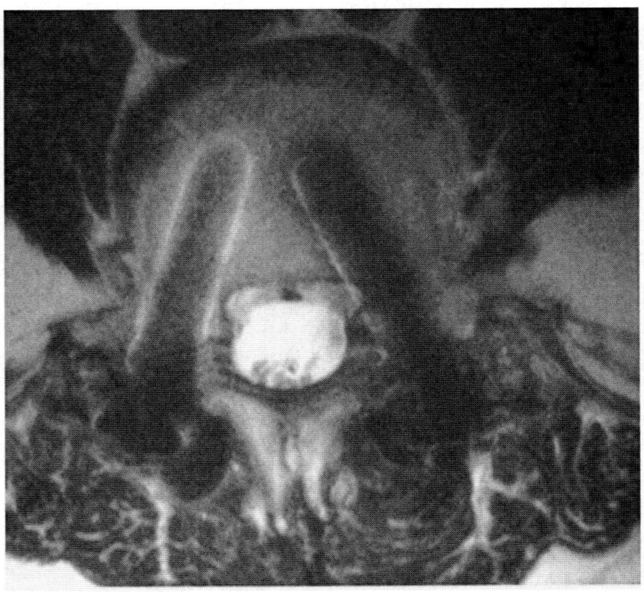

Figure 19.20 *Reduction of Artifact from Screws.* Axial T2-weighted image obtained with the frequency encoding direction parallel to the long axis of the screws results in little artifact and allows for visualization of the spinal canal.

REFERENCES

1. Bundschuh CV. Imaging of the postoperative lumbosacral spine. Neuroimaging Clin North Am 1993;3:499–516.
2. Shafaie FF, Bundschuh CV, Jinkins JR. The posttherapeutic lumbosacral spine. In: Jinkins JR, ed. Posttherapeutic neurodiagnostic imaging. Philadelphia: Lippincott–Raven, 1997:223–244.
3. Henk CB, Brodner W, Grampp S, et al. The postoperative spine. Topics Magn Reson Imaging 1999;10:247–264.
4. Dina TS, Boden SD, Davis DO. Lumbar spine after surgery for herniated disk: imaging findings in the early postoperative period. AJR Am J Roentgenol 1995;164:665–671.
5. Boden SD, Davis DO, Dina TS, et al. Contrast-enhanced MR imaging performed after successful lumbar disk surgery: prospective study. Radiology 1992;182:59–64.
6. Firooznia H, Kricheff II, Rafii M, et al. Lumbar spine after surgery: examination with intravenous contrast-enhanced CT. Radiology 1987;163:221–226.
7. Hueftle MG, Modic MT, Ross JS, et al. Lumbar spine: postoperative MR imaging with Gd-DTPA. Radiology 1998;167:817–824.
8. Ross JS, Masaryk TJ, Modic MT, et al. Lumbar spine: postoperative assessment with surface-coil MR imaging. Radiology 1987;164:851–860.
9. Bobman SA, Atlas SW, Listerud J, et al. Postoperative lumbar spine: contrast-enhanced chemical shift MR imaging. Radiology 1991;179:557–562.
10. Bangert BA, Ross JS. Arachnoiditis affecting the lumbosacral spine. Neuroimaging Clin North Am 1993;3:517–524.
11. McCulloch JA, Young PH. Essentials of spinal microsurgery. Philadelphia: Lippincott–Raven, 1998.
12. Bell, GR. The anterior approach to the cervical spine. Neuroimaging Clinics of North America 1995;5(3):465-479.
13. Hardy RW. The posterior surgical approach to the cervical spine. Neuroimaging Clin North Am 1995;5:481–490.
14. Kalfas IH. Cervical spine stabilization: surgical techniques. Neuroimaging Clin North Am 1995; 5:491–505.
15. Slone RM, MacMillan M, Montgomery WJ. Spinal fixation: part 1. Principles, basic hardware, and fixation techniques for the cervical spine. Radiographics 1993;13:341–356.
16. Karasick D. Anterior cervical spine fusion: struts, plugs, and plates. Skeletal Radiol 1993;22: 85–94.
17. Thompson JE, Smith MM, Castillo M, et al. The posttherapeutic cervicothoracic spine. In: Jinkins JR, ed. Posttherapeutic neurodiagnostic imaging. Philadelphia: Lippincott–Raven, 1997: 193–222.
18. Sloane RM, MacMillan M, Montgomery WJ, et al. Spinal fixation: part 2. Fixation techniques and hardware for the thoracic and lumbosacral spine. Radiographics 1993;13:521–543.
19. Sloane RM, MacMillan M, Montgomery WJ. Spinal fixation: part 3. Complications of spinal instrumentation. Radiographics 1993;13:797–816.
20. Falcone S, Quencer RM, Green BA, et al. Progressive posttraumatic myelomalacic myelopathy: imaging and clinical features. AJNR Am J Neuroradiol 1994;15:747–775.
21. Scavarda D, Peruzzi P, Bazin A, et al. Postoperative spinal extradural hematomas: 14 cases. Neurochirurgie 1997;43:220–227.
22. Albert TJ, Lamb D, Piazza MR, et al. MRI evaluation of fusion mass incorporation after anterior cervical bony fusions: preliminary findings. Paraplegia 1993;31:667–674.
23. Ross JS, Masaryk TJ, Modic MT. Postoperative cervical spine: MR assessment. J Comput Assist Tomogr 1987;11:955–962.
24. Karasick D, Schweitzer ME, Vaccaro AR. Complications of cervical spine fusion: imaging features. AJR Am J Roentgenol 1997;169:869–874.
25. Tartaglino LM, Flanders AE, Vinitski S, et al. Metallic artifacts on MR images of the postoperative spine: reduction with fast spin-echo techniques. Radiology 1994;190:565–569.
26. Frazzini VI, Kagetsu NJ, Johnson CE, et al. Internally stabilized spine: optimal choice of frequency-encoding gradient direction during MR imaging minimizes susceptibility artifact from titanium vertebral body screws. Radiology 1997;204:268–272.

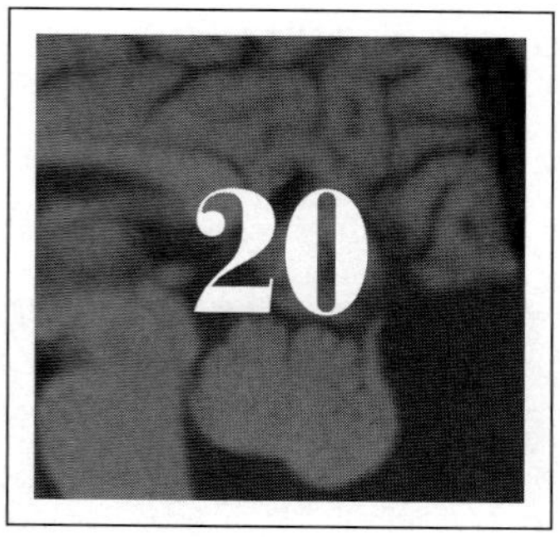

Brachial and Lumbosacral Plexi

- General Considerations
- Anatomy
- Clinical Evaluation

General Considerations

Each brachial plexus (BP) is made up by the anterior components of the C5 to T1 nerve roots (1). Occasionally, it may be formed by the C4 to C7 roots (called a *prefixed* plexus) or by the C6 to T2 roots (called a *postfixed* plexus). Although these variants may slightly alter the physical examination, they are overall of little significance to the clinician and radiologist. The different components of the BP may be recalled by using the following mnemonic (2):

Radiology (roots)
technologists (trunks)
drink (divisions)
cold (cords)
beverages (branches)

I prefer magnetic resonance imaging (MRI) to image the BP (2). To image the BP, we use a large field of view (to include both shoulders) and obtain coronal T1-, axial T1-, and axial T2-weighted images (Fig. 20.1A and B). Using a small field of view, we obtain parasagittal T1-weighted images of each BP (Fig. 20.1C). After contrast is given, we repeat the coronal and axial T1-weighted images. Fat suppression is recommended for T1 images after contrast administration and is helpful when evaluating certain masses, such as lipomas, in the vicinity of the BP.

The proximal aspect of the lumbar plexus courses between the iliacus and psoas muscles inferiorly (3). It then passes anteriorly to its sites of innervation. Occasionally, the lumbar plexus travels within the muscle fascicles of the psoas muscles. The sacral plexus descends laterally to the sacral promontory along the ventral surfaces of the sacral wings. The plexus descends between the iliac vessels and the piriformis muscle and turns back to exit posteriorly through the greater sciatic foramen. We also prefer MRI to image the lumbosacral plexus (LSP). We obtain axial (T1 and T2), sagittal (T1), and coronal oblique (T1) views. After contrast administration, we repeat the axial, sagittal, and coronal oblique T1-weighted sequences, with a least two of these sequences with fat suppression.

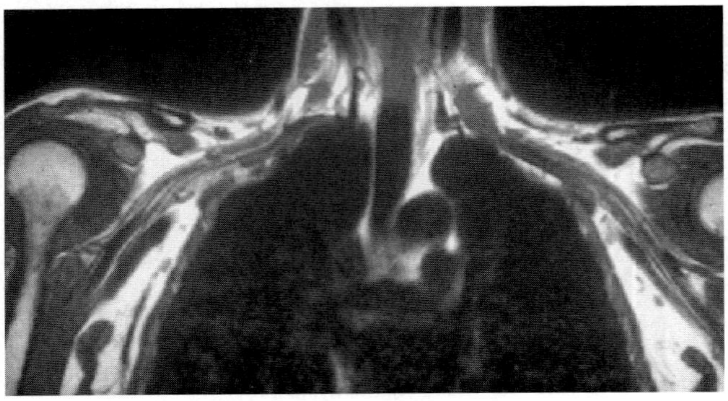
A

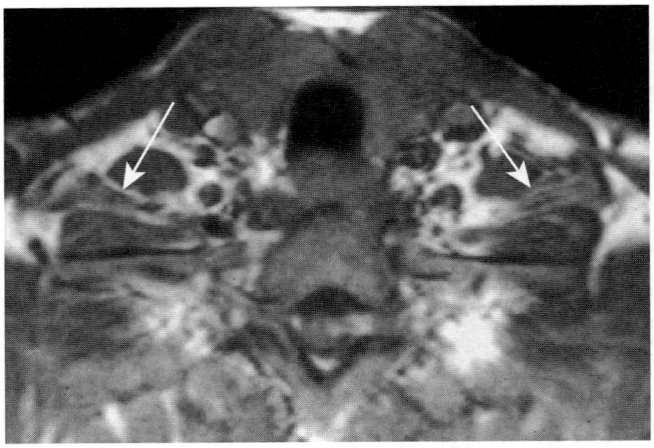
B

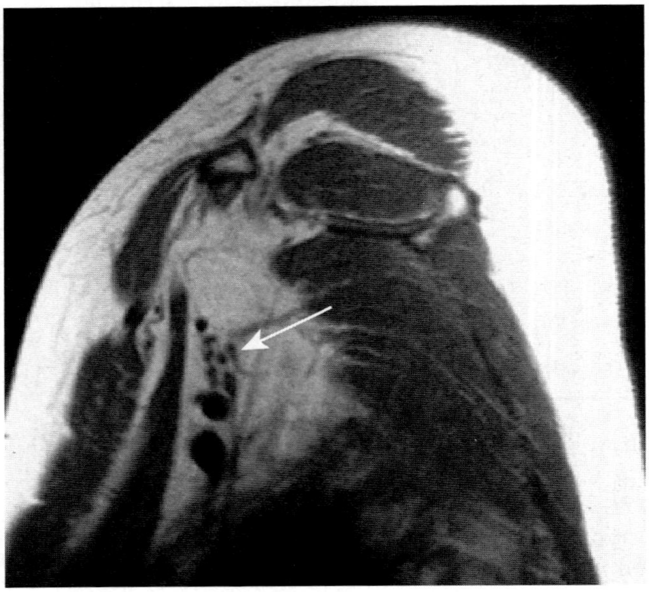
C

Figure 20.1 *Normal Brachial Plexus. A.* Coronal T1-weighted image shows the retroclavicular, infraclavicular, and axillary portions of both brachial plexuses. The study is well centered, and comparison between plexuses is easy. This study was obtained in the body coil, and despite this, it is of good quality and resolution. *B.* Axial T1-weighted image shows the supraclavicular (trunks) of both brachial plexuses *(arrows)* coursing between the anterior and the middle/posterior scalene muscles. C. Parasagittal T1-weighted image shows the distal infraclavicular (cords, *arrow)* located mostly superior and posterior to the subclavian artery. Note that the individual fascicles are well defined and distinct from each other. These fascicles are surrounded by normal fat.

Anatomy

Classic anatomy divides the BP according to the diameter and branching of its components. To understand its configuration, its surgical anatomy is based on external landmarks (mainly the clavicle) (4). The clavicle also dictates the type of surgical approach (supraclavicular or infraclavicular; Tables 20.1 and 20.2).

The imaging anatomy scheme uses easily identifiable landmarks (e.g., the anterior and middle scalene muscles and subclavian artery) to divide the BP (2). From a practical standpoint, it is better to use the surgical anatomy scheme, but it is important to understand its relationship with the imaging anatomy. The innervation provided by the brachial plexus is listed in Table 20.3 (2).

Unlike the BP, which has different anatomic classification schemes, the LSP is classified only according to the traditional anatomic scheme. The sacral plexus is formed by the divisions of the lumbar and sacral roots with a contribution of T12, as follows (5):

Iliohypogastric and ilioinguinal nerves: ventral divisions of T12 and L1
Genitofemoral nerve: the iliohypogastric and ilioinguinal nerves plus a portion of L2
Femoral cutaneous nerve: dorsal divisions of L2 and L3

Table 20.1: Classic Anatomy of the Brachial Plexus Compared with the Surgical Anatomy

Classic Anatomy	*Surgical Anatomy*
C5–T1 roots C5–6 upper trunks C7 mid trunk C8–T1 lower trunks	Supraclavicular
Divisions	Retroclavicular
Posterior cord (posterior division of trunks) Lateral cord (anterior division of superior/middle trunk) Medial cord (anterior division of lower trunks) Branches	Infraclavicular

Table 20.2: Classic Anatomy of the Brachial Plexus Compared with the Imaging Anatomy

Classic Anatomy	*Imaging Anatomy*
C5–T1 roots C5–6 upper trunks C7 middle trunk C8–T1 lower trunks	Bounded by anterior and middle scalene muscles
Divisions (anterior/posterior from each trunk) Posterior cord (posterior division of trunks) Lateral cord (anterior division of superior/middle trunks) Medial cord (anterior division of low trunk)	Adjacent to subclavian artery
Branches	Difficult to identify, distal to humeral head

Table 20.3: Innervation Provided by the Brachial Plexus

Portion of the Brachial Plexus	*Innervation Sites*
Trunks	Supraspinatus, infraspinatus, and teres major muscles
Posterior cords	Latissimus dorsi, subscapularis, and teres minor muscles
Lateral cords	Pectoralis major, biceps, and coracobrachialis
Medial cords	Cutaneous innervation, skin, hand (median/ulnar nerves)

Femoral nerve: ventral divisions of L2 and L3 and dorsal division of L4

Obturator nerve: ventral divisions of L3 and L4

Sciatic nerve: ventral and dorsal divisions of L5, S1, S2, and S3 (the gluteal nerve arises from the superior portion of the sciatic nerve)

Pudendal nerve: from S4 (with some contributions from S2 and S3)

Clinical Evaluation

Brachial Plexus

The Erb-Duchene type of injury accounts for nearly 90% of all brachial plexopathies occurring during birth.

Most patients with brachial plexopathies present with ipsilateral, vague and nonspecific symptoms. Most traumatic avulsions are seen in newborns and young individuals (particularly after motorcycle accidents) (4). The Erb-Duchenne type of palsy involves avulsion of C5 to C6 and the Dejerine-Klumpke palsy, avulsions of C7 to T1 (6). Both usually are due to shoulder dystocia at vaginal delivery. The Erb palsy comprises 80% to 90% of brachial plexopathies in the newborn. The arm is internally rotated and adducted, the elbow extended, the forearm pronated, and the wrist is flexed. Complete recovery may occur but may take months. All supraganglionic avulsions have a poor prognosis. The Dejerine-Klumpke palsy is very rare, comprising only 1% of all brachial plexopathies in the newborn (7). In these patients, the elbow is flexed, the forearm is supinated, the wrist is extended, and there is a clawlike deformity of the hand. The muscles in the involved arm are weak, and Horner's syndrome may be present. Resolution of this plexopathy is possible. The third type of brachial plexopathy in the newborn (accounting for approximately 10% of cases) is a complete avulsion of the BP resulting in absolute weakness and lack of muscle control and tone (4). There is no treatment for this type of injury, and no recovery. In approximately 10% of all neonatal brachial plexopathies, the involvement is bilateral.

About 80% of patients with brachial plexus avulsions will develop pseudomeningoceles and about 80% of them will fill contrast media after myelography.

Avulsion of the BP at its spinal cord origin results in formation of intraspinal or extraspinal cerebrospinal fluid (CSF) collections or hematomas (2) (Figs. 20.2 and 20.3). Eighty percent of patients with avulsions show pseudomeningoceles, but not all of them fill with contrast at myelography (8). The sensitivity and specificity of postmyelogram computed tomography (CT) are 73% to 83% and 87% to 100%, respectively, in avulsions of BP (this is because of the lack of filling of the pseudomeningoceles, which are the most important CT finding in avulsion) (9). Thus, MRI is a better imaging method than postmyelography CT. MR myelography is helpful in identifying the pseudomeningoceles (10) (Fig. 20.4). Establishing the site of injury helps decide the mode of treatment (11–13). For

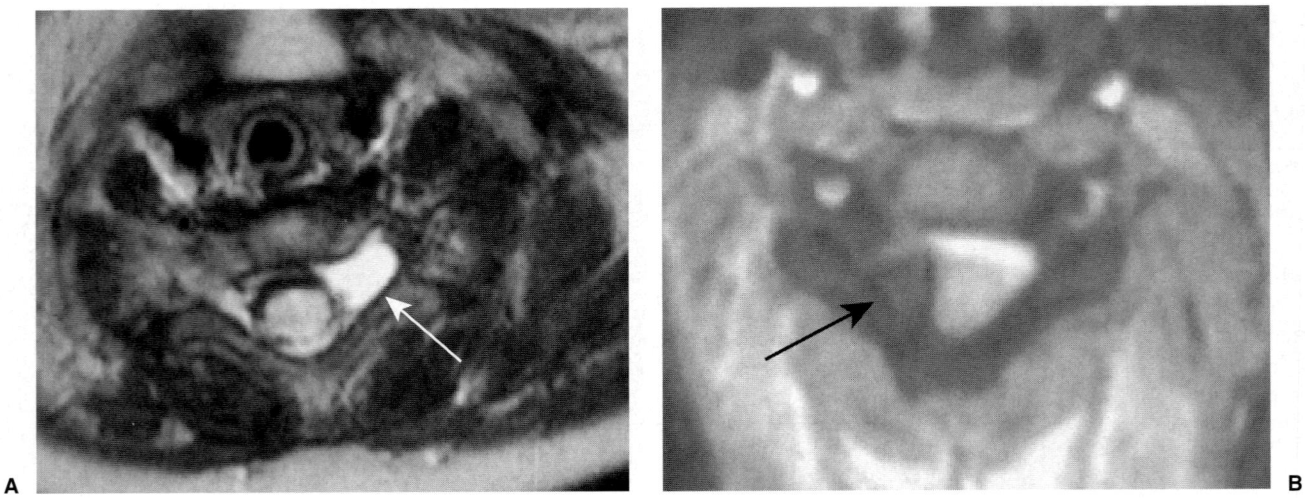

Figure 20.2 *Brachial Plexus Avulsion in Newborns. A.* Axial T2-weighted image in a newborn after a birth complicated by shoulder dystocia shows a left-sided intraspinal bright pseudomeningocele (*arrow*) in the neural foramen and extending into the spinal canal, indicating a supraganglionic avulsion. Note that cerebrospinal fluid surrounding the cord is dark owing to artifact from fast flow. *B.* Axial T2-weighted image in a different patient shows intraspinal dark hematoma (*arrow*) at the root entry zone in a patient with an ipsilateral supraganglionic avulsion.

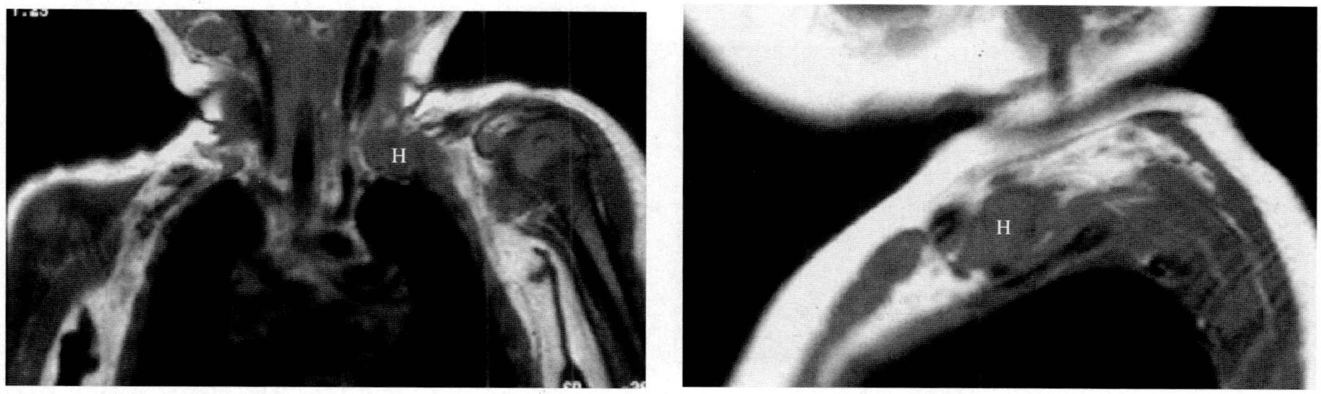

A B

***Figure 20.3** Brachial Plexus Hematoma. A.* Coronal T1-weighted image shows a well defined hematoma *(H)* of intermediate signal intensity in the region of the retroclavicular and infraclavicular portion of the left brachial plexus in this patient whose birth was complicated by a shoulder dystocia. Note elevated left shoulder due to an Erb palsy. *B.* In the same patient, a sagittal T1-weighted image shows the hematoma *(H)* compressing and effacing the fascicles of the brachial plexus. The hematoma was treated conservatively and the symptoms resolved with the aid of physical therapy.

supraganglionic avulsions, there usually is no treatment, whereas intraganglionic or distal avulsions may undergo microsurgical reanastomosis or grafting. Some supraganglionic avulsions may be treated by microsurgical anastomosis. Most of these patients will not recover any significant function, but the procedure decreases their pain. Hematomas in the vicinity of the BP may require decompression to avoid pressure necrosis of the nerves, and subclavian artery aneurysms and pseudoaneurysms may need to be clipped, occluded, or stented (Fig. 20.5). Chronic injuries manifest as atrophy and gliosis of the spinal cord at the level of the avulsion (Fig. 20.6). I have found fat-suppressed images very helpful in

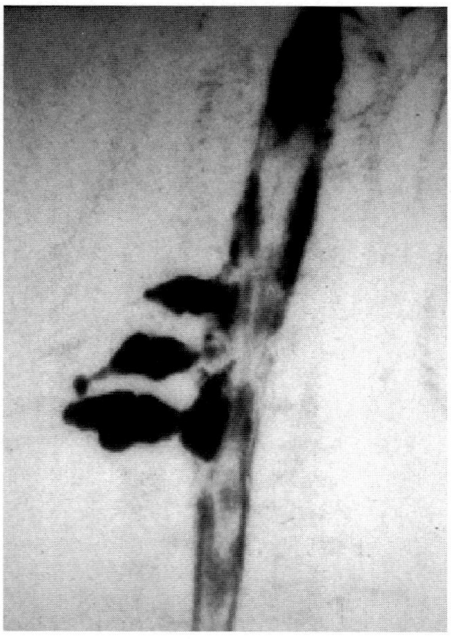

***Figure 20.4** Magnetic Resonance (MR) Myelogram in Avulsion.* Oblique view from an MR myelogram shows several large extraspinal pseudomeningoceles involving the roots of the right brachial plexus. Note that these pseudomeningoceles have an intraspinal component that compresses the spinal cord. (Case courtesy R. Figueroa, Augusta, GA.)

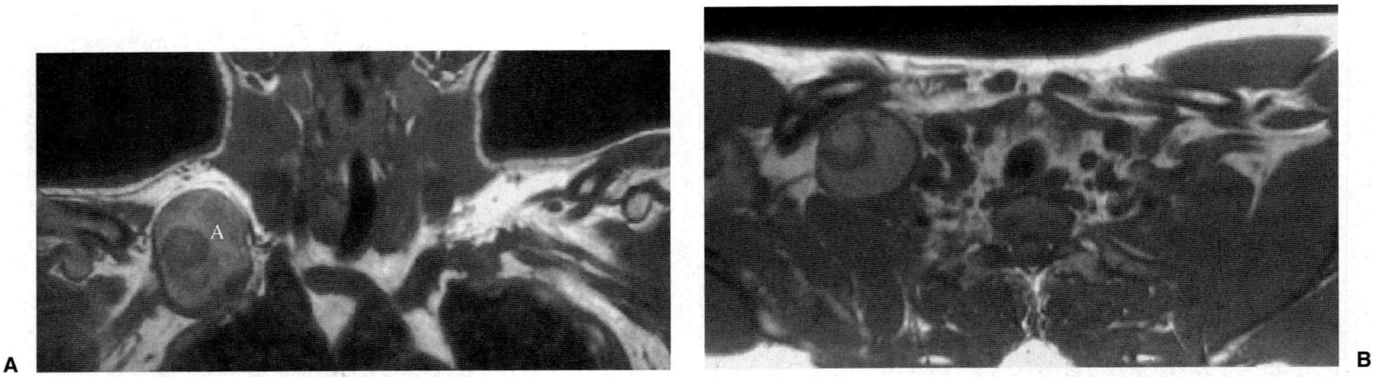

Figure 20.5 *Subclavian Artery Pseudoaneurysm. A.* Coronal T1-weighted image shows a rounded and complex-appearing mass (A) containing peripheral hyperintensity in the right retroclavicular region. The ipsilateral brachial plexus is not seen because it is compressed (compare with the appearance of the normal left brachial plexus). *B.* Axial T1-weighted image clearly shows this post-traumatic pseudoaneurysm to be retroclavicular in location.

evaluating for trauma of the BP. In these images, the injured BP usually is bright. Injury to the BP also may occur if one arm is kept for prolonged periods in an awkward position (14). I have seen this happen in patients waking up with a brachial plexopathy after being in the operating room with one arm hyperextended for a long time (Fig. 20.7).

Sensory symptoms are seen mostly in adults and may follow radiation or indicate the presence of a tumor (15). Tumors commonly produce motor and sensory symptoms. Patients with a BP palsy and Brown-Séquard syndrome usually have an injury at the level of the root entry zone into the cord. Involvement of the phrenic nerve and scapular winging indicate an injury to the supraclavicular BP. A BP palsy with Horner's syndrome indicates an injury to the infraclavicular segment.

A combination of motor and sensory symptoms are common in adult brachial plexopathy and an underlying tumor needs to be excluded in most patients who do not have a history of trauma or irradiation.

After trauma, tumors probably are the most common entity resulting in brachial plexopathies. Primary tumors occur in younger patients and may be nerve related (schwannoma/neurofibroma) or sarcomas (16) (Fig. 20.8). Benign tumors usually are well demarcated and enhance variably. Sarcomas may be either well demarcated or infiltrative.

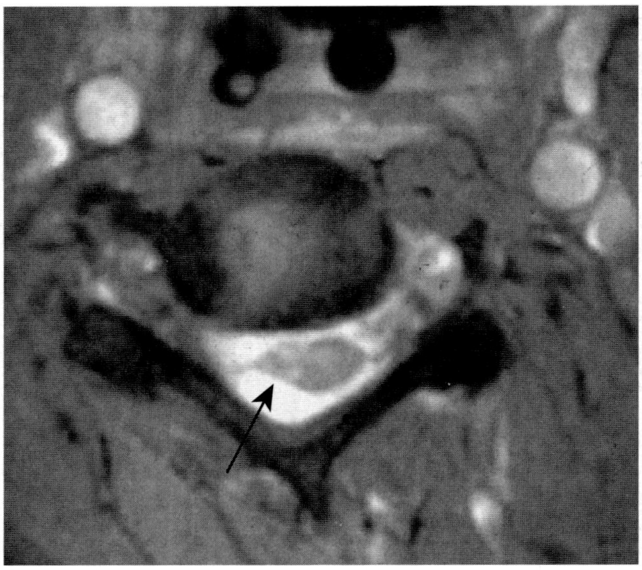

Figure 20.6 *Old Brachial Plexus Injury*. Axial T2-weighted image shows hemiatrophy and increased signal on the right side of the spinal cord *(arrow)* in this patient with an old right brachial plexus injury secondary to a motorcycle accident.

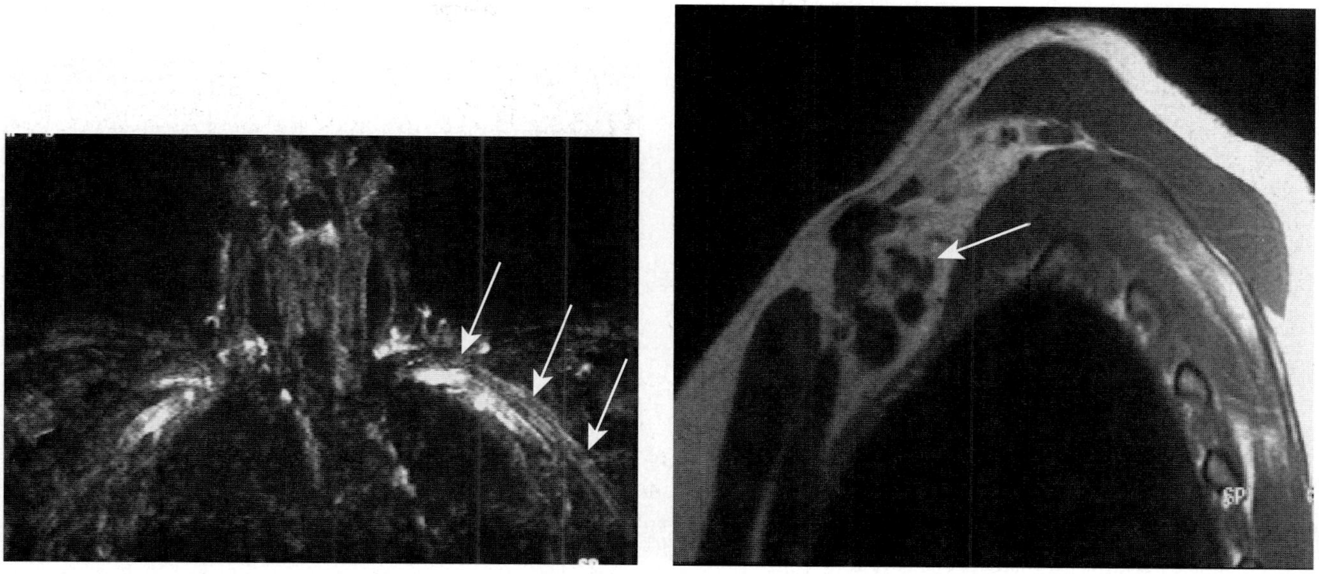

A B

Figure 20.7 *Brachial Plexus Edema. A.* Coronal T2-weighted fat-suppressed image shows diffuse thickening and hyperintensity throughout the left brachial plexus *(arrows)* in this patient who lay with the corresponding arm hyperextended during a kidney harvesting procedure. The patient woke up with a left brachial plexopathy that resolved with conservative treatment. *B.* Sagittal T1-weighted image shows that the infraclavicular fascicles *(arrow)* of the affected brachial plexus are thick and that the fat between them is not well seen (compare with Fig. 20.1C).

Secondary tumors usually are seen in older patients and include lung cancer (Pancoast tumor) and metastases (more commonly from primary breast cancer; Figs. 20.9 and 20.10). In patients with early Pancoast tumor, the only clue as to the presence of disease may be a lesion of intermediate signal intensity effacing the normally bright T1 appearance of the triangular region of fat located superior to the lung apex, medial to the scalene muscles, and lateral to the spine. Larger tumors are easier to identify. In all of these tumors, multiplanar imaging is necessary to exclude invasion of the BP, which may preclude surgery. Occasionally, lymphoma and leukemia (including chloromas) also may

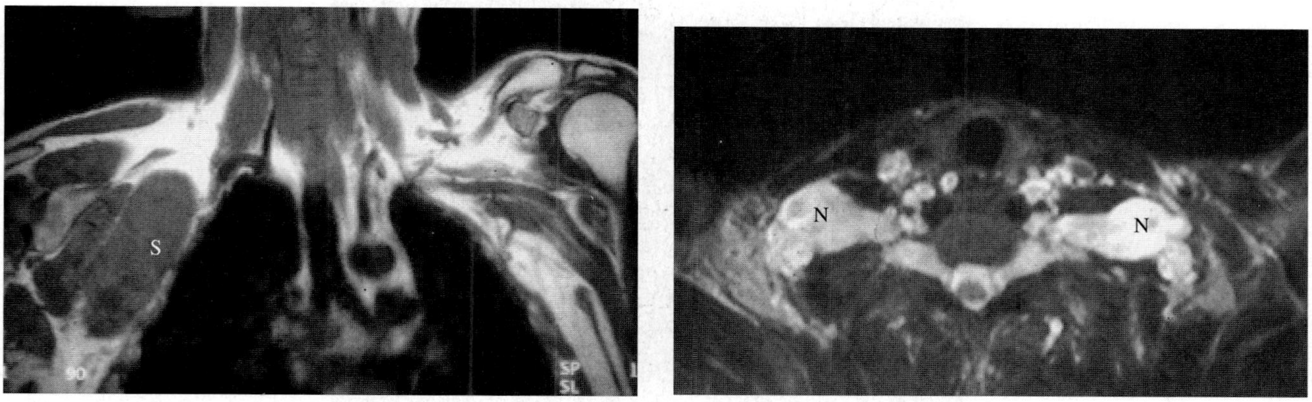

A B

Figure 20.8 *Benign Tumors Affecting the Brachial Plexus. A.* Postcontrast coronal T1-weighted image shows a well defined and mildly enhancing mass (schwannoma, *S*) involving the axillary portion of the right brachial plexus (compare with the left one). *B.* Axial T2-weighted image in a patient with neurofibromatosis type 1 shows plexiform neurofibromas *(N)* involving the supraclavicular portions of the brachial plexuses.

A

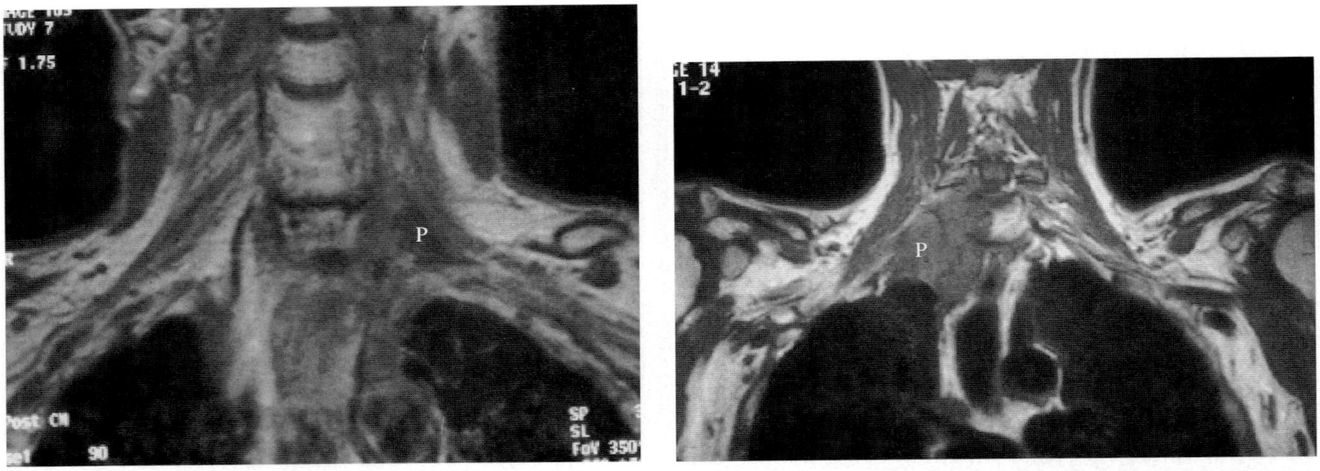

B

Figure 20.9 *Pancoast Tumor. A.* Coronal T1-weighted image shows a left-sided Pancoast tumor *(P)* affecting the proximal brachial plexus. Compare with normal right-side fat at this level. *B.* In a different patient with a more advanced Pancoast tumor, a coronal T1-weighted image shows a large tumor *(P)* involving the right supraclavicular brachial plexus and extending medially to invade the vertebral bodies. The ipsilateral sternocleidomastoid muscle is displaced laterally. Compare with normal left side.

involve the BP (Fig. 20.11). These tumors usually are ill defined and infiltrative, and enhance after gadolinium is given.

Benign masses may result in symptoms by virtue of compression of the BP, whereas malignant ones compress, infiltrate, and destroy it. Chronic pain may be treated by ablation of the plexus. This usually is done by injecting alcohol into the proximal aspect (trunks) of the plexus. The trunks are easily localized by CT because they lie between the anterior and middle/posterior scalene muscles. The lysing material is combined with iodinated contrast so that its distribution can be tracked with CT.

Infection of the BP is very rare and may follow lung disease (fungal, tuberculosis), surgery, or trauma (2). Viral brachial plexitis is very rare, and a postviral inflammatory

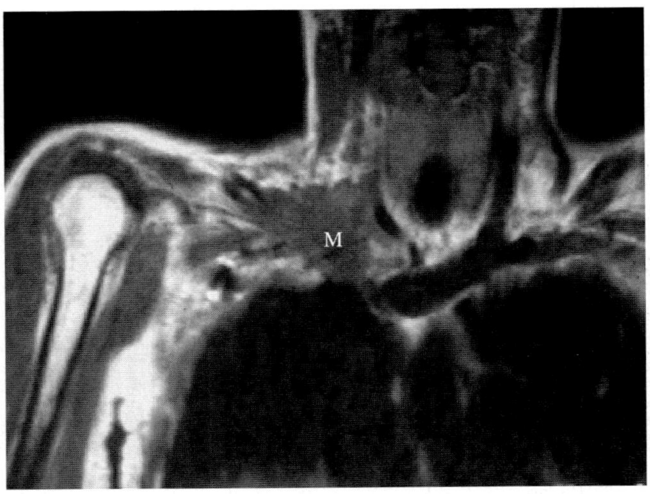

Figure 20.10 *Metastasis to the Brachial Plexus.* Coronal T1-weighted image shows ill-defined mass *(M)* involving the proximal right brachial plexus in this patient known to have metastatic breast cancer.

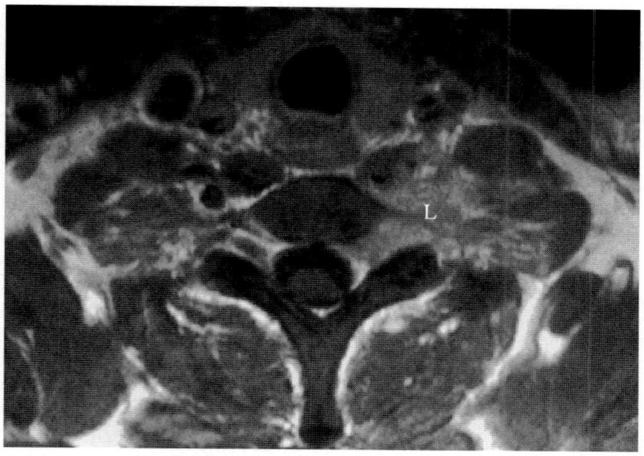

Figure 20.11 *Leukemia Infiltrating the Brachial Plexus.* Postcontrast axial T1-weighted image shows an enhancing and infiltrative lesion *(L)* involving the roots (note extension in a neural foramen) and trunks of the left brachial plexus. The tumor infiltrates the scalene and prevertebral muscles.

process also is known to affect the BP. Both are self-limiting processes and resolve 6 to 12 weeks after onset. A plexopathy also may be a consequence of allergy to drugs. The heredofamilial form of brachial plexopathy is very rare and seen mostly in men. Postradiation plexopathy is seen more often in patients receiving over 6,000 cGy (17). An acute onset correlates with irreversible damage to the BP and permanent sequelae. Patients with a chronic and insidious onset usually are seen 6 months after treatment, and the condition is transient and reversible. In postirradiation plexopathy, the nerves are enlarged diffusely and may be T2 bright. The BP also may show some enhancement after gadolinium administration (17) (Fig. 20.12).

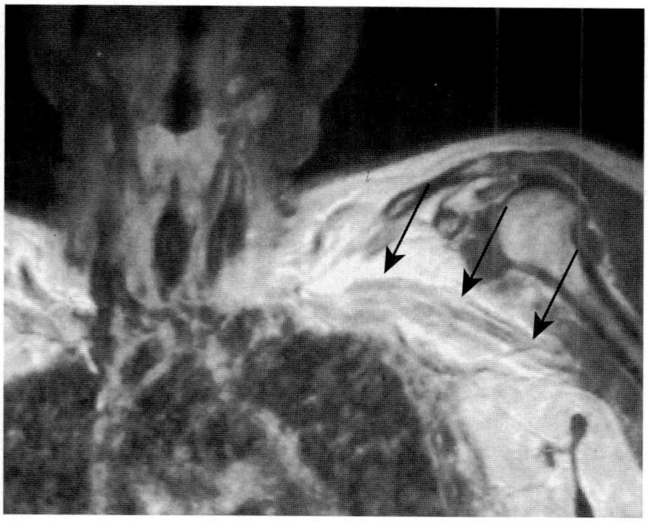

Figure 20.12 *Radiation-Induced Plexitis.* Coronal postcontrast T1-weighted image after irradiation for a left breast cancer shows diffuse thickening and enhancement of the left brachial plexus *(arrows)*.

On sagittal views of the BP, we usually include the cervical spine because disk herniations occasionally result in symptoms mimicking a plexopathy. The cervical rib syndrome also may result in ipsilateral brachial plexopathy (2). It is associated with the presence of an extra rib (cervical rib) and is more common in women. When this is suspected, the presence of the extra rib may be confirmed by radiography. This syndrome tends to be unilateral, but bilateral symptoms occasionally are found.

Lumbosacral Plexus

Similar to the BP, the most common primary tumors of the LSP are nerve sheath tumors (neurofibromas and schwannomas) (18). Tumors of the sacrum, either primary or secondary, also may affect the nerves. CSF-filled cysts (Chapter 16) also may compress the plexus and produce symptoms. Tumors of the piriformis muscle are more commonly metastases or represent direct invasion by a primary neoplasm arising from the pelvis. Abscesses may originate in the pelvis or in the gluteal region and affect the LSP. Blunt trauma is much less common than in the BP. The pelvic bones and sacrum afford a great deal of stability and protect the LSP. Fractures of the pelvis or the sacrum, however, may affect the nerves. Traumatic avulsion of the LSP is rare. One of the most common reasons for a lumbosacral plexopathy is herniated disks. Most lumbar disk herniations (Chapter 17) occur at the L4, L5, and S1 levels, all of which contribute to form the LSP. Other common causes of lumbosacral plexopathy are diabetic neuropathy and vasculopathy. Other neuropathies (hereditary, inflammatory) also may produce symptoms. After irradiation of the pelvis, a lumbosacral plexopathy also may ensue. The piriformis muscle syndrome is a controversial cause of pain. MRI may show enlargement of the muscle on the side of the pain and anterior displacement of the sciatic nerve by the enlarged muscle. The etiology of this syndrome is not known, but it is possible that trauma plays a role in its development. Trauma may lead to intramuscular hematoma and to the formation of adhesions around the piriformis muscle, resulting in tethering and repeated traction to the nerve with development of ischemic injury.

References

1. Posniak HV, Olson MC, Dudiak CM, et al. MR imaging of the brachial plexus. AJR Am J Roentgenol 1993;161:373–379.
2. Mukherji SK, Castillo M, Wagle AG. The brachial plexus. Semin Ultrasound CT MR 1996;17: 519–538.
3. Gebarski KS, Gebarski SS, Glazer GM, et al. The lumbosacral plexus: anatomic-radiologic-pathologic correlation using CT. Radiographics 1986;6:401–403, 424.
4. Guha A, Graham B, Kline DG, et al. Brachial plexus injuries. In: Wilkins RH, Rengachari SS, eds. Neurosurgery, 2nd ed. New York: McGraw-Hill, 1996:3121–3134.
5. Gierada DS, Erickson SJ, Haughton VM, et al. MR imaging of the sacral plexus: normal findings. AJR Am J Roentgenol 1993;160:1059–1065.
6. Kline DG, Hudson AR. Acute injuries of peripheral nerves. In: Youman JR, ed. Neurological surgery, 4th ed. Philadelphia: WB Saunders, 1996:2103–2181.
7. Al-Quatan MM, Clarke HM, Curtis CG. Klumpke's birth palsy: does it really exist? J Hand Surg 1995;20:19–23.
8. Davies ER, Sutton D, Bligh AS. Myelography in brachial plexus injury. Br J Radiol 1966;39: 362–371.
9. Hong SH, Chan KH, Han MH, et al. Cervical root avulsion: magnetic resonance imaging findings and comparison of diagnostic accuracy between magnetic resonance imaging and conventional myelography. Int J Neuroradiol 1996;2:182–187.
10. El-Gammel T, Brooks BS, Freedy RM, et al. MR myelography: imaging findings. AJR Am J Roentgenol 1995;164:173–177.
11. Carlstedt TP. Spinal nerve root injuries in brachial plexus lesions: basic science and clinical applications of new surgical strategies. A review. Microsurgery 1995;16:13–16.
12. Glasby MA, Helms TE. Repairing spinal roots after brachial plexus surgeries. Paraplegia 1995; 33:359–361.

13. Gu YD, Zhang GM, Chen DS. Cervical nerve root transfer from contralateral normal side for the treatment of brachial plexus root avulsions. Chin Med J (Engl) 1991;104:209–211.
14. England JD, Summer AJ. Nontraumatic brachial plexopathy. In Wilkins RH, Rengachari SS, eds. Neurosurgery, 2nd ed. New York: McGraw-Hill, 1996:3245–3250.
15. Dart LH, MacCarthy CS, Love JG, et al. Neoplasms of the brachial plexus. Minn Med 1970;53: 959–964.
16. Lusk MD, Kline DG, Garcia CA. Tumors of the brachial plexus. Neurosurgery 1987;21:439–453.
17. Iyer RB, Fenstermacher MJ, Libshitz HI. MR imaging of the treated brachial plexus. AJR Am J Roentgenol 1996;167:225–229.
18. Gierada DS, Erickson SJ. MR imaging of the sacral plexus: abnormal findings. AJR Am J Roentgenol 1993;160:1067–1071.

SUBJECT INDEX

Numbers followed by "f" indicate figures; numbers followed by "t" indicate tables; and numbers followed by "b" indicate boxes.

A

Abscesses
  of brain
    tubercular, 296
  cerebral, 274
  pseudomonas in postsurgical, 383
Absent pituitary gland, 178–179. *See also* Pituitary gland
Aceruloplasminemia, 87–88
Acetaminophen, toxic epidemics and, 92
Achondroplasia
  communicating hydrocephalus and, 117
  osseous abnormalities and, 122
Acquired hepatocerebral degeneration, hepatic failure and, 81
Acquired immunodeficiency syndrome (AIDS). *See* AIDS
Acute clot, physiology of, 232
Acute demyelinating polyradiculopathy. *See* Guillain-Barre syndrome
Acute disseminated encephalomyelitis (ADEM)
  in comparison to multiple sclerosis (MS), 74
  differential diagnosis of, 362
  FLAIR and, 74
  gadolinium administration for, 361–362
  imaging assessment of, 362–363, 362f–363*f*
  multiple sclerosis (MS) and, 361–362
  spinal cord and, 361–362
  symptoms of, 361–362
  transverse myelitis and, 361–362
Acute disseminated encephalomyelitis (ADEM),
  clinical manifestations of, 74, 75*f*
  demyelination disorders and, 70
Acute hematoma. *See also* Hematoma
  diffusion-weighted imaging (DWI) and, 238, 238*f*
Acute hemorrhage. *See also* Hemorrhage
  magnetic resonance imaging (MRI) and, 232, 232*f*
Acute hemorrhagic leukoencephalopathy, 76*f*
Acute hypertensive hematoma, computed tomography (CT) and, 240*f*
Acute subarachnoid hemorrhage (SAH). *See* Subarachnoid hemorrhage.
Acute transverse myelitis, clinical manifestations of, 362*b*
AD. *See* Alzheimer's disease
ADEM. *See* Acute disseminated encephalomyelitis
Adenohypophysis, hormones produced by, 178*t*
Adenoma, incidental hemorrhagic, 188*f*
Adenomas
  classifications of, 182–183
  hemorrhagic, 180–181
  imaging by MRI for, 183
  pituitary, 180
  producing Cushing's disease, 183
  symptoms produced by, 183*t*
Adrenoleukodystrophy (ALD), 65–66, 66*f*
  FLAIR and, 65*f*
  pathologic zones and imaging correlation in, 67*t*
  symptoms in, 67*t*
adrenomyeloneuropathy, 65
Agenesis of corpus callosum. *See* Corpus callosum
Agyria (lissencephaly-pachygyria complex), 30. *See* also Lissencephaly
AHL. *See* Acute hemorrhagic leukoencephalopathy
AIDS (acquired immunodeficiency syndrome), 278, 280
  anemia and, 87
  CMV myelitis and, 369
  Cryptococcosis neoformans and, 283
  dementia complex, pathologic hallmark of, 278
  progressive multifocal leukoencephalopathy (PML) and, 278, 280
  Treponema pallidum and, 291
Alcohol abuse
  disorders related to, 90
  sequelae of, 90
Alexander's disease (fibrinoid leukodystrophy), 60–61, 60*f*
  manifestations of, 60–61, 60*f*
Alobar HP (holoprosencephaly)
  brain abnormalities in, 20*t*
  facial features and, 17, 18*f*, 18*t*
Alpers syndrome, characteristics of, 81
ALS (amyotrophic lateral sclerosis)
  clinical subtypes of, 97–98, 98*f*
  FLAIR and, 97–98, 98*f*
Alzheimer's disease (AD), 99*f*
  dementia and, 98–99
  MRI and, 98–99
Amino aciduria, 83–85
Amphetamines, cerebral vasculitis and, 217
Amyloidosis
  components of, 102
  hematomas, 102
  hemorrhage related to, 102*f*
  kidneys and brain affected by, 103
Amyotrophic lateral sclerosis (ALS). *See* ALS
AN. *See* Anorexia nervosa
Anaplastic astrocytomas, 153, 153t, 154, 154*f*
Anemias, 87
Aneurysm
  subarachnoid hemorrhage (SAH) and, 234
Aneurysmal bone cyst (ABC)
  anatomical distribution of, 394
  angiography and, 394
  imaging of, 393*f*
  and other lesions associated with, 393
Aneurysmal, pattern of dissection, 225
Aneurysms. *See also* Intracranial aneurysm
  anterior cerebral artery (ACA) infarction and, 211
  anterior communication artery and, 242
  arteriovenous malformations (AVMs) and, 250
  general information about, 239–242
Angiolipoma
  epidural space and, 397
  locations of identity, 397

Angiolipoma (*continued*)
  vascular elements and, 397
Angiomyolipoma
  imaging characteristics, 397–398, 398*f*
  locations of identity, 397
  smooth muscle and, 397
Ankylosing spondylitis (AS)
  complications in adults with, 377
  computed tomography (CT) and, 376–377, 377*f*
  differential diagnosis of, 376–377
  sacroiliac joint involvement in, 376–377
  syndesmophyte formation in adults with, 376–377
Annular tears
  gadolinium enhancement of, 414
  imaging of, 414
Anorexia nervosa (AN), cerebral abnormalities and, 106
Anterior cerebral artery (ACA) infarction, 210–211
  aneurysms and, 211
  causes of, 211
  imaging of, 210*f*
  internal carotid artery occlusion and, 210*f*
Anterior communicating artery
  aneurysms and, 242
Anterior communicating artery aneurysm. *See also* Aneurysm
  bleeding sites of, 242
  computed tomography (CT) of, 243f
Anterior (sincipital) encephaloceles. *See* Sincipital encephaloceles
Anterior occipitoatlantal dislocation
  magnetic resonance imaging (MRI) for, 346
  Powers ratio and, 346
Anterior sacral meningocele, imaging of, 330*f*
Anticysticercal drugs, spinal seizures and, 370
Apparent diffusion coefficient (ADC) maps
  infarctions and, 205
Aqueductal stenosis, congenital noncommunicating hydrocephalus and, 120
Arachnoid cyst, 4, 4*f*
  image of, 167
  imaging modalities and, 166
Arachnoid granulation, imaging of, 118*f*
Arachnoiditis
  adhesions and, 373
  antiinflammatory drugs for, 374
  common causes of spinal, 446*b*
  images of, 374*f*
  imaging features of, 447*f*, 447*t*
  lumbar spine surgery and, 446
  symptoms of, 373, 373*b*, 374
Arteriovenous fistula (AVF)
  dural type of, 250
  vein of Galen malformations and, 250
Arteriovenous malformations (AVMs)
  aneurysms and, 250
  brain and, 248
  calcifications and, 248–249
  catheter angiography for, 249
  clinical importance of, 248
  contrast administration and, 248–249, 249*f*
  external carotid artery (ECA) and, 250
  hemorrhage and, 248
  Osler-Weber-Rendu syndrome and, 248
  seizures and, 248
  treatment of, 250
  Wyburn-mason syndrome and, 248
Ascending transtentorial herniation. *See also* Upward herniation
  cerebellum and, 262
Aspergillosis fumigates
  forms of spread of, 284, 284*f*
  miotic aneurysms and, 285
  T1 weighted image of, 284, 284*f*
Astrocytomas
  anaplastic, 153, 153t, 154, 154*f*
  blood products and, 405
  brainstem, 134–136, 135*f*
  children and, 405
  formation of anaplastic, 156
  formation of grade 2, 156
  gliomatosis cerebri, 153, 153t
  grading of cerebral, 152t
  histologic features of cerebral, 153t
  infiltrative fibrillary, 134
  low-grade, 153, 153t
  magnetic resonance imaging (MRI) of, 405, 406*f*
  midbrain, 153, 153t
  NF-1 and, 41
  optic pathway, 153, 153t
  pontine, 153, 153t
  scoliosis and, 405
  suprasellar, 144
  symptoms of, 405
  (bi)thalamic, 153, 153t
Astrocytomas (intracranial), pleomorphic xanthoastrocytoma, 133
Ataxia
  alcohol consumption and, 90
  olivopontocerebellar degeneration (OPCD) and, 101
  superficial siderosis and, 236
Ataxia-telangiectasia (Louis-Bar syndrome), 41, 56*t*
  relationship of medulloblastoma to, 138
Atherosclerotic disease
  aortic arch and, 223
  arterial territories affected by, 193
  carotid artery bifurcation and, 223
  origin of vertebral arteries and, 223
atlantodental subluxation, juvenile rheumatoid arthritis (JRA) and, 376
Atypical teratoid rhabdoid tumor (ATRT). *See also* Tumors
  histology of, 138, 139*f*
Atypical teratoid rhabdoid tumor. *See* Tumors
Aventriculy, 11, 12*f*
Axonal transport, hormones carried by, 177

B

Basilar artery apex aneurysm, 245, 245*f*
Bacterial meningitis. *See also* Meningitis
  bacteria producing, 273, 274*t*
  complications associated with, 273
  extra axial empyemas and, 274
  imaging studies and, 273
  subdural empyemas and, 275*f*
Bacterial spinal meningitis, disorders of spine in child and, 361
Balo's concentric sclerosis
  MRI features of, 70, 73, 73*f*
  multiple sclerosis (MS) and, 70, 73, 73*f*
  prognosis of, 73–74
Band heterotrophias, 30, 31, 34*f*
Basal ganglia
  calcifications of, 105
  conditions resulting from, 313*b*
  hypoglycemia and, 89, 89*f*
  increased T1 signal intensity and, 79
  lesions of
    Wilson's disease and, 85
  in liver failure, 79, 80*f*
Basilar artery occlusion, cerebellar infarcts and, 213
Basilar artery thrombosis
  DWI images of, 214*f*
  endovascular thrombolysis and, 198
  etiologies for, 213
  images of, 214*f*
  intra arterial thrombolysis and, 213
  MRI and, 213
  types of, 213
Benign compression fractures, on magnetic resonance imaging (MRI), 357*t*
Benign external hydrocephalus. *See also* Hydrocephalus
  children and, 122–123, 123*f*
Bens Jones proteins, multiple myeloma and, 389
Beveled edge sign, eosinophilic granuloma and, 148, 148*f*
Bilateral interfacetal dislocations
  computed tomography (CT) of, 353*f*
Bilateral interfacetal dislocations, indications of, 352–353
Bilaterally locked facets, 353
Bilirubin encephalopathy. *See* Kernicterus
Bilirubin, kernicterus and, 81
Bitemporal hemianopsia, causes of, 186
BI thalamic astrocytomas, 153, 153t, 269
Blastomycosis, nonspecific appearance of, 287*f*
Blindness, ethylene glycol and, 93
Blood blister-like aneurysms, description of, 247
Blood oxygenation level-dependent (BOLD) imaging, capillary telangiectasia and, 253
Blood-brain barrier (BBB), cerebral infarctions and, 107, 195
Bloom of T2 hypointense lesions, differential diagnosis of, 252*b*
Blue rubber bleb syndrome, multiple venous angiomas in, 251
Bone grafts
  abnormalities with, 455
  disk herniation and, 448
  disk herniations and, 455, 455*f*, 456*f*
  kyphosis with, 455

magnetic resonance imaging (MRI) and, 453–454, 455*f*
shapes of, 448–449, 449, 450
spinal canal stenosis and, 455
Bone malignancy, and multiple myeloma, 389
Bone marrow transplantation, neoplasia secondary to, 311
Borrelia burgdorferi, Lyme disease and, 292
Brachial plexopathies
allergy to drugs and, 471
cervical rib syndrome and, 472
Dejerine-Klumpke palsy and, 466
edema in, 469*f*
Erb-Duchenne palsy and, 466
postirradiation of, 471*f*
traumatic avulsions in, 466
tumors in, 468, 469–470, 469*f*
types of, 466
Brachial plexus (BP)
anatomy of, 463, 464*f*
avulsion in newborns, 465*t*, 466*f*
clinical evaluation of, 466
hematoma and, 467*f*
imaging general anatomy vs anatomy of, 465*t*
innervation provided by, 465*t*
leukemia infiltrating, 471*f*
old injury to, 468*f*
surgical anatomy vs anatomy of, 465*t*
Bradykinesia, Parkinson's and, 99
Brain
abscess of
tubercular, 296
zygomycosis and, 285
amyloid and, 102
atrophy with Wilson's disease, 85
classification of traumatic injuries to, 258*t*
Creutzfeldt-Jakob disease (CJD) and, 292
diminished cerebral blood flow and, 194
diseases affecting, 102–104
edema and, 103
effects of liver disease on, 80
effects of miscellaneous systemic disorders on, 106–107
effects of radiation on, 303*t*
human immunodeficiency virus (HIV) infection and, 278–279
lead intoxication and, 93
manganese (Mn) and, 80
metastases to, 165
mucormycosis and, 285
phycomycosis and, 285
radiation injury to, 301
radionuclide scans of, 196
renal disorders affecting, 103*b*
secondary tumors and, 311
technetium-99m-hexamethyl-propylene amine oxime in scan of (TC-HMPAO), 196
thyroid gland disorders affecting, 104–105
Brain atrophy
Acute disseminated encephalomyelitis (ADEM) and, 74
carbon monoxide intoxication and, 92
Menkes' syndrome and, 86
metachromatic leukodystrophy, 67*f*
mucopolysaccharidoses and, 62
in multiple sclerosis (MS), 73
Brain cysts
Alexander's disease and, 51
tuberous sclerosis (TS) and, 51
Brain hemorrhages
hypertensive, 239, 239*t*
posttraumatic, 239, 239*t*
Brain injuries
after child abuse, 267, 267*b*
arteriovenous fistulas and, 262
choroid plexus injuries and, 261
thrombosis and, 262
Brain irradiation
abnormalities associated with, 304
effects of, 301
leukoencephalopathy and, 301
sequela of, 301
transitional malformations and, 253
Brain lesions, carbon monoxide (CO) and, 92
Brain tumors, radiation induced, 304*f*, 304*t*
Brainstem astrocytomas, 134–136, 135*f*
hydrocephalus and, 135
pilocytic type of, 134
Brainstem gliomas
differential association between neurofibromatosis type one and, 134–136
on FLAIR, 135
hydrocephalus and, 135
prognosis of, 134–135
Brainstem infarctions
imaging modalities and, 213
Brainstem shearing injury. *See also* Shearing injuries
axial computed tomography of, 259*f*
Brainstem tumors
midbrain (mesencephalic) gliomas and, 136
in NF-1 and, 42
Breakthrough bleeding, hemorrhagic infarctions and, 211
Brownian motion of water, diffusion magnetic resonance imaging and, 204
Brown-Sèquard syndrome
disks (herniated) associated with, 340
Bulging annulus
in lumbar region, 413–414
spinal canal stenosis and, 413
surgery and, 413–414
tears relative to, 413
Bulging, disk pathology and, 415
Bulk flow, 117
Buphthalmos, neurofibromatosis type 1and, 45
Burst fracture, 356

C

Calcifications, 79
Calcifications, arteriovenous malformations (AVMs) and, 248–249
Calloseptal interface, 72
Calvarial linear fractures, 268–269. *See also* Fractures
Calvarial tuberculosis, pathologic course of, 296
Calvarium
eosinophilic granuloma and, 148
Canalization, 315, 316
Canavan's disease (spongiform leukoencephalopathy), 61–62
basal ganglia and, 61–62, 61*f*
compared to van der Knapp's disease, 61–62
Canavan's disease, differential diagnosis compared to Cree leukoencephalopathy, 62
Capillary telangiectases
brain irradiation and, 304
cavernous angioma and, 253
venous angiomas and, 253
Capillary telangiectasia
blood oxygenation level-dependent (BOLD) imaging, 253
etiology of, 253
image of, 253*f*
in pons, 253
Carbon monoxide (CO) intoxication, 92, 92*f*
Carotid artery
bifurcation of
surgical intervention at, 223
location of dissections in, 225
Carotid artery stenosis, diagnosis of, 223
Catheter angiography, for cerebral vasculitis, 217
Caudal regression syndrome, 317
causes of, 326
forms of, 326
imaging of, 327*f*
levels and incidence of, 326*t*
scoliosis and, 326
systemic syndromes associated with, 326
two types of, 326
Cavernous angioma
capillary telangiectasias and, 253
cerebral vascular malformation and, 251
image of, 439*f*
internal features of, 251
magnetic resonance imaging (MRI) and, 251, 439*f*
symptoms of, 251, 437
temporal lobe and, 111*f*
Cavernous hemangiomas, brain irradiation and, 304
Cavernous malformations. *See* Cavernous angioma, Hemangioma
Cavernous sinus fistula
classifications of, 250
imaging findings of, 250
signs of, 250
Cavernous sinus-internal carotid artery fistula, posttrauma arteriovenous fistula and, 26
Cebocephaly, holoprosencephaly and, 18*t*
Central cord syndrome, disks (herniated) associated with, 340

Central herniation, 262
Central nervous system (CNS), 55*t*
  chemotherapeutic agents for, 308
    complications of, 308
  cysticercosis and, 288
  ethylene glycol and, 92
  hyperglycemia and, 96
  iron metabolism effects on, 87
  Methanol (methyl alcohol) intoxication and, 94
  NF-1 and, 41, 45
  thyroid gland disorders and, 104–105
  tumors in neurobibromatosis type 2, 47*t*
  uncommon fungal infections of, 287*t*
Central neurocytoma
  diagnosis of, 160
  imaging of, 160*f*
Central pontine myelinolysis (CPM), 69*f*
  extrapontine myelinolysis and, 70
  histology of, 69–70
  hypernatremia and, 69
  hyponatremia and, 69
  imaging studies and, 70
  normonatremia and, 69
  osmotic myelinolysis and, 69
Central spinal canal stenosis, 422*f*
Central spinal fluid (CSF)
  encephaloceles and leak of, 28
  open-lip schizencephaly and, 20
Cerebellar artery infarctions, posterior inferior cerebellar artery (PICA) occluded in, 212, 212*f*
Cerebellar atrophy, alcoholics and, 90
Cerebellar calcification
  causes of, 105*t*
Cerebellar herniation, 2113
Cerebellar hypoplasia
  anomalies associated with, 9*t*
Cerebellar medulloblastomas. *See* Medulloblastomas
Cerebellopontine angle lipomas, 56*t*
Cerebellopontine angle, most common masses occurring at, 150*b*
Cerebellopontine angle region, subarachnoid space lipomas and, 24*t*
Cerebellum, embryology of, 1
Cerebral abscesses, 274
  features of, 274–275
  stages in formation of, 277–278*f*, 277*t*
Cerebral astrocytomas. *See* Astrocytomas
Cerebral catheter angiography (CCA)
  information obtained from, 194–195
  risk factors of, 194–195
  signs associated with cerebral infarction obtained from, 194–195
Cerebral edema, shearing injuries and, 262
Cerebral hamartomas
  NF-1 and, 41
Cerebral infarction
  calcification in chronic, 208
  cerebral catheter angiography (CCA) and, 194–195
  in children, 225–226
    etiologies of, 225
    symptoms at presentation, 225
  contraindications for contrast media in, 195
  contrast-enhanced magnetic resonance imaging (MRI) findings in, 201*t*
  definition of, 194
  diffusion-weighted imaging with signal intensity changes of, 209*t*
  embolus and, 207
  incomplete
    definition of, 194
  magnetic resonance imaging (MRI) subfalcine herniation and, 262
Cerebral infarctions
  acute, 194
  blood-brain barrier (BBB) and, 195
  chronic, 194
  common sites of occurrence of, 206
  computed tomography (CT) and, 197
  diffusion-magnetic resonance imaging and, 204
  herniations resulting in, 262
  prognosis of patients with, 194*t*
  sources of emboli that cause, 223
  subacute, 194
Cerebral ischemia
  irreversible, 193–194
  reversible, 193–194
Cerebral vascular malformations
  arteriovenous shunting and, 248
  division according to blood flow of, 248*t*
  divisions according to angiographic appearance, 248
  symptoms of, 248
Cerebral vasculitis
  catheter angiography for, 217
  drugs associated with, 217
  etiology of, 216
  hemorrhage and, 217
  images of, 218*f*
  infectious etiologies for, 216–217, 217*t*
  noninfectious etiologies for, 216–217, 217*t*
Cerebral venous infarction
  in children, 225
  imaging findings of, 225
  seizures in children and, 226
Cerebral venous thrombosis, 221, 221*b*
  etiology for, 221
  images of, 222*f*
  prognosis for, 221
Cerebrospinal fluid (CSF)
  affected by hemorrhage, 121
  affected by infection, 121
  disorders of flow of, 117–131
  empty sella syndrome and, 189
  intracranial hypotension and, 121, 124–125
  overproduction of, 121
  pathophysiology of, 117–118
  subdural hygroma and, 263
  trapped ventricles and, 129–130, 129*f*
  tumors and, 121
Cervical neural foramina
  anatomical examination of, 423
  imaging of, 423
Cervical radiculomedullary arteries, vertebral arteries supplying, 433
Cervical spine
  advantages of surgical posterior approach on, 448
  bright herniation, 419, 419*f*
  bulging annulus in, 414
  disadvantages of surgical posterior approach on, 448
  magnetic resonance imaging (MRI) evaluation of, 417, 418*f*, 419
  microsurgical techniques on, 448
  myelopathy in, 417
  osteophytes and, 419
  symptoms from spondylolysis in, 417
Cervical spine (lower) fractures, 351–354
  classification of, 351
Cervical spine surgery
  complications of, 452–458
  imaging of complications, 452–458
  postoperative magnetic resonance imaging (MRI) evaluation of, 452
CFS. *See* Cerebrospinal fluid
CFS. *See* Chronic fatigue syndrome
Chance fractures
  definition of, 356
  images of, 357*f*
  thoracolumbar region and, 356
Charcot-Bouchard aneurysms
  hypertension and, 239
Charcot-Marie-Tooth disease (CMT)
  hereditary polyneuropathies and, 372–373
  imaging of, 372–373, 372*f*
Chèdiak-Higashi syndrome, 41, 56*t*
Chemotherapeutic agents
  brain perfusion studies and, 309
  effects of, 308–310
  for lymphocytic leukemia
    neuropsychological deficits with, 309
  permanent effects of on central nervous system (CNS), 309
  for treatment of central nervous system (CNS) lesions, 308
Chiari 1
  characteristics of, 5, 6*f*
  symptoms of, 5, 6*f*
  tonsillar herniation and, 5, 6*f*
Chiari 2
  magnetic resonance imaging abnormalities and, 7*t*
  malformation in, 8*f*
  sonography and, 5
  symptoms of, 6
Chiari 3, 8*f*
  hydrocephalus and, 9
  malformation in, 8*f*
  meningoencephalocele and, 9
Chiari 4, 9
Chiari malformations
  chiari 1, 5, 6*f*
  chiari 2, 5–6, 7*t*, 8*f*
Chiasmatic gliomas, optic nerve involvement with, 145
Child abuse
  blood of different ages and, 268*f*

causes of brain injury after, 267*b*
cerebral edema and, 267–268
cerebral infarctions and, 268
cranial traumas in, 257
fractures and, 267
imaging for assessing, 269
subarachnoid hemorrhage (SAH) and, 267
Chordomas, 150, 151
bone tumors and, 396
calcifications in, 151, 152*f*
common sites for, 396
histology of, 396
imaging of, 151, 152*f*, 396, 397*f*
location of, 396*t*
sacral, 150, 151
Choroid plexus
carcinomas, 146–147
differential diagnosis for lesions, 146, 147*t*
hydrocephalus and, 121
injuries
brain injury with, 261
hydrocephalus and, 261
post trauma hemorrhage in, 261
subarachnoid space lipomas and, 24*t*
tumors
choroid plexus papillomas (CPP) and, 145
imaging of, 145–146
Choroid plexus papillomas (CPP)
differential diagnosis of choroid plexus carcinoma and, 145
edema with, 146, 146*f*
hydrocephalus and, 120, 145, 146
image of, 147*f*
Choroidal fissure cysts
imaging and, 166
seizures and, 166
Choroidal vein of galen malformations polymicrogyria, symptoms of, 28
Chronic fatigue syndrome (CFS)
characterizations of, 106
MRI studies and, 106
SPECT studies and, 106
Circle of Willis, intracranial aneurysm and, 242
Clivus, differential diagnosis for masses in, 151
Closed spinal dysraphism, 316, 321–323
associated anomalies in, 322*b*
symptoms of, 321
Closed-lip schizencephaly. *See* Schizencephaly
Clot (acute), physiology of, 232
CO intoxication. *See* Carbon monoxide (CO) intoxication
Cocaine, cerebral vasculitis and, 217
Cockayne's syndrome, 41, 56*t*
Colloid cysts
hydrocephalus with, 168
imaging of, 168, 169*f*
symptoms associated with, 168
Communicating hydrocephalus, 121–122. *See also* Hydrocephalus
achondroplasia and, 117
Complex vascular malformations
spinal
Cobb's syndrome and, 438*f*, 438*t*
syndromes associated with, 438*t*
syndromes associated with, 438*t*
Compound CS (craniosynostosis), 36*t*
Compound fractures
skin lacerations and, 269
Compression fractures
imaging modalities for treatment of, 354
Computed tomographic angiography (CTA)
carotid bifurcations and, 198–199
intercranial aneurysms and, 198–199
study procedure using, 198–199
Computed tomography (CT)
in acute infarction, 198*f*
appearance of subarachnoid blood with, 234, 234*f*
cerebral infarctions and, 197
detecting hemorrhage with, 197
intraaxial hemorrhage and, 231
studies of cerebral infarction using, 199
subdural hematomas and, 235, 235*f*
Congenital
anomalies
infratentorial, 1–15
supratentorial, 15–38
scoliosis
diagnosis of, 336
symptoms of, 336
Congenital white matter disorders. *See* Leukodystrophies
Conjoined nerve roots, vs herniated disk, 423
Contusions
cause of, 260
imaging of, 260, 261*f*
multiple, 260
Conus medullaris, and tight filum terminale syndrome, 329–330
Convexity epidural hematomas, identity of, 265
Copper
metabolism
disorders of, 85–87
Wilson's disease and, 85
Corpectomies, 449
Coronal CS (craniosynostosis), 36*t*
Coronal suture synostosis, 37*f*
Corpus callosum
agenesis of, 16*f*–17*f*
alcohol abuse and, 90
dysgenesis of, 15–17, 16*f*–17*f*
myelination of, 60
myelination of on T1-weighted images, 15*t*
Cortical
dysplasia, 30–38, 32–33, 34*f*
versus mesial temporal lobe heterotopia, 33*f*
Taylor, balloon cell type, 34
dystrophic calcifications
Sturge-Weber syndrome and, 54
organization, 30
PMG and, 32
Cortical contusions, 260–261. *See also* Contusions
Cortisol, anorexia nervosa and, 106
Cowden's syndrome, 41, 56*t*
Lhermitte-duclos disease (LDD) in relation to, 140
CPM. *See* Central pontine myelinolysis
Cranial nerve palsies
brain irradiation and, 305
Cranial neuropathies
multiple sclerosis (MS) and, 70
superficial siderosis and, 236
Cranial traumas, 257–270
child abuse and, 257
classification of, 257
general facts of, 257
Craniopharyngiomas, 143*f*
adult onset of, 144
hemorrhagic adenomas and, 182
histology of, 142–144
imaging features in children, 143*t*
locations for, 142–144, 142*t*
pituitary gland and, 182
rules of 80% for, 142–144
symptoms produced by, 143*t*
Craniosynostosis, 36–38
imaging of, 36*t*
osseous abnormalities and, 122
Crank-case oil, cysts and, 144
Cree leukoencephalopathy
differential diagnosis of Canavan's disease and, 62
Creutzfeldt-Jakob disease (CJD)
brain and, 292
dementia and, 292
histologic features of, 292
T2-weighted image of, 293*f*
Crigler-Najjar disease, kernicterus and, 81
Cryptococcal granulomas (cryptococcomas), immune status and, 283
Cryptococcosis neoformans
AIDS and, 283
brain and, 283
meningitis and, 283
multiple cysts in basal ganglia and, 284*f*
CS. *See* Craniosynostosis, 36–38
CSF-filled cysts
causes of, 401
classifications of, 401
involving nerve roots, 402
locations of, 401–402
mechanism of, 401
origin of, 401
radiculopathies and, 403
symptoms of, 401
Cyclopia, holoprosencephaly and, 18*t*
Cyclosporine
blood pressure and, 306
hypertensive encephalopathy and, 220
manifestations of PRES and, 103
Cyclosporine tacrolimus-induced encephalopathy, imaging of, 307*f*
symptoms of, 306
Cyclosporine toxicity
mechanisms responsible for, 307
symptoms related to, 306

Cystic lesions, imaging and, 283
Cysticercosis
affecting central nervous system (CNS), 370
albendazole for treatment of, 370
anticysticercal drugs for, 370
clinical features of, 288
cysts and, 409
diagnostic tests for, 370
imaging of, 288, 289*f*, 370*f*
immunocompetent population and, 287, 287*t*
praziquantel for treatment of, 370
sites in central nervous system affected by, 288*t*
stages of, 288*t*
types of, 287, 287*t*
Cysts
CSF filled, 401
extramedullary CSF-filled
sites of occurrence, 342
ganglioglioma and, 407
hemangioblastomas and, 149–150
pituitary glands and, 182
Cytomegalovirus, infectious cause of vasculitis and, 439
Cytotoxic edema, 194
cerebral blood flow and, 194
etiology of, 308

D

Dandy-Walker syndrome, 1, 3, 3*f*
posterior fossa arachnoid cysts, 4
Dandy-Walker variant, hydrocephalus and, 1–3, 2*f*
Dawson fingers, 70, 72
Degenerative disk disease, 413
Dejerine-Sottas disease (DS), hypomyelinating neuropathy and, 373
Dementia
amyloidosis and, 102
Creutzfeldt-Jakob disease (CJD) and, 292
Dens fractures
classification (types) of, 350, 350*t*
computed tomography (CT) of, 350*f*
Deoxyhemoglobin, subacute hemorrhage and, 233
Depressed fractures
cause of, 269
clinical results of, 269
Dermal sinus tracts
dermoid tumors and, 323
epidermoid tumors and, 323
goal of imaging, 323
intraspinal abscesses and, 368–369
locations of defects in, 323
procedure for imaging, 325
symptoms related to, 325
Dermoid
cause of, 167
chemical meningitis produced by, 167
common sites for, 167
fourth ventricular, 14, 15*f*
image of fatty, 186*f*
imaging of, 325*f*
imaging of fat droplets spilled from, 169f
tumor
classifications of, 323, 324*t*
etiology of, 13
Desmoplastic medulloblastomas (lateral cerebellar medulloblastomas), 138
Development venous anomalies, 251. *See also* Venous angioma
Devic's disease (neuromyelitis optica), 74
diagnosis of, 367
gadolinium and, 367
histologic process of, 367
magnetic resonance imaging (MRI) and, 367, 367*f*
MRI findings for, 74
nerves affected with, 367
Diabetes insipidus
posterior ectopic lobe and, 179
transection of pituitary stalk and, 269
Diastatic fractures
cranial suture(s), 269
Diastema, 333
Diastematomyelia, 333
computed tomography (CT) of, 334*f*
etiology for, 333
types of, 333, 334*t*
Diethylene glycol
clinical manifestations of, 92–93
toxicity of, 92
Diffuse axonal injuries
mechanisms for associated damage with, 260
shearing
common locations for, 257
head trauma and, 257
Diffuse brain anoxia
etiologies for, 213
Diffuse brain edema
child abuse and, 267
subarachnoid hemorrhage (SAH) and, 266
Diffuse brain hypoxia
etiologies for, 213
MRI and, 213
neonatal
periventricular leukomalacia (PVL) and, 226
white matter and, 226
Diffuse neonatal hypoxia, periventricular leukomalacia and, 226
Diffusion-weighted magnetic resonance imaging (DWI)
acute infarction and, 205*f*
Brownian motion of water and, 204
cerebral infarctions and, 204
compared to conventional MRI, 204
dermoids and, 13
epidermoids and, 13, 14*f*
physiologic information from, 204
posterior reversible encephalopathy syndrome (PRES) and, 103
stratification of infarctions *vs.* TIAs with, 204
thrombolytic therapy and, 204
water and, 238
Diplococcus pneumoniae, causative agent for diskitis (infectious) in children, 378
Diplomyelia, split cord syndrome and, 335
Disjunction
ectodermal elements and, 315
Disk herniations. *See also* Herniated disks
with bone grafts, 455
Brown-Sèquard syndrome and, 340
central cord syndrome and, 340
internuclear cleft and, 415
residual or recurrent, 446
surgical anterior approach on, 448–449, 449*f*
Diskitis. *See also* Osteomyelitis
fungal
infection in disk space in, 380
infectious
cervical spinal involvement in, 378
clinical diagnosis of, 378
differential diagnosis of, 378
imaging of, 378*f*
mechanism of infection spread in, 378
predisposing factors in, 378
Staphylococcus aureus and, 378
thoracic spinal involvement in, 378
various healing stages in, 380*t*
Dissection of extracranial blood vessels, 224–225
causes for, 224–225
evaluations with catheter angiography, 224–225
MRA and, 225
MRI and, 224–225
Doppler sonography. *See* Transcranial Doppler sonography (TCD)
Dowel (Cloward fusion)
bone grafts and, 449
Downward herniation, 262
Duplicated pituitary gland, 180
imaging of, 181*f*
Duplicated pituitary gland. *See also* Pituitary gland
Dural arteriovenous fistula (AVF), 436*f*
Duret hemorrhages, downward herniations and, 262
Dysautonomia, 41
Dysembryoplastic neuroepithelial tumor (DNET), of temporal lobe, 110*f*
Dysgenesis of corpus callosum. *See* Corpus callosum
Dysplasia of Taylor, 35*f*
Dysraphism. *See also* Open spinal dysraphism
diagnosis of, 318
sonography and, 318
in utero repair of, 318

E

Ecchorndrosis physaliphora, 151
chordoma and, 396
Ectopic (translocated) posterior pituitary lobe, images of, 181*f*
Edema
in brachial plexopathies, 469*f*
brain, 103

metastases and, 166
vasogenic, 194
Emboli, arterial territories affected by, 193
Embryonic development, alcohol and, 91
Empty sella syndrome
causes of, 189
cerebral spinal fluid (CSF) and, 189
pseudotumor cerebri and, 189
visual field deficits with, 189
Encephalitis
chronic fatigue syndrome and, 106
temporal lobe epilepsy and, 111
Encephaloceles. *See also* Occipital encephaloceles
anteriorly located, 28
ethmoidal, 28*f*
nasofrontal, 27*f*
nasoorbital, 27*f*
posterior, 11, 12*f*
Encephalopathy
uremic, 103
Encephalotrigeminal angiomatosis. *See* Sturge-Weber syndrome (SW)
Endolymphatic sac tumor (cystadenoma), 56*f*
Endoscopic ventriculostomies
hydrocephalus treatment using, 130–131, 130*f*
nonfunctioning third, 131*f*
MRI and, 131
Endplate. *See* Vertebral endplate
Eosinophilic granuloma (EG)
calvarium and, 148
histiocytosis and, 148*f*, 148*t*
Langerhans cell histiocytosis and, 392
spinal cord involvement with, 392
thoracic region involvement with, 392
vertebra plana and, 392, 392*f*
Ependyma injury, 261
Ependymomas, 140*f*
clinical symptoms of, 138–139
imaging of, 138–139
NF-2 and, 46
spinal cord and, 403
Ependymomas (spinal)
differential diagnosis of, 405
division of, 403
magnetic resonance imaging (MRI) appearance of, 403, 404*f*
subclinical bleeds and, 403
symptoms of, 403
Epidermoid, fourth ventricular, 14, 15*f*
Epidermoid tumors
classifications of, 323, 324*t*
etiology of, 13
images of, 324*f*
Epidermoids
images of, 168*f*
imaging used for differentiating cysts from, 166–167
MRI sequences and, 13, 14*f*
Epidural abscess
causative organisms for, 383
etiology of, 383
findings on postcontrast magnetic resonance imaging (MRI), 383, 384*f*
infectious spread with, 383
and neurologic signs in children, 383
predisposing factors for, 383
regions affected, 383
symptoms of, 383
Epidural fibrosis (scar), images of, 445
Epidural hematomas, 265
arterial *vs.* venous, 341
brain herniations and, 265
computed tomography (CT) and, 236*f*
diagnosis of, 265
image of, 341*f*
imaging modalities used for, 265, 265*f*
from lumbar puncture, 341
magnetic resonance imaging (MRI) and, 237–238
middle meningeal artery and, 265
from spinal surgery, 341
Epidural lipomatosis
appearance on magnetic resonance imaging (MRI) of, 398, 399*f*
exogenous steroid therapy and, 398
morbidly obese patients and, 398
Epidural scar
etiology of, 446
imaging with contrast and, 446
Epilepsy
heterotopia and, 30
seizures and, 107
sites of epileptogenic foci with, 107
Erdheim-Chester disease, pituitary gland and, 189*t*
Ergot derivatives, cerebral vasculitis and, 217
Escherichia coli, causative agent for diskitis (infectious), 378
Ethanol abuse. *See* Alcohol abuse
Ethmocephaly, holoprosencephaly and, 18*t*
Ethmoidal encephalocele, 28*f*
Ethylene glycol intoxication, treatment for, 92, 93*f*
External carotid artery (ECA), arteriovenous malformations (AVMs) and, 250
External herniation. *See also* Transcalvarial herniation
brain and, 262
Extraaxial empyemas
with bacterial meningitis, 274
in children, 274
Extraaxial hemorrhage, 234–237
appearance of by computed topography (CT), 235*t*
Extracerebral injury
epidural hematoma and, 265
Extracerebral injury, epidural hematomas and, 263
Extracranial arterial disease, 223–224
Extradural lesions
classification of, 387
metastases and, 388
multiple, 388
Extrapontine myelinolysis, central pontine myelinolysis (CPM) and, 70
Eye of the tiger, Hallervorden-Spatz disease and, 88, 88*f*

F

Facet joints, changes in, 422
Facial dysraphism, sincipital encephaloceles and, 28
Failed back surgery syndrome
etiologies for, 444*b*
recurrent symptoms and, 443, 444*b*
FAS. *See* Fetal alcohol syndrome
Fetal alcohol syndrome (FAS), alcohol abuse and, 90, 91
Fibrinoid leukodystrophy. *See* Alexander's disease
Fibromuscular dysplasia (FMD)
stroke like symptoms and, 195–196
view from catheter angiogram of, 224*f*
Filar lipoma, 327–328
Filum terminale
differential diagnosis of mass from, 405
lipomas of, 327
paragangliomas and, 407
Fistula, 335
FLAIR
acute disseminated encephalomyelitis (ADEM) and, 74
Adrenoleukodystrophy (ALD) and, 65*f*
ALS (amyotrophic lateral sclerosis), 97–98, 98*f*
brainstem gliomas on, 135
bright cerebrospinal fluid (CSF) on, 236
MELAS syndrome (mitochondrial myopathy, encephalopathy, lactic acidosis and strokes) and, 83*f*
subarachnoid hemorrhage (SAH) imaged on, 236
ventilation devices and, 236
FLAIR images brainstem infarcts and, 201
FLAIR imaging multiple sclerosis (MS) and, 70–73*f*
Flocculonodular lobule, 1
Focal cerebral edema, causes of, 262
Focal ischemia, herniation and, 262
Focal lesions
Graft-*versus*-host disease (GVHD) and, 310
Foramina
lateral, 1
midline, 1
Foramina of Monro, giant cell astrocytoma (GCA) and, 51
Fracture-dislocations, etiology of, 354–355
Fractures
calvarial linear, 268
complex, 269
of petrous temporal bone, 269
pneumocephalus and, 269
Free fragment (sequestered fragment), 415, 417*f*
Friedreich's ataxia
characterizations of, 373
iron metabolism and, 88–89
neuropathies and, 373
Frontonasal region, formation of, 25
Functional MRI (blood oxygenation level-dependent technique), seizure foci and, 107–108

Fungal infections, 283–290
  spinal cord and, 369–370
Fungi
  less common
    nonspecific imaging finding of, 285, 287*t*
Fusion
  degenerative changes in, 455*f*
  kyphosis at site of, 455

G

Gadolinium chelates
  for acute disseminated encephalomyelitis (ADEM), 361–362
  Devic's disease (neuromyelitis optica) and, 367
  differentiation of herniated disk post, 443
  enhancement in neurofibromas, 400
  enhancement in schwannomas, 400
  magnetic resonance imaging (MRI) and, 200
  MRA artifact and, 202
  osteoblastomas (giant osteoid osteomas) with, 395
  postsurgical spinal infection and, 453
  subdural hematomas and, 237
Gangliocytoma, 140–142
  desmoplastic infantile, 142*f*
Ganglioglioma
  central nervous system (CNS) and, 407
  characteristics on MRI, 140, 141*f*
  diagnosis of, 407
  imaging of, 407, 408*f*
  locations of, 407
Ganglion cell tumors. *See also* Tumors
  seizures and, 140
Ganglion cysts, 424
Ganglioneuroma, 140–142
Gelastic seizures, hamartoma of tuber cinereum (hypothalamic hamartomas) and, 171
Gelatinous pseudocysts
  cystic lesions and, 283
Genes, affecting spinal formation, 317
Germinal matrix
  location of, 239
  pregnancy and, 239
  premature infants and, 239
Germinal matrix hemorrhage, 239
  four classifications of, 239, 240*t*
  four grades of, 239
  periventricular leukomalacia, 239
Germinoma, image of, 162*f*
Giant aneurysms
  common sites for, 247
  magnetic resonance imaging (MRI) characteristics of, 247*f*
Giant cell astrocytoma (GCA), 133
  hydrocephalus and, 51, 145
  tuberous sclerosis (TS) and, 51, 52*f*, 145
  ventricular shunt and, 145
Giant cell granulomas
  pituitary gland and, 189*t*
  in sella turcica post surgically, 190
Giant cell tumor (GCT)
  common locations of, 394, 394*f*
  magnetic resonance imaging (MRI) and, 394, 394*f*
  metastasis and, 394
Giant disk herniation
  imaging of, 418*f*, 419
Giant heterotopias, 30, 33*f*
Giant oral pyogenic granulomas
  Sturge-Weber syndrome and, 51
Gilbert's disease
  kernicterus and, 81
Glioblastoma multiforme (GBM), 152, 152*t*
  cerebral gliomas and, 154
  histologic features of, 154
  imaging studies of, 154, 155*f*
  primary type of, 155
  secondary type of, 155
Gliomatosis cerebri, 153, 153t
  diagnosis of, 156
  image of, 157*f*
  imaging studies of, 156
Gliosis, temporal lobe epilepsy and, 111
Globi pallidi
  carbon monoxide intoxication and, 92, 92*f*
  Huntington's disease and, 96
Globoid cell leukodystrophy. *See* Krabbe's disease
Glutamate, thiamine depleted brain regions and, 90
Glutaric aciduria, 84
Glutaric aciduria type 1, 84, 84*f*
Gorlin's syndrome (basal cell nevus syndrome), 41, 56*t*
  relationship of medulloblastoma to, 138
Grafts. *See also* Bone grafts
  disk herniations and, 448
Graft-*versus*-host disease (GVHD)
  bone transplantation and, 310
  contrast enhancement with, 310
  focal lesions and, 310
  organs affected, 310
Granulomatous angiitis
  clinical symptoms with, 439–440
  spinal cord and, 439–440
Gray matter, hypoglycemia and, 89
Gray matter malformations, 30*t*
Guillain-Barre syndrome (GB)
  causes of, 371
  histologic description of, 371
  magnetic resonance imaging (MRI) findings for, 371, 371*f*
  symptoms of, 371
  treatment of, 371
GVHD. *See* Graft-*versus*-host disease
Gyral enhancement
  subacute MCA and, 207

H

Haemophilus influenza type B, meningitis and, 274
Hallervorden-Spatz disease (HS), 88, 88*f*
  eye of the tiger and, 88, 88*f*
  genetic defects in, 88
Hamartin, tuberous sclerosis (TS) and, 48
Hamartoma of tuber cinereum (hypothalamic hamartomas)
  imaging studies of, 171, 171*f*
  symptoms of, 171
Hamartomas, 42
  FLAIR images and, 44, 44*f*
Hand-Schuller-Christian disease
  exophthalmos and, 148*t*, 149
  histiocytosis and, 148*t*, 149
Hangman's fracture (traumatic spondylolysis of C2)
  computed tomography (CT) of, 348, 348t, 349*f*
  grades of, 348, 348t, 349*f*
  hyperextension and, 348
Hardware
  complications from, 456
  fractures of, 456–457, 458*f*
  lumbar region, 456
  plate dislodgement of, 458*f*
  pseudoarthrosis and, 456
  radiographs for misplaced, 456, 457*f*
  thoracic spine, 456
Harrington rods
  laminectomies and, 451–452
Headache, hamartoma of tuber cinereum (hypothalamic hamartomas) and, 171
Heart failure, hypoglycemia and, 89
Hemangioblastomas (HB)
  cysts and, 149–150, 406
  histology of, 149–150
  image of, 149*f*
  imaging of, 406, 407*f*
  origination in spinal cord of, 405
  pial based tumors and, 57
  symptoms of, 405
  Von Hippel-Lindau disease (VHL) and, 54, 149, 405
Hemangioma. *See* Vertebral hemangioma
Hematoma. *See also* Spinal epidural hematoma; Spontaneous epidural hematoma
  brachial plexus (BP) and, 467*f*, 468*f*
  hemosiderin and, 237
    amyloidosis and, 102
    epidural, 237
    subdural, 237, 264*f*
Hemichorea-hemiballism (HH)
  clinical manifestations of, 96–97
  hyperglycemia and, 96–97
  MRI studies and, 96–97
Hemicord, split cord syndrome and, 333
Hemimegalencephaly, 35, 36*f*
Hemimyelocele
  anatomy of, 321
  open dysaphisms and, 315
Hemispheric astrocytomas
  in children, 145
  symptoms of, 145
Hemochromatosis, intestinal iron absorption and, 87
Hemoglobin
  computed tomography (CT scan and moiety of, 231

Hemolytic-uremic syndrome
hypertensive encephalopathy and, 220
kidneys and brain affected by, 103
tomography and, 104*f*
Hemophilus influenzae, bacterial meningitis and, 273
Hemorrhage
amyloidosis-related, 102*f*
cerebral vasculitis and, 217
in choroid plexus injuries, 261
chronic sequelae of, 231
on diffusion-weighted imaging (DWI), 238, 238*f*
magnetic resonance imaging (MRI) of hematoma in, 232*f*
MCA infarctions with, 207
measurement of clot in, 231
pituitary, 187, 188, 189
venous thrombosis and, 239
Hemorrhages, Duret, 262
Hemorrhagic infarction, 211*f*
Hemorrhagic infarctions
acute blood in, 211
CT imaging and, 211
etiology of, 211
imaging preferences for, 211, 211*f*
laminar necrosis and, 211
septic embolism and, 211
venous infarcts and, 211
Hemosiderin, hematomas and, 237
Heparinization
cerebral infarctions and, 197
Hepatic encephalopathy
manganese (Mn) and, 80
proton MR spectroscopy (MRS), 80–81
Hepatic failure, Wilson's disease and, 85
Hepatic insufficiency, abnormalities on brain MRI and, 79
Hepatolenticular degeneration, 85–86. *See* Wilson's disease
Hepatorenal syndrome, kidneys and brain affected by, 103
Hereditary polyneuropathies
Charcot-Marie-Tooth disease (CMT) and, 372–373
disorders associated with, 372–373
symptoms of, 372–373
types of, 372–373
Herniated disks
cause of, 415
common sites for, 415–416
computed tomography (CT) of, 416*f*
location and incidence of lumbar, 417*t*
lumbosacral plexus (LSP) and, 472
magnetic resonance imaging (MRI) evaluation of, 417, 418*f*
radial tears and, 413, 414*f*
surgical open door technique for, 450
surgical posterior approach for, 449–450
symptoms of, 415
Herniations
causes of, 262
disk pathology and, 415
subfalcine, 262
transtentorial, 262
Heroin, cerebral vasculitis and, 217
Herpes simplex (viral infection)
encephalitis and, 281
etiology of, 281
FLAIR image and, 282*f*
histologic findings, 281
imaging studies of, 281
symptoms of, 281
Herpes zoster
magnetic resonance imaging (MRI) findings of, 369, 369*f*
myelitis and, 369
symptoms of, 369
Heterotopias
epilepsy and, 30
nodular gray matter, 32*f*
seizures and, 30
subcortical, 30
subependymal, 30
Hexamethylpropylene amine oxime (HMPAO), seizure evaluation with, 107
Hippocampal developmental anomalies, temporal lobe epilepsy and, 109, 110*f*
Hippocampal sclerosis (mesial temporal sclerosis), 107–112
diagnosis of, 109, 110*f*
Hippocampi
common pathologic processes affecting, 109–111
imaging and, 108
Histiocytosis, 148–149, 149*t*
T1-weighted image of, 190*f*
Holoprosencephaly, 17–20
brain abnormalities in, 20*t*
facial features and, 17
Homeobox genes (Hox A-D, Gbx, Dbx)
chiari 1 and, 5
Homocystinuria, amino aciduria and, 83
Homonymous hemianopsia
medial occipital lobe and, 211
Hormones, produced by adenohypophysis, 178*t*
Hox gene, spine formation and, 317
Human immunodeficiency virus (HIV), infectious cause of vasculitis and, 439
Hunter's disease, 64*f*, 65*t*
Huntington's disease, 96, 96*f*
Hurler's syndrome, spinal abnormalities in, 64*f*, 65*t*
Hydrocephalus
astrocytomas and, 42
bacterial meningitis, 273
benign external, 122–123
cerebellar infarcts and, 213
Chiari 1 and, 5
Chiari 2 and, 6
Chiari 3 and, 9
choroid plexus
injuries of, 261
choroid plexus and, 121
papillomas and, 120
papillomas (CPP) and, 145, 146
colloid cysts causing, 168
communicating, 117
Dandy-Walker variant and, 3
diagnosis of normal-pressure, 121–122
endoscopic ventriculostomies and, 130–131, 130*f*
etiologies of, 118*t*, 119*t*
features on imaging studies of, 118, 119*t*
giant cell astrocytoma (GCA) and, 51, 145
Menkes' syndrome and, 86
midbrain (mesencephalic) gliomas and, 136
middle cerebral artery aneurysm and, 244
noncommunicating, 117, 119*f*
etiologies of, 120*t*
in utero repair and, 7
ventricular diverticula and, 118–119*t*, 120*t*
Hypenatremia, central pontine myelinolysis (CPM) and, 69
Hyperammonemia, liver failure and, 80
Hyperextension dislocation, 351
magnetic resonance imaging (MRI) and, 351, 351*f*
Hyperextension injuries
herniated disks and, 351
ligamentous disruption in, 351
Hyperextension teardrop fracture, 351
osteoporosis and, 351
Hyperflexion injuries
diagnosis of, 352
disrupted ligaments in, 352
imaging of, 352
Hyperflexion teardrop fractures, indications of, 354
Hyperglycemia
affects on CNS and, 96
hemichorea-hemiballism (HH) and, 96–97, 97*f*
Hypernatremia, osmotic myelinolysis and, 68, 69
Hypertelorism
duplicated pituitary gland and, 180
hypothalamus and, 180
Sincipital encephaloceles and, 26, 28
Hypertension
brain abnormalities and, 103
Charcot-Bouchard aneurysms and, 239
Hypertensive encephalopathy
etiologies for, 220, 220*f*
lesions in, 220
images of, 220, 220*f*
seizures and, 220
Hypertensive hemorrhages
Charcot-Bouchard aneurysms and, 239
location and frequency of, 239, 239*t*
Hypertrophied ligamentum flavum, 422
Hypoglycemia, 89, 89*f*
sequelae of, 89, 89*f*
symptoms of, 89, 89*f*
Hypoglycemia, microcephaly and, 89
Hypogonadotropic hypogonadism, iron (Fe) and87
Hypomelanosis of Ito, 41, 56*t*
Hyponatremia
central pontine myelinolysis (CPM) and, 69

Hyponatremia (*continued*)
neurologic symptoms of, 69*t*
osmotic myelinolysis and, 68, 69
Hyponatremia encephalopathy, clinical systems of, 69*t*
Hypoplasia of optic nerves, septooptic dysplasia (SOD) and, 22
Hypoplasia, T1-weighted image of, 179*f*
Hypothalamic hamartomas. *See also* Hamartoma of tuber cinereum, 171
Hypothyroidism
effects of, 104
hormone replacement and, 104–105, 105*f*
panhypopituitarism and, 104–105
pituitary gland and, 104–105, 105*f*
pituitary hyperplasia and, 187
white matter calcifications and, 104–105, 105*t*
Hypoxia, gray matter involvement in, 213
Hypoxic encephalopathy, watershed zones affected by, 193

I

Idiopathic scoliosis, types of, 336*t*
Idiopathic transverse myelitis, imaging of, 363*f*
Imaging
abnormalities associated with hypoglycemia, 89
artifact and, 459
pathophysiology of stroke and, 193–194
Incidental filar lipomas, etiology of, 327
Incontinentia pigmenti, 41, 56*t*
Infection, 278, 279*f*
after spinal surgery, 452–453
indications for gadolinium administration with, 453
intraventricular septation secondary to, 129*f*
perforation of trachea and, 457–458, 459*f*
predisposing factors postsurgically for, 452–453
Infectious diskitis. *See* Diskitis (infectious)
Infratentorial aneurysms
imaging of, 246*f*
intracranial aneurysms and, 245
Infratentorial congenital anomalies, 1–15
Infundibular tilt, pituitary gland and, 178
Inhalant abuse
substances used in, 95, 96
symptomatic similarities to b12 deficiency and, 96
teenagers and, 95
Injuries (penetrating)
of brainstem, 269, 270*f*
extracranial compartment and, 269
intracranial compartment and, 269
Interfacetal dislocations, imaging features of, 355*t*
Interhemispheric fissure
subarachnoid space lipomas and, 24*t*
Interhemispheric fusion, anomaly of, 20
Interhemispheric lipomas. *See* Lipomas
Intermediary shearing injuries, 259, 260, 260*f*
Internal carotid artery
affected by fibromuscular dysplasia (FMD), 195
stenoses of, 195
Internuclear cleft, 415
Interpeduncular cistern, subarachnoid space lipomas and, 24*t*
Interventional procedures
in arterial circulations, 206
thrombolysis and, 206
in venous circulations, 206
Intervertebral disk, physiology of, 413
Intraaxial hematomas
posttraumatic aneurysms and, 247
Intraaxial hemorrhage
appearance of
on 1.5-T magnetic resonance imaging (MRI), 234*t*
computed tomography (CT) and, 231
Intracanalicular tumor, definition of, 150, 151*f*
Intracerebral hematomas
signal characteristics of, 231
significance of water contents of, 231–232
Intracranial aneurysms, 239–242. *See also* Aneurysms.
associated disorders with, 242
bleeding risk relative to size of, 242
catheter angiography and, 247–248
circle of Willis and, 239–242
detection of, 247–248
rupture risks of, 242
subarachnoid hemorrhage (SAH) and, 239
Intracranial gangliogliomas, rule of 50s for, 140
Intracranial hypotension
MRI and, 124, 124*f*
Intracranial hypotension, cerebral spinal fluid (CSF) and, 124–125
Intracranial lesions. *See also* Brain
primary injuries, 257–262
Intracranial neuroenteric cysts, 13
Intradural extramedullary lesions, 399–403
Intramedullary lesions, 403–410
Intramedullary microcysts, spinal cord cysts and, 409
Intraspinal epidermoids, causes of, 325
Intraspinal lipoma
myelopathy and, 323
spinal cord and, 321
T1-weighted image of, 323*f*
Intraventricular hemorrhage, Moyamoya and, 218–220
Invertebral fusion cages
images of, 444*f*
Invertebral fusion cages, discussion of, 443
Iron (Fe)
metabolism
disorders of 87,87*t*
overload
disorders of, 88
Irradiation. *See also* Brian irradiation; Radiation
effects of, 301–306
Ischemia
blood flow and, 194
causes of, 262
gray matter and, 213

J

JC virus, progressive multifocal leukoencephalopathy (PML) and, 279
Jefferson burst fractures
axial loading and, 346
computed tomography (CT) images of, 348*f*
symptoms of, 346–347
Joubert's syndrome
findings on imaging of, 9, 10*f*
symptoms of, 9, 10*f*
Juvenile pilocytic astrocytoma (JPA). *See also* Tumors
clinical findings of, 133–134
histology of, 133–134
imaging appearance of, 133–134, 134*f*
Juvenile rheumatoid arthritis (JRA)
atlantodental subluxation in, 376, 376*f*
calcifications in ligaments in, 376
diagnosis of, 376
imaging abnormalities with, 376, 376*f*
spine involvement in, 376
symptoms of, 376

K

Kayser-Fleischer rings, Wilson's disease and, 85
Kernicterus (bilirubin encephalopathy)
hyperbilirubinemia and, 81
neonates and, 81–82, 82*f*
Kernohan notch, uncal herniation and, 262
Kinky hair syndrome, 87
Klippel-Trenaunay syndrome, 41, 56*t*
Korsakoff psychosis, 90
Krabbe's disease (globoid cell leukodystrophy)
characterizations of, 62, 63*f*
diagnosis of, 62
late-onset variant of, 62
neuropathies and, 373
Kyphoscoliosis
closed spinal dysraphism and, 321
Kyphosis
with bone grafts, 455
in tuberculosis (spinal), 380

L

Lactic acid, and mitochondrial encephalopathies, 82
Laminar necrosis
cortex of cerebellum and, 214
cortex of cerebrum and, 214
diffuse anoxia and, 214
hypoglycemia and, 89
MRI and, 214–215, 216*f*
watershed (border zone) infarcts and, 213
watershed zones affected by, 214
Laminoplasties
advantages of procedure, 450

spinal canal stenosis, 450
Langerhans cell histiocytosis
disorders of, 148*t*
eosinophilic granuloma (EG) and, 392
L-Asparaginase
central nervous system (CNS) complications with
symptoms of toxicity in, 308
Lateral cerebellar medulloblastomas (desmoplastic), 138
Lead intoxication
brain changes and, 93
children and, 93
CT scans and, 93
Lesionectomy, surgical procedure for seizure and, 109
Lesions
adult, 182–191
childhood, 178–182
chronic, 270
differential diagnosis of on gradient-echo images, 252*b*
edematous
T2-weighted images and, 259
epidural, 397–399
intracranial, 257–262
Leukodystrophies, generalized brain enlargement and, 35
Leukemia
central nervous system (CNS) and, 166, 166*t*
complications of, 166*t*
Leukodystrophies, 60–68
Leukoencephalopathy
brain irradiation and, 301
as complication methotrexate treatment, 308, 309*f*
magnetic resonance imaging (MRI) and, 301
radiation-induced, 303*f*
Lhermitte-Dulcose disease (LDD)
imaging studies of, 140
in relation to Cowden's disease, 140
Ligaments
evaluation of, 339
injury of, 340*f*
magnetic resonance imaging (MRI) and assessing, 339–340
Limbic encephalitis, epilepsy and, 111
Linear fractures. *See* Fractures
Lipomas
imaging of, 171, 172*f*
interhemispheric, 22–23
intracranial, 22–23, 24*f*, 24*t*
linear (tubular), 22–23
locations of, 171
nodular, 22–23
Lipomyelocele, closed neural tube defects and, 321
Lipomyelomeningoceles
closed neural tube defects and, 321
imaging of, 322*f*
Lipophilic. SPECT for seizures and, 107
Lissencephalia, differences between, 31*f*, 31*t*
Liver failure, 79, 80*f*
Alper's syndrome and, 81
basal ganglia in, 80*f*
chronic, 79, 80*f*
effects of chronic, 312*f*
Lobar HP (holoprosencephaly), 18, 19*f*
brain abnormalities in, 20*t*
septooptic dysplasia (SOD) and, 18
Lobectomy
selective temporal, 109
complications of, 109
standard temporal, 109
Lordosis, 336
Low-grade astrocytomas, 153, 153t, 154
Lumbar herniated disk
epidural hematoma and, 419
imaging of, 419
Lumbar puncture
epidural hematoma from, 341
intraspinal epidermoids and, 325
Lumbar radiculomedullary arteries, lumbar arteries supplying, 433
Lumbar spine
disorders affiliated with surgery of, 443
surgical complications of, 443, 444, 446
surgical procedure on, 443
Lumbosacral plexus (LSP)
abscesses affecting, 472
herniated disks affecting, 472
radiation and, 472
tumors in, 472
Luque rods, laminectomies and, 451–452
Luxury perfusion
195
Lyme borreliosis
cerebral on differential studies, 292
clinical stages of, 292*t*
Lymphocytic hypophysitis
adenohypophysis and, 191
imaging studies of, 191
pituitary gland and, 189*t*
pregnancy and, 191
symptoms of, 191
Lymphoma
acquired immunodeficiency syndrome (AIDS) and, 157, 158, 160
bone lesions and, 398
distinguishing between types of, 398–399
Hodgkin's, 398
imaging of, 159*f*
non-Hodgkin's, 398
spinal invasion of, 398

M

Macroadenoma
figure of eight image and, 185*f*
T1-weighted image for, 185*f*
Macroadenomas. *See also* Pituitary macroadenomas
symptoms by mass effect of, 183
Macrocephaly
Alexander's disease and, 60–61
disorders with, 60–65
Magnetic resonance angiography (MRA), 201–203
circle of Willis evaluation with, 202
overestimate of stenosis and, 201
stroke viewed with, 203*f*
time of flight (TOF) with, 201
Magnetic resonance imaging (MRI)
Alpers syndrome and, 81
appearance of hyperacute blood on, 232, 232*f*
Balo's concentric sclerosis and, 70, 73, 73*f*
benign *vs.* malignant compression fractures on, 357*t*
carbon monoxide (CO) intoxication and, 92
cerebral infarctions seen on, 200, 200*f*, 201, 201*b*
of children's spine, 317–318, 318*t*
classification of spinal cord injuries with, 342 343*f*, 343*t*
correlation between prolactin levels and findings of, 184*t*
differentiating tumefactive MS from neoplasia, 70
differentiation of pediatric and adult spine in, 17–318
for evaluating disk abnormalities, 340
evaluation of spine in children and, 318
findings for Devic's disease (neuromyelitis optica) and, 74
gadolinium chelates and, 200
Hemichorea-hemiballism (HH) and, 97
intracerebral blood in hemorrhage and, 231–232
metallic hardware artifacts by, 459, 460*f*
parenteral nutrition and, 80
Parkinson's disease and, 99
phases in Paget's disease, 431*t*
pituitary portal system and, 178
postoperative cervical spine surgery evaluation using, 452
protocol for imaging partial complex seizures with, 107
reduction of artifacts in, 460*f*
sequelae of kernicterus and, 81–82
spinal trauma and, 340
T2 weighted images on
hepatic insufficiency and, 79
Wilson's disease and, 85, 86
Magnetic resonance imaging abnormalities, Chiari 2 and, 7*t*
Magnetic resonance (MR) myelogram, in avulsion, 467*f*
Magnetic resonance venography
in venous thrombosis, 203*f*
Malacia, hypoglycemia and, 89
Malignant compression fractures
on magnetic resonance imaging (MRI), 357*t*
Manganese (MN)
chronic liver failure and, 312, 312*f*
cirrhotic patients and, 79–80
in enzymatic cell cycles, 80
neurotoxic properties, 79–80
occupational toxicity and, 312
physiological transport of, 312
poisoning, 79–80
toxicity of, 312

Maple syrup disease, amino aciduria and, 83
Marchiafava-Bignami syndrome (MB), alcohol abuse and, 90
Marfan syndrome
cervical venous epidural plexus and, 434
MB. *See* Marchiafava-Bignami syndrome
MCM (mega cisterna magna), 1–2*f*
arachnoid cysts and, 4
vermis and, 1
Meckel's cave, subarachnoid space lipomas and, 24*t*
Medial occipital lobe
affected by PCA infarction, 211
Medications (anticonvulsant), 311–312, 311f. *See also* specific drugs
Medications (immunosuppressive)
effects of, 306–308
Medulloblastomas
adult, 138
childhood, 138
lateral cerebellar (desmoplastic), 138
in relation to primitive neuroectodermal tumors (PNET), 136
relationship of Gorlin's syndrome to, 138
rule of 90s for, 136*t*
WHO grade 4, 136–137*f*
Mega cisterna magna (MCM), 1–2, 2*f*
Megalocephalia, 35
MELAS syndrome (mitochondrial myopathy, encephalopathy, lactic acidosis and strokes), 82–83, 83*f*
FLAIR and, 83*f*
Proton magnetic resonance spectroscopy and, 83*f*
T2 weighted image and, 83*f*
Meningeal disease, with neurosarcoidosis, 293
Meningeal diverticulum, 403
Meningeal fibrosis, shunt placement and, 126, 126*f*
Meninges
disorders affecting, 371–375
post operative pseudomeningocele and, 452
Meningiomas
in children, 165
histologic grades of, 401
histologic types for, 163
image of, 187*f*
imaging of, 401*f*
locations of, 400
MRI of, 163, 164*f*
neurofibromatosis type 2 (NF-2), 47*f*
NF-2 and, 46
sites for appearance of, 163
symptoms of, 400
Meningitis. *See also* Bacterial Meningitis
bacteria producing, 274*t*
cerebrospinal fluid (CFS) finding and, 273
cerebrospinal fluid (CFS) in different types of, 274*t*
clinical symptoms of, 295
complications of, 273–278
Cryptococcosis neoformans, 283
imaging of ventriculitis and, 276*f*
pathologic course of, 295
pneumocephalus and, 266
subdural empyema secondary to, 276*f*
subdural sterile collections secondary to, 275*f*
uncomplicated, 275*f*
Meningoencephalocele, Chiari 3 and, 9
Meninx primitiva
arachnoid cysts in relation to, 4
Menkes' syndrome, 86–87, 86*f*
genetic defects of, 86–887
Mercury intoxication, symptoms of, 95
Merlin
neurofibromatosis type 2 (NF-2) and, 46
Mesial temporal lobe heterotopia, vs cortical dysplasia, 33*f*
Metabolic disorders, kidneys and brain affected by, 103
Metachromatic leukodystrophy, 67*f*
brain atrophy and, 67*f*
juvenile form of, 67
symptoms of, 67
Metastasis, 151
to brain, 165
imaging of, 165*f*, 166, 388–389
to pituitary gland, 187
presumed breast, 186*f*
prostate, 389
sclerotic, 389
spinal, 389
of tumors in adults, 165
types of, 388–389
vertebral
images of, 388*f*
Methanol (methyl alcohol) intoxication
CNS and, 94
ingestion and, 93–94, 94*f*
MRI and, 93–94, 94*f*
Methotrexate
calcification on CT with, 308
induced focal necrosis, 308, 309*f*
induced leukoencephalopathy, 308, 309*f*
neurotoxicity and, 308
symptoms associated with, 308
Methylmalonic acidemia, 84
propionic aciduria compared to, 84
Methylmalonic aciduria, 84
Metopic CS (craniosynostosis), 36*t*
Metopic suture synostosis, 38*f*
Microabscesses, in spine infection, 378
Microadenomas, 183, 183*t*. *See also* Pituitary microadenomas
Microcephaly
disorders with, 68
hypoglycemia and, 89
Midbrain astrocytomas, 153, 153t
Midbrain (mesencephalic) gliomas, 136
hydrocephalus and, 136
parinaud's syndrome and, 136
symptoms of, 136
Middle cerebral artery (MCA)
contrast medium and, 195
intracranial aneurysms and, 244
Middle cerebral artery aneurysm
computed tomography (CT) of, 244*f*
etiology of, 244
hydrocephalus and, 244
Middle cerebral artery (MCA) infarctions
acute, 206–210
causes of occlusions with, 206–207
CT scan and, 206–207
FLAIR and, 206–207
mortality rate of, 206
MRI and, 206–207
preferred modalities for imaging, 206–207
treatment for, 206–207
hemorrhagic CT image, 208*f*
subacute
computed tomography (CT) in, 207*f*
CT sensitivity and, 207–210
gyral enhancement and, 207–210
parenchymal contrast enhancement and, 207
pseudonormalization of, 207*f*
Midline spinal hamartoma, 325
Minamata disease, ingestion of mercury and, 95
Mineralizing angiopathy, 306*f*
Mitochondrial encephalopathies
lactic acid and, 82
oxidative respiratory mechanism and, 82
Mitochondriopathies, 82
Morquio's syndrome, 65*t*
Moyamoya disease (idiopathic progressive arteriopathy of childhood), 218
disorders associated with, 218
etiology of, 218
imaging of, 218–220, 219*f*
intraventricular hemorrhage and, 218–220
MR spectroscopy
gliomas and, 45
hamartomas and, 45
viral pontomesencephalitis and, 136
MRI. *See* Magnetic resonance imaging
MRI T2-weighted images
Wernicke's encephalopathy and, 90
MRS. *See* Proton MR spectroscopy
MS. *See* Multiple sclerosis
Mucopolysaccharidoses
cerebrospinal fluid-containing spaces and, 62, 65
etiology of, 62, 65
generalized brain enlargement and, 35
genetics and biochemical defects in, 62, 64*t*, 65
imaging abnormalities in, 65*t*
Mucormycosis
disorders associated with, 285
imaging results showing, 285, 286*f*
pathological process of, 285
Multiple aneurysms
criteria for assessing bleeding of, 246
subarachnoid hemorrhage (SAH) and, 246
view from angiogram of, 246*f*
Multiple myeloma
bone malignancy and, 389
common affected bones in, 389
diagnosis of, 389

imaging of, 389, 390*f*
peripheral neuropathy and, 389
Multiple Schmorl's nodes
Scheuermann's disease and, 429
Multiple sclerosis (MS), 70–74
Balo's concentric sclerosis and, 70
brain atrophy and, 73
chronic-progressive type of, 70
cranial neuropathies and, 70
FLAIR imaging and, 70–73*f*
magnetic resonance imaging (MRI) of, 363–364, 364*f*
MRI and, 70
optic neuritis and, 70
pathology of, 70
relapsing/remitting type of, 70
symptoms of, 363
variants of, 73
Myalgic encephalomyelitis. *See* Chronic fatigue syndrome
Mycobacterium avium-intracellulare, immunosuppressed patients and, 295
Mycobacterium tuberculosis
infections caused by, 295
in tuberculosis (spinal), 380
Myelin, amino acid disorders and, 83
Myelination, normal, 59–60
Myelinolysis, alcohol abuse and, 90
Myelocele
clinical features of, 318
open dysaphisms and, 315
spinal dysraphism and, 318
Myelocystocele, open dysaphisms and, 315
Myelomalacia, spinal cord infarction and, 452, 454*f*
Myelomeningoceles
Chiari type 2 malformation and, 318
clinical features of, 318
imaging of spine post surgical after repair of, 320
open dysaphisms and, 315
repaired, 320*f*
unrepaired, 318, 319*f*
in utero repair of, 7
Myelopathy, intraspinal lipoma and, 323

N

Nasal dermoids, 26*f*
Nasal gliomas, 25, 26*f*
Nasoethmoidal encephalocele, 25
Nasofrontal encephalocele, 27*f*
National Cancer Institute, classification for Von Hippel-Lindau disease, 54, 55*t*
National Institutes of Health (NIH)
criteria for diagnosis of neurofibromatosis type 1, 42, 42*b*
criteria for diagnosis of neurofibromatosis type 2, 46*t*
criteria for diagnosis of tuberous sclerosis, 42
Necrosis, induced by stereotactic radiosurgery, 302*f*
Neisseria meningitidis, meningitis and, 274
Neonates
hypoglycemia and, 89
periventricular leukomalacia and, 226*f*
phenylketonuria (PKU) and, 84
Neoplasia, secondary to bone marrow transplantation, 311
Nerve roots
disorders affecting, 371–375
radiculopathy and damage to, 452
Nerve sheath tumors
neurofibromas and, 399–400
schwannomas and, 399–400
Neural placode
myelocele and, 319
myelomeningocele and, 319, 319*f*
Neural tube
defects of
two types of, 321
Neurocutaneous diseases, neuroimaging of, 56*t*
Neurocutaneous melanosis, 41, 56*t*
Neurocutaneous syndromes, rare, 36, 56*t*
Neuroenteric cyst, imaging of, 335
Neurofibrin, neurofibromatosis type 1 and, 41
Neurofibromas
gadolinium enhancement in, 400
malignant degeneration of, 399–400
nerve sheath tumors and, 399–400
Neurofibromatosis, 41
differential association between brainstem gliomas and, 134–136
schizophrenia and, 17
type 1(NF-1), 41, 42*b*
type 2 (NF-2), 41, 46*b*
volume of corpus callosum and, 17
Neurofibromatosis type 1, 79
areas of presumed vacuolar myelin and, 43*f*
buphthalmos and, 45
clinical finding associated with, 45
dysplasia of the sphenoid bone and, 42, 42*f*
generalized brain enlargement and, 35
genetic anomalies and, 41
less common lesions associated with, 45
neurofibrin and, 41
optic pathway astrocytomas and, 43*f*
protein truncation test for, 42
spinal involvement and, 45*f*
and tectum astrocytoma, 43*f*
Neurofibromatosis type 2 (NF-2)
lesions and, 46
meningiomas and, 47*f*
merlin and, 46
spinal tumors and, 47, 48*f*
vestibular schwannomas and, 46*f*
Neuroimaging, features of rare neurocutaneous diseases, 56*t*
Neurologic disorders, relationship of renal failure and, 103*b*
Neuronal necrosis, kernicterus and, 81
Neurosarcoidosis
causing meningeal disease, 293
etiology of, 293
Neurotuberculosis
imaging of, 295*f*
meningitis and, 295
Neurulation congenital spinal anomalies and, 315
Nevus flammeus, Sturge-Weber syndrome and, 51
Newborns
brachial plexus avulsion in, 466*f*
Nidus, arteriovenous malformations (AVMs) and, 249
Noncommunicating hydrocephalus. *See also* Hydrocephalus
aqueductal stenosis and, 120
congenital, 120
Nonlissencephalic focal cortical dysplasia, 34*f*
Nonneoplastic masses, 166–171
Nonocclusive cerebral vascular disease, 231–253
Normal-pressure hydrocephalus. *See also* Hydrocephalus
diagnosis of, 121–122, 122*f*
Normocephaly, disorders with, 65–67
Normonatremia, central pontine myelinolysis (CPM) and, 69
North American Symptomatic Carotid Endarterectomy Trial (NASCET, measurements of stenosis set by, 195

O

Occipital encephaloceles, syndromes with presentation of, 11
Occipital lobes, hypoglycemia and, 89
Occipitoatlantal dissociation, injury causing, 346
Occipitoatlantal injuries
images of, 347*f*
types of, 346
Oligoastrocytoma, 156
Oligodendroglioma
calcification in, 156
image study of, 158*f*
imaging of, 156
symptoms of, 156
Olivopontocerebellar atrophy. *See* olivopontocerebellar degeneration
Olivopontocerebellar degeneration (OPCD; olivopontocerebellar atrophy), 101
ataxia and, 101
MRI and, 101, 101*f*
Opalski cells, Wilson's disease and, 85
OPCD. *See* Olivopontocerebellar degeneration
Open lip schizencephaly. *See* Schizencephaly.
Open spinal dysraphism, 315
complications after repair of, 320*b*
diagnosis of, 318
locations of, 319
Optic nerve gliomas (bilateral), neurofibromatosis type 1 and, 42, 43*f*
Optic nerves, chiasmatic gliomas and, 145
Optic neuritis
cisplatin and, 308
multiple sclerosis (MS) and, 70
radiation-induced, 305–306*f*

Optic pathway astrocytomas, 153, 153t
  neurofibromatosis type 1, 43*f*
Optoinfundibular hypoplasia, small pituitary gland and, 179
Optoinfundibular hypoplasia, imaging of, 180*f*
Osler-Weber-Rendu syndrome, arteriovenous malformations (AVMs) and, 248
Osmotic myelinolysis
  central pontine myelinolysis (CPM) and, 69
  hyponatremia and, 68, 69
  and patient profile, 69
Ossification of posterior longitudinal ligament (OPLL)
  etiology of, 427
  images of, 428*f*
  radiculopathies and, 427
  symptoms of, 427, 428, 429
  three types of, 427–428
Osteoblastomas (giant osteoid osteomas)
  computed tomography (CT) of, 396*f*
  gadolinium administration with, 395
  spine and, 395
  symptoms of, 395
Osteoid osteoma. *See also* Osteoblastomas
  anatomical distribution of, 395
  classification according to bone location of, 395
  differential diagnosis for, 395
  imaging of, 395, 395*f*
  pain with, 395
Osteomyelitis
  acquired immunodeficiency syndrome (AIDS) and, 378*f*
  imaging of endplate erosion in, 379*f*
  imaging of vertebral, 379*f*
  vertebral
    infection in disk space in, 380
Osteophytes, surgical open door technique for (*see* laminoplasty), 450
Osteophytosis, surgical anterior approach for, 449–450
Otomastoiditis, tuberculosis and, 296

P

Pacchionian granulations, cerebral spinal fluid (CSF and, 117
Paget's disease
  characterized by, 430
  imaging and, 430, 430*f*
  magnetic resonance imaging (MRI) of phases in, 431*t*
  multiple bone involvement with, 430
  sites of involvement in, 430*t*
Pancreatic islet cell tumors, Von Hippel-Lindau disease (VHL) and, 57
Panda sign, Wilson's disease and, 85*f*, 86
Panhypopituitarism, and hypothyroidism, 104–105
Pantopaque, myelography and, 13
Paragangliomas
  bleeding and, 407
  in filum terminale, 407
  imaging of, 407, 408*f*
Paraplegia, spinal cord infarction and, 437
Parasite, pituitary gland and, 189*t*
Parenteral nutrition
  T1 signal intensity and, 80
Parinaud's syndrome, midbrain (mesencephalic) gliomas and, 136
Parkinson's disease, 99–100, 100*f*
  MRI and, 99
  symptoms of, 99
Parkinson's plus syndrome, 101
Pars intermedia, role in pregnancy, 177
Partial complex seizures
  vascular malformations and, 111
Pax gene, spine formation and, 317
Pelizaeus-Merzbacher disease (PMD), myelin and, 68, 68*f*
Perfusion magnetic resonance imaging
  compared to MRI, 205–206
  hyperacute cerebral infarctions and, 205–206
  parameters obtained with, 205–206
Peripheral neuropathy
  alcohol abuse and, 90
  inhalant abuse and, 96
  in multiple myeloma, 389
Perishunt cysts, shunt misplacement and, 127–128, 127f
Perisylvian syndrome, 35*f*
Periventricular edema, development of, 118
Periventricular leukomalacia (PVL), 17, 17*f*
  changes in white matter and, 226
  chronic changes on CT or MRI in, 226, 226*f*
  cranial sonography and, 226
  diffuse neonatal hypoxia and, 226
  imaging of, 226*f*
  in neonates, 226
  watershed infarction and, 226
PET
  regional cerebral metabolism and, 107
  seizures and, 107
Petrous temporal bone
  fractures of, 269
    facial nerve palsy and, 269
    hearing loss and, 269
Phakomatoses pigmentovascularis, Sturge-Weber syndrome and, 41, 51
Phenylketonuria (PKU), 84*f*
  amino aciduria and, 83
  neonate and, 84
Phenylpropanolamine, cerebral vasculitis and, 217
Phenytoin (Dilantin), 311
  antiepileptic drugs and, 311
  complications of
    dermatologic, 311
    hematologic, 311
    neurologic, 311
  effects on brain, 311
  folate deficiency related to, 311
Phycomycosis, brain and, 285
Pial based tumors, hemangioblastomas and, 57
Pick's bodies, pick's disease and, 101
Pick's disease
  MRI and, 101
  PET and, 101
  SPECT and, 101
  symptoms of, 101
  T2-weighted image of, 100*f*
Pilocytic astrocytoma, 133. *See also* Juvenile pilocytic astrocytoma (JPA)
  WHO grade 1, 134*f*
Pineal gland
  cysts in
    hydrocephalus and, 170
    image of, 170*f*
    MRI brain examinations and, 170
  tumors in
    classification related to origin, 161*t*
    classifications of, 161*t*
    symptoms related to, 161
Pineocytoma, 162*f*, 163*f*
Pioneering neurons, 30
Piriformis muscle syndrome
  etiology of, 472
  magnetic resonance imaging (MRI) and, 472
Pituitary adenomas. *See also* Adenomas
  in children, 180
  Cushing's syndrome-producing, 180
  symptoms of, 180
Pituitary apoplexy
  causes of, 187
  characterizations of, 187
  hemorrhage in, 187, 188*f*, 189
Pituitary gigantism, generalized brain enlargement and, 35
Pituitary gland
  abnormalities related to, 182
  absent, 178–179
  anatomy of, 177–178, 177*t*
  craniopharyngioma and, 182
  cysts and, 182
  duplication of, 180
  empty sella syndrome and, 189
  histiocytic disorders of, 189, 189*t*, 190
  hypothyroidism and, 104–105
  incidental abnormalities of, 178
  inflammatory lesions of, 189, 189*t*, 190
  infundibular tilt and, 178
  malfunctioning of, 179
  origin of, 177*t*
  physiology of, 177–178
  pituitary portal system surrounding, 178
  Rathke's cleft cyst and, 182
  reasons for shrinkage of, 179
  studies assessing function of, 178
  symptoms of metastases to, 187
  tumors of
    secretion of thyroid-stimulating hormone and, 183
Pituitary hemorrhage, MRI for evaluation of, 187, 188, 189
Pituitary hyperplasia
  conditions presenting in conjunction with, 187
Pituitary macroadenomas
  symptoms by mass effect of, 183
Pituitary microadenomas, 183
  dynamic sequences in imaging of, 183
  T1-weighted image of, 184*f*

types of, 183*t*
Pituitary portal system
MRI and, 178
pituitary gland and, 178
Pituitary stalk, injury to, 269
Pituitary tumors, secretion of thyroid-stimulating hormone and, 183
Plasmacytoma, 151
multiple myeloma and, 389
Platinum agents, central nervous system complications with, 308
Pleomorphic xanthoastrocytoma, 133
Plug (Smith-Robinson procedure), bone grafts and, 449, 450
Pneumatoceles, emergent treatment and, 266
Pneumocephalus
imaging of, 267*f*
treatment of, 266
Poliomyelitis
clinical presentation of, 365
diagnosis of, 365
imaging in child, 366*f*
paralytic type of, 365
risk of development of, 365
Polymicrogyria (PMG), 20, 34*f*
Pons, capillary telangiectasia and, 253
Pontine astrocytomas, 153, 153t
Pontomedullary junction, subarachnoid space lipomas and, 24*t*
Porphyria
characterizations of, 106–107
MRI and, 106–107
Porphyrins, porphyria and, 106
Posterior cerebral artery (PCA) infarction, 210–211
on FLAIR image, 210*f*
Posterior communicating artery aneurysm
angiograms and, 242
intracranial aneurysms and, 242, 244*f*
symptoms of, 242
Posterior ectopic pituitary lobe
absence of, 179, 180
adenomas and, 179
diabetes insipidus and, 179
translocation of neurohypophysis, 179
tumor invasion of, 180
Posterior encephaloceles, 11, 12*f*
Posterior fossa arachnoid cysts, 4*f*. *See also* arachnoid cysts
Dandy-Walker syndrome and, 4
Posterior inferior cerebellar artery (PICA), Wallenberg's syndrome and, 212–213
Posterior pituitary lobe, effects of hydration on, 177
Posterior reversible encephalopathy syndrome (PRES)
cerebral vascular autoregulation and, 103
characterizations of, 103
diffusion-weighted imaging and, 103
Posterior reversible leukoencephalopathy syndrome (PRES), 220
Posterior thoracic approach
laminectomies and, 451
stabilization of thoracic spine and, 451
Postfixed plexus, brachial plexus and, 463
Posttransplantation lymphoproliferative disorder (PTLD)
imaging of, 310*f*
immunosuppression and, 310
Posttraumatic aneurysms
causes of, 247
intraaxial hematomas and, 247
pseudoaneurysms and, 247
Postvaccination myelitis
imaging findings of, 366
tetanus vaccine and, 366
and vaccines known to induce, 365
Powers ratio, measurement establishing diagnosis of dislocation, 346
Precocious puberty, hamartoma of tuber cinereum (hypothalamic hamartomas) and, 171
Prednisone, neurotoxicity and, 308
Pregnancy
hypertensive encephalopathy and, 220
vertebral hemangioma and, 391
Prenasal heterotopia (nasal glioma), 25, 26*f*
Prenasal space, malformation related to, 25
Prepontine region, achrachnoid cysts and, 4
PRES. *See* Posterior reversible encephalopathy syndrome
Presyrinx state, cysts and, 409
Primary sarcomas, 151
Prions, disorders caused by, 292*t*
Progeria, 41, 56*t*
Progressive multifocal leukoencephalopathy (PML)
AIDS and, 278, 280, 280*f*
conditions predisposing to, 279*b*
JC virus and, 279
Prolactin, etiologies of elevated, 183, 184*t*
Propionic aciduria, methylmalonic acidemia compared to, 84
Propylene glycol, toxicity of, 92
Prosencephalic vein, vein of Galen malformations (VGM) and, 28
Protein truncation test, for diagnosis of neurofibromatosis type 1, 42
Proton magnetic resonance (MR) spectroscopy (MRS)
acute infarction and, 204*f*
brain sequelae of chemotherapy using, 310
hepatic encephalopathy and, 80–81
hippocampi and, 108
identification of lactate using, 203–204
MELAS syndrome (mitochondrial myopathy, encephalopathy, lactic acidosis and strokes) and, 83*f*
Pseudo delta sign, subarachnoid hemorrhage (SAH) and, 266
Pseudoaneurysms
mucormycosis and, 285
posttraumatic aneurysms and, 247
Pseudoephedrine, cerebral vasculitis and, 217
Pseudomeningoceles
brachial plexus avulsions and, 466
establishing mode of treatment, 466–477
MR myelography in identification of, 466
Pseudomonas, causative agent for diskitis (infectious), 378
Pseudosynovial cysts, description of, 424
Pseudotumor cerebri, empty sella syndrome and, 189
Pseudotumor, hydrocephalus and, 122
Pseudoarthrosis, fracture of hardware and, 456
Pseudomeningoceles
injury to meninges and, 452, 454*f*
syndrome of intracranial and intraspinal hypotension and, 452
Purkinje cells, alcohol abuse and, 90
Pyogenic diskitis
disorders of spine and, 361
imaging of, 379*f*

Q

Quadrigeminal plate region, subarachnoid space lipomas and, 24*t*

R

Radiation necrosis, late radiation induced, 303*f*
Radiation. *See also* Brain irradiation
effects on brain and, 301
Radiation-induced myelitis
sites of involvement in, 368
symptoms of, 368
tumors and, 368
Radiculopathy, damage to nerve roots and, 452
Radiographs, for misplaced instruments, 456
Rasmussen's encephalitis
clinical signs of, 281
histologic findings, 281
imaging studies of, 281
T2-weighted image of, 283
temporal lobe epilepsy and, 111
Rathke's cleft cyst
hemorrhagic adenomas and, 182, 182*f*
MRI and, 182, 182*f*
Rectangle (Bailey-Badgley procedure), bone grafts and, 449, 450
Recurrent residual disk herniation
images of, 445
Reduced arterial pulsation hydrocephalus, diminished arterial pulsations and, 118
Refsum's disease, 41, 56*t*
symptoms of, 373
variations of, 373
Renal cell carcinoma, Von Hippel-Lindau disease (VHL) and, 57
Renal disorders
affect on brain, 103*b*
Renal failure, diseases affecting, 102–104
Retrogressive differentiation, 315
Rheumatoid arthritis (RA)
affected spinal sites in, 375
etiology of, 375
image of, 375*f*
spinal involvement in, 375
symptoms of, 375

Rhomboencephalosynapsis, characterizations of, 10, 11*f*
Rosai-Dorfman disease, pituitary gland and, 189*t*
Rosenthal fibers, macrocephaly and, 61
Rule of 50s, for intracranial gangliogliomas, 140
Rule of 90s,for medulloblastoma, 136*t*

S

Sacral plexus, anatomy of, 464–465
Sacrococcygeal teratoma, imaging studies and, 331, 332*f*
Sacrococcygeal teratoma, types of, 331, 331*t*
Sagittal CS (craniosynostosis), 36*t*
Sagittal suture synostosis, 37*f*
SAH. *See* Subarachnoid hemorrhage
Salmonella, causative agent for diskitis (infectious), 378
Sanfilippo's syndrome, 65*t*
Sarcoidosis. *See also* Neurosarcoidosis
  central nervous system (CNS) and, 293, 367
  differential diagnosis of, 367
  images of, 294*f*, 368*f*
  pituitary gland and, 189*t*, 190
  spinal cord and, 367
Scar. *See* Epidural scar
Scheie's syndrome, 65*t*
Scheuermann's disease
  diagnosis of, 429
  etiology of, 429
  juvenile dyphotic disorder and, 429
  kyphosis and, 429
  symptoms of, 429
Schizencephaly (SC), 20, 21*f*
  closed lip, 20, 22*f*
  open lip, 20, 21*f*
Schizophrenia, volume of corpus callosum and, 17
Schmorl nodes, endplate fractures and, 340–341
Schwannomas, 150, 150*b*
  gadolinium enhancement in, 399–400, 400*f*
  nerve sheath tumors and, 399–400
  vestibular, 150, 150*b*
Scoliosis
  caudal regression syndrome and, 326
  congenital, 336
  ganglioglioma and, 407
  idiopathic, 336
  osteoid osteoma and, 395
Secondary tumors, 311
Segmental CS (craniosynostosis), 36*t*
Seizures
  Alper's syndrome and, 81
  applications of imaging in patients with, 107
  arteriovenous malformations (AVMs) and, 248
  cerebral venous infarction in children and, 226
  ganglion cell tumors and, 140
  heterotopia, 30
  hypertensive encephalopathy and, 220
  partial complex
    roles of neuroimaging in, 107
  protocol for MRI with partial complex, 107
  techniques in surgery for, 109
  tuberculosis, 296
Selective vulnerability, 213
Semilobar HP (holoprosencephaly), 18, 19*f*
  brain abnormalities in, 20*t*
Senile plaques, Alzheimer's disease (AD) and, 98
Sepsis, kernicterus and, 81
Septic embolism, hemorrhagic infarctions and, 211
Septooptic dysplasia (SOD)
  clinical manifestations of, 22
  alobar HP and, 18
  septum pellucidum, 22
  two types of, 22
Septum pellucidum, septooptic dysplasia (SOD) and, 22
Serratia, causative agent for diskitis (infectious), 378
Shearing injuries, 258*f*, 259, 260*f*
  of brainstem, 258*f*, 259
  computed tomography (CT) of, 258*f*
  of corpus callosum, 258*f*, 259
  diffuse cerebral edema and, 262
  imaging modalities for assessing, 259
  intermediary, 259, 260*f*
Sheehan's syndrome
  diagnosis of, 189
  etiology of, 189
  necrosis of pituitary gland in, 189
Shine-through phenomenon, 214*f*
Shunt
  arteriovenous
    vascular malformations with, 248
  calcification of, 127
  complications of ventricular, 125, 125*f*, 126*t*
  degeneration of, 128*f*
  malfunction of, 127–128
  meningeal fibrosis after placement of, 126, 126*f*
  perishunt cysts secondary to, 127–128, 127f
  placement of intraventricular, 126
  skull changes after ventricular, 128*f*
  subdural hematomas after
  symptoms of infections related to, 127
  trapped ventricles and, 130
Shy-Drager syndrome, multisystem atrophy syndromes and, 101
SIH. *See* Spontaneous intracranial hypotension
Sincipital encephaloceles. *See also* Encephaloceles, 25, 26, 27
  facial dysraphism and, 28
  hypertelorism and, 26, 28
Sinus dermal tract, 25
Sjögren-Larson syndrome, 41, 56*t*
Skull base fractures
  classification of, 268–269
  complex, 269
  description of, 269
  pneumocephalus and, 269
Slit ventricle syndrome, diagnosis of, 124
Somnolence syndrome
  brain radiation and, 306
Sonic hedgehog gene, spine formation and, 317
SPECT
  defects of brain scans with, 196
  seizures and application of, 107
Spectroscopy
  Adrenoleukodystrophy (ALD) and, 65
Spinal anomalies (congenital)
  classification of, 315–317
  embryology of, 315
Spinal arteriovenous fistulas (AVFs)
  catheter angiography and, 437
  classification of, 435
  Foix-Alajouanine syndrome and, 435
  histologic review of, 435
  imaging of, 435, 436*f*
  surgery and, 435
  trauma and, 437
Spinal arteriovenous malformations. *See* Spinal AVMs
Spinal AVMs
  classifications of, 434*t*
  magnetic resonance imaging (MRI) and, 434, 435*f*
Spinal bone lesions
  with fluid levels
    differential diagnosis of, 394
Spinal brucellosis, 381, 382*f*
Spinal canal stenosis
  with bone grafts, 455
  laminoplasties and, 450, 450*f*
Spinal chordomas. *See* Chordomas
Spinal cord
  anterior spinal artery and, 433
  categorization of acute injuries to, 342, 343*t*
  disorders affecting, 361–370
  evaluation of, 342
  Human immunodeficiency virus (HIV) infection and, 278–279
  inflammatory disorders affecting, 367
Spinal cord abscesses
  antibiotic therapy and, 368
  common organisms involved in, 368
  disorders associated with, 368
Spinal cord cysts, 409
  histology of, 409
  imaging studies of, 409, 409*f*
Spinal cord ependymomas. *See* Ependymomas
Spinal cord infarction
  associated diseases with, 437
  images of, 440*f*, 452, 453*f*
  paraplegia and, 437
  postsurgical myelomalacia and, 452
  secondary to occlusion of spinal artery, 437
  surgery in cervical region and, 452, 453*f*
  vascular injury and, 452
Spinal cord vasculitis, image of, 441
Spinal disk. *See* Herniated disk

Spinal epidural hematoma
differentiated from subdural hematoma, 341
evaluation of, 341
trauma and, 341
Spinal injury, types of, 346–358
Spinal lymphoma
bony lesions and, 390
imaging of, 390, 390*f*
Spinal myelomeningocele, Chiari 2 and, 5
Spinal stenosis, variations of, 422
Spinal subdural hematomas, complications from, 342
Spinal surgery, epidural hematoma from, 341
Spinal trauma
diagnostic evaluation of, 339–344
imaging techniques for evaluating, 339
Spinal tumors, classification of, 387
Spine, 315
cervical region
involvement in diskitis (infectious), 378
forming of, 315
genetic mechanisms affecting, 317
normal dimensions of, 417
postsurgical imaging artifact and, 459, 459*f*
post surgery and, 443–460
Split notochord syndrome
embryonic development anomalies and, 315
etiology of, 335
spinal malformations related to, 333, 333t, 335–336
vertebral body anomalies in, 336
Split spinal cord syndrome, malformations related to, 333*t*
Spondylolisthesis
causes of, 425
grades of, 425–426
imaging of, 426*f*
Spondylolysis
cervical, 427*f*
congenital defects and, 427*f*
etiology of, 427
imaging of, 426
Spontaneous epidural hematomas, location of, 341
Spontaneous intracranial hypotension (SIH)
etiology of, 124–125, 124*f*
Tarlov cysts and, 125
Staphylococcus aureus, causative agent for diskitis (infectious), 378
Stenoocclusive, 225
Stenosis, common sites of, 202
Stereotactic radiosurgery, necrosis induced by, 302*f*
Streptococcus, causative agent for diskitis (infectious), 378
Streptococcus pneumoniae, meningitis and, 274
Strionigral degeneration, multisystem atrophy syndromes and, 101
Stroke
aim of imaging in, 193
cortical edema and, 207
definition of, 193
fibromuscular dysplasia (FMD) and, 195–196
magnetic resonance angiography (MRA) in, 203*f*
pathophysiology of, 193–194
treatment of, 194
Sturge-Weber syndrome (SW) and encephalotrigeminal angiomatosis, 41
etiology of, 51, 53–54*f*
Subacute hemorrhage
magnetic resonance imaging of, 233, 233*f*
oxidation of deoxyhemoglobin in, 233
Subacute middle cerebral artery (MCA) infarctions. *See* Middle cerebral artery (MCA) infarctions
Subarachnoid hemorrhage (SAH)
aneurysm and, 234
child abuse and, 267
common causes for, 239
computed tomography (CT) and, 234, 234*f*, 266, 266*f*
diffuse brain edema and, 266
imaging by FLAIR, 236
magnetic resonance imaging (MRI) and, 236, 237*f*
multiple aneurysms and, 246
pseudo delta sign and, 266
superficial siderosis, 236
volume of blood and, 234
Subarachnoid space
lipomas
locations of, 24*t*
meningitis and, 273
Subarachnoid spaces
differential diagnosis in children of enlarged, 123
Subcallosal striations, 72
Subdural empyemas, with bacterial meningitis, 268*f*, 275*f*
Subdural hematomas
blood of different ages, 267
chronic (low density), 263
computed tomography (CT) and, 235, 235*f*
differential diagnosis of, 263
extracerebral injury and, 263
fat in epidural space and, 341, 342*f*
gadolinium and, 237
imaging of, 263, 264*f*
magnetic resonance imaging (MRI) and, 237–238, 237*f*
physiology of, 263
Subdural hygroma, 263, 265
cerebrospinal fluid (CSF) and, 263
head trauma and, 263
imaging of, 263
lesions of brain with, 263, 265
Subependymoma, 139
Subfalcine herniation. *See also* Herniations
cerebral infarction and, 262
Subligamentous herniations, 415
Sudanophilic leukodystrophies, 68
Sunflower cataract, Wilson's disease and, 85
Superficial siderosis
ataxia and, 236
cranial neuropathies and, 236
subarachnoid hemorrhage (SAH) and, 236
Suprasellar astrocytomas
histology of, 144–145
imaging of, 144f
symptoms of, 145, 145*t*
Suprasellar cistern, subarachnoid space lipomas and, 24*t*
Suprasellar mass, diagnosis of on MRI, 25
Supratentorial anomalies, Chiari 3 and, 9
Supratentorial astrocytomas
in children, 146*f*
Supratentorial congenital anomalies, 15–38
Supratentorial tumors, 142–149, 152–172
hemispheric gliomas and, 145
Supravermian cistern, arachnoid cysts and, 4
SW. *See* Sturge-Weber syndrome
Sylvian regions, subarachnoid space lipomas and, 24*t*
Syndesmophyte formation, in ankylosing spondylitis (AS), 377
Synovial cysts
differential diagnosis of, 424
imaging of, 424, 425*f*
locations in spine, 424
types of, 424
Syphilis
clinical stages of, 291, 291*t*
hydrocephalus and, 291
treponema pallidum and, 291
Syringomyelia
Chiari 1 and, 5
cysts from, 402

T

T1 signal intensity
parenteral nutrition and, 80
T1 weighted images
Alzheimer's disease and, 99*f*
T2-weighted images
MELAS syndrome (mitochondrial myopathy, encephalopathy, lactic acidosis and strokes) and, 83*f*
myelin and, 59
Tacrolimus toxicity, 308
Target sign calcifications, seen in tuberculosis, 296
Tarlov cysts
diagnosis of, 403
etiology of, 403
spontaneous intracranial hypotension (SIH) and, 125
surgical resolution of, 403
Technetium-99m-hexamethyl-propylene amine oxime (HMPAO)
nuclear studies of brain and, 196
Tectum astrocytoma, neurofibromatosis type 1, 43*f*
Tela choroidea (vascularized pia), 1
Temporal lobe
dysembryoplastic neuroepithelial tumor (DNET) of, 110*f*

Temporal lobe epilepsy
developmental anomalies and, 109
encephalitis and, 111
Temporal lobe seizure
imaging and, 107
tumors and, 109
Tensor imaging
Krabbe's disease and, 62
unmyelinated white matter tracts and, 60
Teratomas, images of, 13, 161*t*, 162*f*
Terminal myelocystoceles, 320
imaging studies of, 331
Thalamic astrocytoma, radiation and chemotherapy -induced after treatment for, 302*f*
Thalamotomy
complication of, 100*f*
Thiamine, deficiency of, 90
Thoracic compression fracture
computed tomography (CT) of, 356*f*
Thoracic disk herniations
images of, 420*f*
incidence of, 419–420
locations of, 419–420
symptoms of, 419–420
Thoracic radiculomedullary arteries, intercostal arteries supplying, 433
Thoracic spine. *See also* Cervical spine surgery
complications of surgery and, 452
indications for surgery of, 451, 451*f*
injuries
etiology of, 354
surgical approaches used in, 451
Thoracolumbar junction injuries
etiology of, 356
Thrombolysis, as interventional procedure, 206
Thrombolytic drugs, stroke prognosis using, 197
Thrombolytic therapy
Diffusion-weighted magnetic resonance imaging and, 204
Thrombosis, mucormycosis and, 285
Thrombotic thrombocytopenic purpura (TTP)
characterizations of, 103–104
hypertensive encephalopathy and, 220
imaging findings for, 103–104
kidneys and brain affected by, 103
neurologic symptoms of, 103–104
Thyroid gland
disorders affecting the brain and, 104–105
secondary tumors and, 311
Thyrotrophs, hyperplasia of, 105
TIA. *See* Transient ischemic attacks
Tight filum terminale
etiology for, 329
image of, 329*f*
symptoms of, 329
Time of flight (TOF), evaluation of vessels with, 201
Tolosa Hunt syndrome
pituitary gland and, 189*t*, *190*
Tonsillar herniation, Chiari 1 and, 5
Top-of-the-basilar syndrome
etiologies for, 213
Torcular inversion, 3
Total parenteral nutrition, 79
increased T1 signal intensity and, 312
neurotoxic effects of, 312
Toxicity, occupational, 79
Toxoplasmosis gondii
AIDS and, 290
differentiation between lymphoma and, 291*t*
imaging studies of, 290, 290*f*
immunocompromised population and, 287
sites of focal lesions with, 290, 290*f*
Transcalvarial herniation. *See also* External herniation
brain and, 262
Transcranial Doppler sonography (TCD)
extracranial carotid arteries and, 196
study results using, 196–197
Transfusional siderosis, 87
Transient ischemic attacks (TIA)
cerebral infarction and, 193
cerebral thrombolytic therapy and, 193
increased T2 signal and, 223
Transitional vascular malformations
bleeding of, 253
Transmantle heterotopias, 30
Transtentorial herniation, bilateral PCA infarctions and, 210
Trapped ventricles
cerebrospinal fluid (CSF) and, 129–130, 129*f*
shunt and, 130
Trauma
arteriovenous fistula (AVF) and, 250
complication of, 342
epidural hematomas and, 452
subarachnoid hemorrhage (SAH) and, 239
Treponema pallidum
AIDS and, 291
syphilis and, 291
Trichothiodystrophy, Pelizaeus-Merzbacher disease (PMD) and, 68
Trigonocephaly, 38*f*
TSC2 gene, 48
TTP. *See* Thrombotic thrombocytopenic purpura
Tuberculosis
computed tomography of, 295–296*f*
differential diagnosis of, 295–296
infectious cause of vasculitis and, 439
otomastoiditis and, 296
pituitary gland and, 189*t*
reasons for incidence increase of, 295
seizures and, 296
tubercular pituitary abscesses with, 190, 190*f*
Tuberculosis (spinal)
clinical manifestations of, 380
differential diagnosis, 380, 381
frequent sites for, 380
kyphosis and, 380
mycobacterium tuberculosis in, 380
noncontrast image of, 381*f*
paraplegia in, 380
spinal cord abscess in, 382*f*
Tuberin, tuberous sclerosis (TS) and, 48
Tuberous sclerosis (TS), 41, 48–51, 49*b*
brain cysts and, 51
criteria for diagnosis of, 48, 49*t*
giant cell astrocytoma (GCA) and, 51, 52*f*, 145
hamartin and, 48
hamartomas and, 50*f*, 51
tuberin and, 48
Tumefactive MS, Balo's concentric sclerosis and, 73
Tumors
in adult, 149–172
in brachial plexopathies, 468, 469–470, 469*f*
brain, 165
classifications of pineal gland, 161*t*
contrast material doses, 186
hemispheric astrocytomas, 145
imaging of atypical teratoid rhabdoid, 136
infratentorial, 133–142
intracranial, 133–149
lumbosacral plexus (LSP) and, 472
pituitary gland, 182–183
of primitive cells
atypical teratoid rhabdoid tumor (ATRT), 136
medulloblastoma, 136
radiation induced, 301, 304, 304*t*
supratentorial, 152–172
temporal lobe seizures and, 109
types of secondary, 311
Von Hippel-Lindau disease (VHL) and, 149

U

Uncal transtentorial herniation. *See also* Herniations
cerebral infarction and, 262
Unilateral interfacetal dislocation, imaging of, 355*f*
Unilateral megalencephaly, generalized brain enlargement and, 35
Upward herniation. *See also* Ascending transtentorial herniation
cerebellum and, 262
Urinary anomalies, caudal syndrome and, 326

V

Vacuum phenomenon, in lumbar region, 422
Vagal nerve stimulator, seizure disorder and, 108
Van der Knapp's disease, Canavan's disease (spongiform leukoencephalopathy) compared to, 61–62
Vascular age-related changes
of increased T2signal in white matter of older population, 223
proposed etiologies for, 223
Vascular anatomy, 433–444

Vascular malformations
divisions according to angiographic appearance, 248
partial complex seizures and, 111
radiation-induced, 304, 305*f*
Vascular malformations. *See* Cerebral vascular malformations
Vasculitis
infectious causes, 439
involving spinal cord, 439
sarcoidosis and, 439
Vasogenic edema, 194
etiology of, 308
Vasopressin
brightness in T1 weighted image signal and, 177
Vein of Galen, arteriovenous fistula (AVF) and, 250
Vein of Galen malformations (VGM), 28–30, 29*f*
Venous angiomas
brain irradiation and, 304
capillary telangiectasias and, 253
imaging of, 251, 251*f*
symptoms of, 251
Venous infarctions, subacute necrotizing myelopathy and, 439
Venous occlusions, 221–223
Venous sinus thrombosis
dural arteriovenous fistula and, 250
etiologies for, 221*t*
images of, 222*f*
Venous thrombosis
hemorrhage and, 239
magnetic resonance venography for, 203*f*
Venous thrombosis. *See* also Cerebral venous thrombosis
Venous thrombus
imaging for, 202
infections and, 202
Ventricular diverticula, hydrocephalus and, 118–119*t*, 119*f*
Ventricular shunt. *See* Shunt
Ventriculitis
abscesses and, 278*f*
hydrocephalus and, 278
imaging of meningitis and, 276*f*
Ventriculitis (ependymitis), studies for documentation of, 127
Ventriculostomies. *See* Endoscopic ventriculostomies
Ventriculus terminalis
cyst in conus medullaris related to, 409
image of, 329*f*
spinal magnetic resonance imaging studies (MRI) and, 328
spinal sonograms and, 328
symptoms of, 328
Vermis, 1
Dandy-Walker syndrome and, 1
Dandy-Walker variant and, 1
Mega cisterna magna (MCM) and, 1
Vertebra plana, differential diagnosis of, 393
Vertebrae, tumors in, 394
Vertebral artery
ascending cord deficits and, 345
injury of on MRI, 344–345, 345*f*
location of dissections in, 225
occluded, 345
Vertebral column agenesis, caudal regression syndrome and, 326
Vertebral endplates
changes in, 420–422
differential diagnosis in, 422
Modic changes in, 421*t*
preferred imaging techniques for, 421*f*, 422
Vertebral hemangioma
imaging of, 391, 391*f*
locations for tumors in, 391
Vertebral metastases. *See also* Metastases
images of, 388*f*
Vertical compression injuries, indications of, 354
Vestibular schwannomas
neurofibromatosis type 2, 46*f*
VHL. *See* Von Hippel-Lindau disease
Vigabatrin
damage to white matter tracts and, 312
lesions associated with, 311
Vincristine
neurologic complications with, 308
neurotoxicity and, 308
Viral pontomesencephalitis
differentiated from brainstem gliomas, 136
MR spectroscopy and, 136
Vestibular schwannomas
imaging of, 150
symptoms of, 150
Visual deficits, hamartoma of tuber cinereum (hypothalamic hamartomas) and, 171
Von Hippel-Lindau disease (VHL)
hemangioblastomas and, 54, 149
National Cancer Institute classifications of, 41, 54–57, 55*f*, 55*b*
hemangioblastoma and, 54, 55*f*
tumors and, 149

W

Wada test
procedure for, 107–108
purpose of, 107–108
Wallenberg's syndrome, symptoms of, 213
Wallerian degeneration (WD)
etiology of, 216
image of, 202*f*
MRI vs CT imaging of, 216
T-2 signal intensity and, 201
Warehouse worker's headache, carbon monoxide intoxication and, 92
Water
diffusion-weighted imaging (DWI) and, 238
Watershed (border zone) infarcts
hypoxia and, 213
laminar necrosis and, 213
in periventricular leukomalacia, 226
Watershed zones
ischemia affecting, 193
hypoxic encephalopathy affecting, 193
laminar necrosis affecting, 214
Wedge fractures
classification of, 356
etiology of, 352
lateral radiograph of, 352*f*
Wegener granulomatosis, pituitary gland and, 189*t*
Werner's syndrome, 41, 56*t*
Wernicke-Korsakoff syndrome (WK), alcohol abuse and, 90
Wernicke's encephalopathy, MRI T2-weighted images and, 90, 91*f*
White matter
acquired disorders of, 68–76
acute disseminated encephalomyelitis (ADEM) and, 74
AIDS dementia complex and, 278
amino acid disorders, 83–84
calcifications of, 105, 105*t*
diffuse hypoxia and, 226
disorders of
classification of, 59
gliomatosis cerebri and, 156
hypoglycemia and, 89
periventricular leukomalacia (PVL) and, 226
progressive leukoencephalopathy and, 308
Wilson's disease (hepatolenticular degeneration), 85–86, 85*f*
basal ganglia lesions and, 85
proton MR spectroscopy (MRS) and, 81
WK. *See* Wernicke-Korsakoff syndrome, 90
Wormian (intrasutural) bones, 86, 87
World Health Organization (WHO)
classification of juvenile pilocytic astrocytomas and, 133
Wyburn-Mason syndrome, arteriovenous malformations (AVMs) and, 248

X

Xenon computed tomography (CT), measurement of blood perfusion using, 199
Xeroderma pigmentosa, 41, 56*t*

Z

Zygomycosis, brain and, 285